Pediatric Skeletal Trauma

Ingo Marzi • Johannes Frank
Stefan Rose

Pediatric Skeletal Trauma

A Practical Guide

Springer

Ingo Marzi
Department of Trauma
Hand & Reconstructive Surgery
University Hospital Frankfurt
Goethe University
Frankfurt am Main, Germany

Johannes Frank
Department of Trauma
Hand & Reconstructive Surgery
University Hospital Frankfurt
Goethe University
Frankfurt am Main, Germany

Stefan Rose
University Hospital Frankfurt
Goethe University
Frankfurt am Main, Germany

ISBN 978-3-030-93683-9 ISBN 978-3-030-93685-3 (eBook)
https://doi.org/10.1007/978-3-030-93685-3

This Springer imprint is published by the registered company Springer Nature Switzerland AG
The registered company address is: Gewerbestrasse 11, 6330 Cham, Switzerland

Preface

Even with great care and every possible preventive measure, accidents in childhood are unavoidable. The result is stress for each affected child, their parents, friends, and not least, for all persons involved in treating the resulting injuries. Parents are generally anxious and insecure in these circumstances, and their expectations can be extraordinarily high. A thorough understanding of pediatric traumatology is needed to master these situations safely and successfully, providing each injured child with age-appropriate care and the best possible outcome.

This book has been designed with this in mind to offer solid preparation for the treatment of injured children. Its pragmatic structure should provide rapid orientation when needed for immediate situations as well as an overall treatment concept and approaches to therapy and follow-up. This manual is composed of two parts: one focused on general topics and the other on specifics.

The general sections offer a systematic presentation of the unique features of pediatric fractures and injuries overall, as well as typical developmental phenomena. These are essential for a fundamental understanding of clinical and radiological diagnosis along with conservative and operative therapeutic approaches.

The specialized sections first discuss the normal developmental regional anatomy and radiographic presentation in childhood. This is followed by a detailed introduction of the most foreseeable injuries to the extremities, with many case studies and examples. Injuries to the soft tissues, the pelvis, and the spine are also specifically addressed. These sections are carefully structured. A short, informative text is offered for each injury localization, followed by a comprehensive tabular presentation listing specific features as well as the indications for conservative and/or operative treatment. Immediately following these tables, the most characteristic injuries are demonstrated with radiographs, including treatment and follow-up images. Emphasis has been placed on clear diagrams, treatment instructions, and unambiguous recognition of injuries on imaging. The chapters are replete with practical treatment tips.

The book also has three special chapters discussing the treatment of unrecognized injuries and post-traumatic deformities resulting from growth disturbances and other complications.

This comprehensive presentation of pediatric traumatology is based on the experience of the collaborating authors Ingo Marzi, Johannes Frank, and

Stefan Rose treating injured children in large academic medical centers for over thirty years. Most cases presented were treated and documented by the authors themselves, and the treatment algorithms used correspond to the current guidelines and consensus discussions.

The work itself, in parts, introduces treatment developments to those initially presented in Ingo Marzi's German-language textbook that was first published in 2006: Kindertraumatologie. The original text included contributions from numerous well-known traumatology, pediatric surgery, and orthopedic specialists of national and international renown, for which the current authors are very grateful. The 2nd edition from 2010 and especially the 3rd edition from 2016 have been extensively edited by the authors and supplemented with their own case studies and treatment experience; thus, the current Pediatric Skeletal Trauma Manual also reflects the authors' individual long-term clinical experience.

The authors would like to thank their colleagues at the University Hospital Department of Traumatology: Dr. Maren Janko, Dr. Katharina Mörs, and Dr. Maika Voth, for their support in compiling case studies. Special thanks to Dr. Sarah Hamilton for her English-language assistance in the drafting of the text. We would like to thank Springer Nature Publishers London for the attractive implementation of the book.

We also sincerely thank our wifes Petra Marzi, Dorothea Frank, and Birgit Rose for their continued support throughout the time-consuming preparation of this book.

- Marzi I (ed) (2006) Kindertraumatologie, 1st ed. Springer, Heidelberg, p 468
- Marzi I (ed) (2010) Kindertraumatologie, 2nd ed. Springer, Heidelberg, p 423
- Marzi I (ed) (2016) Kindertraumatologie, 3rd ed. Springer, Heidelberg, p 572

Frankfurt am Main, Germany — Ingo Marzi
Frankfurt am Main, Germany — Johannes Frank
Frankfurt am Main, Germany — Stefan Rose
August 2022

Contents

Part I General Considerations

1 Bone Growth and Healing . . . 3
1.1 Bony Growth . . . 3
Diametric Growth . . . 3
Longitudinal Growth . . . 3
Epiphyseal Plate Structure . . . 4
Suspension of Growth: Physiological Plate Fusion . . . 4
1.2 Bone Healing . . . 5
Callus Formation and Consolidation Times . . . 5
Consolidation Times . . . 6
1.3 Healing and Growth Abnormalities . . . 6
Diametric Growth . . . 6
Longitudinal Growth . . . 7
1.4 Spontaneous Correction . . . 9
Recommended Literature . . . 11

2 Injury Patterns and Diagnostics . . . 13
2.1 Fractures . . . 13
Articular Region . . . 14
2.2 Dislocations . . . 18
Shoulder . . . 18
Elbow . . . 19
Hips . . . 20
Knee . . . 20
2.3 Radiological Examination . . . 20
Radiography . . . 20
Ultrasound . . . 20
Computed Tomography (CT) . . . 21
Magnetic Resonance Imaging (MRI) . . . 21
Other Approaches . . . 21
2.4 Radiological Development of the Pediatric Skeleton . . . 21
Coned Epiphysis . . . 24
Pseudoepiphysis . . . 24

2.5 Radiological Diagnostic Clues. 25
Harris Lines 25
Fat Pad Sign 25
Battered Child Syndrome (Child Abuse) 26
2.6 Pediatric Fracture Classifications. 30
AO Pediatric Comprehensive Classification of Long Bone Fractures (PCCF) 30
Li-La Classification for Pediatric Long Bone Fractures 35
Recommended Literature 35

3 Treatment Principles. 37
3.1 Conservative Treatment Options 37
Basic Principles 38
3.2 Technical Features of Conservative Treatment 42
Basic Casting Principles. 42
Cast Wedging 42
Special Casting Techniques 44
3.3 Conservative Fracture Treatment 47
Radiographic Controls 48
Follow-Up 49
Consolidation 49
3.4 Operative Treatment Options 50
Reduction 50
Fixation Procedures 52
Further Techniques. 64
Recommended Literature 64

4 Soft Tissue Injuries 67
4.1 Vascular Injuries. 67
Causes, Mechanism of Injury. 67
Classification 67
Diagnostic Assessment. 67
Primary Treatment 68
Therapy 69
Complications, Growth Disturbances 69
Follow-Up 70
4.2 Nerve Injuries. 70
Causes, Mechanisms of Injury 70
Classification 70
Diagnostic Assessment. 71
Primary Treatment 72
Treatment 73
Complications, Growth Disturbances 73
Follow Up. 74
4.3 Tendon Injuries 74
Causes, Mechanism of Injury. 74
Classification 75
Diagnostic Assessment. 78

Primary Treatment ... 79
Therapy ... 79
Complications, Growth Disturbances ... 82
Follow Up ... 82
Recommended Literature ... 82

Part II Specific Injuries

5 Shoulder ... 87
5.1 Shoulder Girdle ... 87
Physiological Findings ... 87
Clavicle Fractures ... 87
Injuries of the Acromioclavicular Joint ... 98
Injuries of the Sternoclavicular Joint ... 99
Scapular Fractures ... 102
5.2 Shoulder Joint ... 106
Glenohumeral Shoulder Dislocation and Rotator Cuff Injuries ... 106
Recommended Literature ... 113

6 Humerus ... 115
6.1 Physiological Findings ... 115
Ossification Centers and Growth Plate Fusion ... 115
6.2 Proximal Humerus Fractures ... 117
Incidence, Mechanism of Injury and Clinical Picture ... 117
Classification ... 123
6.3 Diaphyseal Humeral Fractures ... 123
Incidence, Mechanism of Injury and Clinical Picture ... 123
Recommended Literature ... 129

7 Elbow ... 131
7.1 Physiological Findings ... 131
Age-Dependent X-ray Findings ... 131
7.2 Supracondylar Humerus Fractures ... 134
Incidence, Mechanism of Injury, and Clinical Presentation ... 134
Classification and Treatment Concept ... 134
7.3 Distal Humerus Transcondylar Fractures ... 150
Incidence, Mechanism of Injury, and Clinical Presentation ... 150
7.4 Elbow Dislocation ... 160
Incidence, Mechanism of Injury, and Clinical Presentation ... 160
7.5 Distal Humerus Epicondylar Fractures ... 167
Incidence, Mechanism of Injury, and Clinical Presentation ... 167
Recommended Literature ... 173

8 Proximal Radius and Olecranon ... 175
8.1 Physiological and Radiological Findings ... 175
8.2 Fractures and Dislocations of the Proximal Radius ... 177
8.3 Fractures of the Proximal Ulna ... 186
Recommended Literature ... 195

9 Forearm 197
9.1 Physiological Findings 197
9.2 Fracture Types and Localisation of the Forearm 197
9.3 Forearm Fractures 202
9.4 Monteggia Injuries 226
9.5 Galeazzi Injuries 230
9.6 Technical Considerations 234
Recommended Literature 243

10 Hand 245
10.1 Carpal Fractures and Dislocations 245
Incidence, Mechanism of Injury and Clinical Picture 246
10.2 Metacarpal Fractures 258
Incidence, Mechanism of Injury and Clinical Picture 258
10.3 Finger Fractures and Dislocations 270
Incidence, Mechanism of Injury and Clinical Picture 270
Recommended Literature 279

11 Hip 281
11.1 Physiological Findings 281
11.2 Proximal Femur Fractures 283
Incidence, Mechanism of Injury, and Clinical Presentation 283
Classification 283
Type I Fractures 284
Type II Fractures 284
Type III Fractures 286
Type IV Fractures 287
Treatment Objective 290
11.3 Apophyseal Avulsions 297
11.4 Traumatic Hip Dislocations 298
11.5 Transient Synovitis, Legg–Calvé–Perthes Disease (LCPD), and Slipped Capital Femoral Epiphysis (SCFE) . . . 300
Recommended Literature 311

12 Femur 313
12.1 Physiological Findings 313
12.2 Femoral Shaft Fractures 314
Incidence, Mechanism of Injury and Clinical Picture 314
Subtrochanteric Fracture 319
Transverse Fractures 326
Oblique and Spiral Fractures 330
Compound Femur Fractures 334
Distal Femur Fractures 338
Technical Tipps Femur Fractures 344
Recommended Literature 348

13 Knee 349
13.1 Physiological Findings 349

13.2 Fractures around the Knee 352
Incidence, Mechanism of Injury, and Clinical Presentation 352
Distal Femur Fractures around the Knee 354
Proximal Tibia Fractures around the Knee 358
Proximal Tibial Avulsion Fractures 362
13.3 Patellar Injuries 370
Patella Fracture 371
Patellar Dislocation 378
13.4 Pediatric Knee Ligament Injuries 385
Intercondylar Eminence (Tibial Spine) Avulsion Fractures. 387
Ligamentous Cruciate Ligament Lesions 391
Femoral Collateral Ligament Avulsions 397
13.5 Meniscus Injuries 399
Recommended Literature 402

14 Tibia and Fibula 405
14.1 Physiological Findings 405
Fascial Compartments of the Lower Leg 405
14.2 Fractures of the Tibial Shaft 406
Incidence, Mechanism of Injury, and Clinical Presentation 406
Classification 413
Fractures of the Proximal Tibia 414
Fractures of the Tibia Shaft 416
Fractures of the Distal Tibia 422
Technical Aspects 426
Recommended Literature 427

15 Ankle Joint 429
15.1 Physiological Findings 429
15.2 Distal Tibia Fractures 431
Incidence, Mechanism of Injury, and Clinical Presentation 431
Classifications 433
15.3 Epiphysiolysis and Epiphyseal Fractures of the Distal Tibia. 434
15.4 Transitional Fractures 444
15.5 Ankle Distortion Trauma 453
Incidence, Mechanism of Injury, and Clinical Presentation 453
15.6 Osteochondritis Dissecans of the Talus 456
Incidence, Mechanism of Injury, and Clinical Presentation 456
Recommended Literature 463

16 Foot 465
16.1 Physiological Findings 465
Ossification Centers and Growth Plate Fusion 465
16.2 Bony Foot Injuries 467
Incidence, Mechanism of Injury and Clinical Presentation. 467
16.3 Talus Fracture 468
Incidence, Mechanism of Injury and Clinical Presentation. 468

16.4 Calcaneus Fracture . . . 474
Incidence, Mechanism of Injury and Clinical Presentation. 474
16.5 Tarsal Fracture: and Hindfoot Injuries . . . 482
Incidence, Mechanism of Injury and Clinical Presentation. 482
16.6 Metarsal and Phalangeal Injuries . . . 485
Recommended Literature . . . 496

17 Pelvis . . . 497
17.1 Physiological Findings and Classifications . . . 497
Age-Dependent X-Ray Findings . . . 498
Classification . . . 499
17.2 Avulsion Injuries (Apophyseal Avulsion Fractures) . . . 501
Incidence, Mechanism of Injury and Clinical Picture . . . 501
17.3 Pelvic Rim and Pelvic Ring Fractures . . . 504
Incidence, Mechanism of Injury and Clinical Picture . . . 504
Classification . . . 505
A-type pelvic fractures . . . 506
B-type pelvic fractures . . . 512
C-type pelvic fractures . . . 516
17.4 Acetabular Fractures . . . 519
Incidence, Mechanism of Injury and Clinical Picture . . . 519
Classification . . . 519
17.5 Complex Injuries . . . 524
Incidence, Mechanism of Injury and Clinical Picture . . . 524
Classification . . . 524
Recommend Literature . . . 528

18 Spine . . . 529
18.1 Physiology, Anatomy and Development of the Spine . . . 529
18.2 Injuries to the Spine: General . . . 531
Incidence . . . 531
Neurological Complications . . . 531
Diagnostic Assessment . . . 531
Differential Diagnosis of Growth-Related Findings . . . 534
Classification . . . 535
Treatment . . . 537
18.3 Injuries to the Cervical Spine . . . 538
Incidence, Mechanism of Injury and Clinical Picture . . . 538
Classification . . . 538
Particulars . . . 538
Diagnosis . . . 538
Occipital Fracture . . . 539
Occipitoatlantal Dislocation . . . 540
Atlas Fracture . . . 541
Atlantoaxial Dislocation (AAD) . . . 543
Axis and Dens Fractures . . . 545
Os Odontoideum . . . 548

Injuries to the C2/C3 Segment and Pseudosubluxation.... 549
Injuries to C3–C7. 551
18.4 Injuries to the Thoracic Spine 558
Incidence, Mechanism of Injury and Clinical Picture 558
Classification 558
18.5 Injuries to the Lumbar Spine 562
Incidence, Mechanism of Injury and Clinical Picture 562
Classification 562
18.6 Spinal Cord Injuries. 569
Incidence, Mechanism of Injury and Clinical Picture 569
Diagnostic Assessment 569
Treatment and Prognosis 570
Recommended Literature 570

Part III Secondary Reconstructions

19 Secondary Reconstruction of the Elbow. 573
19.1 Mechanism of Injury 573
19.2 Deformities of the Distal Humerus 573
Treatment. 574
Operative Therapy 574
19.3 Deformities of the Proximal Forearm 580
Treatment. 581
Operative Therapy 582
19.4 Complications 585
19.5 Practical Conclusions. 587
Recommended Literature 587

20 Secondary Reconstruction of the Forearm and Wrist. 589
20.1 Epidemiology. 589
20.2 Deformities of the Forearm 589
Therapy 589
Corrective Procedures 589
20.3 Deformities at the Wrist Level. 595
Treatment. 596
Operative Therapy 597
20.4 Complications 607
20.5 Conclusions 607
Recommended Literature 608

21 Secondary Reconstruction of the Lower Leg: Femur, Tibia and Ankle 611
21.1 Epidemiology. 611
Differential Diagnosis 611
21.2 Deformities of the Femur. 611
Therapy 612
Corrective Procedures 612

21.3 Deformities of the Tibia and Ankle 618
Therapy 618
Corrective Procedures 619
21.4 Complications 625
21.5 Conclusions 625
Recommended Literature 625

About the Authors

Prof. Dr. Ingo Marzi is Director of the Department of Trauma, Hand-, and Reconstructive Surgery, University Hospital Frankfurt, Goethe-University since 20 years. He is past President of the European Society for Trauma and Emergency Surgery, past President of the German Orthopedic and Trauma Society, and Editor-in-Chief of the European Journal of Trauma and Emergency Surgery. Prof. Marzi has written several books on Trauma and Pediatric Trauma Surgery. Prof. Marzi has published intensively in the field of pediatric trauma and organized numerous pediatric trauma courses.

Prof. Dr. Johannes Frank leads the Section for Hand, and Reconstructive Surgery of the University Hospital Frankfurt, Goethe-University in Frankfurt since 20 years. He is a well-recognized Hand- and Pediatric Orthopedic-Trauma Surgeon including complex reconstructive hand, and tumor surgery. Prof. Frank is a well-established active board member of various hand and trauma societies organizing teaching courses including pediatric trauma. In addition, he has published extensively in trauma care and written practical surgical books.

Prof. Dr. Stefan Rose is working as a trauma surgeon including pediatric trauma at a trauma center in Luxemburg. Prof. Rose is a faculty member of the Goethe-University in Frankfurt, where he was attending earlier. He is an active course instructor for pediatric trauma and general orthopedic trauma and has contributed to various books.

Part I

General Considerations

1 Bone Growth and Healing

1.1 Bony Growth

Diametric Growth

The growth plates are responsible for longitudinal bone growth and the periosteal/endosteal system for diametric increases. While fresh bone is added along the periosteum, older bone is degraded along the endosteal surface, maintaining thickness and weight and preserving the tubular nature of the long bones according to Roux's law: optimum resilience with the minimum material. This dynamic equilibrium is also responsible for fracture healing and correction of angulation and callus remodeling.

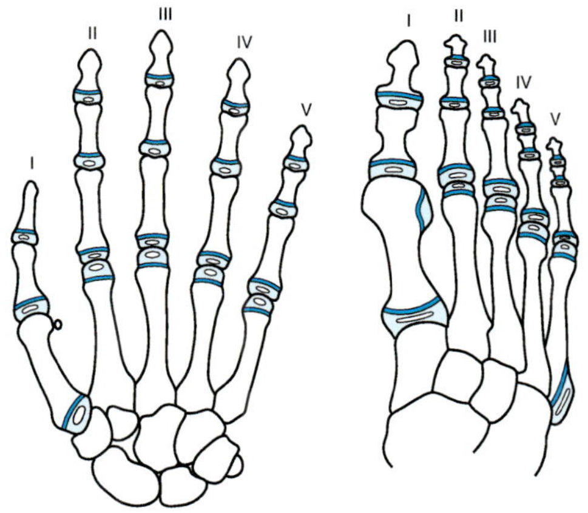

Fig. 1.1 Growth plates of the hand and foot. Phalanges, MCs, and MTs each have a single growth plate. The growth plates of all phalanges and the MC/MT of the first ray are located proximally and of the remaining MCs/MTs distally

Longitudinal Growth

The epiphyseal plates are the origin of longitudinal bone growth and are located at each end of the large long bones. The phalanges, metacarpals (MCs), and metatarsals (MTs) each have a single growth plate. These are located proximally in the phalanges and the MCs/MTs of the first ray. The growth plates of the remaining MCs and MTs are located distally (Fig. 1.1).

The growth plates of the large long bones have disproportionate effects on longitudinal growth (Fig. 1.2), which are more pronounced in the upper versus lower extremities. Most longitudinal growth of the upper extremity occurs in the proximal humerus and distal forearm, and that of the femur occurs near the knee joint.

I. Marzi et al., *Pediatric Skeletal Trauma*, https://doi.org/10.1007/978-3-030-93685-3_1

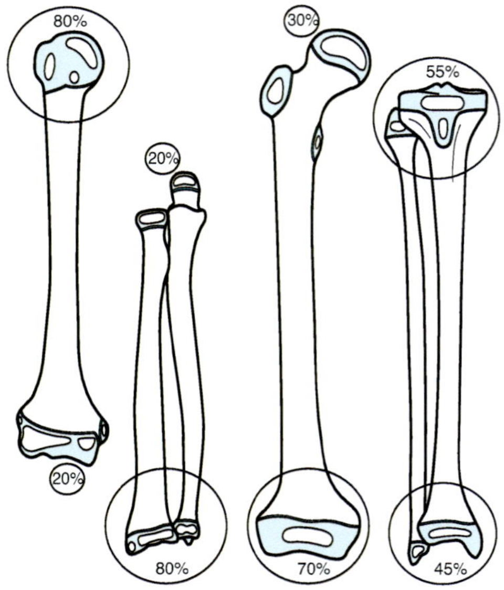

Fig. 1.2 Growth distribution of individual growth plates of the long bones. Epiphyseal plates are located at each end of the large bones, contributing unequally to longitudinal growth. The proximal humerus plate accounts for up to 80%, those around the elbow up to 20% each, and those of the distal forearm again, up to 80%. Growth is less lopsided in the lower extremities, with the proximal and distal femur plates accounting for 30% and 70% and the proximal and distal tibia plates for 55% and 45%, respectively

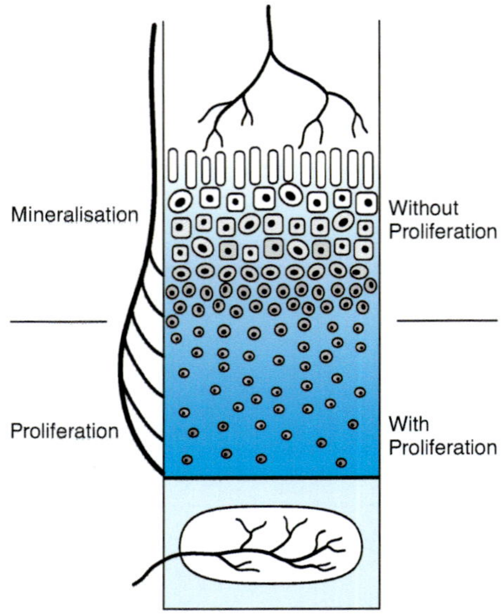

Fig. 1.3 Diagram of growth plate structure. Clinically, the epiphyseal portion with proliferative potential (the zone of proliferation and the early layer of maturation) must be distinguished from the metaphyseal portion without it (hypertrophy and mineralization). The plate is supplied by three vascular systems: the epiphyseal, metaphyseal, and periosteal systems, which communicate with one another

Epiphyseal Plate Structure

The epiphyseal plate separates the epiphysis and metaphysis. Longitudinal growth begins with multiplying chondrocytes in the zone of proliferation on the epiphyseal side. Moving towards the metaphysis, the proliferating chondrocytes stack in columns. The cells begin to hypertrophy, accumulating elements of the extracellular matrix, which correspondingly shrinks. The matrix and cells are increasingly mineralized and then ossified in the zone adjacent to the metaphysis. The growth plate is vascularized through three systems: periosteal, epiphyseal, and metaphyseal, which communicate with one another.

The plate is divided functionally into two essential parts: the epiphyseal portion undergoing proliferation and the metaphyseal portion undergoing mineralization (Fig. 1.3). These systems are in equilibrium during growth. From a clinical perspective, the key is to differentiate the epiphyseal portion with proliferation potential from the metaphyseal portion without it.

Suspension of Growth: Physiological Plate Fusion

There are three phases of growth within the plates, each of variable duration. During active growth, depending on the individual plate, until around 10–12 years, the proliferative and mineralizing processes are in equilibrium, and the bone grows. Hormonal and humoral influences then lead to a short dormant phase during which there is still growth potential, but proliferation and mineralization have ceased. This short recovery phase rapidly transitions to the fusion phase, when the proliferation potential gradually ebbs, and mineralization works its way through the plate. This typically begins excentrically as known from the distal tibia epiphysis (Fig. 1.4).

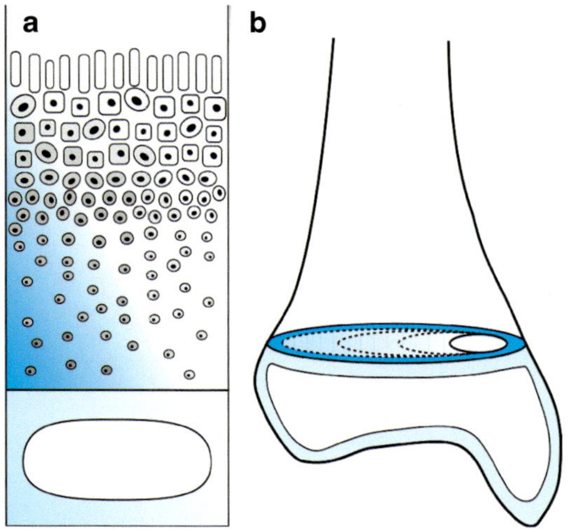

Fig. 1.4 (**a**, **b**) Physiological growth plate fusion. (**a**) Mineralization begins in the metaphyseal portion of the growth plate and moves through to the epiphyseal region in small discrete areas. (**b**) From there, it spreads gradually throughout the growth plate. In the distal tibia, closure begins eccentrically in the anterior area of the medial malleolus, moving posteriorly and anteriorly, with the lateral quadrant of the growth plate last to ossify

The time of closure depends on several individual factors, including gender and the growth potential of the respective plates.

1.2 Bone Healing

Callus Formation and Consolidation Times

Pediatric fractures heal almost exclusively through callus formation, even when there is stable internal fixation. The initial soft callus is formed of connective tissue, into which osteoblasts migrate and begin the process of mineralization and fracture stabilization. The fracture first stabilizes to movement and then to loading. Remodeling to the original shape occurs gradually according to the child's age and use—reshaping is affected by functional demand. Depending on the callus formed, the process can last for months or even years when angulation is present (see below).

Various factors affect the amount of callus formed. The more angulation present, the larger the callus, especially on the concave side of the fracture. The more unstable the fracture and the younger the child, the more callus results (examples: clavicle fractures, apophyseal avulsions of the pelvis, newborn femur fractures).

Fracture location and surface area affect healing time. Oblique fractures heal almost twice as quickly as transverse fractures; metaphyseal almost twice as rapidly as diaphyseal fractures.

Tenderness to palpation of the soft callus decreases with increasing mineralization. Once the recommended immobilization period has ended, and there is no tenderness to percussion, the fracture is stable for splint-free mobilization. Radiological confirmation is generally unnecessary. However, if performed, the x-ray will confirm with periosteal callus bridging of the fracture gap in three cortices (of four, shown in two planes) (Fig. 1.5).

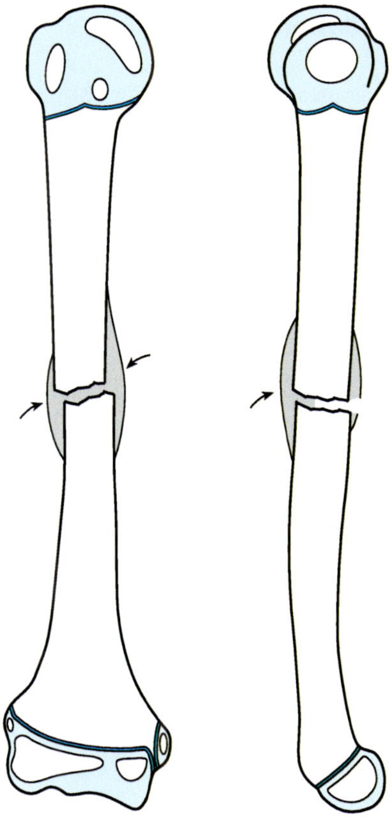

Fig. 1.5 Assessment for fracture stability on x-ray. If the fracture gap shows periosteal bridging along 3 of 4 cortices on A.P. view and lateral x-rays, the fracture is stable for mobility

Table 1.1 Guide values for average consolidation times

Fracture localization	Consolidation time (weeks)
Clavicle	2–3
Proximal humerus	2–3
Humeral shaft	3–6
Distal humerus	3–4
Proximal forearm	3–4
Ulnar shaft, radial shaft	4–6
Distal forearm	3–4
Carpal fractures	6–12
Femoral neck	4–12
Femoral shaft	3–6
Distal femur	3–4
Proximal tibia	3–4
Tibial shaft	4–5
Distal tibia	3–4
Metacarpals and metatarsals	3–4
Fingers and toes	1–2

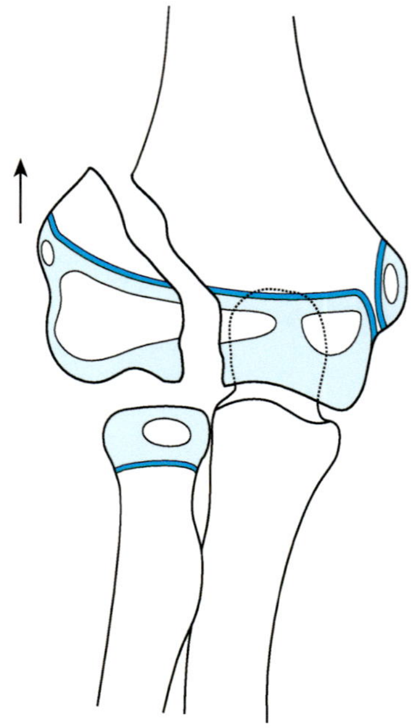

Fig. 1.6 Non-union of a fractured lateral condyle of the humerus. There is a considerable risk for non-union in displaced fractures treated conservatively. The deformity continues to develop until growth is complete, mainly deviating posterolaterally and resulting in considerable joint deformity, usually valgus

Consolidation Times

Typical consolidation times for the most common fractures are shown in Table 1.1.

1.3 Healing and Growth Abnormalities

Diametric Growth

Abnormal diametric growth is evident when fracture consolidation is absent or incomplete, i.e., complete or partial non-union.

Both hypertrophic and atrophic complete non-unions of diaphyseal fractures are rare and occur exclusively from pathological or iatrogenic etiologies. The prognosis is good, especially for hypertrophic non-union. Two metaphyseal/epiphyseal fracture locations of the distal humerus are more likely to result in non-union due to muscle tension-induced instability: displaced fractures of the lateral condyle treated conservatively (iatrogenic) and fractures of the medial epicondyle (iatrogenic and/or idiopathic). The consequences of the latter example are relatively minor. Only around 10% of medial epicondyle non-unions are symptomatic, requiring treatment. In contrast, non-unions of the lateral condyle result in a severe deformity (Fig. 1.6). Almost every case will become symptomatic, and treatment options are limited (secondary joint reconstruction is no longer possible).

Partial non-union and consolidation disruptions or delays typically appear in classic greenstick fractures of the diaphysis that are not "completed" during treatment. There is rapid healing along the intact cortex that prevents periosteal bridging on the disrupted side (Fig. 1.7). Genuine refracture (within 1 year and after inadequate trauma) occurs in 20–30% of cases. A similar situation occurs after greenstick fractures of the proximal tibial metaphysis. There is always a certain amount of valgus angulation in these injuries, promoting rapid lateral healing with markedly delayed consolidation of the medial side. The adjacent growth plate is unilaterally stimulated, resulting in medial overgrowth (see below) and, thus, reinforced primary valgus (Fig. 1.8).

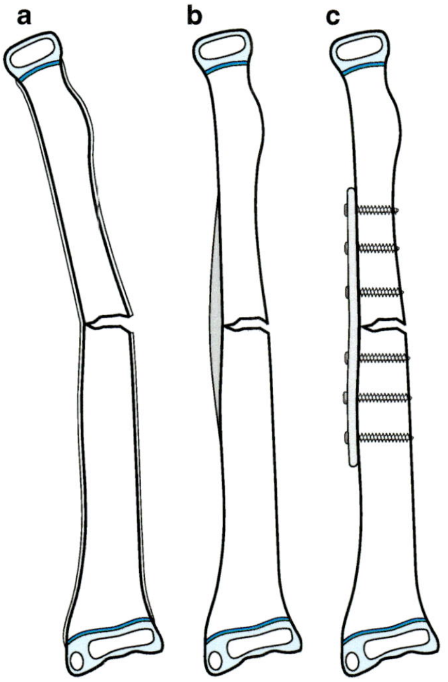

Fig. 1.7 (**a**–**c**) Delayed union in a diaphyseal greenstick fracture. (**a**) In greenstick fractures, one cortex is intact and the other completely disrupted. (**b**) If this situation is left during reduction, without compression of the disrupted fracture side, the intact cortex will heal rapidly, and consolidation will not occur on the opposite side. This risks refracture. (**c**) The same problem is seen in adolescents when there is a "blocking" plate fixation

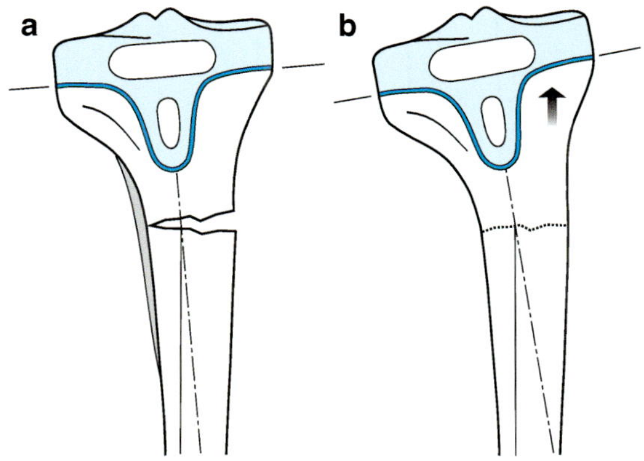

Fig. 1.8 (**a**, **b**) Delayed union of a metaphyseal greenstick fracture. Flexion fractures of the metaphysis can develop the same problems as diaphyseal fractures (◉ Fig. 1.7). (**a**) The intact cortex heals rapidly, while healing of the opposing, disrupted side is lacking. (**b**) The consequences are different for the metaphysis. Instead of refracture, partial overstimulation of the nearby growth plate occurs due to protracted healing, worsening the primary angulation. Clinically, this problem is significant at the proximal tibia

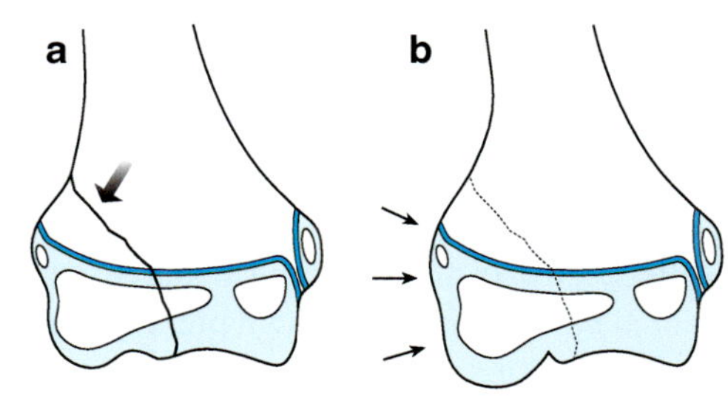

Fig. 1.9 (**a**, **b**) Stimulative growth disturbance, partial growth plate stimulation. (**a**) Partial stimulation of the lateral growth plate always occurs after fractures to the humeral lateral condyle. (**b**) Stable immobilization decreases time to fracture consolidation, decreasing the duration of lateral stimulation and thus, results in a less pronounced variation of the elbow axis

Longitudinal Growth

All problems with longitudinal growth and the repercussions depend on the child's age at the time of injury: the younger the patient, the more pronounced the consequences.

Hyperstimulation of growth plates is expected after every pediatric fracture. The resulting issues depend on patient age and duration of fracture healing. Bony overgrowth should be expected after fractures suffered during active plate growth until approximately 10 years of age. Shortening is more likely after injuries during the dormant and fusion phases. The more angulation, lateral translation, and need for callus remodeling, the longer the time of stimulation and, thus, the more pronounced the consequences (lengthening or shortening). Limb length discrepancies rarely exceed the average 1 cm, and only discrepancies of the lower extremities affect spinal balance. To assess for clinical repercussions, measurements must always be carried out functionally!

Partial stimulation occurs rarely and is only clinically relevant in the proximal tibia and the humeral lateral condyle. In the humeral condyle, lateral overgrowth always occurs, resulting in variation of the elbow axis. Stable treatment shortens the time to consolidation and thus, reduces deformity (Fig. 1.9).

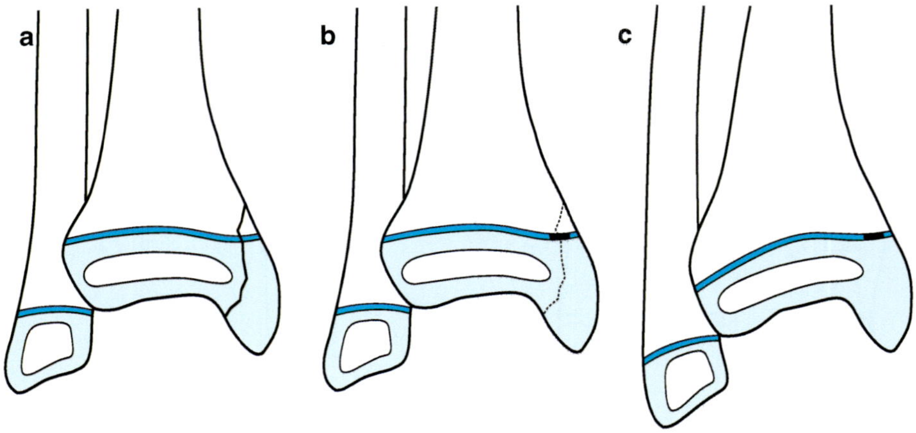

Fig. 1.10 (**a–c**) Inhibitory growth disturbance, premature partial growth plate fusion. (**a**, **b**) In epiphyseal fractures with wide-open physes and epiphyseal separations, partial ossification of the growth plate can occur with epiphyseal/metaphyseal bridging. (**c**) While the rest of the plate continues to grow normally, growth ceases at each point of bridging. This results in increasing deformity, e.g., of the distal tibia, with medial fusion leading to increasing varus deformity, which the fibula invariably follows

In summary, stimulative growth disorders are expected after all fractures during growth. The consequences depend on patient age at the time of injury, and duration is limited (to a maximum of 2 years).

Inhibitory growth disturbances are only expected after fractures that are adjacent to or cross the growth plates. They can affect the entire plate or isolated regions, although premature partial closure occurs much more commonly than complete fusion. Angulation results from partial fusion, and overall shortening from complete fusion. Growth abnormalities continue until growth of the affected area is completed (Fig. 1.10).

There are various etiologies of inhibitory growth disturbance. In wide-open growth plates, bony ingrowth of typical epiphyseal fractures (Salter-Harris III and IV) can reach the physis, including the zone of proliferation. The size of the resulting "healing bridge" depends on fracture width. Depending on patient age, the bridge can disrupt spontaneously or remain and lead to increasing deformity.

Bony ingrowth of the fracture gap does not occur in epiphyseal separations (Salter-Harris I and II) or fractures adjacent to the growth plate. In these cases, vascular injury leads to varying levels of growth cartilage destruction, with subsequent ossification of necrotic areas in the proliferation zone. This process can also occur in epiphyseal fractures (Salter-Harris III and IV). These necrosis-spanning bridges are too wide for spontaneous disruptions during growth.

The prognosis regarding growth does not differ fundamentally between epiphyseal fractures and separations. The latter are more common in the lower extremities, but usually in older-aged children, when growth disturbances are less likely to produce clinically relevant complications.

Factors besides patient age affect the development of inhibitory growth abnormalities. Growth plate age is important. Plates responsible for higher proportions of longitudinal growth spend more time growing and thus, have more time to generate distortions. Another factor is the extent of displacement. Growth disturbances are much more common after displaced (versus nondisplaced) fractures. For an unknown reason, inhibitory disturbances are also much more common in the lower extremities (about 30% of cases) than in the upper extremity (about 5%).

Both stimulative and inhibitory growth disorders are unpredictable and cannot be avoided entirely regardless of treatment. Treatment can, however, create better conditions. For stimulative disturbances, the need for remodeling can be reduced. For inhibitory disturbances, the fracture gap width can be decreased. For epiphyseal separations, the prognosis cannot be improved with treatment but can be worsened with rough and/or repeated reduction attempts or other interventions that might damage vascular supply to the physis.

1.4 Spontaneous Correction

Theoretically, angulation in all three spatial planes should correct over the course of growth without the need for intervention. There are various mechanisms involved, but like growth disturbances, they vary according to several factors. The reliability and magnitude of correction increase with younger age, increased proportion (and duration) of growth expected from the closest physis, multi-directionality of the closest joint, and more pronounced angulation. Other fundamental rules include that varus deformities correct better than valgus overall. Angulation in the sagittal plane corrects better than the frontal plane. Dynamic simulation has more effect than static.

The periosteal/endosteal system is entirely responsible for the remodeling of side-to-side translation (Fig. 1.11). Frontal and sagittal plane angulation is corrected with combined periosteal/endosteal remodeling and targeted asymmetrical corrective growth of the epiphyseal plates. Although diaphyseal remodeling is directly responsible for correcting angulation, the epiphyses adjust gradually from oblique to orthograde in the plane of loading. These mechanisms appear to be interdependent (Fig. 1.12) but how they are regulated remains unclear.

Correction of shortening through a stimulative growth response is indiscriminate and unreliable. Reliable length correction is seen only in the paired bones (and not compared to the contralateral limb). There is no internal regulation of symmetrical growth in humans, and thus, post-traumatic length discrepancies are not corrected spontaneously during growth.

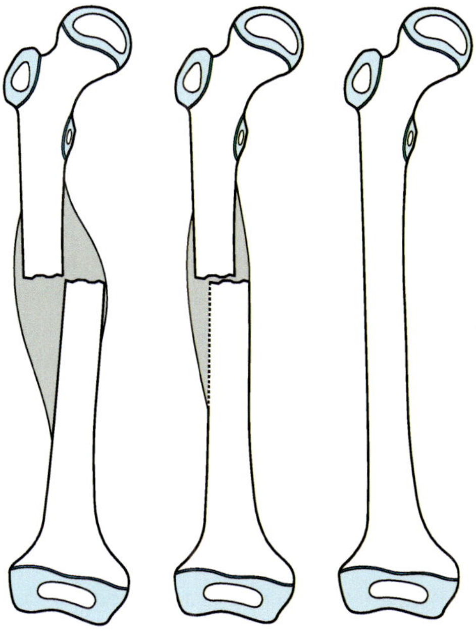

Fig. 1.11 Spontaneous correction of side-to-side translation. Periosteal and endosteal formation/destruction remodel the callus with increasing structural changes depending on the fracture until the original shape is restored

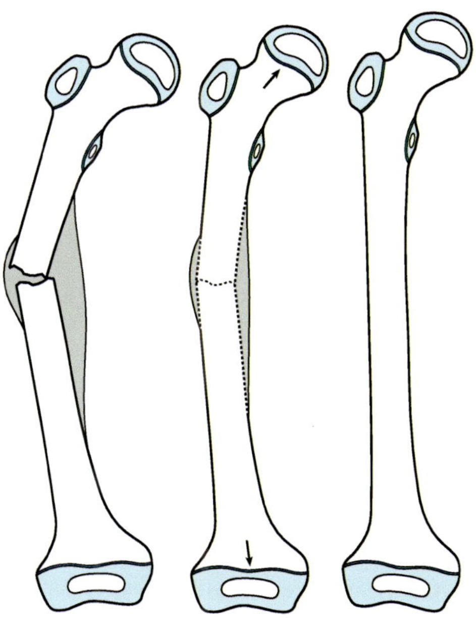

Fig. 1.12 Spontaneous correction of angulation. Periosteal/endosteal correction occurs through shaft remodeling. The epiphyses are initially oblique to the angulation but slowly adjust through asymmetrical growth so that they are orthograde to the loading plane

Rotational deformity can also correct over time indiscriminately according to physiological derotational processes, but little is known about this phenomenon for various bones. To date, there are reports of spontaneous correction for rotational deformities of the humerus and femur (Fig. 1.13). Such deformities are well compensated functionally, and patients are asymptomatic during the relatively long period of correction. Rotational deformities near hinge joints, e.g., on the leg or finger phalanges, are not functionally compensated and are more likely to be symptomatic.

Thus, deformities that are functionally well-compensated are challenging to identify and measure (both radiologically and clinically) and do not require interventive correction. In contrast, poorly compensated deformities are more easily measured clinically and should also be addressed on presentation.

The potential for spontaneous correction can be integrated into treatment. Although the periosteal/endosteal and epiphyseal systems correct for length discrepancies, they cannot influence rotational correction. Thus, extensive angulation of the lower extremities should not generally be left to natural corrective forces. The primary treatment goal should be to minimize the scope of required repair and remodeling and limit post-traumatic leg length discrepancies to idiopathic limits, which are up to 1 cm in 25–30% of the population.

Post-traumatic length discrepancies of the upper extremities are clinically unimportant. The expectation of spontaneous correction is wholly integrated into primary and secondary treatment. For children up to 11 or 12 years, proximal humerus correction is expected for varus up to 50° and angulation in the sagittal plane (Fig. 1.14). In children up to 10 years, the proximal radius corrects tilt to about 50° (Fig. 1.15). The distal radius corrects dorsal and radial tilt to about 40° (Fig. 1.16). Limits of plausibility and tolerance are discussed individually in the corresponding chapters as well as the reconstruction options in separate chapters.

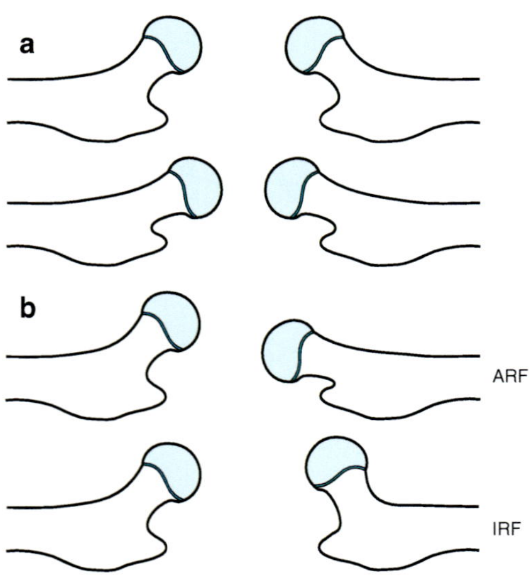

Fig. 1.13 (**a**, **b**) Spontaneous correction of rotational errors; example: femur. Rotational deformity of the femur appears in the anteversion difference of the femoral neck. (**a**, **b**) Anteversion decreases physiologically from birth to the end of growth from about 35° to 15°. The external rotation deformity of the distal fragment (ERD), evidenced by reduced anteversion of the affected side, practically prefers this anteversion. Increased unilateral derotation enables the internal rotation deformity (IRD) of the distal fragment, evidenced by increased anteversion of the affected side, to diminish over the course of growth and thus, become clinically meaningless

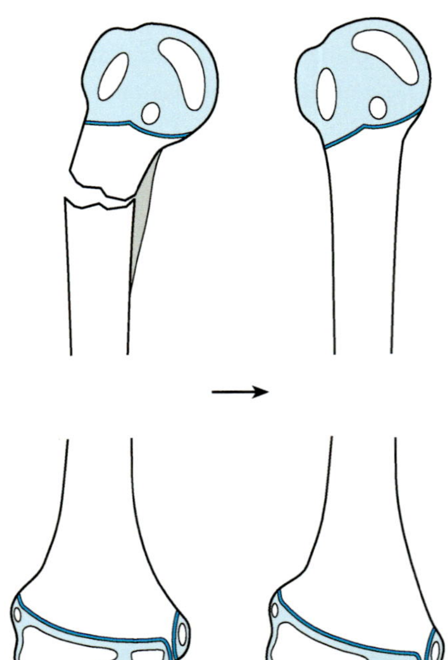

Fig. 1.14 Integration of spontaneous correction into treatment. Reliable correction can be expected and integrated into primary and post-primary treatment. For example, in children up to 12 years, varus angulation up to 50° will correct spontaneously

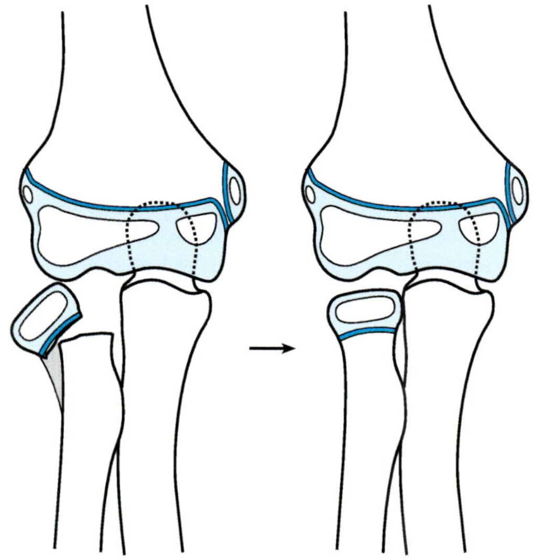

Fig. 1.15 Integration of spontaneous correction into treatment. Reliable correction can be expected and integrated into primary and post-primary treatment. For example, in children up to 10 years, tilt of the radial head up to 50° will correct spontaneously

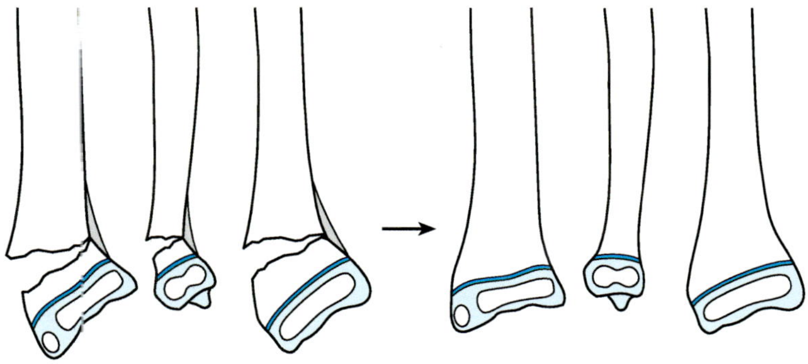

Fig. 1.16 Integration of spontaneous correction into treatment. Reliable correction can be expected and integrated into primary and post-primary treatment. For example, in children up to 12 years, dorsal and radial tilt of the distal radius up to 50° will correct spontaneously

Recommended Literature

Auner B, Marzi I (2013) Oberes Sprunggelenk: Frakturen und Übergangsfrakturen im Kindesalter (Übersichten). Trauma und Berufskrankheit 15(2):217–223

Beck A, Kinzl L, Ruter A, Strecker W (2001) Frakturen mit Beteiligung der distalen Femurepiphyse. Langzeitergebnisse nach Wachstumsabschluss bei primär operativer Versorgung. Unfallchirurg 104:611–616

Berson L, Davidson RS, Dormans JP, Drummond DS, Gregg JR (2000) Growth disturbances after distal tibial physeal fractures. Foot Ankle Int 21:54–58

Buchholz IM, Bolhuis HW, Broker FH, Gratama JW, Sakkers RJ, Bouma WH (2002) Overgrowth and correction of rotational deformity in 12 femoral shaft fractures in 3-6-year-old children treated with an external fixator. Acta Orthop Scand 73:170–174

de Sanctis N, Della Corte S, Pempinello C (2000) Distal tibial and fibular epiphyseal fractures in children: prognostic criteria and long-term results in 158 patients. J Pediatr Orthop B 9:40–44

Frank J, Sander AL, Voth M, Marzi I (2016) Sekundäre Rekonstruktionen am Ellenbogengelenk im Kindesalter. Trauma und Berufskrankheit.

Hasler CC, von Laer L (2000) Pathophysiologie posttraumatischer Deformitäten der unteren Extremität im Wachstumsalter. Orthopäde 29:757–765
Hasler CC, von Laer L (2001) Prevention of growth disturbances after fractures of the lateral humeral condyle in children. J Pediatr Orthop B 10:123–130
Hell AK, von Laer L (2014) Growth behaviour after fractures of the proximal radius: differences to the rest of the skeleton. Unfallchirurg 117(12):1085–1091
Landin LA (1997) Epidemiology of children's fractures. J Pediatr Orthop B 6:79–83
Laurer HL, Sander AL, Wutzler S, Walcher F, Marzi I (2009 Jul 8) Therapy principles of distal fractures of the forearm in childhood. Chirurg 80(11):1042–1052
Lieber J (2014) Growth behavior after fractures of the distal forearm: reasons for the high rate of overtreatment. Unfallchirurg 117(12):1092–1098
Maier M, Maier-Heidkamp P, Lehnert M, Wirbel R, Marzi I (2003) Ausheilungsergebnisse konservativ und operativ versorgter kindlicher Femurfrakturen. Unfallchirurg 106:48–54
Marzi I, Maier B, Laurer HL (2002) Ab wann wird die kindliche Fraktur zur Fraktur des Erwachsenen? Zeitpunkt und Bedeutung des Fugenschlusses. Kongressbd Dtsch Ges Chir Kongr 119:699–702
Rockwood CA, Wilkins KE, Beaty JH (1996) Fractures in children, 4th edn. Lippincott-Raven, New York
Schneidmüller D, Kraft C, Bühren V, von Laer L (2014) Growth behavior after femoral shaft fractures. Unfallchirurg 117(12):1099–1104
Schneidmüller D, Sander AL, Wertenbroek M, Wutzler S, Kraus R, Marzi I et al (2014 Feb) Triplane fractures: do we need cross-sectional imaging? Eur J Trauma Emerg Surg 40(1):37–43
Vogt B, Schiedel F, Rödl R (2014) Guided growth in children and adolescents. Orthopäde 43(3):267–284
von Laer L (2014 Nov 26) Growth behavior after epiphyseal plate injury. Unfallchirurg 117(12):1071–1084
von Laer L, Kraus R, Linhart WE (2012) Frakturen und Luxationen im Wachstumsalter, 6th edn. Thieme Verlag, Stuttgart
Zimmermann R, Gabl M, Angermann P, Lutz M, Reinhart C, Kralinger F, Pechlaner S (2000) Spätfolgen nach Frakturen im distalen Unterarmdrittel im Wachstumsalter. Handchir Mikrochir Plast Chir 32:242–249

2 Injury Patterns and Diagnostics

2.1 Fractures

Unlike adult injuries, pediatric fractures are consistent in presentation more according to patient age and less according to direction and mechanism of injury. Because the growth plate is more commonly injured than the nearby joint, articular fractures are rare. Metaphyseal fractures and epiphyseal separations occur more frequently, and diaphyseal fractures less. Children do not suffer the more complex comminuted articular fractures seen in adults, except complex fracture-dislocations, e.g., of the elbow.

The rare articular fractures conform strongly to patterns. The stereotypical articular fracture of the upper extremity is the lateral condyle fracture of the humerus, which always occurs in the main loading area of the joint. In the lower extremity, articular fractures of the medial malleolus are always external to the main loading area, along the edge of the articular surface. These patterns change only as the physes begin to fuse, with the emergence of transitional fractures. Transitional fractures also conform to typical age-dependent patterns and do not appear like adult injuries.

Pediatric fracture classifications have focused on injuries to the epiphyseal plates. Unfortunately, it is impossible to glean information regarding the prognosis for post-traumatic growth and development based on these systems. Too many external factors affect growth. Therapeutic guidelines are also impractical as a means of classification because treatment is based on individual, social and economic factors in addition to fracture location and displacement. Thus, classifications are limited to morphological description so that there is at least a common understanding of the injury.

In this chapter, pediatric fractures and characteristics will be briefly introduced, and classifications will be discussed at the end. The aim is practicality rather than completeness to ensure accurate documentation and care quality.

I. Marzi et al., *Pediatric Skeletal Trauma*, https://doi.org/10.1007/978-3-030-93685-3_2

Articular Region

Physeal fractures are classified according to a general system (e.g., Salter-Harris, Aitken). This system considers the morphological structure of the growth plate and bone and not the anatomical region involved. However, it is essential to distinguish articular from shaft fractures, regardless of the fracture type and location of physeal damage.

In articular fractures, the state of the growth plate (wide open versus fusing) must be evaluated because this determines the type of injury (classic versus transitional). Articular fracture of the distal tibia is an example. In a classic injury (before plates begin to fuse at the age of 10–12 years), the fracture line is located along the medial edge of the articular surface, running perpendicular to but not involving the loading area. There are two variations of this injury (with and without metaphyseal involvement) described by Aitken (Types 2 and 3) and Salter-Harris (III and IV).

With the start of physiological plate fusion, the transitional fracture line usually runs oblique to the articular surface, into the lateral aspect of the joint and the main loading area. Depending on the mechanism of injury, there can also be a metaphyseal wedge fragment. These fractures are usually subsumed within the category of typical malleolar fractures, which is misleading because they require different treatment and have a different prognosis regarding growth. Unlike classic articular fractures, transitional fractures are no longer expected to produce relevant growth disorders from partial physeal closure. For this reason, the two should be differentiated and aptly designated.

In terms of classification, articular fractures crossing the physis should be distinguished from those not affecting it. When the injury has crossed the plate, classic versus transitional fractures are assessed. Epiphyseal fractures, classic or transitional, must be divided into those with and those without metaphyseal involvement. Transitional fractures typically run laterally and in two planes. A metaphyseal wedge does not always continue past the growth plate in a triplane I presentation. Instead, it can present as a discretional triplane II fracture, i.e., the wedge fragment supplementing the primary anterior epiphyseal fracture (Figs. 2.1 and 2.2).

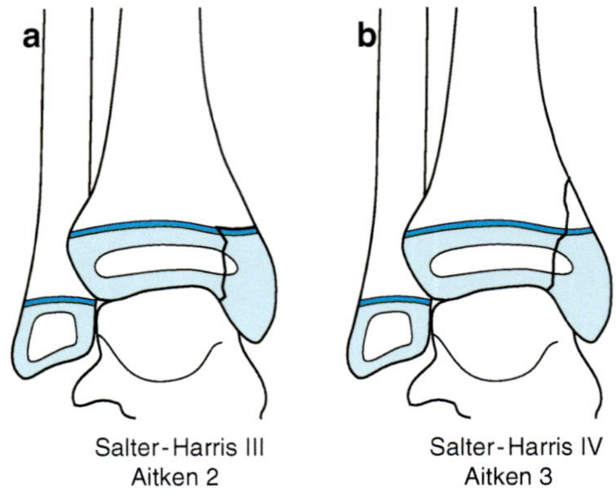

Fig. 2.1 Fracture across the open growth plate. (**a**) Epiphyseal fracture, (**b**) Epi-metaphyseal fracture

Articular fractures not affecting the epiphyseal plate are bony ligament avulsions (e.g., tibial intercondylar eminence fractures or fibulotalar ligament ruptures avulsing the fibular tip) and osteochondral or chondral flake fractures after dislocation (e.g., patellar dislocation). Osseous, chondral, or periosteal ligament tears are common until the ages of 10–12 years because the ligaments are more stable than their attachments. Ligament ruptures are far more common over this age, but this does not mean that ruptures do not occur before age 10 nor that avulsions do not occur in patients over 12 (Fig. 2.3).

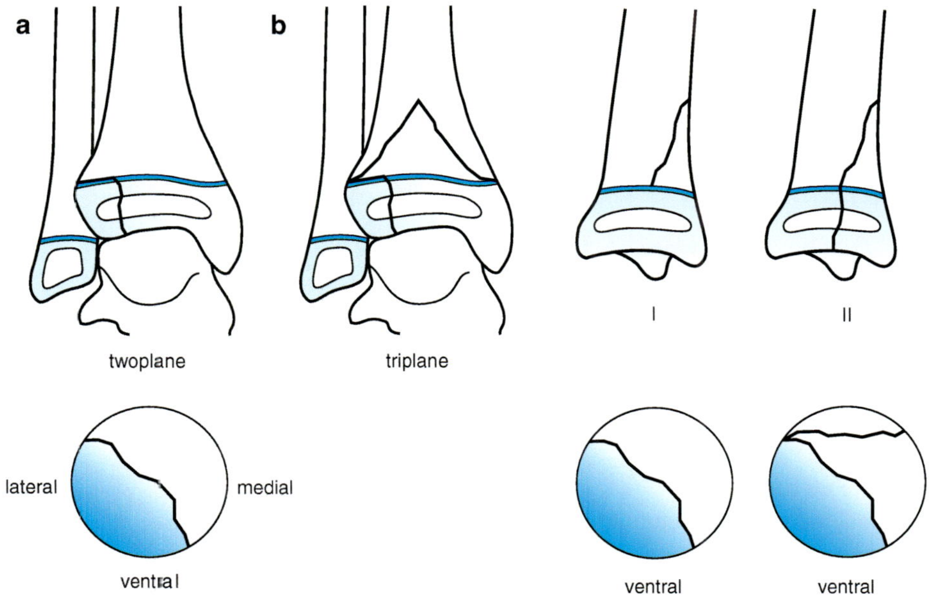

Fig. 2.2 Fracture across the fusing growth plate. Transitional fractures: (**a**) Epiphyseal fracture, (**b**) Epi-metaphyseal fracture

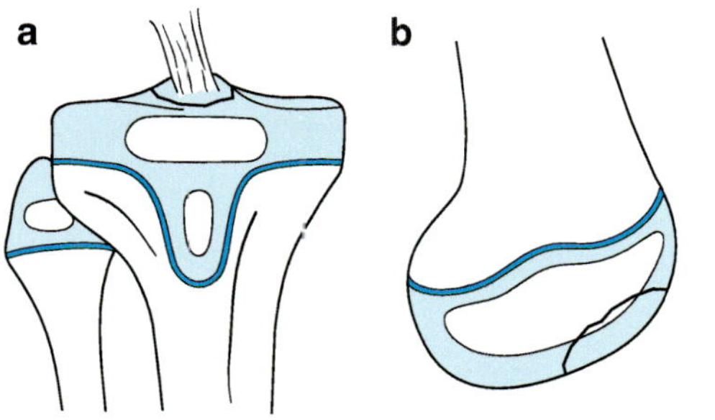

Fig. 2.3 (**a**) Epiphyseal osteochondral ligament rupture, (**b**) "Flake fractures"

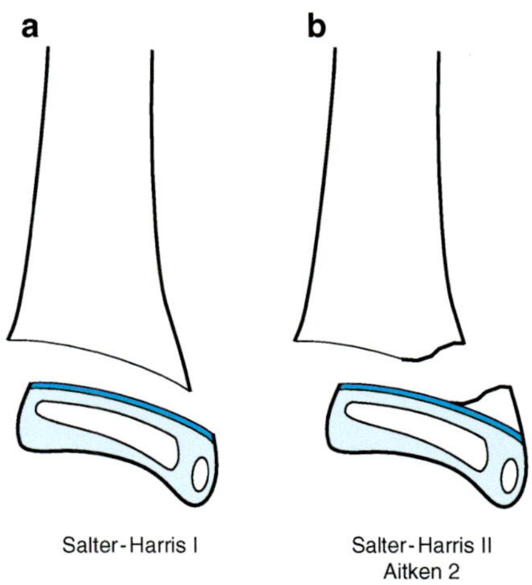

Fig. 2.4 Epiphysiolysis. (**a**) No metaphyseal fragment (Salter-Harris I), (**b**) With epi-metaphyseal fragment (Salter-Harris II)

Epiphysis/Metaphysis

Epiphyseal Separation

Epiphyseal separation is the most peripheral fracture of the metaphyseal shaft. Although the epiphysis protects the joint, it is not directly affected. Separation occurs within the zone of hypertrophy, the structurally weakest area of the plate. Epiphyseal separations occur more often around puberty due to hormonal influences, especially in the lower extremities. They are among the most common pediatric injuries and occur four times more frequently in the upper versus lower extremities (e.g., finger phalanges, distal radius, proximal radius, proximal humerus (Fig. 2.4).

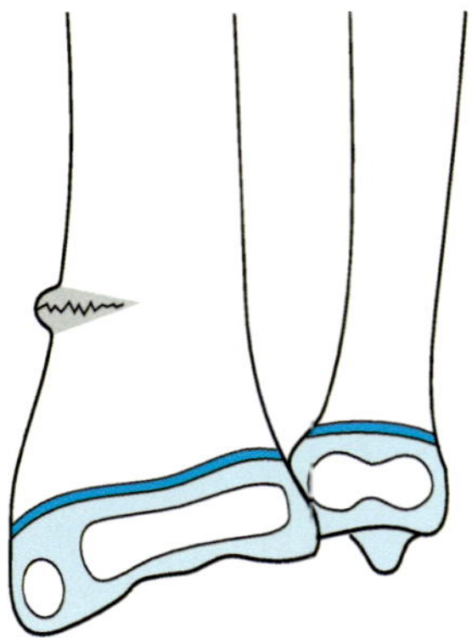

Fig. 2.5 Metaphyseal compression fracture

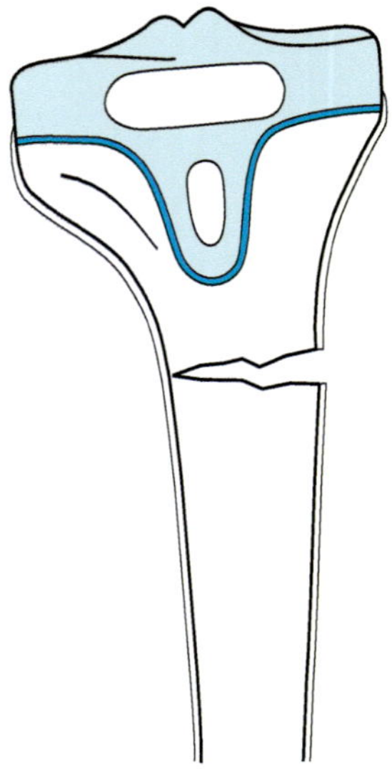

Fig. 2.6 Metaphyseal greenstick fracture

Compression Fractures

Metaphyseal compression fracture is a classic contusion injury occurring somewhat further along the shaft. In most cases, a single cortex is compressed, and the other remains intact. These fractures are painful but harmless. They can be found in all metaphyses but most commonly in the distal forearm (Fig. 2.5).

Greenstick Fractures

Greenstick (bending) fractures are also found in the metaphysis. They are only clinically relevant in the proximal tibia with a stimulative growth disorder (Fig. 2.6) and sometimes in the distal radius. Regardless of location (shaft or metaphysis), greenstick fractures are flexion fractures and not subperiosteal compression fractures!

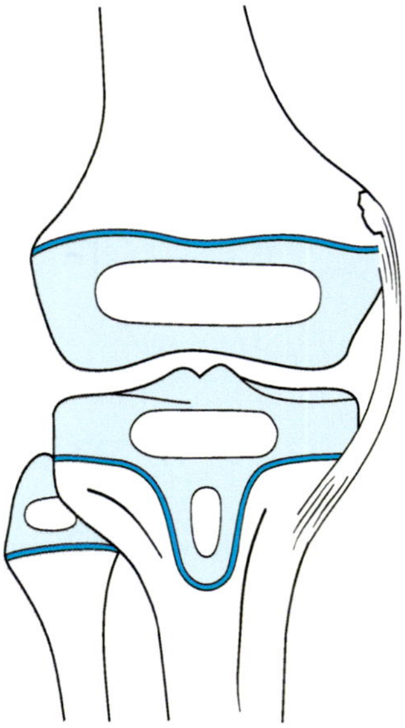

Fig. 2.7 Metaphyseal ligament avulsion

Metaphyseal Fractures

Complete fractures of the metaphysis are also important. Typical examples are supracondylar humerus fractures, types III and IV.

Stress Fractures

There are two peak age incidences for stress fractures in children: between 2 and 4 years and around puberty. Small children learning to walk and run can often "overdo" it, resulting in recurrent mini traumas and bony overload. Common sites of invisible fissures or "toddler's fracture" are in the tibia, fibula, tarsus, and femur. Around puberty, excessive sports activity is the typical cause of stress fractures in the proximal tibia or the metatarsals.

Collateral Ligament Avulsions

Isolated osseous, chondral, or periosteal metaphyseal collateral ligament avulsions of the distal femur can occasionally occur (Fig. 2.7).

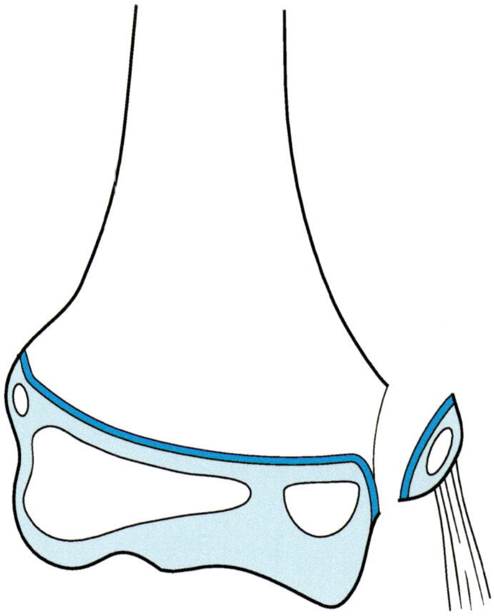

Fig. 2.8 Metaphyseal rupture (apophyseal avulsion) at the medial collateral ligament

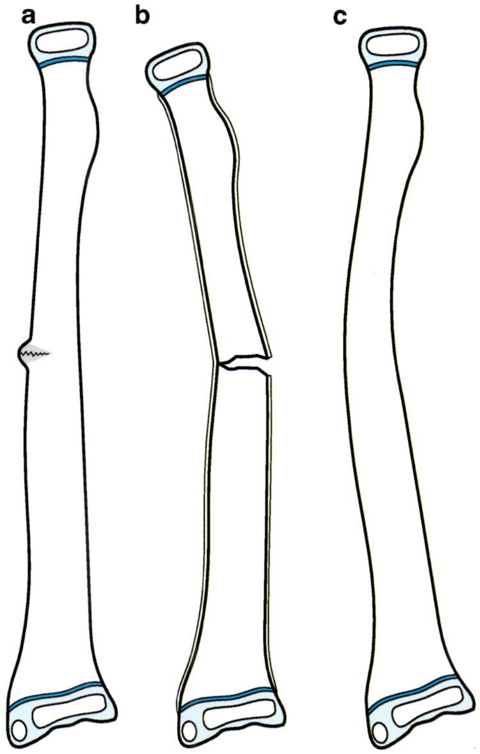

Fig. 2.9 Diaphyseal greenstick fracture. (**a**) Compressed greenstick fracture, (**b**) Classic greenstick fracture, (**c**) Bowing fracture

Tendon Avulsion

Muscle tendon tears avulsing the bony attachment occur mainly in the elbow region and the pelvis (humeral medial epicondyle, anterior iliac spines, lesser trochanter (Fig. 2.8)). Hormones and sports stress are contributing factors and explain why this occurs most often in adolescents. Apophyseal growth plates are structured like epiphyseal growth plates. However, because the functional loading differs (tensile versus compressive force), they do not contribute to longitudinal bone growth.

Diaphysis

Greenstick Fractures

Greenstick fractures are stereotypical pediatric injuries of the shaft and are most common in the forearm. They are flexion injuries and not subperiosteal compression fractures! Thus, there is always some angulation. The three main presentations are the classic greenstick fracture, compressed greenstick fractures in toddlers, and bowing fractures (Fig. 2.9). One cortex (on the concave side) remains intact in classic greenstick fractures while the opposite is completely disrupted. If left to heal spontaneously, the intact cortex heals quickly but prevents callus bridging (and thus, healing) on the opposite side. The risk of refracture is high, with about 20–30% of cases. A compressed greenstick fracture presents almost exclusively in children under age five and does not have the healing problem described above. **Bowing fractures**, which occur later in childhood and adolescence, also do not have healing problems and are difficult to detect. The issue may result from function-limiting angulation, similar to certain Monteggia injuries.

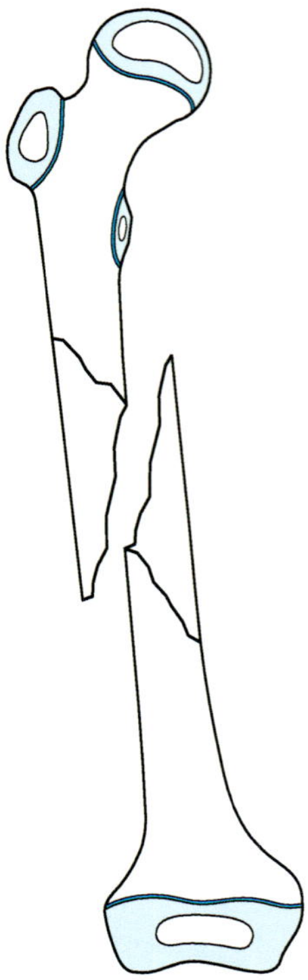

Fig. 2.10 Diaphyseal oblique and compound fractures

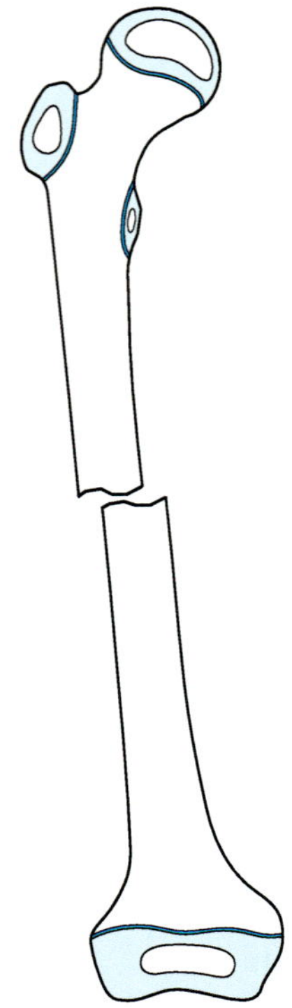

Fig. 2.11 Diaphyseal transverse fractures

Oblique Fractures

Oblique fractures include those with partial or complete rotational wedges and comminuted fractures. They are longitudinally unstable, except isolated tibia fractures, because there is no anchoring of the fragments. The large fracture surface facilitates rapid healing, achieving consolidation in almost half the time of transverse diaphyseal fractures (Fig. 2.10).

Transverse Fractures

Because of the smaller surface area, these fractures heal more slowly than oblique fractures. The fractures are longitudinally stable when the fragments are aligned (Fig. 2.11).

2.2 Dislocations

Dislocations become more common than completely displaced metaphyseal fractures as the ligament attachments become more stable than the ligaments themselves (see also ligament lesions). In other words, they increase just before the involved skeletal region reaches maturity.

Shoulder

Shoulder dislocations typically occur after the age of 10–12 years. Like in adults, anterior dislocations can have associated labral injuries,

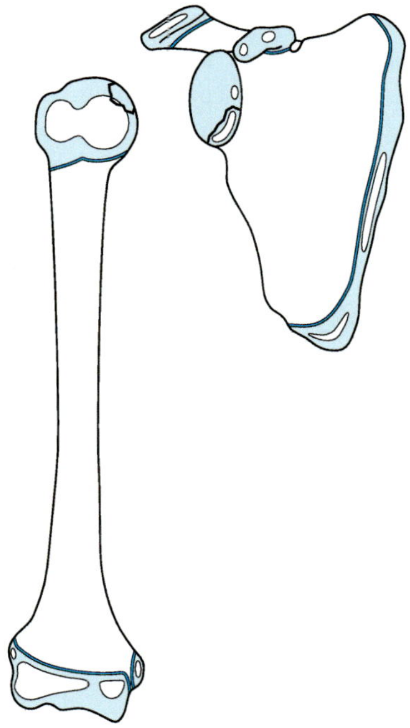

Fig. 2.12 Shoulder dislocation with the osteochondral flake of the human and “Bankart” lesion

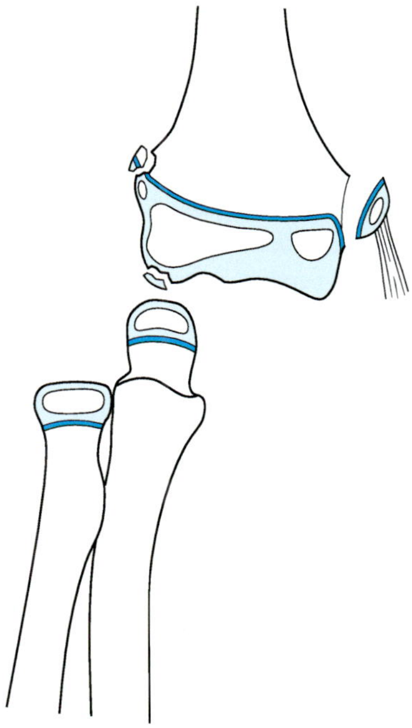

Fig. 2.13 Elbow dislocation with apophyseal rupture of the medial epicondyle

flake fractures, direct injury to the humeral head, and anterior osteochondral glenoid injuries (Fig. 2.12).

Elbow

Elbows generally dislocate posteriorly. Associated injuries include avulsions of the medial epicondyle, lateral collateral ligament tears, and osteochondral flake fractures from the lateral condyle (Fig. 2.13).

Radial head dislocations are often overlooked in either isolated or Monteggia lesion contexts. Monteggia lesions include the classic fracture and proximal and mid-ulnar fractures combined with radial head dislocations or fracture-dislocations. Every elbow radiograph should be checked for the correct position of the radial head within the humeral capitellum (Fig. 2.14).

A pulled elbow (“nursemaid’s elbow”) is neither a dislocation nor a subluxation. It is a painful blocking of the radial head in extreme pronation and can be released with a quick, targeted maneuver.

a

b

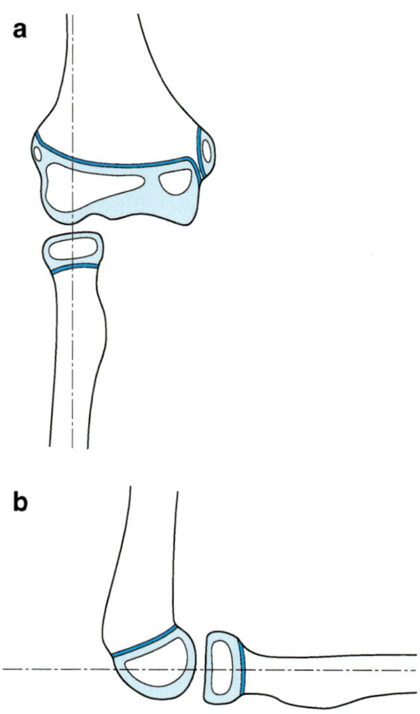

Fig. 2.14 Radial head and capitellum humeri should be in a straight line in (**a**) A.P. view and (**b**) lateral view

Hips

Traumatic posterior hip dislocation is rare and always the result of high-speed trauma. Thus, there are often associated injuries such as flakes, acetabular avulsions, etc. MRI is necessary to diagnose concomitant acetabular injury so that the indication for a possible operative intervention can be seen.

Knee

Patellar dislocations are not usually traumatic, but congenital patellar dislocation occurs after trauma in one-third of cases and habitually in two-thirds. Traumatic patellar dislocations are associated with flake fractures of the patella or lateral femoral condyle as retinaculum avulsions.

2.3 Radiological Examination

A thorough clinical examination of the patient must be performed in a skillful and child-focused manner. This means that potential injuries must be targeted right away.

Imaging pediatric fractures requires experienced radiologists and technical equipment. The radiologist must be familiar with the developing skeleton as well as typical injury presentations and mechanisms. Radiation hygiene demands that diagnostic imaging be kept to a minimum with low-dose protocols whenever possible. An indication for imaging follows clinical examination. Theoretically, the same radiological techniques and settings are used for children and adults. However, the choice of procedure and the extent of imaging should be based on age and the specific diagnostic question.

If an initial image shows an evident fracture or dislocation requiring surgery, further imaging should be delayed until the child is under anesthesia. If findings are unclear, splint immobilization and analgesia can also be optimized before completing diagnostic imaging. In select cases, when gross displacement and deformity are ruled out, more thorough diagnostic imaging can be completed over the subsequent days, provided the patient is immobilized and clinical findings are typical. In rare cases, sedation may be necessary (CT, MRI), but the indication for the examination must be clear. Specific diagnostic approaches and criteria are detailed in the corresponding chapters.

Radiography

Standard exposures are the anterior-posterior (AP) and lateral (as precise as possible). Images usually include the adjacent joint to evaluate the complete osteochondral unit. For an accurate fracture assessment, images should be centered on the injury (no overview images in two planes). Oblique views may be necessary in some cases to determine displacement (e.g., assessment of the distal humerus or ankle mortise). Non-standard projections may be necessary in cases of fracture or severe pain.

The timing of follow-up films depends on the specific injury. The typical protocol is initial trauma images followed by reduction/fixation films and an eventual consolidation check. Fractures with a tendency for secondary displacement (e.g., humeral lateral condyle fractures) will have targeted follow-up checks scheduled within defined time windows. Stable and compressed fractures do not require further x-ray controls.

Ultrasound

Ultrasound is well suited to assess soft-tissue injuries, including tendons, ligaments, and joint effusions, and is highly sensitive in detecting sternum and rib fractures. Fractures are identified directly and indirectly through subperiosteal hematoma or post-traumatic hemarthrosis. Injuries to the non-ossified epiphyses can be diagnosed in infants by examining the position related to the metaphysis and evidence of joint effusion. Some clinics use it to follow up conservatively treated fractures, e.g., of the distal forearm. Ultrasound enables dynamic assessment coupled with clinical examination, as well as guided aspiration.

Computed Tomography (CT)

Computed tomography (CT) is used to assess pediatric polytrauma, complicated fractures, and surgical planning, and particularly for traumatic brain injuries (TBI), thoracoabdominal injuries, and pelvic and vertebral fractures. Although there are many individual assessment tools for mild TBI, CT is the gold standard for diagnosing severe and moderate injuries.

Dose-reducing protocols are implemented for children; particularly the thyroid, neck area, and eyes should be protected. Current data shows that ultra-low dose protocols keep voltages within 20–80 kV with minimal current time and comparable radiation exposure to conventional radiographs. Multi-slice CT is superior to conventional techniques and is particularly suitable for special surgical planning and trauma diagnosis because it is performed rapidly and enables 3D reconstructions along with lower radiation.

Magnetic Resonance Imaging (MRI)

Magnetic resonance imaging (MRI) is used to visualize non-ossified parts of the skeleton like epiphyses, physes, cartilage, and soft-tissue structures like ligaments, tendons, and muscles. It is used in trauma surgery to diagnose spine injuries and occult fractures and detect injuries to the structures listed above. It is useful in diagnosing articular injuries when x-ray findings are unclear, especially of the knee, ankle, and sternoclavicular joints. Relevant pediatric knee and shoulder injuries require MRI before operative intervention. For other locations such as the elbow, it rarely provides therapeutically relevant information.

MRI can reliably distinguish stress fractures from bone tumors. Conventional radiographs are less reliable for this as the periosteal reaction can be misinterpreted. MRI gives no radiation load; however, it is a relatively complex process. It is expensive and often requires sedation in smaller children with a relatively long examination time. The new sequence protocol with diffusion and strongly T2-weighted sequences is important today. It is often superior to CT for diagnostic imaging of the upper extremities.

Other Approaches

Other techniques such as bone scintigraphy, angiography, or arthrography are not used for routine diagnosis and are only available for less common and special cases. Special stress recordings are no longer indicated, e.g., for diagnosis of a fibular collateral ligament tear. As yet, there has been no conclusion regarding the need for contralateral x-ray comparisons for the diagnosis of pediatric fractures. A comparison should not be necessary for fracture diagnosis when the radiologist is familiar with pediatric x-ray anatomy. There are a few select indications for contralateral comparison, e.g., congenital deformities and previous injuries or post-traumatic deformities.

2.4 Radiological Development of the Pediatric Skeleton

Familiarity with the timeline of epiphyseal plate fusion and the development of ossification centers is essential for accurate diagnosis and determination of bone age (Tables 2.1 and 2.2; Figs. 2.15 and Fig. 2.16). There are two visible epiphyses in the newborn at term: the distal femur and the proximal tibia. Other ossification centers develop according to age. Apophyseal centers arise during adolescence and fuse with the bones by age 25. The iliac crest apophysis fuses in girls

Table 2.1 Ossification centers of the elbow and age of development

Humeral capitellum	1 year
Radial head	5 years
Medial epicondyle	7 years
Olecranon	10 years
Lateral epicondyle	11 years

Table 2.2 Ossification centers of the carpal bones

Capitate	3 months
Hamate	3 months
Triquetrum	3 years
Lunate	3–4 years
Trapezium	5 years
Scaphoid	6 years
Trapezoid	6 years
Pisiform	10 years

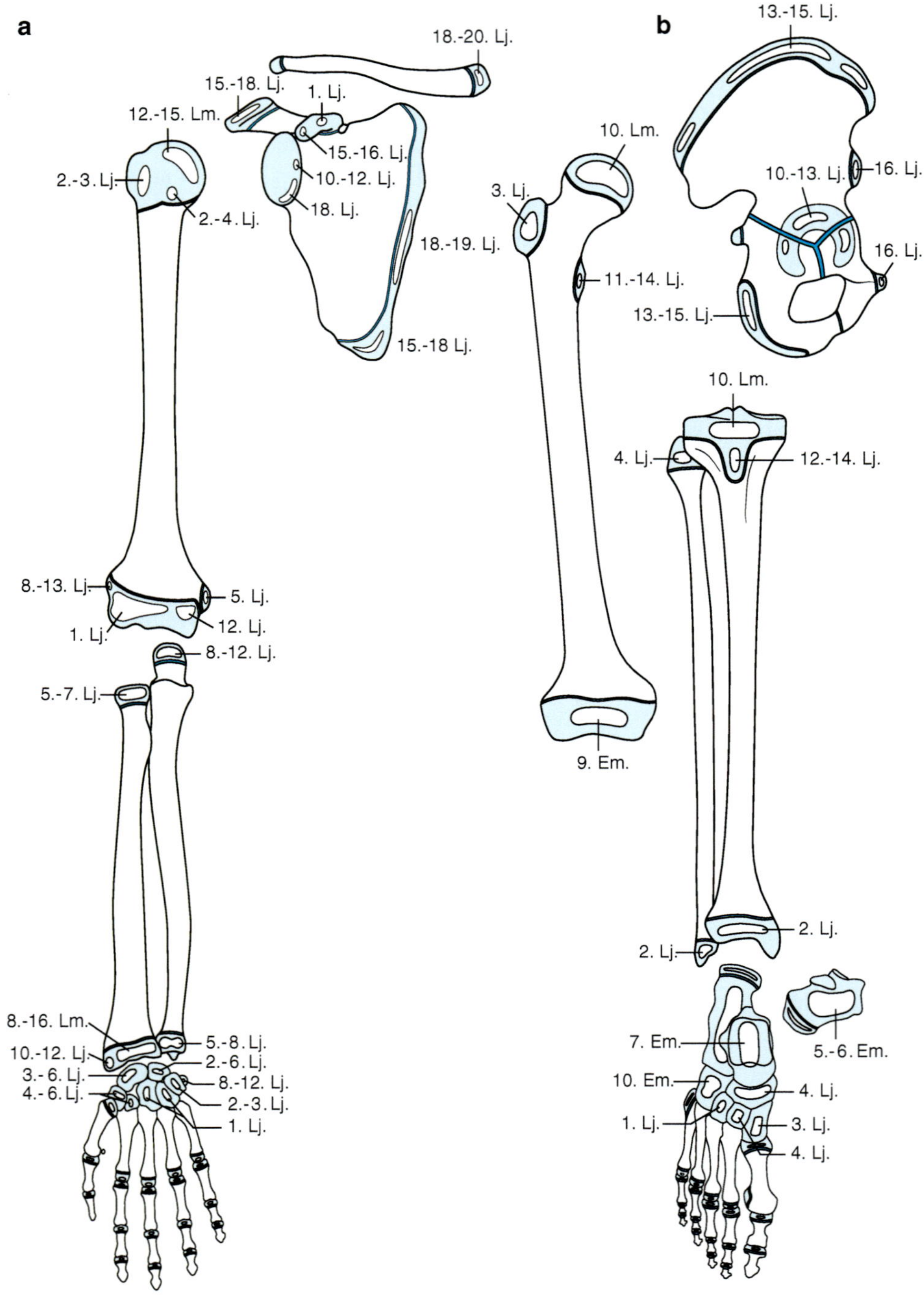

Fig. 2.15 Ossification centers of the skeleton and age. (**a**) Upper extremity, (**b**) Lower extremity. (*Lj*) life year; (*Lm*) life month; (*Em*) embryonal month

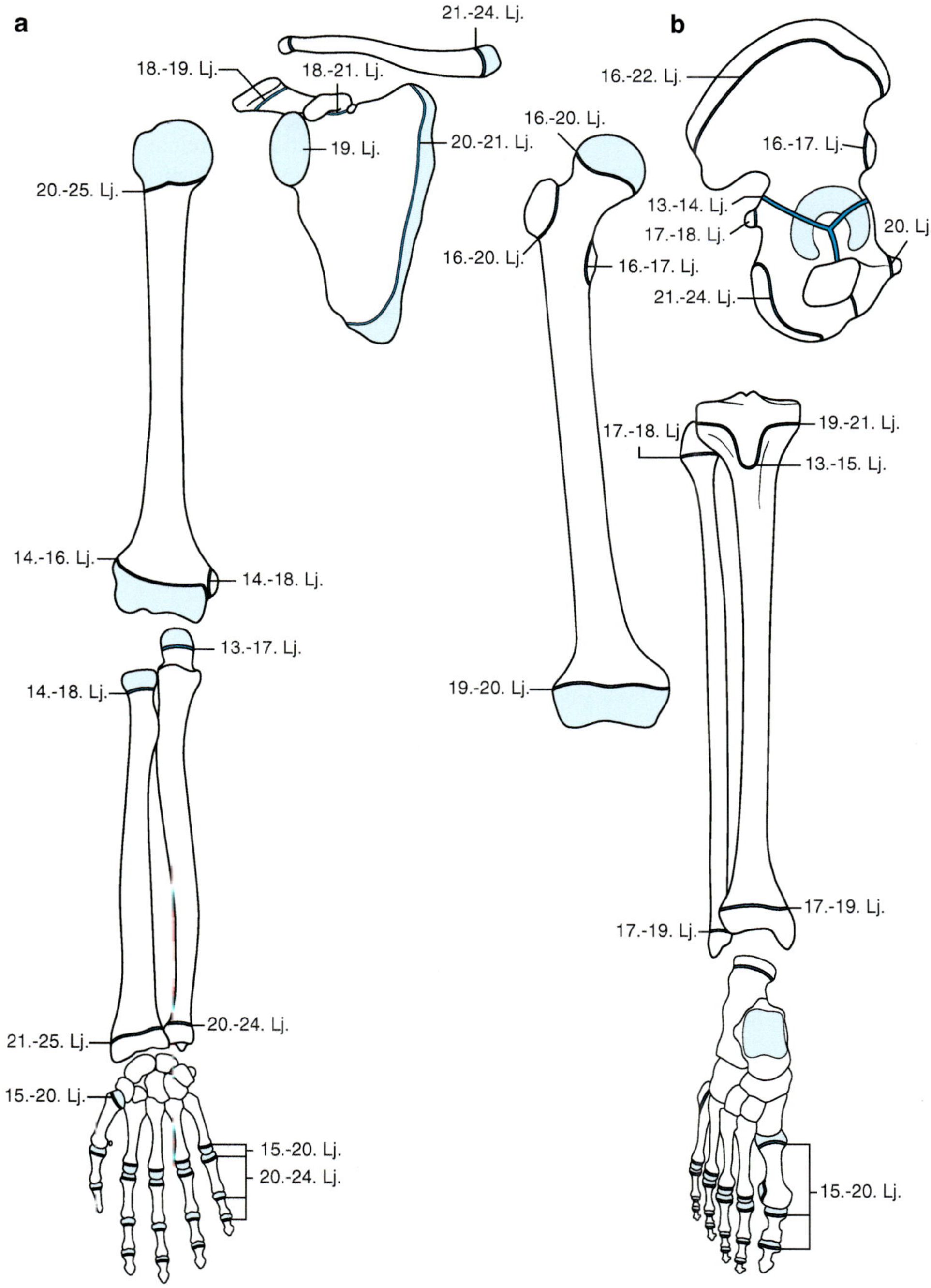

Fig. 2.16 Complete fusion of the growth plate. The beginning of closure depends on age and sex. (**a**) Upper extremity, (**b**) Lower extremity. (*Lj*) life year; (*Em*) embryonal month

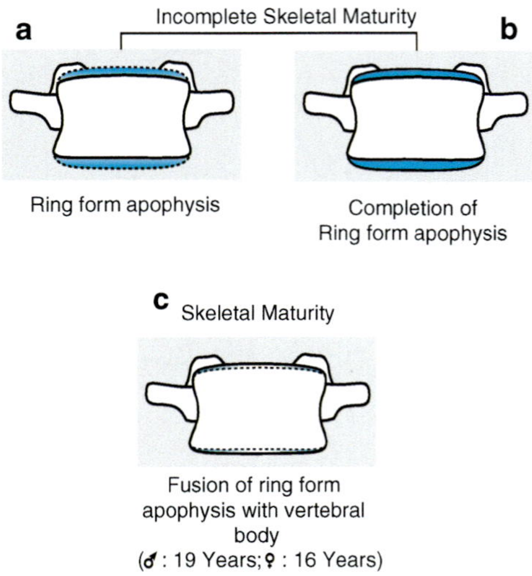

Fig. 2.17 Determination of bone age by the vertebral body ossification. (**a**) The ring apophysis begins to be visible. (**b**) The ring apophysis is completely developed but not yet fused with the vertebral body. (**c**) Complete skeletal maturation: the ring apophysis is fused with the vertebral body (boys 19 years, girls 16 years)

Table 2.3 Risser sign

Stage 0	Apophysis not visible
Stage 1	Starting lateral ossification
Stage 2	Ossification over half of the circumference of the iliac crest
Stage 3	Starting fusion of the apophysis with the iliac crest
Stage 4	Apophysis is fused over half of the ilium
Stage 5	Apophysis is completely fused with the ileum

around age 13 and later in boys, around 14.5 years. The physis of DII in the hand fuses shortly before menarche. Vertebral growth can continue until age 30.

A determination of skeletal maturity is essential when selecting treatment and helps to assess prognosis. Hand radiographs are commonly compared to standardized atlas images to determine bone age. Other indicators are vertebral ring apophyses (Fig. 2.17) and the iliac crest apophysis (Risser sign; Table 2.3 and Fig. 2.18).

There is considerable variability in the appearance of ossification centers to be distinguished from pathological findings. They can emerge as multiple centers, have irregular borders, or be fragmented. There are also physiological variants that are more common in skeletal dysplasias.

Coned Epiphysis

Coned epiphysis is found in approximately 4% of normal hand skeletons but is frequently present in chromosomal abnormalities and skeletal dysplasias.

Pseudoepiphysis

Pseudoepiphysis can be a physiological variant in the proximal MCs II–IV and distal MC I; it is increased in skeletal dysplasias.

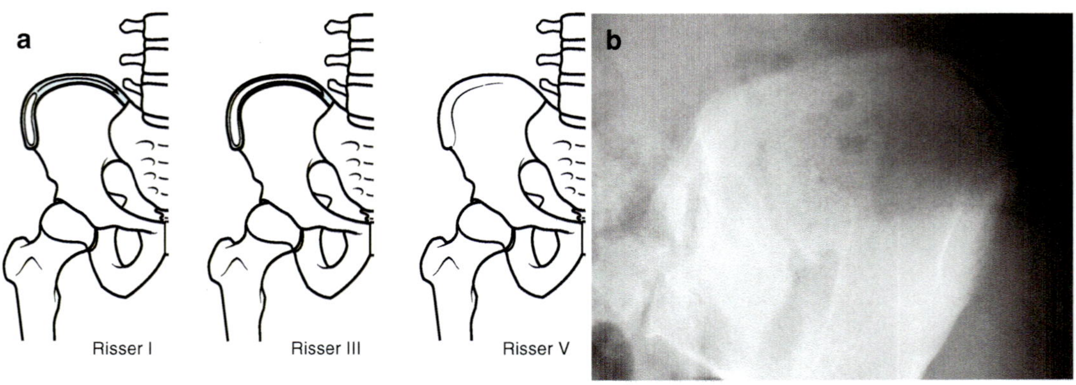

Fig. 2.18 Risser sign: Skeletal development can be determined from the iliac crest apophysis. (**a**) Illustration, (**b**) X-ray Risser II

2.5 Radiological Diagnostic Clues

Periosteal callus reactions and fracture line compression are indications of fractures not detected on primary x-ray. These are generally seen on MRI. However, there is no therapeutic benefit to performing MRI specifically to identify occult fractures since these are treated the same as suspected occult fractures: conservatively with immobilization. MRI is useful to diagnose osteochondral or chondral fractures or flakes. Knee MRI has gained particular importance as it replaces purely diagnostic arthroscopy procedures and enables better preoperative planning.

Harris Lines

Harris lines (growth arrest lines) are radiopaque lines in the metaphysis parallel to the growth plate. They usually form because of a systemic illness, e.g., a viral or bacterial infection. They can be useful in diagnosing partial growth plate disturbances, evident when the growth plate no longer runs parallel to the line (Fig. 2.19).

Fat Pad Sign

A fat pad sign indicates joint effusion (Fig. 2.20) and is a valuable diagnostic clue. In the elbow, it occurs in the olecranon fossa and is not visible on

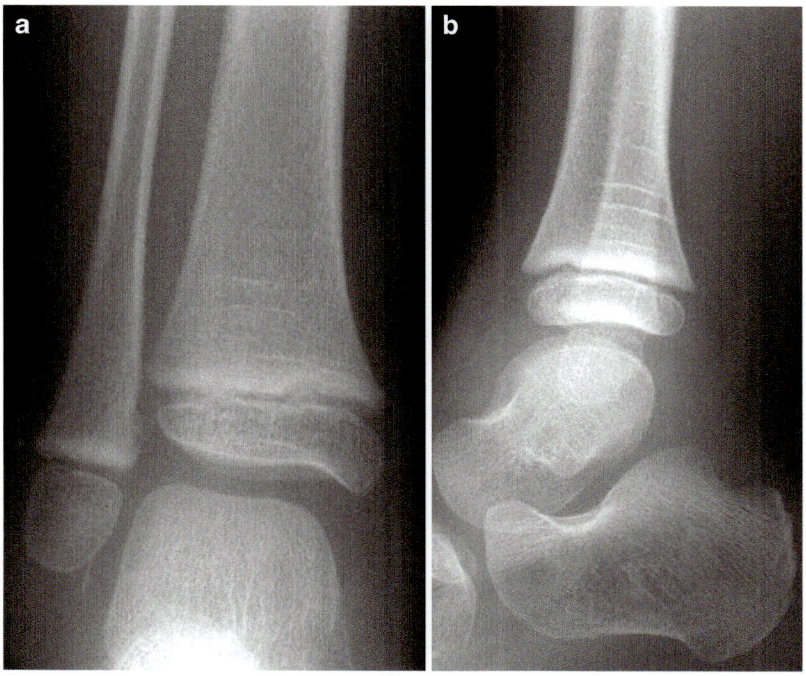

Fig. 2.19 Harris line. (**a**) A.P. view, (**b**) Lateral view

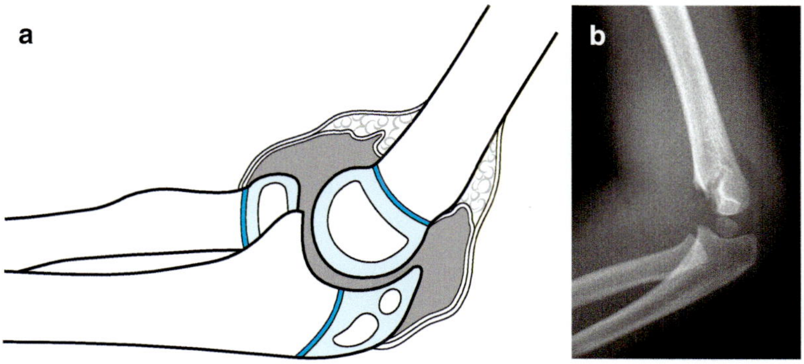

Fig. 2.20 Fat pad sign. (**a**) Illustration, (**b**) X-ray

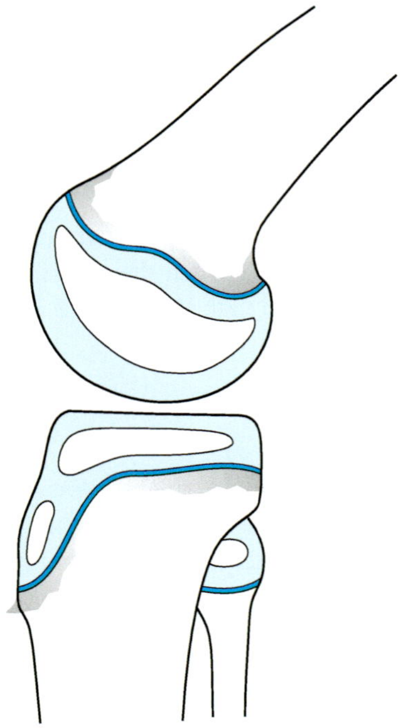

Fig. 2.21 Metaphyseal corner sign

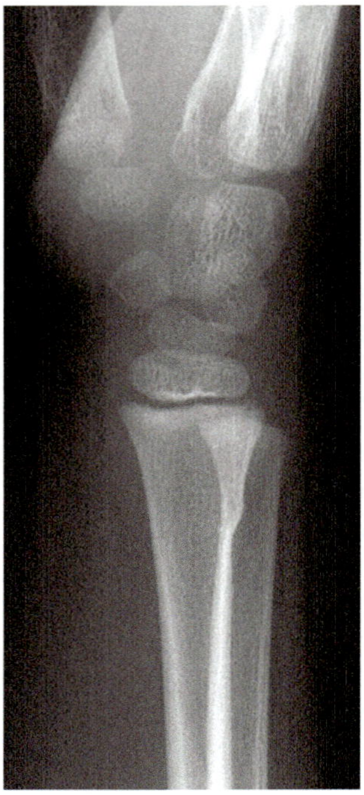

Fig. 2.22 Buckle fracture

x-rays of uninjured joints. The anterior fat pad is found in the coronoid and radial fossae and can be visualized on normal films as a narrow border along the anterior humerus. Stretching of the joint capsule from effusion displaces this anteriorly or posteriorly, making it more radiographically obvious. This sign is often associated with fractures of the distal humerus, but not every fracture has a positive fat pad sign.

Battered Child Syndrome (Child Abuse)

The following radiological findings can indicate child abuse:

- multiple fractures of different ages with pronounced callus formation
- fractures that rarely occur in children such as rib, scapula, sternum, spinous process fractures
- periosteal bone reaction from subperiosteal hematoma
- blurry metaphyseal contours, especially in infants and toddlers (Fig. 2.21), indicating metaphyseal avulsion fractures with simultaneous epiphyseal separation, resulting from tension on the joint capsule.

If battered child syndrome is suspected, complete body x-rays should be carried out in a single plane to rule out further injuries.

Special Pediatric Fracture Forms

The pediatric skeleton has unique qualities compared to adults, including epiphyseal plates, thicker cortices, and high elasticity, which enables reversal of deformity. The pediatric periosteum has a higher fat content, increased vascularization and is thicker than that of adults so it often remains intact after injury (greenstick fracture).

Buckle (Torus) Fracture

Typical bulging compression fracture, predominantly of the distal radial metaphysis. The periosteal tube remains intact (Fig. 2.22).

Greenstick Fracture

Flexion fracture with complete disruption of one cortex and incomplete disruption of the other side. Inadequate treatment leads to an increased deformity (Fig. 2.23).

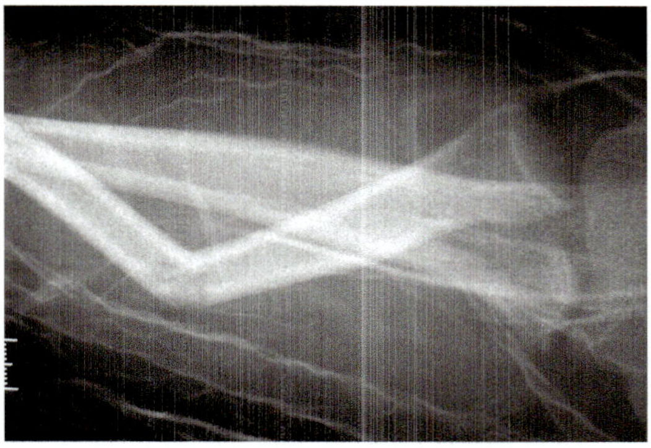

Fig. 2.23 Diaphyseal greenstick fracture

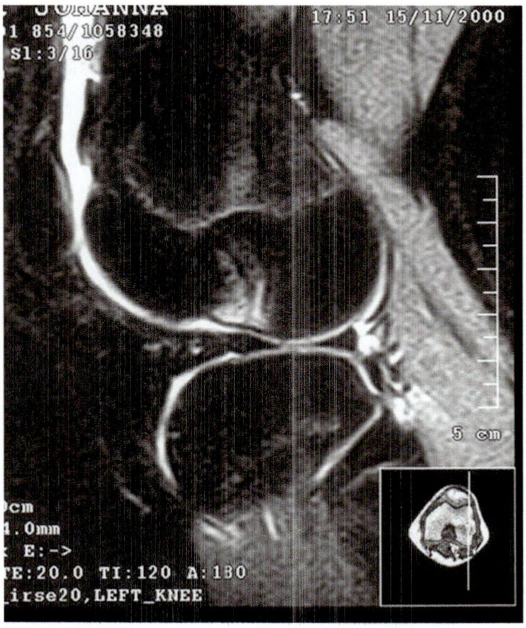

Fig. 2.24 Chondral and osteochondral fracture ("flake fracture") of the knee

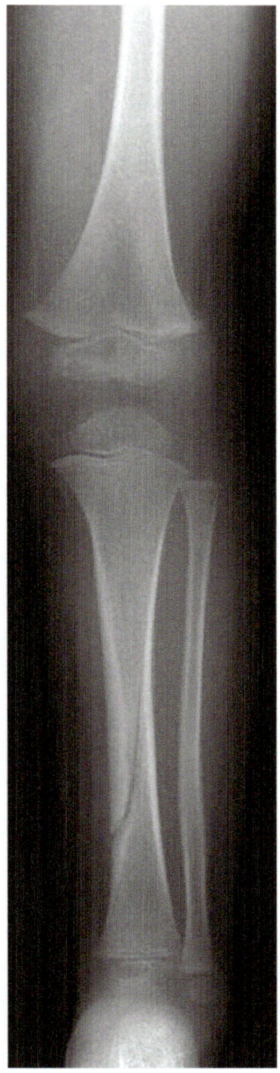

Fig. 2.25 "Toddler's fracture," 2-year-old boy. Typical in the age when children begin walking

Bowing Fracture

No detectible fracture line. Multiple microfractures of the convex side lead to bending and are only recognized indirectly during recovery and by clinical symptoms.

Chondral and Osteochondral Fractures (Flake Fractures)

In children, chondral fractures predominate, most common in the ankle mortise and the knee joint, including the patella. X-ray often provides only indirect indications of fracture. Diagnosis is confirmed, e.g., during diagnostic arthroscopy or on MRI (Fig. 2.24).

Apophyseal Avulsions and Epiphyseal Ligament Tears

These are the result of rotational trauma and generally do not affect bony growth. Familiarity with the apophyses and ossification centers is essential.

Toddler's Fracture

This fracture occurs typically in toddlers who are learning to walk. It is a barely discernible oblique or spiral stress fracture of the tibia (Fig. 2.25).

Vertebral Fractures

Vertebral fractures are rare in children. They occur most commonly in the thoracic, followed by the lumbar spine. Severe cervical spine injuries can occur from sufficient trauma. Characteristics of the pediatric spine, e.g., the apical ossification center of the dens and the secondary ossification centers of the transverse and spinous processes, can make diagnosis challenging.

The posterior ring of the Atlas ossifies around age 4 years, and complete fusion occurs between 7 and 10 years. In the Axis, the posterior arches ossify at 2–3 years and fusion with the vertebral body occurs at age 7. The Os terminale of the Dens fuses with the body at 11–12 years.

The pediatric spine has greater elasticity. This can result in physiological anterior displacement of C2 on C3 or C3 on C4 with the potential for pseudo-subluxation up to age 8. Alignment of the spinolaminar line is maintained regardless. Evaluation of spinal alignment can be assisted by tracking imaginary lines following the edges of the anterior and posterior vertebral bodies, along the facet joints and the spinous processes (Fig. 2.26). Vertebral bodies can also show typical growth region injuries analogous to those of the extremities, e.g., separation of the vertebral endplate from the growth zone.

Conventional radiography is the first-line approach. Along with AP and lateral projections for the spine and prevertebral soft tissues, oblique views of the facet joint, functional views, transoral views, conventional tomography (dens), and special projections (e.g., swimmer's views) can be performed. CT is superior to conventional radiographs for fracture diagnosis, and targeted CT should be used early when indicated (because of the radiation dose, indications are strict).

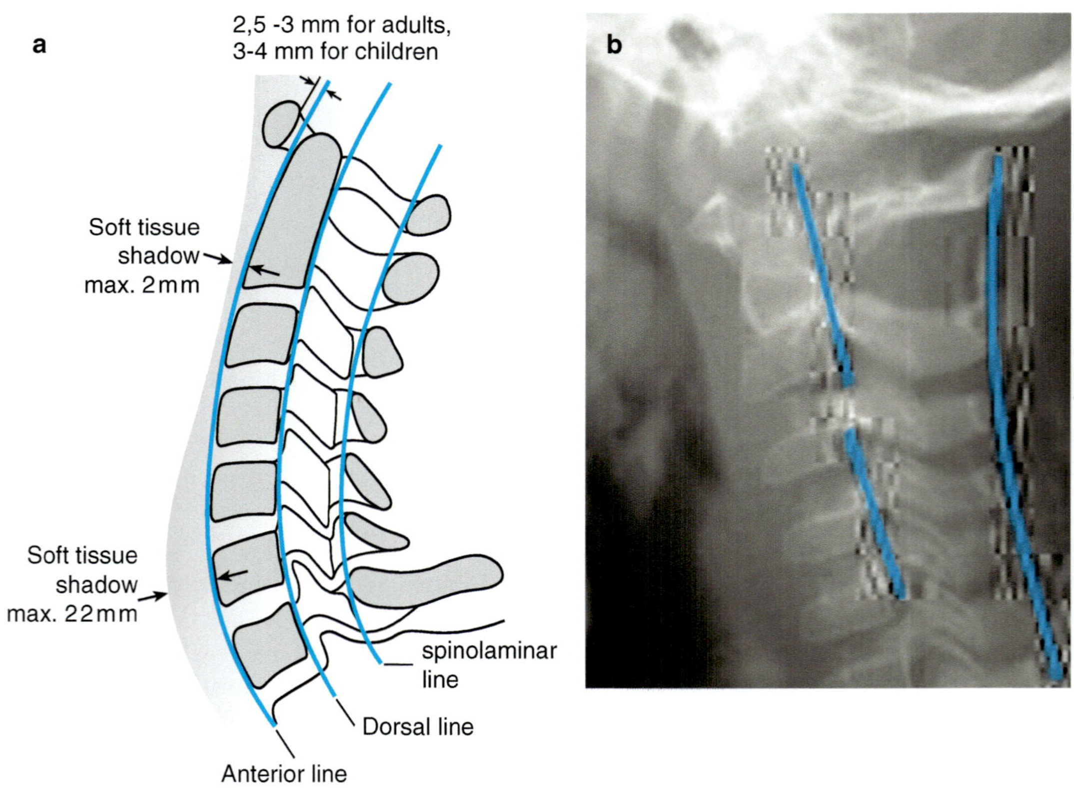

Fig. 2.26 Assessment of spinal alignment. (**a**) Schematic demonstration of a line. The distance between the dens and atlas can be up to 4 mm in children. (**b**) Pseudo-subluxation in a 4-year-old boy

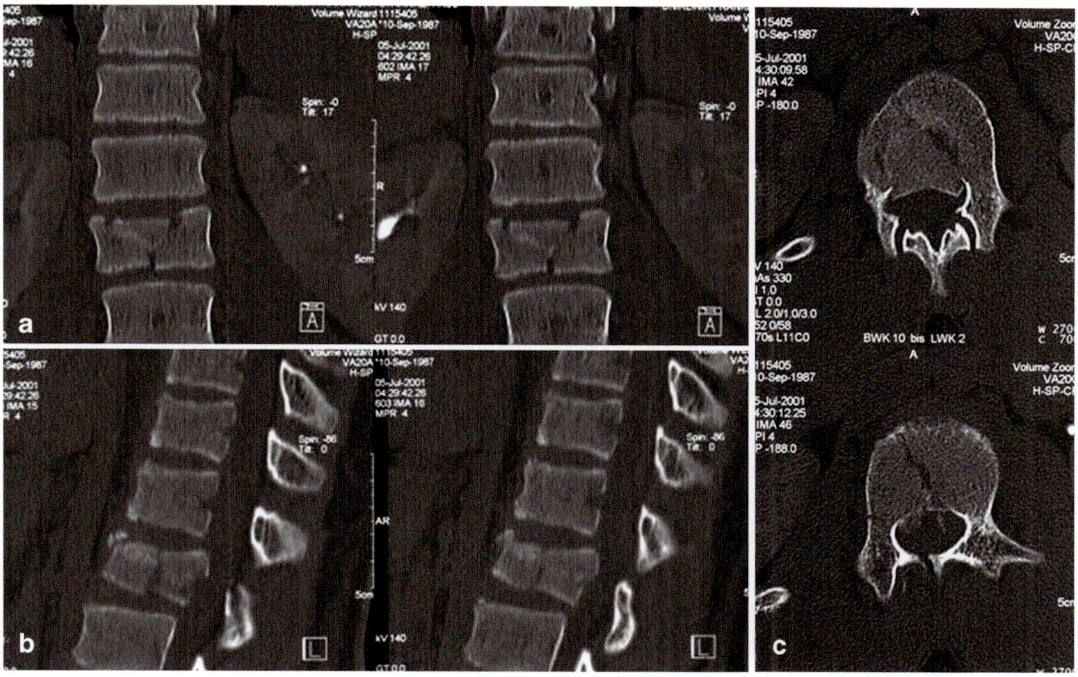

Fig. 2.27 Compression and compression fracture of the first lumbar vertebra. The posterior bony fragment substantially narrows the spinal canal. (**a**) Coronal reconstruction, (**b**) Sagittal reconstruction, (**c**) Axial image at the fracture site

Spiral CT enables multi-dimensional reconstructions of the fractured vertebrae and thus, facilitates both diagnosis and operative planning (Fig. 2.27).

MRI can be performed when symptoms are present and there are no native-film findings. It is especially good at detecting occult vertebral fractures ("bone bruises"). MRI also offers an accurate diagnosis of spinal cord, intervertebral disc, and ligamentous injuries. When symptoms persist without evidence of bony injury, MRI may be needed to identify discoligamentous injury or soft tissue damage.

Pathological Fractures

Pathological fractures occur principally after inadequate trauma in systemically or locally damaged bone cysts are the most common cause of pathological fractures in children. Juvenile bone cysts tend to occur in the proximal metaphysis of the femur, tibia, and humerus (Fig. 2.28). A cyst appears as a sharply delineated lucency with marginal sclerosis on radiographs. The most important differential diagnosis is the aneurysmal bone cyst, which grows rapidly, is located eccentrically, and is often associated with pain. Benign fibrotic change is generally asymptomatic and visible in 30% of normal skeletons in the first 20 years of life. Fibrous cortical defects are radiolucent, usually with a narrow sclerotic border, and they are located close to the cortex in long bone metaphyses. When they spread to the medullary canal, they are referred to as a non-ossifying fibroma.

In fibrotic dysplasia (Jaffé-Lichtenstein syndrome), the bone marrow is replaced with connective tissue. It occurs in (predominantly) monostotic and (also) polyostotic forms and commonly affects the femur, tibia, facial skull, ribs, and/or pelvis. Radiographically, there are protrusions of the flat bones and cyst-like projections of the long bones (mostly diaphyseal) with varying transparency, but typically with a frosted

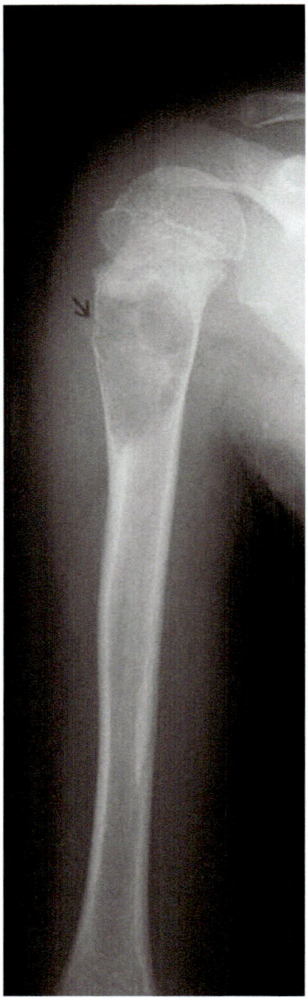

Fig. 2.28 Pathological fracture of the lateral wall of a juvenile bone cyst of the proximal humerus (8 years girl)

glass appearance. Other causes of pathological fractures are various metabolic disorders, which will not be discussed further here.

2.6 Pediatric Fracture Classifications

In children, differences in anatomy, physiology, and biomechanics create different fracture patterns and introduce challenges for diagnosis and treatment that are not present in adults. Categorization and documentation of injuries must be carried out using appropriate classification systems to reach meaningful conclusions regarding prognosis or treatment outcomes. The adult AO Classification has been applied to children due to the lack of a comprehensive, specific system for pediatric fractures, but it is not practical for the reasons stated above.

Classifications must be based on morphological criteria and have a sound system for documentation that enables comparison and collection of prospective data as well as proper follow-up and assurance of care quality. Because final assessment cannot be performed before the end of growth and the variety of injuries present in different age groups, it is challenging to integrate classification-oriented treatment recommendations. However, this is a goal when developing new systems.

The following will introduce two current pediatric fracture classifications of the long bones, which have evolved in recent years.

AO Pediatric Comprehensive Classification of Long Bone Fractures (PCCF)

This classification was developed by the Pediatric Expert Group (PAEG) of the Association for Osteosynthesis/Association for the Study of Internal Fixation (AO/ASIF) in collaboration with AO Clinical Investigation and Documentation (AOCID) and the International Association for Pediatric Traumatology. It underwent a strict validation process with the AO Classification Supervisory Committee and is currently recognized worldwide, also by the OTA (Orthopedic Trauma Association of North America).

The proposed classification is based on the Müller AO Classification for adults and accounts for pediatric fracture features (Fig. 2.29). Assessment is based on conventional anterior-posterior and lateral trauma images.

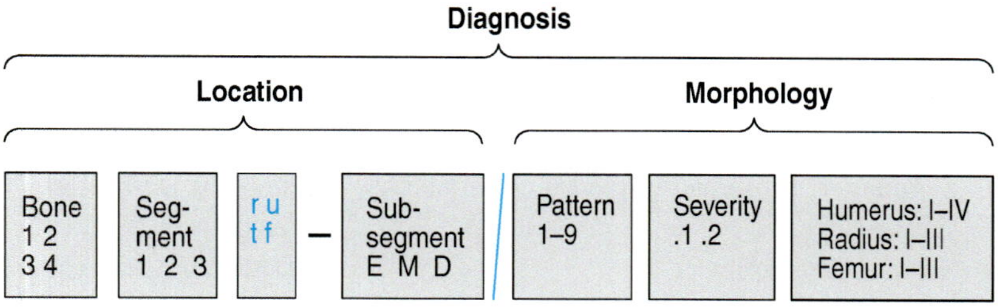

Fig. 2.29 Principles of pediatric fracture classification

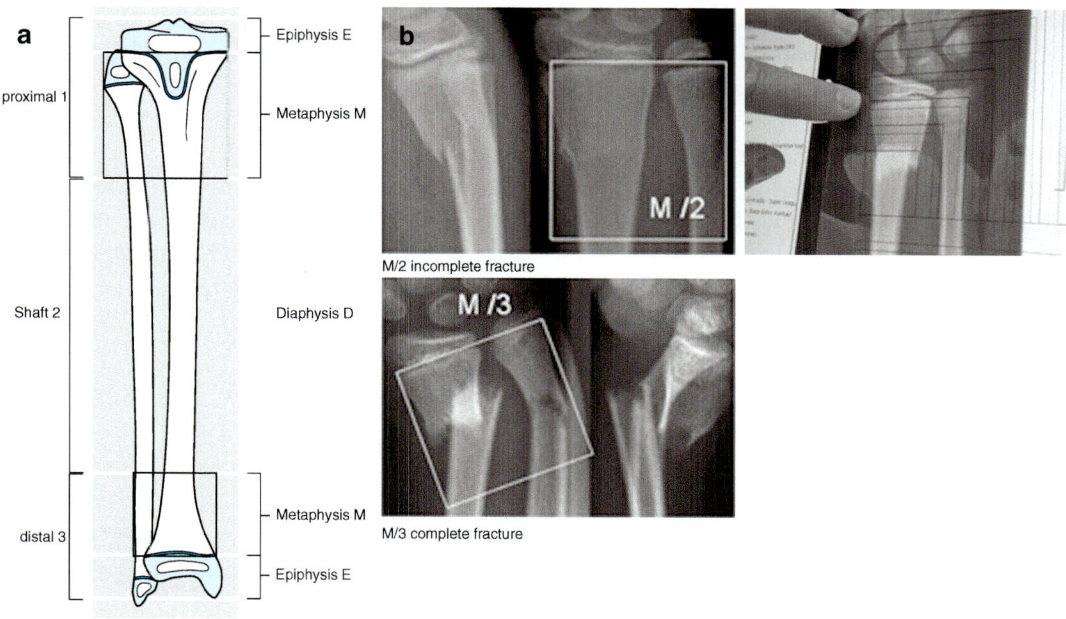

Fig. 2.30 (**a**) The metaphysis is defined as a square of which each side measures the maximal width of the bony epiphyseal plate (on A.P. view x-ray). For paired bones, both physes are included in the width measurement. (**b**) A transparent "squares" template can be placed over the corresponding radiograph for more accurate and reliable diagnosis

Bone and Segment

Like in the Müller AO Classification for adults, individual bones are numbered as Humerus = 1, Radius/Ulna = 2, Femur = 3, and Tibia/Fibula = 4. Except for Monteggia and Galeazzi injuries, paired bony injuries with the same pattern (pediatric code) are classified with a fracture code indicating injury severity. If a single bone is affected, a letter suffix (r,u,t,f) is added to the segment code (e.g., 22u describes an isolated ulnar shaft fracture). If both bones are injured with different patterns (e.g., complete radius fracture with bowing ulnar fracture), each bone must be designated separately with the respective letter suffix.

Bony segments are designated as proximal = 1, diaphyseal = 2, and distal = 3, and these are defined differently than in adults. The metaphysis is the area of bone covered by a square of which each side measures the maximal width of the bony epiphyseal plate (Fig. 2.30a). For the paired bones (ulna/radius and tibia/fibula), both physes must be included in the measurement of width. Thus, the following three segments can be distinguished:

- Segment 1: proximal epiphysis and metaphysis (square)
- Segment 2: diaphysis
- Segment 3: distal epiphysis and metaphysis (square).

Pediatric malleolar fractures are considered distal tibia fractures (e.g., typical Salter-Harris III and IV fractures of the distal tibia are 43).

Fracture Subsegment Code

Severity grade A-B-C used in adults has been replaced with the designations for diaphysis (D), metaphysis (M), and epiphysis (E). The most common injuries in children are shaft fractures (segment 2) and epi/metaphyseal fractures (segments 1 and 3). The designation of E-M-D clearly distinguishes intraarticular and extraarticular fractures because epiphyseal fractures are intraarticular by definition. An injury is designated as metaphyseal when the fracture center is within the metaphyseal square (Fig. 2.30b). An exception is the proximal femur, where the metaphysis is defined as the area between the femoral head and the intertrochanteric line. The square definition of metaphysis can yield misclassification from imprecise AP images or angulation in the frontal plane.

Pediatric Code

Specific childhood features were transferred into a pediatric code. These are specific to the different fracture subsegments E, M, and D, and each fracture is classified accordingly.

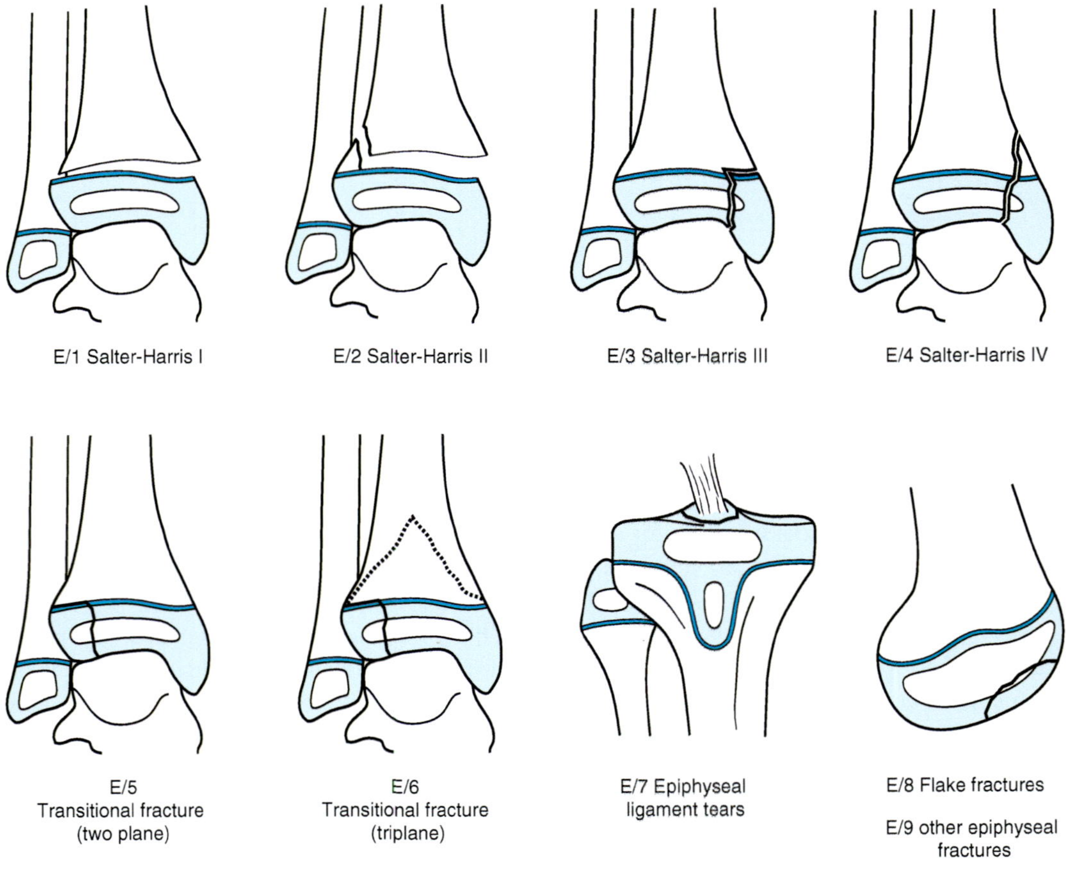

Fig. 2.31 Classification of epiphyseal fractures (E)

Epiphyseal fractures are assigned codes as following (Fig. 2.31):

- Salter-Harris I to IV = E/1 to E/4
- E/5 = Tillaux (twoplane) fracture
- E/6 = triplane fracture
- E/7 = intraarticular avulsion fracture
- E/8 = flake fracture
- E/9 = other fractures

Metaphyseal fractures are designated as (Fig. 2.32):

- M/2 = incomplete (buckle/torus, spiral, and greenstick) fracture
- M/3 = complete fracture
- M/7 = avulsion injury (osteoligamentous, musculoligamentous, simple)
- M/6 = proximal metaphyseal ulnar fracture with radial head displacement (most proximal Monteggia injury)

The pediatric code for diaphyseal fractures (of segment 2) is shown in Fig. 2.33 and includes:

- D/1 = bowing fracture
- D/2 = greenstick fracture
- D/3 = Toddler's fracture
- D/4 = complete transverse fracture angle ≤30°

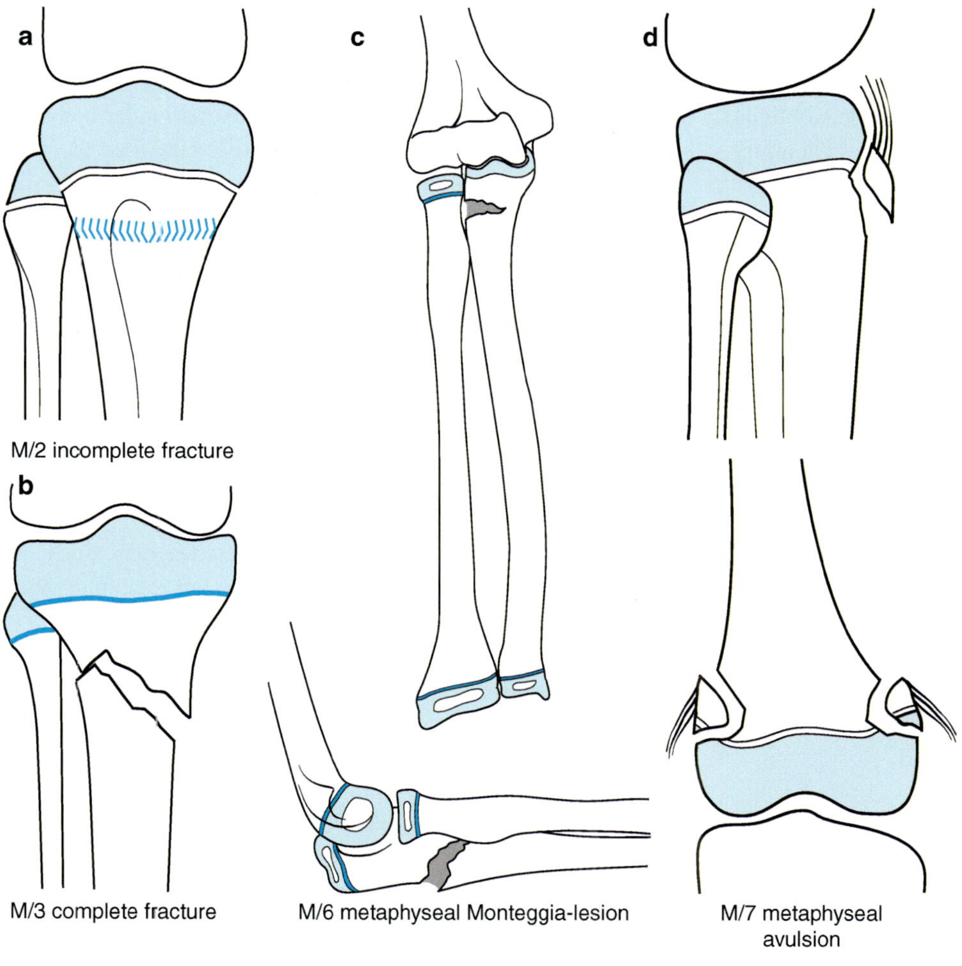

Fig. 2.32 Classification of metaphyseal fractures (M). (**a**) M/2; (**b**) M/3; (**c**) M/6; (**d**) M/7

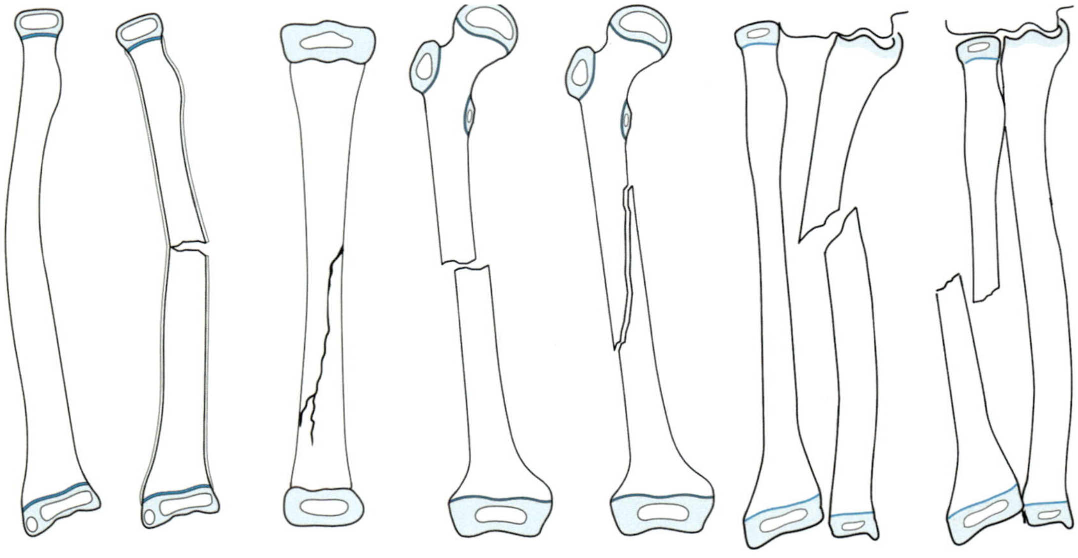

Fig. 2.33 Classification of diaphyseal fractures (D)

- D/5 = complete oblique or spiral fracture
- D/6 = Monteggia injury
- D/7 = Galeazzi injury
- D/9 = other fracture

For more reliable classification, a 30° angle should be used in radiographs.

Fracture Severity Code

A subdivision indicating the degree of severity is needed for identifying indications for different methods of internal fixation. This code distinguishes simple (.1) and multi-fragmentary (.2) fractures.

Exceptions and Displacement Codes

Because not all pediatric fractures can be classified according to the above system, the following supplemental definitions and rules have been established:

- Apophyseal fractures are classified as metaphyseal fractures.
- Transitional fractures with or without a metaphyseal wedge are classified as epiphyseal fractures.
- Intraarticular and extraarticular bony ligament tears are respectively classified as epiphyseal and metaphyseal fractures.
- Supracondylar humerus fractures (code 13-M/3) are supplementally classified using the von Laer system (grades I-IV):
  - Type I: incomplete fracture. On the true lateral view, Rogers' line intersects the capitellum, AND the varus/valgus gap is ≤2 mm on AP.
  - Type II: incomplete fracture. On true lateral, Rogers' line no longer intersects the capitellum OR the varus/valgus fracture gap is >2 mm on AP.
  - Type III: complete fracture. Cortical continuity is disrupted but remaining bony contact of the fracture surfaces.
  - Type IV: complete fracture. No cortical continuity and no bony contact.
- Radial Head Fractures (21-M/2 or /3; or 21-E/1 or /2) are also classified according to angulation and the extent of displacement:
  - I = no angulation and no displacement,
  - II = angulation with displacement up to half the width of the shaft,
  - III = angulation with displacement more than half the width of the shaft.

- Femoral Neck (epiphyseal):
  - E/1 = epiphyseal separation without metaphyseal wedge,
  - E/2 = epiphyseal separation with a metaphyseal wedge.
- Femoral Neck Fractures (metaphyseal):
  - I = midcervical
  - II = basicervical
  - III = transtrochanteric.
- The femoral intertrochanteric line delimits the metaphysis. The complete fracture code is thus, composed of 5 or 6 codes, depending on whether a supplemental code is applied.

Li-La Classification for Pediatric Long Bone Fractures

The non-profit Li-La Association (Light and Laughter for Sick Children, Efficiency in Medicine Association) and the Institute for Evaluative Research in Orthopaedic Surgery at the University of Bern developed a documentation system. They validated it with the associated classification in a multicenter study of 2308 fractures. The documentation and classification version 2.1 can be viewed online at the Institute for Evaluative Research in Bern and on the Li-La website (www.li-la.org).

Recommended Literature

Ackermann O (2015 Jul 7) Bone fracture ultrasound. 2015:1–17

Bohndorf K, Imhof H (1998) Radiologische Diagnostik der Knochen und Gelenke. Thieme, Stuttgart

Colonna PC (1928) Fracture of the neck of the femur in childhood. A report of six cases. Ann Surg 88:902

Greenspan A (1990) Skelettradiologie: Orthopädie, Traumatologie, Rheumatologie, Onkologie. VCH, Weinheim

Greulich WW, Pyle SI (1959) Radiographic atlas of skeletal development on the hand and wrist. University Press, Stanford

Heuck F, Bast BRG (1994) Radiologische Skizzen und Tabellen. Peripheres Skelett. Thieme, Stuttgart

Keats TE (1992) Normvarianten im Röntgenbild: Befunde ohne Krankheitswert. Ullstein Mosby, Berlin

Köhler A, Zimmer EA (1989) Grenzen des Normalen und Anfänge des Pathologischen im Röntgenbild des Skeletts. Thieme, Stuttgart

Moritz JD, Hoffmann B, Sehr DH, Eggerking J, Keil K, Caliebe A, Dischinger J, Heller M, Bolte H (2012) Pediatric fracture diagnosis – ultra-low-dose CT with an effective dose equal to that of radiographs. Rö Fo 184(11):1026–1033

Müller ME, Allgöwer M, Schneider R, Willenegger H (1991) Manual of internal fixation, 3rd edn. Springer, Heidelberg

Nau C, Marzi I, Ziebarth K, Berger S (2015) Fractures in children and adolescents. In: Rommens PM, Hessmann MH (eds) Intramedullary nailing. Springer, Heidelberg

Norell HG (1954) Roentgenologic visualization of the extracapsular fat. Acta Radiol 42:205–210

Ogden JA (2000) Skeletal injury in the child. Springer, New York

Slongo T, Audigé L, Schlickewei W, Clavert J-M, Hunter J (2006 Jan) International Association for Pediatric Traumatology. Development and validation of the AO pediatric comprehensive classification of long bone fractures by the Pediatric Expert Group of the AO Foundation in collaboration with AO Clinical Investigation and Documentation and the International Association for Pediatric Traumatology. J Pediatr Orthop. 26(1):43–49

Sommerfeldt DW, Dietz HG (2011a) Pediatric and adolescent traumatology - lower extremities. Unfallchirurg 114(5):380

Sommerfeldt DW, Dietz HG (2011b) Pediatric and adolescent traumatology - upper extremity. Unfallchirurg 114(4):284

Stöver PDB, Rogalla P (2008) CT-Untersuchungen bei Kindern. Radiologe 48(3):243–248

Strohm PC, Uhl M, Hauschild O, Stankovic Z, Reising KJ, Lesniak M, Südkamp NP (2008) Welchen Stellenwert hat das Ganzkörper-Spiral-CT in der Primärdiagnostik polytraumatisierter Kinder? Z Orthop Unfall 146(01):38–43

von Laer L, Gruber R, Dallek M, Dietz HG, Kurz W, Linhart W, Marzi I, Schmittenbecher P, Slongo T, Einberg A, Wessel L (2000) Classification and documentation of children's fractures. Eur J Trauma 1:2–14

von Laer L, Kraus R, Linhart W (2012) Frakturen und Luxationen im Wachstumsalter, 6th edn. Thieme, Stuttgart

Treatment Principles

3

3.1 Conservative Treatment Options

The approach to pediatric fractures differs from adults and must be understood for appropriate care. Non-invasive treatment methods are still most frequently used. The costs of treatment (financial and otherwise) for both patients and caregivers and the risks and potential therapy changes must be considered individually. Fracture-related criteria like location, articular or physeal involvement, and stability remain essential, but broader biopsychosocial criteria like age, gender, physeal maturity, family resources, logistics, caregiver competence, and financial considerations also influence treatment.

All potential treatment methods should be mastered, and each case evaluated individually (Table 3.1). The ultimate selection is made in consultation with the patient and parents. Any treatment requiring anesthesia should be definitive; further interventions (re-reduction, changes in treatment plan) should be avoided, since recurrent interventions are more likely to yield undesirable outcomes. Stability, follow-up capability, and the likelihood of further procedures/anesthesia should be assessed before opting for conservative immobilization.

The goals of fracture treatment are to:

- Minimize pain
- Stabilize the fracture
- Minimize functional restriction
- Offer definitive treatment
- Minimize effort/complexity
- Heal rapidly
- Avoid growth disturbances.

Many patients and parents have more resistance to anesthesia than to surgical interventions. Thus, conservative treatment must always be considered when selecting treatment. Unfortunately, there is little data that is well-founded and without methodological problems.

Injuries for which conservative treatment are indicated are:

- Stable fractures: greenstick, torus (buckle), mildly displaced fractures of the distal metaphysis of Salter types I and II, non-displaced articular fractures with fracture gap ≤2 mm
- Unstable fractures: with adequate stability after reduction, or if they can be converted into a stable fracture (e.g., greenstick fractures in small children).

I. Marzi et al., *Pediatric Skeletal Trauma*, https://doi.org/10.1007/978-3-030-93685-3_3

Table 3.1 Considerations for optimal fracture management

Fracture	Biological	Social	Complexity	Benefits for
Displacement?	Age	Family situation?	For the patient?	Patient?
Articular involvement/proximity?	Growth plate maturity?	Technical skills?	For caregivers?	Caregivers?
Growth plate involvement?	Sex?	Resources/costs?	Risks?	Payor (insurance)?

Basic Principles

Little experimental data backs up the broad clinical application of plaster casts. The basic principles of conservative treatment have not been thoroughly evaluated. Available conclusions, e.g., regarding the callus-promoting and fracture-stabilizing effects of circumscribed interfragmentary motion, are mostly assumptions derived indirectly from other research results.

The two main forms of conservative treatment are passive retention and active redression (noninvasive reduction/retention techniques).

Retention

Simple retention usually involves the adjacent joints. The primary goal is pain management, and the secondary goal is to reduce the risk of fracture displacement. It reduces "false mobility."

Plaster Casts

The most common form of retention by far is cast immobilization using unilateral, semicircular, and (mostly) circular splints. To avoid compartment syndrome, circular casts should always be split immediately and completely, including all cushioning material. Fractures at risk of displacement require precise radiological controls with the option to change approach until days 8–10.

Traditional plaster of Paris has been increasingly displaced by artificial casting materials with various desirable properties (semi-rigid, semi-elastic, rigid, colored, water-repellent, lightweight, x-ray permeable). Most of the time, non-medical properties (ease of cleaning, logistics, faster processing) have driven this change. Traditional plaster is more versatile for experienced casters regarding modeling, correcting, and wedging (redression techniques, see below). A circular plaster cast with strip reinforcements retains its modeled shape during setting. In contrast, artificial materials spontaneously resume a tubular diameter while hardening. For successful wedging, an appropriate form must be modeled and held during application to avoid gaps between the cast and skin as swelling decreases. These gaps interfere with desired results.

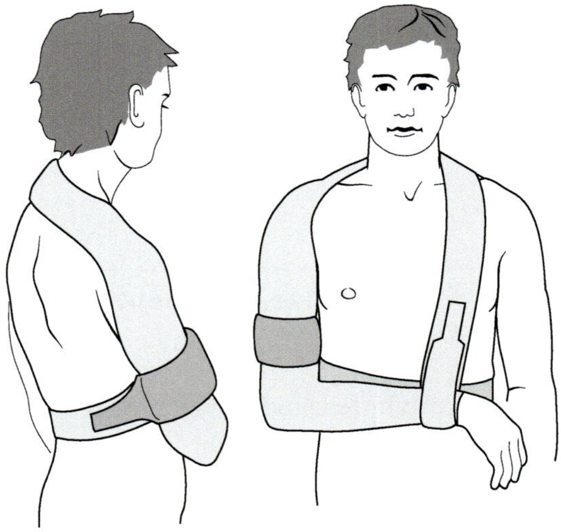

Fig. 3.1 Gilchrist bandage

The word "cast" is used in this book for both materials with more precise details as needed.

Bandages: Gilchrist, Desault, Velpeau

The Gilchrist bandage is a long tube slipped over the arm and chest to immobilize the upper arm close to the thorax. The tube has one hole in the approximate middle, through which the arm is inserted, and a second hole at the wrist, leaving the hand free. The distal tube end is run posteriorly around the thorax, looped around the distal upper arm, and usually fastened. The proximal end is run behind the neck and brought down anteriorly on the uninjured side, tied around the wrist of the injured arm and fastened, usually with a safety pin (Fig. 3.1). This immobilizes the upper arm with sufficient pain reduction so that the patient will no longer require analgesics after a few days.

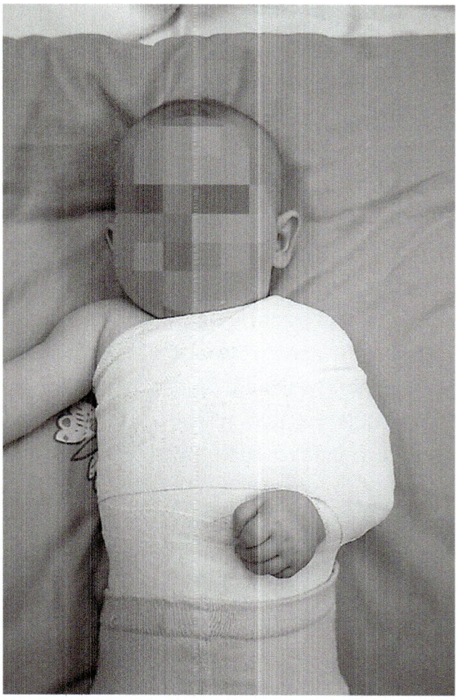

Fig. 3.2 Customized Desault dressing

Desault and Velpeau bandages are based on the same immobilization principle but in the form of a vest or bandage surrounding the thorax (Fig. 3.2). Commercially available, ready-made materials are often too big or too small in young children, but they can be easily adapted and are less risky than a figure-of-eight bandage (see below).

These bandages are applied for epiphyseal separations of the proximal humerus, subcapital humerus fractures, and humeral shaft fractures.

Cast Wedging

Cast wedging can correct or prevent angulation in the frontal and sagittal planes. It is used mainly in the forearm and tibial shaft for angulated, greenstick, and distal metaphyseal fractures, especially isolated injuries of one of the paired bones.

Angulated tibial shaft and distal forearm fractures are now the rare injuries for which cast wedging is still performed. The indication is noted during initial treatment, and wedging is planned as a non-invasive procedure. The relative stability of the soft callus makes manipulation

Table 3.2 Timing of plaster wedging

Indication and planning	Day of injury/primary treatment
Immobilization	Day 1
Casting	Day 8 (4–8)
Wedging	Day 8–10
Redression	>Day 8
Cast removal	Day 28 (with consolidation)

considerably less painful, so it can be performed with the conscious patient's cooperation, thus enabling active correction without anesthesia. The key to successful wedging is an accurate indication and good communication with the patient and parents.

This communication begins on the day of injury with a discussion of diagnosis, treatment plan alternatives (retention, reduction, or fracture completion under anesthesia), and consequences (Table 3.2). The wedging approach is outlined along with the treatment goals and the protocol for wedging failure, i.e., waiting for spontaneous healing versus definitive fracture treatment under anesthesia as an elective procedure on the same or following day.

Essential for this discussion:

- Explanation and description of the wedging approach
- Establishment of treatment goals:
  - Pain control: short-term
  - Functional restoration: medium-term
  - Cosmetics, anatomic restoration: long-term
- Alternatives, Problems, Options

Traction

Only skin traction is a genuinely conservative (non-invasive) treatment. This technique stems from a different (non-operative) era and was a traditional treatment of choice, especially for fractures of the femur and tibia before social factors and cost-efficiency gained prominence in clinical decision-making. Overhead Traction remains the treatment of choice in certain regions, especially before age 2 years, and the duration can be lessened to 7–10 days with a hip

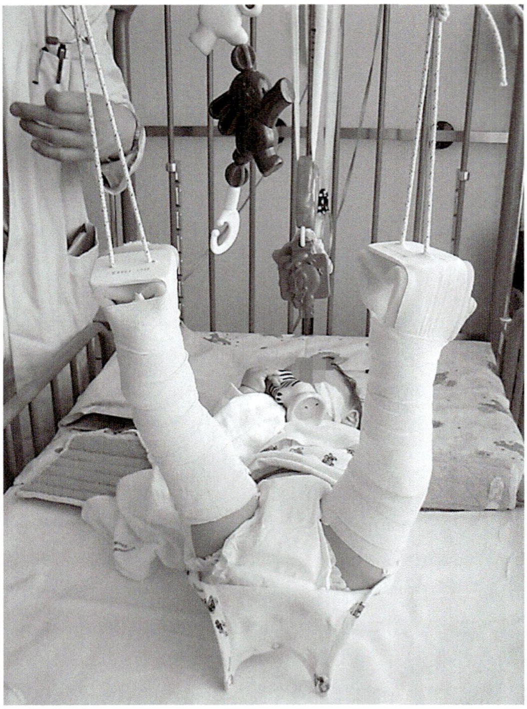

Fig. 3.3 Overhead traction

spica cast (Fig. 3.3). It can also be used as a bridge to definitive treatment. The disadvantages are long-term high-grade immobilization and with it, exclusion from the social environment. In addition, not all children tolerate this procedure well and then, a surgical stabilization with ESIN or external fixation should be considered. It needs to be understood and mastered—in particular the skin and rotation—, but in the context of child-centered treatment concepts, traction remains a bridge or fallback method for exceptional cases.

A hanging cast (upper arm cast with additional axial weight on the elbow) is a type of traction and, thus, redression. However, the instability (fractures are usually above or at the level of the cast edge), lever-arm on lying down, and overall heaviness make it unsuitable for children.

Figure-of-Eight Bandage

The figure-of-eight bandage (Fig. 3.4) reduces shoulder movement and, thus, the pain of a fresh clavicle fracture by pulling the shoulders slightly back. Some consider this a dynamic fracture treatment to correct fragment position. However, because of the three-dimensional shear effects on the clavicle, this is at best only theoretically possible. In practice, achieving correction would require powerful traction that would cause pain at the fracture site and constriction in the axilla with associated neurovascular consequences. Ready-made products not always fit, so a self-assembled stockinette bandage customizable to individual patients within minutes might be used. It is padded with cotton along two-thirds of its length, guided behind the neck and under the armpits, then tied between the shoulder blades. It can be easily repositioned as needed.

Cuff and Collar (Blount) Sling

In supracondylar humerus fractures that are non-displaced or displaced only in anteversion, the pull of the triceps tendon can be used to stabilize or achieve dynamic fracture redression by bringing the elbow progressively (over days) into the most acute angle tolerated. The increasing tension-band effect immobilizes and adjusts fracture position as the swelling decreases. Sometimes it is better to apply an upper arm cast the first days and no later than day 4, a padded wrist sling (cotton-padded stockinette) is hung from a sling around the neck and tightened daily to decrease the angle as tolerated until the wrist is tight to the jugulum and the hand is practically lying on the opposite shoulder (Fig. 3.5). In addition to reliable correction, the advantages are better mobility and easier hygiene than with a long-arm cast. However, there is a level of compliance required from both patient and parents because daily tensioning must be performed despite reservations. It works reliably if the

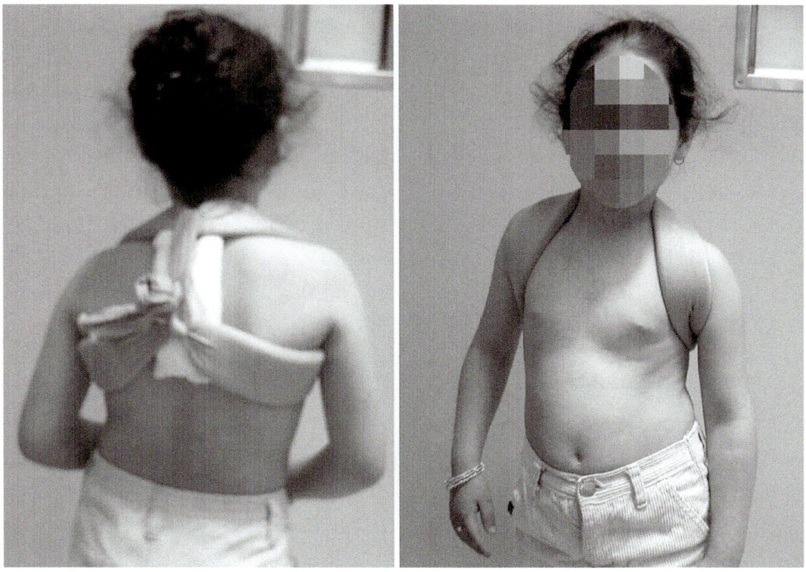

Fig. 3.4 Figure-of-eight bandage with padded stockinette

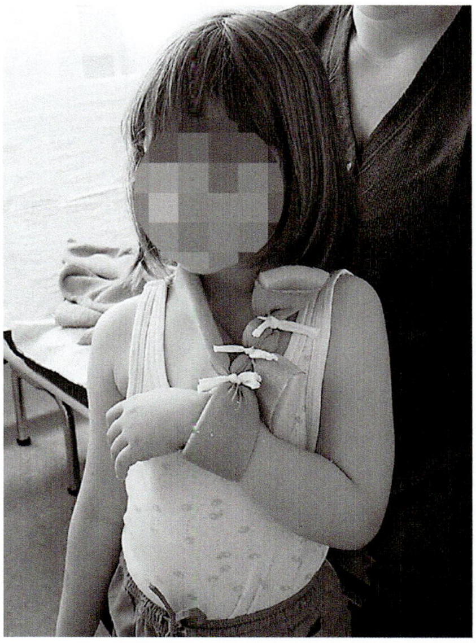

Fig. 3.5 Cuff and collar (Blount) sling

process is well explained. Radiographs might be necessary after a few days and to check consolidation.

Sarmiento Brace

Functional fracture treatment with a Sarmiento brace is more active immobilization than true redression. It is an anatomically modified circular splint that is split and adaptable with Velcro fasteners, indicated for moderately displaced diaphyseal humerus, tibia, and complete lower leg fractures. It surrounds the adjacent joints but does not rigidly bridge them. The continual adaptation of the brace to limb musculature as swelling decreases enhances the splinting effect. Early functional mobilization maintains or restores the anatomical relationships. The minimal shearing movements are thought to promote callus formation.

Tape

The concept of conservative early functional treatment of fibulotalar ligament injuries, including rupture, has proven itself many times and has replaced fibulotalar ligament repair as primary therapy. Numerous techniques and artificial materials compete in this market. They are all based on the principle of allowing rolling tibiotalar movements of the ankle joint while preventing fibulotalar stress with supination during the first 6 weeks of healing.

3.2 Technical Features of Conservative Treatment

Basic Casting Principles

Extremity (splint) immobilization is a team effort provided by the physician, cast technician, and an assistant or two for larger casts. The physician is present and responsible for appropriate immobilization (position, shape, specific guidelines such as planned wedging, etc.). The cast technician is responsible for good technical execution, the assistant for providing and promptly handling materials, and the second assistant for positioning, e.g., holding the femur.

The patient should be as relaxed as possible, with adequate analgesia, distraction from fear, and comfortable positioning. Tense muscles during casting lead to complaints in the cast!

Plaster or artificial materials should never directly touch the skin. A reversed stockinette works well (threads toward the cast for better binding of plaster and decreased itching), with additional padding only over the ends and at the lever point if wedging is planned. Tubular gauze is placed along the primary splitting line; this enables splitting with scissors rather than an oscillating saw. Next, the first circular layer of semi-rigid synthetic casting tape or white plaster is applied. Reinforcement strips of rigid synthetic or plaster are placed bilaterally, then covered with more circular wrapping, followed by a wet elastic bandage. After binding (material is no longer sticky) and removing the outer bandage, the cast is completely split and fixed with an elastic bandage to avoid compartment syndrome.

The responsible physician instructs the patient and family about cast hygiene. Written information regarding follow-up and neurovascular checks is recommended, with the telephone number of the physician on call. Cast checks with neurovascular assessments should be performed after the cast is hardened and dry, either a few hours later or on day 1, and at each radiological position and consolidation control.

Practical Guide

- Before casting, allocate tasks among the technician and assistants.
- Explain the steps quietly and calmly with the patient before casting.
- Do not change joint positions while casting (wrinkles → pressure ulcers).
- Hold only with the flat palm of your hands (avoid pressure points in the cast).
- Pressure is only permitted/necessary for supracondylar thigh splints.
- The assistant holds the reinforcement strips.
- Fix with a water-dipped elastic bandage. This accelerates the setting process (only with cold water; exothermic reaction).

Cast Wedging

Cast wedging is shown in Fig. 3.6 an example of plaster wedging for a tibial shaft fracture. When wedging is planned, extra cotton padding is applied in the areas of the fracture and three contact points: the proximal and distal concavities and the convex fulcrum (Numbers 1–3 in Fig. 3.7). The circular cast is applied as usual, although the side to be wedged (the fracture concavity) must be twice as thick as the convex side (4 and 2 layers of rigid synthetic reinforcements instead of 3 and 3, or 2 and 1 plaster reinforcement strips instead of 1 and 1). Modeling pres-

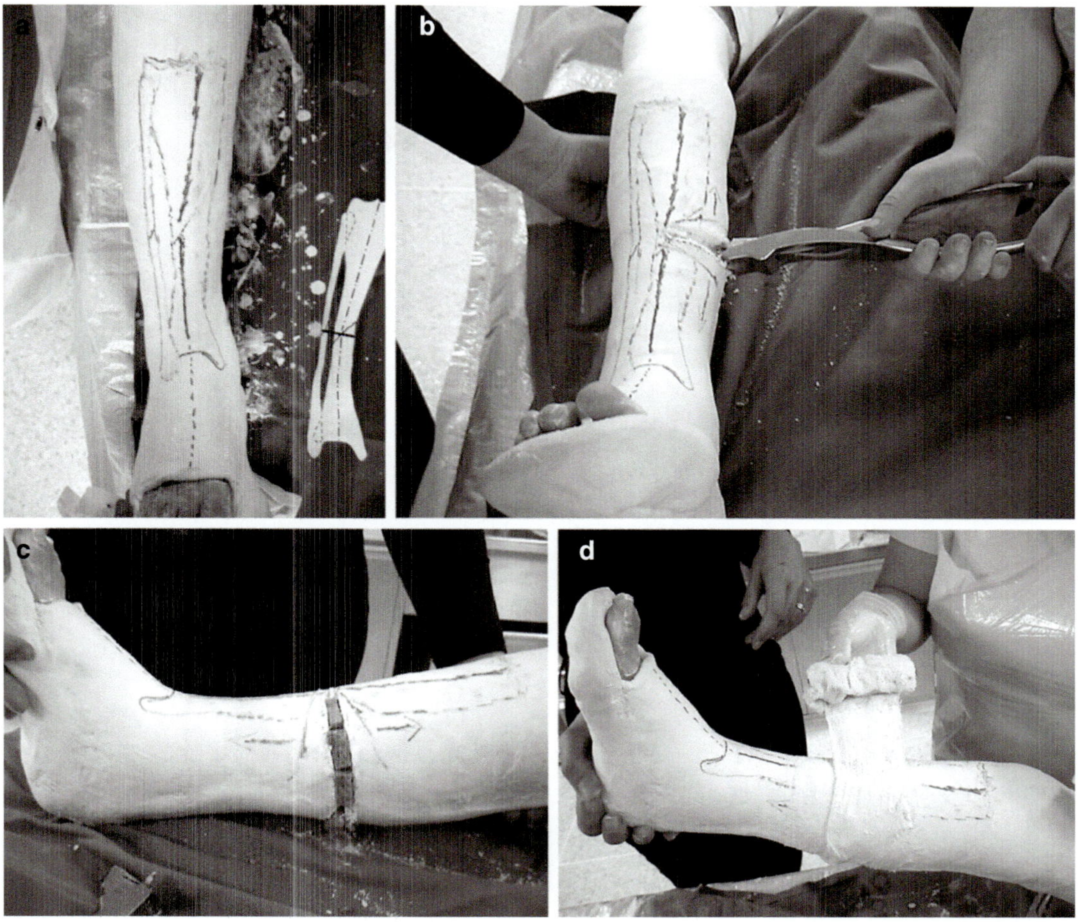

Fig. 3.6 Cast wedging in a tibial shaft fracture with varus deformity. (**a**) Indication: isolated tibial shaft fracture, distal forearm fracture, (**b**) Semicircular splitting of the cast (about two-thirds of the circumference). Wedging in the concavity of angulation (observing patient reactions). Caution: Pressure ulcers! (**c**) Filling with cork, (**d**) Wrapping the cast

sure just under the pain tolerance threshold must be applied to the distal contact point (number 4 in Fig. 3.7) until the setting process is complete to avoid wedging protrusion into the padding. Finally, cast splitting is performed on the side of the primary fracture, on the lower leg, anterior paramedian.

Wedging should be planned around day 8 since soft callus has formed and the initial swelling has decreased. First, the previously split cast is closed. Once it has set (with plaster, possibly on the following day), the wedging plane is marked using the trauma images and an image intensifier, and the wedge cut is made (approximately 2/3 of the circumference). The wedge is placed at the concave apex (note combined deformities in multiple planes). The more distal the fracture, the more proximal the wedging area should be to improve leverage. Redression is performed slowly using a plaster

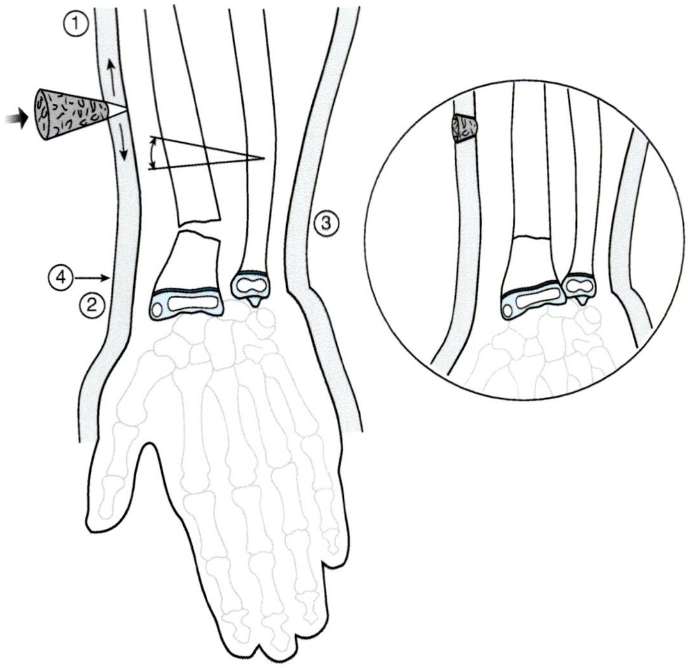

Fig. 3.7 Plaster wedge: The wedge must always be introduced at the concave apex. Note combined deformities in multiple planes. To achieve the desired leverage effect, the further distal the fracture, the more proximal the wedge must be placed

spreader or by bending the casted extremity proximally and distally while observing the patient. Stop at the first complaint and wait or gradually reverse as needed until the patient signals a lack of discomfort. This is repeated until the desired position is attained. If the patient has persistent complaints, the distance must be reduced. A piece of cork or wood is cut to size and then inserted over some additional cotton padding material and clamped to the cut cast edges. Once the desired result has been documented with an image intensifier, the wedge area is closed with a synthetic or plaster wrap. Intrusion of the wedge within the cast should be carefully checked to avoid pressure necrosis. A cast check is performed at 24 h. If the patient has symptoms not requiring analgesia, the cast can be split into two half-shells and temporarily fixed with an elastic bandage, replaced in several days with semi-rigid synthetic casting.

Complications

The only potential complication of wedging is pressure ulcer formation on the opposing side. If discomfort is present, the cast is windowed and re-padded. If the patient is then symptom-free, the cast can be closed again with circular casting. Thus, the anesthesia-free nature of this approach enables reliable avoidance of complications. Secondary displacement and/or delayed consolidation are not expected because soft callus stability is not disrupted by redression.

Special Casting Techniques

Because plaster of Paris technique is well established overall, the following will detail only casting techniques implemented in our clinic using synthetic materials. Casts are consistently applied as composites combining limited transverse elasticity with accommodations for swelling.

Long-Arm Splint

Indications
Elbow lesions, refractory pulled elbow, forearm injuries with painful pronation.

Special Features
Fingers should be freely moveable.

- A reversed terrycloth stockinette is placed from the fingertips to the axilla. The cast ends before the MCP joints.
- Elbow in 90° flexion (or in a comfortable position).
- Wrist in intrinsic-plus position: 30° extension, MCP joints in 90° flexion.
- Tubular gauze is placed along the splitting line.
- Semi-rigid synthetic casting tape (Caution: no edges in the elbow crease) hold onto the fingers or the palm (or use a finger-trap device).
- Rigid synthetic splints (forearm): 3 layers of reinforcements each posterior and anterior on the forearm with a U-shape around the elbow (exception: for wedging, 4–5 on the concave and 2 on the convex side).
- Rigid synthetic splints (upper arm): 3 layers of reinforcement lateral and medial each with a U-shape around the elbow.
- Semi-rigid synthetic cast tape wrap, fix with a water-dipped bandage.
- During the setting process, model the desired regions (interosseous, wedging fulcrum).
- Split (cut) along the lateral side (to the last fiber). In case of elbow lesions, cut out a diamond shape.
- Fix with elastic bandages.

Forearm Splint

Indications
Wrist, metacarpal, forearm injuries with painful pronation.

Special Features
Fingers should be freely moveable.

- Reversed terrycloth stockinette from the fingertips to the axilla. The cast ends before the MCP joints. Elbow in 90° flexion (or in a comfortable position).
- Wrist in intrinsic-plus position: 30° extension, MCP joints in 90° flexion.
- Tubular gauze is placed along the splitting line.
- Rigid synthetic splints: 3 layers each posterior and anterior on the forearm.
- Semi-rigid synthetic casting tape wrap (attention: no edges in the elbow crease), fix with a water-dipped elastic bandage.
- During the setting process, model the desired regions (interosseous, wedging fulcrum).
- Split along the lateral edge (to the last fiber). In case of elbow lesions, cut out a diamond shape.
- Fix with an elastic bandage.

Posterior Forearm Splint
Posterior, anterior, immobilization of the long finger.

Indications
Wrist, metacarpal, finger injuries.

Special Features
Fingers should be freely moveable.

- Elbow on a mat, forearm oblique.
- Wrist in intrinsic-plus position: 30° extension, MCP joint in 90° flexion (except for finger

splints!). Interdigital padding for long finger splints!

- Cut a rigid synthetic reinforcement strip, possibly including a long finger. Wet and wring out extra water.
- Cover with a terrycloth stockinette and pull smooth.
- Apply posteriorly or anteriorly to the forearm and wrap with paper tape until it has set or fix immediately with an elastic bandage.

Upper Leg Splint

Indication

Lower leg injuries.

Special Features

Toe protection is generally more comfortable.

- An assistant is responsible for the thigh!
- Reversed terrycloth stockinette to the groin. The cast ends a maximum of three finger-widths below the groin, angled to the hip.
- Padding strips over the front edge of the tibia from the superior patellar edge to the toes, over malleoli, heel, and fibular head.
- Tubular gauze should lie under the end areas, passed around the patella.
- Knee joint in 15° flexion, ankle in neutral position: 90° dorsiflexion, no supination, no pronation.
- Toes free (all five mostly visible).
- Semi-rigid synthetic casting tape, unwind in the direction of pronation (attention: no edges in the ankle crease).
- Rigid synthetic splints: 3 layers each lateral and medial, U-formed from the thigh around the foot sole.
- For walking cast: soles of rigid synthetic casting (possibly with toe protector).
- Semi-rigid synthetic casting tape, fix with a water-dipped bandage.
- Bilateral modeling of the supracondylar thigh (palmar pressure until it sets).
- Split (cut) anteriorly (to the last fiber), around the patella.
- Fix with an elastic bandage.

Knee Tutor

Indication

Knee joint injuries.

Special Features

Make sure there is sufficient distance to the malleoli! Slipping leads to pressure points.

- An assistant is responsible for the thigh!
- Reversed terrycloth stockinette to the groin. The cast ends a maximum of three finger-widths below the groin, angled to the hip.
- Padding strips edge to edge over the patella and fibular head, felt wrapping along the upper and lower edges.
- Knee joint in 0–15° flexion, ankle free.
- Tubular gauze along the splitting line.
- Semi-rigid synthetic 7.5 cm casting tape, begin at least two finger-widths proximal to the ankle. Fix with a water-dipped bandage.
- Rigid synthetic splints laterally and medially, 3 layers each from the thigh to the lower edge.
- Bilateral modeling of the supracondylar thigh (palmar pressure until it sets).
- Split (cut) anteriorly (to the last fiber), around the patella.
- Fix with an elastic bandage.

Lower Leg Splint

Indication

Injuries of the ankle, tarsal, and metatarsals.

Special Features

Also for primary treatment of fibulotalar ligament injuries.

- An assistant is responsible for the knee!
- Reversed terrycloth stockinette to the groin. The cast ends a maximum of three finger-widths below the groin, angled to the hip.
- Padding strips edge to edge over the anterior tibial edge and ankle.
- Thin tubular gauze along the splitting line.
- Ankle in neutral position: 90° flexion, no supination, no pronation.
- Semi-rigid synthetic 7.5cm casting tape, begin one finger-width proximal to the MTP joint (wrapping in the direction of pronation). Fix with a water-dipped bandage.
- Rigid synthetic splints: 3 layers each lateral and medial, U-formed from the knee around the sole of the foot.
- Sole of the foot (3-5 layers of rigid synthetic reinforcement) without (in mid/forefoot lesions always with) toe protection.
- Model the plantar arch.
- Split (cut) anteriorly (to the last fiber), around the patella.
- Fix with an elastic bandage.

Tape (Ankle Boot)

Indication

Fibulotalar ligament injuries.

Special Features

The wrap should be as thin as possible, so that it fits in the shoe, is not split, and can be simply unwound for removal.

- An assistant holds the foot by the toes. Alternatively, the patient can sit on the edge of the plaster table.
- Stockinette from the toes to above the malleoli (third of the lower leg).
- Ankle in neutral position: 90° flexion, no supination, no pronation.
- Padding strip anteriorly from malleolus to malleolus.
- Semi-rigid synthetic 7.5 cm casting, begin one finger-width proximal to the MTP joint (wrapping in the direction of pronation).
- Once the supramalleolar end is reached, flip the stockinette over and return from anterolateral → anteroplantar → lateral malleolus → anterior → medial malleolus → heel, several times if necessary. Finish distally after flipping the gauze stockinette.
- Fix with a water-dipped bandage.
- The patient should stand on both feet to model the plantar arch.

"Geisha Shoe" Cast

Indication

Metatarsal and Toe Injuries.

Special Features

- Reversed terrycloth stockinette from the tips of the toes to above the ankle, padding at the MTP joints and ankle.
- Tubular gauze is placed along the cutting line.
- Ankle in neutral position: 90° flexion, no supination, no pronation.
- Semi-rigid synthetic 7.5 cm casting tape, begin one finger-width proximal to the MTP joint (wrapping in the direction of pronation).
- Rigid synthetic reinforcement strip with 4 layers from the tip of the big toe to the heel (toe protection).
- Semi-rigid synthetic cast tape wrap, fix with a water-dipped bandage.
- Model the plantar arch.

3.3 Conservative Fracture Treatment

Indications and treatment options are shown in Table 3.3 and the advantages and disadvantages of plaster and synthetic in Table 3.4.

Table 3.3 Indications and treatment options for retention and redression

Type	Form		Indications
Retention (passive)	Bandage	Desault/Velpeau, Gilchrist Splints Circular cast	Proximal (possibly diaphyseal) humerus fracture Humerus shaft fractures Non-displaced stable fractures
Redression (active dynamic)	Cast wedging		Isolated tibial shaft fracture Distal forearm fracture
	Bandage	Figure-of-eight Sling (Blount) (Skin) traction	Clavicle fracture Supracondylar humerus fracture (Laer grades I and II) Displaced femur fracture in toddlers <3 years.
		Sarmiento brace Tape	Diaphyseal humerus fracture Lower leg fracture Fibulotalar injury

Table 3.4 Advantages and disadvantages of plaster and synthetic material

	Advantages	Disadvantages
Plaster of Paris	Modeling capacity Correctible Redression simpler Residues more easily removed Can be decorated	Heavy Cleaning is challenging
Synthetic	Lightweight Radiolucent Colored	Redression complex Residue removal Sharp edges possible

Radiographic Controls

X-rays are an invasive diagnostic instrument and should be limited as much as possible. Before each examination, the potential and anticipated results (secondary displacement, consolidation, etc.) should be considered and the clinical repercussions discussed with the patient/family. Protecting the patient from radiation is an obligation, including limiting the number of images and protective gear for the sensitive thymus, thyroid, bone marrow, and gonads. There is a summation of radiation, and thus, the need for each image must be weighed.

X-rays are performed as documentation immediately after active treatment, followed by the first position check within the first week after intervention. At this point, swelling has subsided, secondary displacements might have occurred, and the soft callus has significantly reduced pain. This is an ideal time to correct angulation since the callus remains sufficiently malleable. In adolescents and exceptional cases of conservative treatment for diaphyseal fractures, an additional position check might be necessary on day 14.

Consolidation checks are needed for all fractures treated actively (through reduction, completion, or redression), for articular fractures, fractures with accepted misalignment, or those at increased risk for disordered consolidation. These films should be performed cast-free in two planes, for each fracture at 4–6 weeks.

Non-displaced metaphyseal buckle, or metaphyseal phalangeal fractures do not necessarily require consolidation radiographs. Clinical assessment is generally sufficient in an asymptomatic patient showing indolent callus and signs of cast-wear indicating painless use. A functional follow-up visit is recommended 3–4 weeks after cast removal.

Controls for long-term growth are primarily clinical, with optional photographic documentation up to 2 years post-injury when needed. Radiological controls are performed only when there is suspected growth disturbance with consequent deformity. MRI can visualize post-traumatic growth plate bridging and assist in further treatment planning.

Follow-Up

There is generally no need for specific follow-up once the fracture has consolidated and immobilization is removed. Children regain full functionality within a short time through normal play activities. They react intuitively to restricted mobility and pain and thus, determine the extent to which the affected limb can be used. Requirements or prohibitions are usually unnecessary.

Physical therapy is rarely needed during childhood. Because the therapist (rather than the child) chooses the extent of movement and loading, "over-therapy" can result, especially when the therapist does not have pediatric experience. However, targeted therapy is indicated (and necessary) in cases of delayed recovery or specific symptoms, e.g., joint stiffness.

There are always questions about when a child can resume sports. The patient's attitude and sport-specific requirements (contact, jumping, etc.) must be considered. In most cases, it is best if the patient decides when to resume practice. An exception is competitive and high-performance athletes, who might feel pressured. These activities should wait until consolidation is confirmed.

Consolidation

Table 3.5 shows the mean consolidation times for the most common pediatric injuries with recommendations of the time needed to immobilize or until movement stability.

Table 3.5 Recommendations for time (in weeks) to immobilize or until movement stability for the most common pediatric fractures after conservative treatment

		<5 years	5–10 years	>10 years
Clavicle fractures		1	2	2–3
Humerus	Proximal	1	2–3	3
	Diaphyseal	2	3–4	4–6
	Supracondylar	1–2	2–3	3–4
	Condyle	3	3–4	4
	Y-fracture	2–3	3	3–4
	Medial epicondyle (and elbow dislocation)	2–3	2–3	2
Olecranon		1	2–3	3–4
Proximal radius		1	2	2
Forearm diaphysis		3	4	4–6
Distal radius		2	3–4	4
Epiphyseal separation distal radius		2	2–3	3–4
Carpal bones		–	4–6	6–12
Metacarpals basal and subcapital		–	2	2–3
Metacarpals diaphysis		–	3–4	4–6
Finger		1–2	2–3	2–3
Femoral neck		–	4–6	6–12
Femur	Subtrochanteric	3–4	4–5	4–6
	Diaphysis	1–3	4–5	4–6
	Condyles including epiphyseal separations	2–3	3–4	4
	Eminence	–	3–4	4
Tibia	Proximal metaphysis	2–3	3–4	4
	Diaphysis	–	3–5	4–6
Ankle joint		2–3	3–4	4–5
Metatarsals and calcaneus		–	4–8	6–12
Metatarsals		2–3	3	3–4

3.4 Operative Treatment Options

Reduction

Before deciding on an open or closed approach, the need for reduction must be considered. Various criteria (age, location, displacement, correction potential) are part of these decisions. Risks include unnecessary anesthesia and operative procedures with remaining risks. On the other hand permanent deformity or complex secondary reconstructions should not happen.

Reduction Criteria

No reduction for:

- Stable, non-displaced fractures of the upper or lower extremities, regardless of age (Fig. 3.8)
- Stable compression fractures or metaphyseal greenstick fractures within acceptable limits
- Unstable humerus fractures, provided the initial angulation is within acceptable limits (primary fixation only, x-ray control at 4–7 days).

Reduction for:

- All fractures, stable and unstable, outside the age and location-dependent limits, especially forearm shaft fractures since angulation here can lead to significant functional deficits (Fig. 3.9). In the lower extremity, maintenance of length, axis, and rotation is essential.

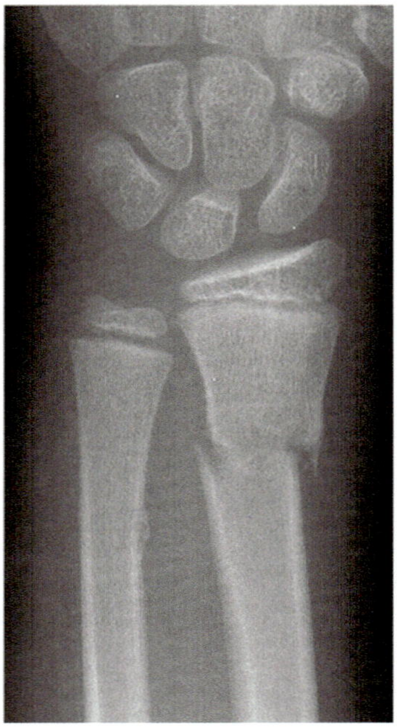

Fig. 3.8 Stable radius fracture, fixation only in cast

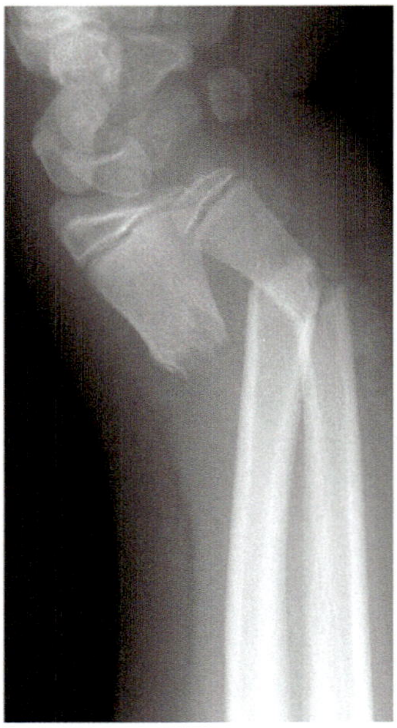

Fig. 3.9 Unstable distal forearm fracture, reduction and operative stabilization necessary

Open or Closed?

The need for open versus closed reduction depends not only on fracture morphology but also on the experience of the treating surgeon. Several aspects must be considered:

- Before treatment, there is a thorough evaluation of the fracture considering reducibility, stability, healing behavior, and prognosis.
- The first treatment should be the last. In other words, it should be definitive and not require re-reduction or secondary stabilization. This means that critical fractures should be treated in the operating room or be prepared for surgery.
- Each reduction should be performed with sufficient analgesia, usually under general anesthesia or with a plexus block in older children.

Most modern stabilization procedures, conservative or operative, allow closed treatment. Even plate fixation could usually be minimally invasive. In cases when open reduction is necessary, however, stable internal or external fixation could be performed whenever possible. There is hardly a point in performing open surgical reduction with conservative immobilization because secondary displacement can always occur in closed casts. The exceptions are articular fractures, which should be visualized (arthroscopically or open) and anatomically reduced and fixed.

Open Reduction

Open reduction is rarely necessary for pediatric fractures. Two types require it:

- Fractures that fail initial closed reduction attempts to provide stable treatment. Here, secondary open reduction is performed.
- Fractures that are intended for open reduction or for which open reduction must be planned.

Secondary Open Reduction

Most common fracture types:

- Transverse diaphyseal fractures from direct trauma → fragments in various compartments
- Diaphyseal multi-level fractures
- Articular fractures with secondary displacement more than 2 mm at the cast-free day 5 control.

  Most common locations:

- Distal humerus, supracondylar
- Forearm fractures
- Femoral shaft fractures (transverse)
- Fractures of the distal and proximal tibia

Primary Open Reduction

Most common fracture types:

- Articular fractures with displacement greater than 2 mm (Fig. 3.10)
- Partially open fractures
- Defect fractures, e.g. with soft tissue injury

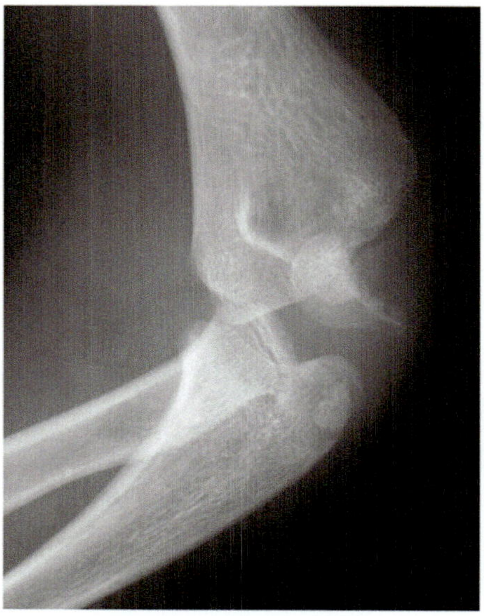

Fig. 3.10 Most of the joint fractures must be reduced open in order to control the joint surface, as in the completely displaced radial condyle fracture

Most common locations:

- Fractures of the lateral humeral condyle or the medial epicondyle, Y-fractures of the distal humerus with primary displacement greater than 2 mm,
- SCFE (slipped capital femoral epiphysis) with slipping over 10°
- Displaced femoral neck fractures
- Fractures of the distal femoral condyles
- Tibial plateau fractures with displacement over 2 mm
- Fractures of the distal tibia (two plane and tri-plane fractures), if cannulated screw correction is not possible; there is the option of targeted closed reduction, practically the only exception in an articular fracture
- Displaced or comminuted fractures of the talus and calcaneus
- Displaced fractures of the distal radial forearm

A primary open approach is not indicated for radial head or neck fractures because there is an exceptionally high risk for growth disturbances (Fig. 3.11).

These points offer a foundation for a thorough consideration of treatment strategy. In individual cases, the procedure must be adapted to the injury, your specialty and technical competence, and treatment conditions. Today, it is essential to factor in socio-economic aspects, including the need to resume sports or school, or for home care.

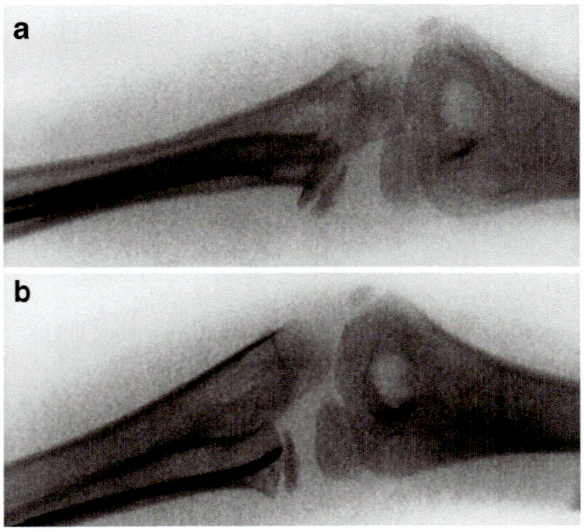

Fig. 3.11 Closed reduction and fixation of a displaced radial head fracture with retrograde ESIN. (**a**) Trauma image, (**b**) Reduction and fixation

Fixation Procedures

The following will introduce individual fixation procedures, briefly discussing the main principles and tricks of implementation and pointing out contraindications or limiting factors to application. For more detailed descriptions, please refer to the respective technical literature.

Successful fixation of pediatric fractures is based on familiarity with the variety of fixation techniques used according to age and the availability of various materials adapted for children.

Transfixion Wire Fixation

Transfixion wire fixation is an adaptive fixation, which is maxima stable regarding movement but not under loading. It usually requires supplemental cast immobilization. The advantages are that it can be performed percutaneously, and anesthesia is not required for removal, as the K-wire can in most cases remain above the skin. It is available almost anywhere and anytime.

Indications

- Open or closed reduced metaphyseal fractures of all long bones, practically regardless of age
- Articular fractures in younger children (<10 years)
- Fractures of the hand and foot, also open fractures with soft tissue injury

Contraindications

- Diaphyseal fractures should not be fixed with transfixion wires!

Typical Fractures

- Subcapital humerus fractures, or ESIN
- Supracondylar humerus fractures
- Lateral humeral condyle fractures (only in younger children; screws are more stable in the metaphyseal part)

- Medial humeral epicondyle fractures (only in small children, otherwise screws)
- Distal radius
- Distal epiphyseal/metaphyseal femur fractures
- Proximal epiphyseal/metaphyseal tibia fractures
- Distal epiphyseal/metaphyseal tibia/fibula fractures (alternatively cannulated screws)
- Fractures of the metacarpals/metatarsals
- Phalangeal fractures (hand/foot)

Technique

- Before transfixion wires are drilled, the fragments must be reduced.
- Whenever possible, the wires should be inserted percutaneously, even if open reduction is necessary, to enable anesthesia-free removal (Fig. 3.12)
- Wire diameters are: Fingers 1.0–1.2 mm; Metacarpal bones 1.2–1.4 mm, Upper arm

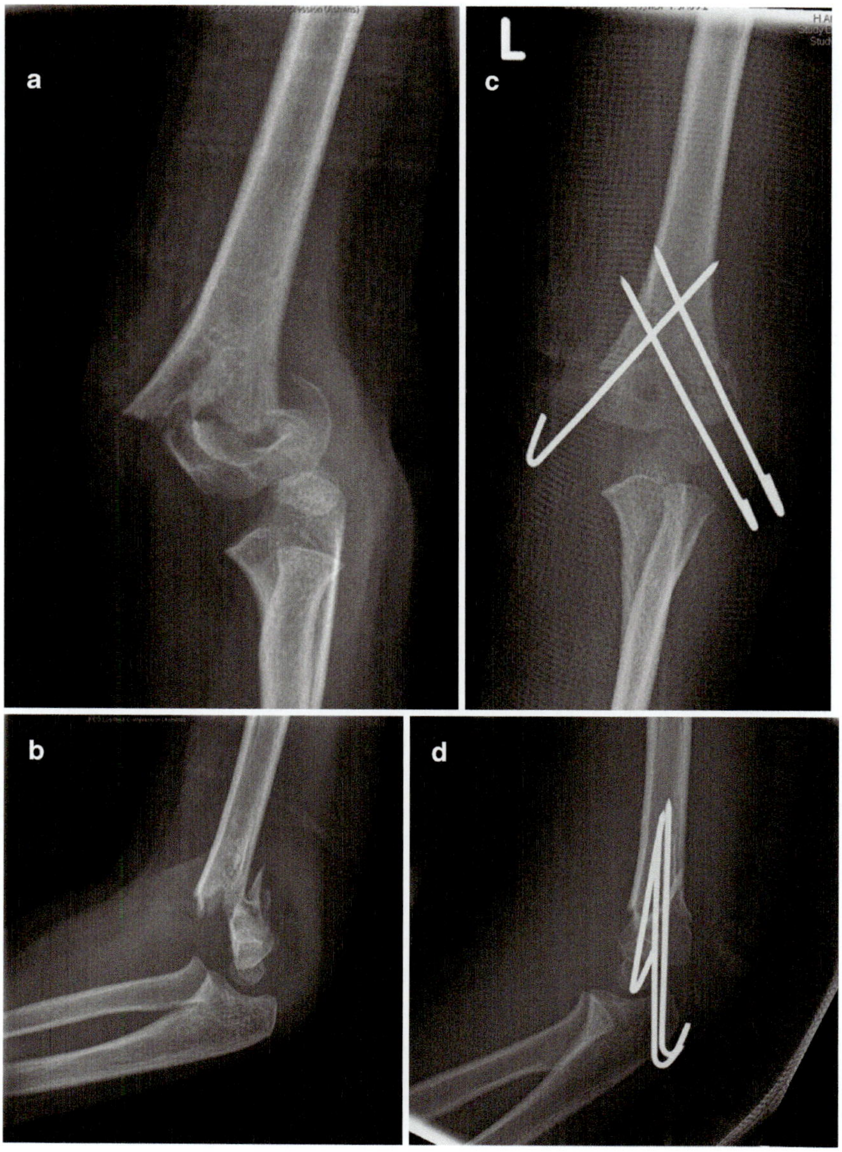

Fig. 3.12 Displaced supracondylar humerus fracture Type III. (**a**, **b**) Trauma image. (**c**, **d**) After reduction of fixation with K-wires. The K-wires should stay outside the skin to make the metal removal easier. Note: The ulnar nerve must be controlled by a short open incision

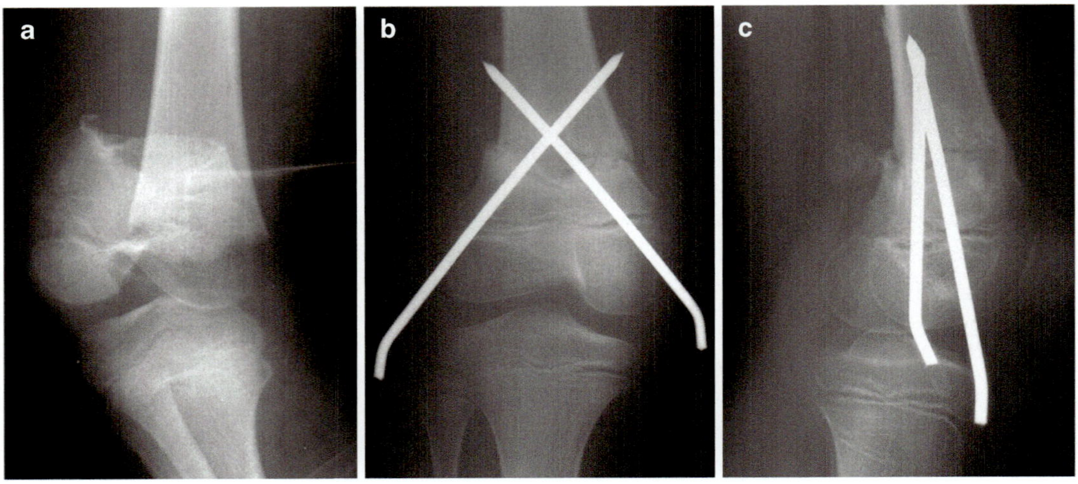

Fig. 3.13 Reduction and fixation of a distal femur fracture of a 9 years old child with 2 crossed K-wires of 2.5 mm; additional cast necessary. (**a**) Trauma image, (**b**) After osteosynthesis A.P. view and (**c**) Lateral view

joints 1.4–1.8 mm, Shoulder, Hip, Knee 1.6–2.5 mm
- The wires should always cross proximal to the fracture line (Fig. 3.13).
- If the physis must be crossed, repeated drilling should be avoided.
- The wire tips must just perforate the opposite cortex.
- Pin care is necessary and does reduce the risk of infection.

Tricks
- A good anesthesia and relaxation allows a smooth reduction
- A good reduction requires less subsequent manipulation.
- Stable holding of the reduction is important for good Wire-Positioning
- Plot the wire vectors in a single plane, so you do not need to rotate the image intensifier often

Hardware Removal
- According to age and fracture, at earliest 3 and latest 5 weeks.
- Ambulant in hospital or outpatient clinic.
- In younger children, with light sedation or oral analgesia 20 min before the procedure.

Problems
- Instability if the fixation is not good enough with the risk for secondary dislocation
- Non-union in instability
- Superficial or deep infections, if unstable or pin care not adequate
- Low compliance

Screw Fixation
Much of what applies to transfixion wires also applies to screw fixation. However, while screw fixation is adaptive, it also adds compression to the fragments and thus, offers better stabilization. A cast is still necessary, and it should be functional (i.e., can be removed to move joints, to care the pins), especially in older children. Cancellous screws are generally used, preferably cannulated, self-drilling, self-tapping steel or titanium (Fig. 3.14). These modern screws are also ideal for closed fixation, especially of the lower extremities. The screws should be reverse-cutting to simplify removal.

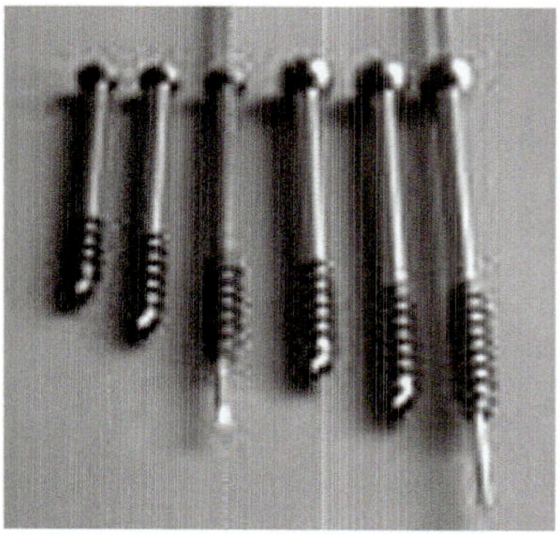

Fig. 3.14 Perforated, cannulated self-drilling and self-cutting titaneum screws

Indications

- Reduced (open or closed) epiphyseal/metaphyseal fractures in all locations, predominantly in children over 10 years
- Articular Fractures

Contraindications

- Diaphyseal fractures.

Typical Fractures

- Y-fractures of the distal humerus
- Lateral humeral condyle (older children)
- Medial humeral epicondyle (older children; caution: small fragments can be split!)
- SCFE (slipped capital femoral epiphysis)
- Femoral neck fractures in younger children
- Distal epiphyseal/metaphyseal femur fractures (Salter-Harris II, III and IV)
- Proximal epiphyseal/metaphyseal tibia fractures
- Distal epiphyseal/metaphyseal tibia/fibula fractures
- Carpal and tarsal bone fractures

Technique

- Before the screws can be placed, the fragment(s) must be reduced.
- Articular fractures should be reduced anatomically, open if indirect maneuvers are unsuccessful.
- Screw dimensions are usually 3.5, 4.0, 4.5, and 6.5 mm.
- Drill one or two guidewires (1.2/1.6 mm) perpendicular to the fracture line at the optimal position or parallel to the physis.

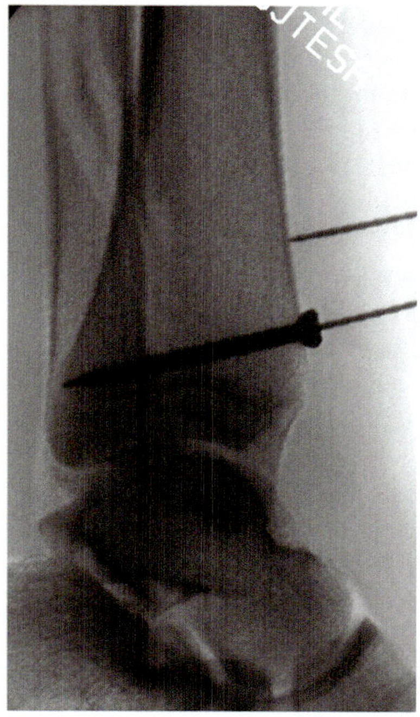

Fig. 3.15 Closed reduction and percutaneuous screw osteosynthesis of a Salter-Harris II fracture of the distal tibia. Note first the insertion of a wire and control in 2 x-ray view. Then overscrweing without drilling of a cannulated screw

- Measure the screw length along the protruding transfixion wire (length 15 cm minus protruding segment).
- Free insertion of the screws. If cannulated screws are not used, a glide hole must be predrilled (lag-screw technique).
- In older children, the physis may also be perforated with the screw, especially before growth is complete.
- Fixation should be documented intraoperatively with x-ray or fluoroscopy.

Tricks

- Closed approach. If the extremity is placed directly on the image intensifier, the result is a better image with less radiation.
- Reduce the fracture under fluoroscopy and adjust the fracture line image to orthograde (Fig. 3.15).
- Hold a free guidewire over the fracture to find optimal placement per fluoroscopy.

- Drill the guidewire parallel to this through a stab incision, in the second plane exactly parallel to the surface of the image intensifier.
- Visualize the screw insertion and indirect fracture reduction/compression on fluoroscopy.

Hardware Removal

This is performed after full consolidation regardless of age and fracture type. Removal is performed in day surgery under short general or local anesthesia.

- Under fluoroscopy, visualize the screw axially so the drilling position is evident.
- Insert the guidewire, make a stab incision, and remove the screw over the guidewire.

Problems

- Hardware removal
- Screw heads can be turned around, especially titanium screws; inform parents of this in advance.
- Small fragments can break off when threads are "aggressive."

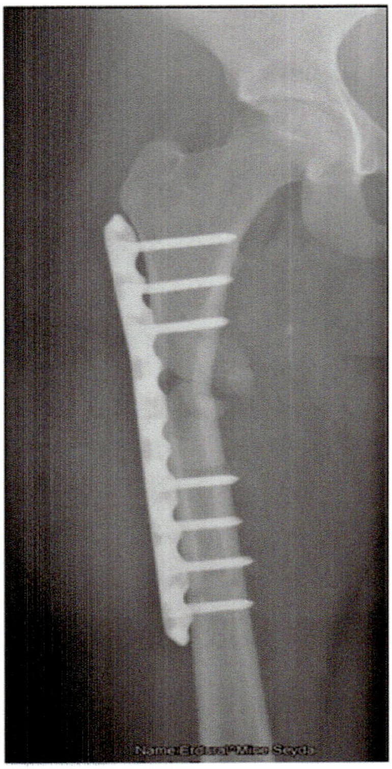

Fig. 3.16 Proximal femur fracture in an adolescent. Plate osteosynthesis during polytrauma management

Plate Fixation

The indications for plate fixation are reduced due to the variety of more child-friendly procedures. Plates should only rarely used in patients under 12 or 13, but in polytrauma patients with ongoing other surgeries it might be appropriate as in these situations fluoroscopy might be limited. However, they are a good option for young adolescents and mostly grown, somewhat overweight children, especially with newer application techniques and modern angular stable plate types. Thus, if plate fixation is indicated, the recommendation is to use low compression dynamic compression plates or low-contact plates (LCP) (Fig. 3.16). If possible, these plates should be inserted using a minimally invasive technique.

Indications

- Diaphyseal or proximal or distal fractures of the large long bones

- Phalangeal fractures (mini plates, rare)
- Completely unstable, multi-fragment fractures in overweight children and those over 12, as alternative to a standard nail
- Refractures of the femur and tibia with closed medullary canal
- Diaphyseal fractures in adolescents, fractures along the metaphyseal-diaphyseal junction of the radius in those over 12

Contraindications

- Joint-adjacent fractures with risk to disrupt growth plate circulation

Typical Fractures

- Long spiral shaft fractures with or without a wedge fragment
- Comminuted femur and tibia fractures
- Lateral femoral neck fractures (various angled plates)

Technique

Follow the respective manufacturer's guidelines for plate fixation. Plate fixation should be biological: i.e., no extensive exposure of the bone, no periosteal stripping, no meticulous adaptation and fixation of free fragments. If possible, this might be performed with a minimally invasive technique. Fixation of the plate with at least 2 (3) proximal and 2 (3) distal screws, preferably apart from the fracture, so that the plate can swing internally like a fixator, when angular stable screws are used.

Problems

- Hardware removal is laborious
- Invasive
- The greatest incidence of femoral overgrowth, especially in younger children

Hardware Removal

This is performed after full consolidation regardless of age and fracture type.

Tension Band Fixation

Tension banding is reserved for very special fractures and, as the name suggests, is used when a fragment needs to be stabilized with tension. It is performed through an open approach and neutralizes large tensile forces from strong tendon/muscle attachments.

Indications

- Olecranon fractures (practically every age)
- Patellar fractures
- Lateral clavicle fractures or non-unions of the distal clavicle
- Possible avulsions of the greater trochanter

Contraindications

- Articular Fractures
- Epiphyseal/metaphyseal fractures or diaphyseal fractures

Technique

- Open visualization of the fracture and fragment reduction
- Two transfixion wires are inserted perpendicular to the fracture plane through both fragments. Care must be taken that the wires are as far as possible from the surface, i.e., as far away from the direction of tension as possible so that they can counteract the pull of the cerclage (Fig. 3.17)

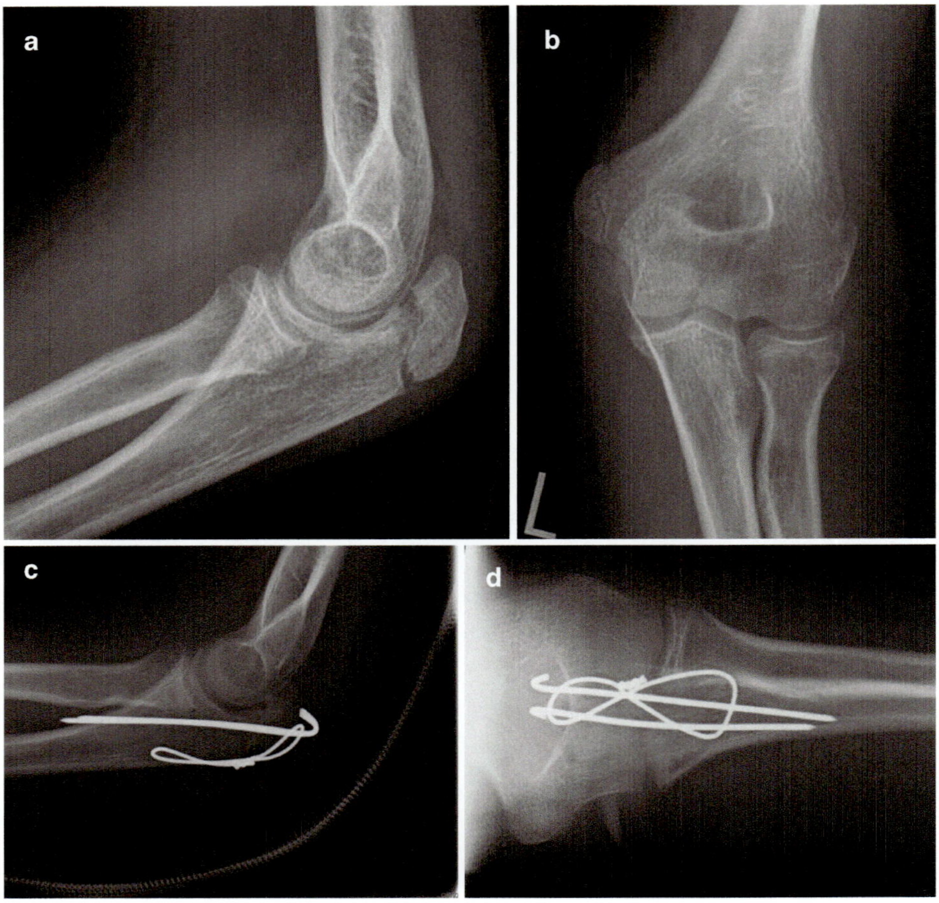

Fig. 3.17 Tension bend wiring of an intra-articular olecranon fracture. (**a**, **b**) Trauma image, (**c**, **d**) Tension bend wiring

Patella

- Both transfixion wires protrude about 5 mm proximal and distal, with the ends bent to right angles. 8 or O-shaped cerclage is applied since wire on the interior patellar surface is irritating.
- Turn the transfixion wires so that the bent ends secure the cerclage and point towards the patella.
- Alternative technique: Use cannulated screws instead of transfixion wires and feed the wires through the screws. Advantage: less soft tissue compression.

Olecranon

- Drill two parallel wires as close to the joint as possible from the tip of the olecranon so they are anchored in the distal cortex of the ulna.
- Drill a 2.0 mm canal approximately 3 cm distal to the fracture, perpendicular to the long axis, and pull the cerclage through. Create a figure-of-eight sling, with the whorl on the lateral (radial) side (more soft tissue, no nerve).
- Alternative technique: Use of screws instead of cerclage.

Problems

- Cutting through the transfixion wires or the cerclage.
- Necrosis of the muscle/tendon attachments. Guide the cerclage wire without tension through the muscle/tendon attachments!

Tricks

- Tighten the whorl slowly, so the wire can stretch and thus, is better applied to the fragments and soft tissues.

Hardware Removal

Cerclage should always be removed, especially in children, since it irritates once the swelling decreases, especially the whorl. Thus, cerclage wires are placed so they can be removed without completely opening the primary incision.

Intramedullary Nailing: ESIN

ESIN (elastic stable intramedullary nailing) is a minimally invasive, motion and partial-load stable, biological, and pediatric-adapted fixation for transverse, oblique, and short spiral diaphyseal fractures using elastic intramedullary nails (titanium or steel). The goal of ESIN is to obtain adequate reduction and stabilization for each respective age. Since it is generally a closed procedure, an anatomical reduction is not expected. Instead, non-angulated fixation is achieved.

The biomechanical principle is the symmetrical tensioning of two elastic nails inserted in the metaphysis, each of which has three support points within the bone; this must be respected to achieve optimal results.

Indications

ESIN is used primarily to treat diaphyseal and metaphyseal fractures in children, and its use depends on patient age, fracture, and localization. The age limit has to do with physiological development. Experience has yielded a lower limit around 3 years and an upper limit at 13–15 years. For lower extremity fractures, a body weight above 40–50 kg is also critical.

- **Fracture Type:** transverse fractures, short oblique or transverse fractures with a wedge fragment, long oblique fractures with possible cortical bracing, spiral fractures, multi fragment, and bifocal fractures, pathological fractures with juvenile bone cysts.
- **Fracture Localization:** Femoral diaphysis, distal and subtrochanteric metaphysis; lower leg diaphysis and distal metaphysis; humeral diaphysis, subcapital, and supracondylar; radial and ulnar diaphysis, radial neck or head.
- **Extended indication range with dedicated consideration:** Polytrauma and traumatic brain injury, both also above the age limits mentioned above, pathological fractures from benign bone cysts and prophylactic stabilization in juvenile bone cysts, osteogenesis imperfecta, humerus and forearm in adults

Contraindications

- Articular fractures
- Complex, totally unstable femur fractures or lower leg fractures lacking cortical bracing, especially with increasing age and/or overweight

Technique for Femur Fractures

Careful preoperative planning, choice of appropriate implant, and precise rotation check compared to the non-injured extremity are essential for a good operative result.

- **Child positioning:** The child is supine on a radiolucent table. The assistant extends the injured extremity, and the image intensifier is set to visualize the entire femoral length on both AP and lateral projections
- **Fracture reduction:** Free positioning of the child enables reduction during the procedure. In complex fractures, both legs should be prepped to enable comparison of rotation.
- **Nail diameter selection:** Measure the canal isthmus on x-ray. Individual nail diameter should be at least one-third the diameter of the canal. Select nails with identical diameters to avoid varus or valgus misalignments.
- **Nail entry point determination:** To protect femoral growth, the entry point should be 1–2 cm proximal to the distal epiphyseal plate. In children, this corresponds to approximately one finger-width proximal to the superior

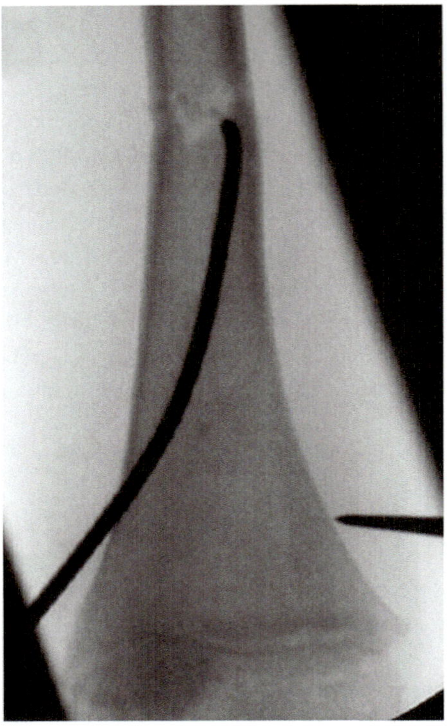

Fig. 3.18 Radiological control of the nail insertion point. Both insertions and opening of the medullary canal should be on the same level and the distance ot the growth plate should be at least 2 cm

patellar pole. If it is unclear, check the intended entry point under fluoroscopy (Fig. 3.18).

- **Incision:** The opposing medial and lateral skin incisions are placed approximately 3–4 cm distal to the planned entry point, depending on the child's size.
- **Open canal:** The bilateral openings of the medullary canal must be congruent to optimize symmetrical tensioning. Split the fascia lata sufficiently. At the proximal end of the incision, insert the awl perpendicular to the bone and punch it firmly. The cortical opening must be slightly larger than the selected nail diameter.
- **Pre-bend nails:** The nails are pre-bent to three times the canal diameter; the curve apex ends up within the fracture zone. The tip is a continuation of the arch. Pre-bend both nails (Fig. 3.19). Note: Bending increases the internal contact pressure and shifts the nail crossing point towards the metaphysis. This increases stability in complex fractures.
- **Insert the first nail:** Insert the nail into the medullary space with the tip perpendicular to

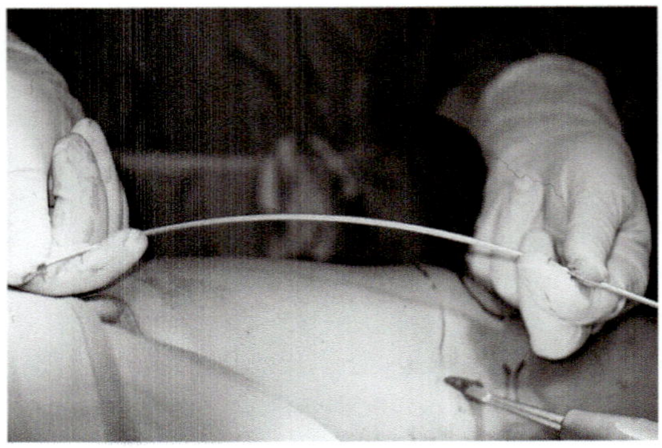

Fig. 3.19 The center of the prebending should be exactly at the fracture site

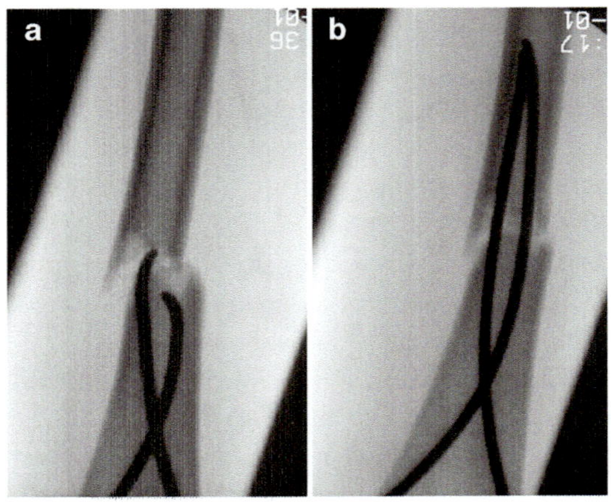

Fig. 3.20 Depending from the type of the fracture, one of the nails must be pushed first over the fracture site. (**a**) Advancement of nails, (**b**) Passing the fracture site

the shaft. Rotate the insertion tool 180° and align the nail tip to the canal axis. If necessary, check nail position with fluoroscopy.

- **Advance the first nail to the fracture zone:** Advance the nail to the fracture zone manually with twisting movements or light hammer taps.
- **Insertion of the second nail:** Repeat the previous two steps for the second nail at the other entry site, with the first crossing of the nails within the metaphysis.
- **Advance nails further:** Indirectly reduce the fracture definitively by turning the nails and advancing the tips several centimeters past the fracture to hold the fragments securely. If necessary, reduction can also be achieved using axial leg traction or with a lever. Finally, advance the nails reciprocally through the fracture zone (Fig. 3.20). Note: Twisting a nail more than 180° around its axis and the "cork-

screw" phenomenon (more than two nail crossing points) are critical to avoid (Fig. 3.21) Nails deformed during reduction maneuvers must be replaced and discarded.

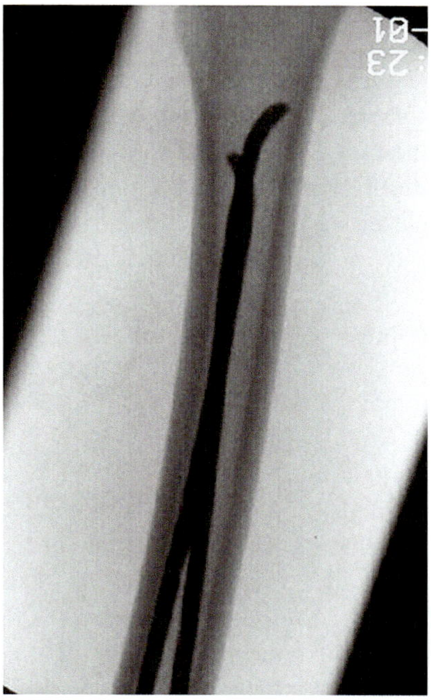

Fig. 3.21 Turning of the nail of more than 180° may lead to the cork puller phenomenon as visible her. This has to be avoided in order to maintain stability

- **Check the nail tips:** Check the position of the nail tips in the proximal fragment with fluoroscopy in two planes and align the tips in the canal on the frontal plane. Before adjustment, take care that the tip of the medial nail will not perforate the calcar.
- **Check rotation:** Once provisional fixation is secured, before the nails are definitively anchored in the proximal metaphysis, rotation must be controlled, and the nail tips correctly aligned. If an extension table is used, detach the leg (sterile) from the table to check rotation. This also enables axial fluoroscopy of the proximal femur.
- **Shorten nail:** Clip the extra nail protruding from the distal end according to the planned anchoring position. Take care that the end protrudes about 1 cm from the entry point for later removal. Note: Ends that are too long lead to pseudobursa formation and impede free knee flexion. They can also perforate the skin and cause infections (Fig. 3.22).
- **Definitive nail positioning and anchoring:** Secure the nail in position with gentle hammer taps to the anchoring pin. Bend the nail tips slightly with a suitable instrument to facilitate later removal of the implant.

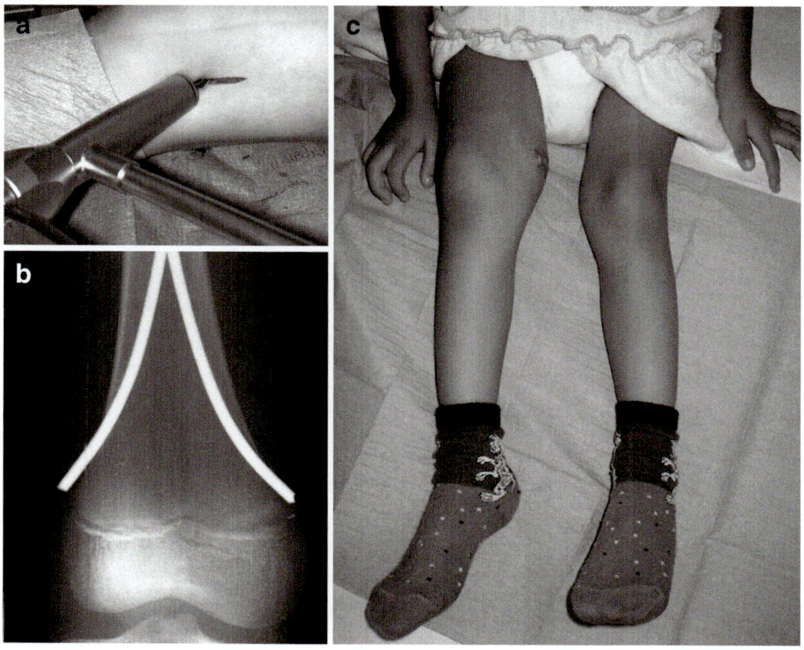

Fig. 3.22 (**a**) Correct bending and sharp cutting of the nails is necessary. (**b**) The correct length is important. (**c**) Otherwise this may result in pain and skin irritations

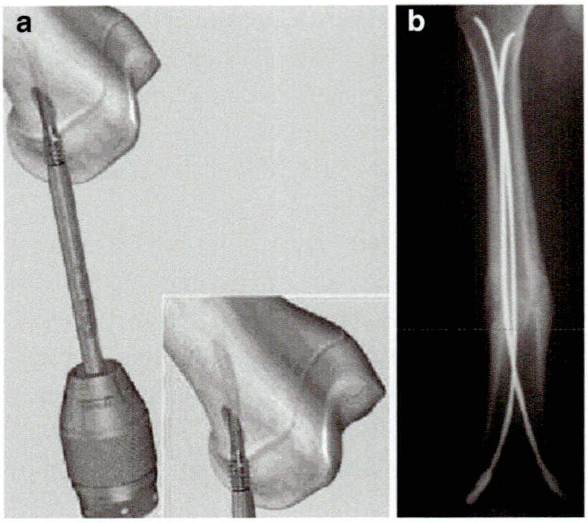

Fig. 3.23 With the "end cap", the nail stays in the position. (**a**) Schematic view of the concept. (**b**) X-ray of a healed fracture with an end cup

Problems

- **Stability:** With long oblique fractures, spiral fractures, and multi-fragment fractures, end caps can be used to increase stability (Fig. 3.23). Their application is simple and does not require additional intervention.
- **Corkscrew Phenomenon:** Turning the second nail more than 180° around the first nail can lead to intertwining. As a result, nails are pushed away from the cortex, and support is lost.
- **Nail perforation of the proximal femur:** The medially inserted nail can easily perforate the calcar because of femoral anteversion. Thus, axial fluoroscopy must be performed.
- **Injury to the physis:** Appropriate distance to the physis must be respected when choosing the entry point. Injury to the growth plate leads to growth disorders.
- **Skin irritation/infection:** Nails that have not been sufficiently shortened lead to skin irritation, and the exit point can produce local infection. On the distal femur, it can also block knee flexion.
- **Incorrect nail diameter:** Too-small diameter nails lead to instability and secondary deformity.
- **Eccentric entry point heights:** This leads to unequal nail tensioning, which results in varus or valgus deformities.

Tricks

- **Femur:** Better reduction is possible by inserting both nails to the fracture level and then advancing the fragment using a "joy-stick" method for better control.
- **Radial Head:** Closed reduction of completely displaced fractures with a percutaneous K-wire as "joy-stick" before advancement of the retrograde ESIN.
- **Tibia:** After definitive placement of the nail, the tips are rotated posteriorly to avoid recurvation of the tibia.

Hardware Removal

The advantage of ESIN is that healing occurs rapidly due to the relatively fine implants. Thus, regardless of fracture location, complete radiological consolidation should be verified before implant removal. This applies particularly in femur and forearm fractures. If this is evaluated appropriately, refractures are not expected.

Conventional Intramedullary Nailing

Because of expected growth disturbances, fixation with conventional intramedullary nails is indicated only in adolescents with fused or fusing epiphyseal plates. In markedly obese children, stable intramedullary nail fixation might also be necessary while the growth plates are fusing. The procedure and indications correspond to those in adults. Small diameter intramedullary nails are available with lateralized entry points for the proximal femur to protect the growth plate. In principle, humeral, femoral, and tibial nails can be used for the respective shaft fractures.

External Fixator

After ESIN, the second most common surgical approach to pediatric shaft fractures is external fixator application. Age-appropriate fixators and implants must be selected. Children generally tolerate external fixators well. Nevertheless, it is always important to consider pain, especially at the time of removal. Short anesthesia or sedation is often required. Because of the rapid healing, the fixator can be left until complete consolidation, without procedure change. This is a complementary alternative to ESIN, especially in 3° open, unstable fractures and older children.

Indications

- Completely unstable, multi-fragment fractures, especially in older children, of the femur, tibia, and forearm
- Polytrauma and traumatic brain injury
- Long spiral femur fractures ± a wedge fragment
- Open fractures with tissue defect (Fig. 3.24)

Contraindications

- Practically no contraindications if an appropriate device is available.

Typical Fractures

- Complex femoral diaphyseal fractures, distal, metaphyseal fractures
- Complex lower leg and tibia fractures, diaphyseal and proximal/distal metaphysis
- Complex forearm fractures, non-retainable distal radius fractures
- Open fractures (3°)

Technique

- Normally closed, for lower extremity with or without extension table.
- Free fluoroscopy must be ensured.
- As in ESIN, a preoperative provisional reduction is recommended to achieve a relatively non-angulated start.
- Schanz screws are set under fluoroscopy. In the case of "monotube" systems, the distance between entry sites is specified. In "tube-to-tube" systems, screws can be placed freely.
- One screw should be placed close to the fracture, and the other more distant.
- For the reduction, all clamps and screws must be open for free fragment manipulation.
- Daily pin care is a prerequisite to stay infection-free.

Problems

- Pin tract infections (good pin care is required)
- High refracture rate, especially when removed early for infection
- Deformity
- Delayed healing
- Schanz screw avulsion

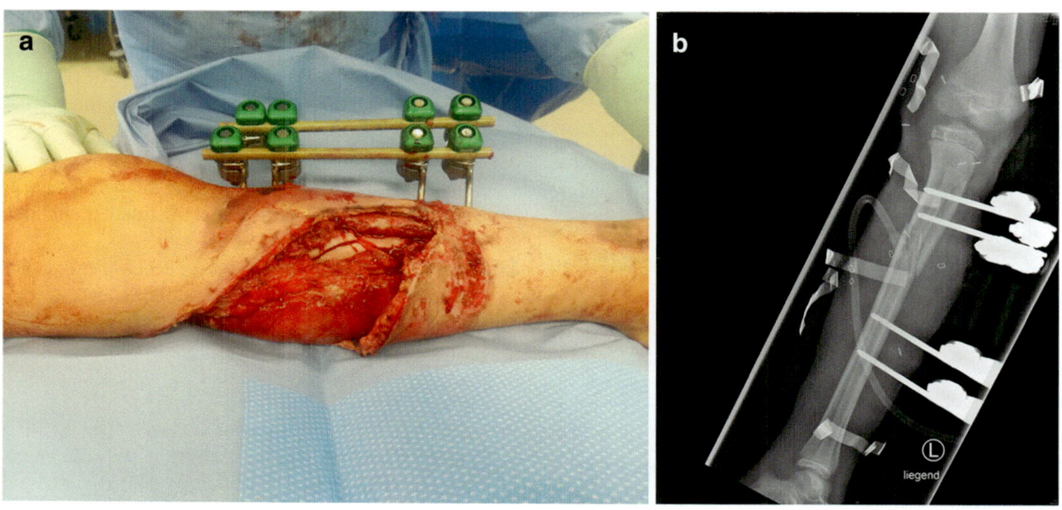

Fig. 3.24 Open lower leg fracture. (**a**) Debridement and stabilization with an external fixateur. (**b**) X-ray of stabilized fracture of the tibia

Tricks

- Pay attention to the soft tissues when placing the Schanz screws (better with "free" systems).
- "Stab" incisions should be large enough to allow secretions to drain.
- Showering/bathing makes care easier, followed by good cleaning and minimal disinfection.

Hardware Removal

The fixator should not be removed before clearly visible callus, generally at 4–8 weeks, depending on fracture type and child age. Suitable sedation or short anesthesia is recommended. The procedure can always be performed as an outpatient.

Further Techniques

There are no other relevant operative alternatives for pediatric fracture fixation than those described here. In cases where anesthesia is required for fracture reduction, the choice of fixation and operative versus conservative approach should always be considered ahead of time.

Hardware Removal

When the fractured bone is healed, the question of hardware removal emerges. This represents another invasive procedure, potentially requiring anesthesia and procedural risks like infection, wound healing disorders, neurovascular injury, and refracture. One clear indication is symptoms in the treated region (pain, functional limitations, skin irritation, etc.). External fixation materials should always be removed. This can often be done as an outpatient, with analgesia or sedation as needed.

Internal fixation materials such as screws or plates can be covered in bone quickly, especially in children, making delayed hardware removal more challenging. Persistent tensile forces that can occur because of osteosynthesis (especially in the diaphyseal region) should be avoided during remodeling. Materials left behind (especially steel plates) can corrode with increasing metal abrasion, leading to reactive granulation tissue and the risk of later infection. Thus, despite newer titanium implants, which can theoretically be left in place, early hardware removal is carried out in children. Radiological and clinical controls are always performed ahead of time. The timing of removal is given in the corresponding chapters.

Recommended Literature

Beaty J, Kasser J (2001) Rockwood and Wilkin's fractures in children. Lippincott Williams & Wilkins, Philadelphia

Blount WP (1957) Knochenbrüche bei Kindern. Thieme, Stuttgart

Böhler L (1929) Die Technik der Knochenbruchbehandlung. Mandrich, Wien

Dietz HG, Schmittenbecher PP, Illig P (2001) Intramedulläre Osteosynthese im Wachstumsalter. Urban & Schwarzenberg, München

Dietz HG, Schmittenbecher PP, Slongo T, Wilkins KE (2006) Elastic Stable Intramedullary Nailing (ESIN) in children. Thieme, Stuttgart

Joeris A, Lutz N, Wicki B, Slongo T, Audigé L (2014 Dec 20) An epidemiological evaluation of pediatric long bone fractures—a retrospective cohort study of 2716 patients from two Swiss tertiary pediatric hospitals. BMC Pediatr 14(1):314

Ladenhauf HN, Schaffert M, Bauer J (2014) The displaced supracondylar humerus fracture: indications for surgery and surgical options: a 2014 update. Curr Opin Pediatr 26(1):64–69

Lieber J (2014) Growth behavior after fractures of the distal forearm: reasons for the high rate of overtreatment. Unfallchirurg 117(12):1092–1098

Ligier JN, Metaizeau JP, Prvot J, Lascombes P (1988) Elastic stable intramedullary nailing of femoral shaft fractures in children. J Bone Joint Surg 70-B: 74–77

Maier M, Maier-Heidkamp P, Lehnert M, Wirbel R, Marzi I (2003) Results of femoral shaft fractures in childhood in relation to different treatment modalities. Unfallchirurg 106(1):48–54

Metaizeau JP (1988) Ostosynthese chez l'enfant par E.C.M.E.S. Sauramps Medical, Montpellier

Metaizeau JP, Lascombes P, Lemelle JL et al (1993) Reduction and fixation of displaced radial neck fractures by closed intramedullary pinning. J Pediatr Orthop 13(3):355–360

Prevot J, Lascombes P, Ligier JN (1993) The ECMES (Centro-Medullary Elastic Stabilising Wiring) osteosynthesis method in limb fractures in children. Principle, application on the femur. Apropos of 250 fractures followed-up since 1979. Chirurgie 119(9):473–476

Rang M (1983) Children's fractures. Lippincott, Philadelphia

Rüedi TP, Buckley RE, Moran CG (2007) AO principles of fracture management, 2nd edn. Thieme, Stuttgart

Schmittenbecher PP, Dietz HG, Linhart WE (2000) Complications and problems in intramedullary nailing of children's fractures. Eur J Trauma 6: 287–293

Slongo TF (2008a) Ante- and retrograde intramedullary nailing of humerus fractures. Oper Orthop Traumatol 20(4–5):373–386

Slongo TF (2008b) Correction osteotomy of neglected "monteggia" lesion with an external fixator. Oper Orthop Traumatol 20 (4–5): 435–449

Slongo T (2014) Radial external fixator for closed treatment of type III and IV supracondylar humerus fractures in children. A new surgical technique. Oper Orthop Traumatol 26(1):75–96

von Laer L, Kraus R, Linhart WE (2012) Frakturen und Luxationen im Wachstumsalter, 6th edn. Thieme, Stuttgart

Weinberg A-M, Hasler C-C, Leiner A, Lampert C (2000) External fixation of pediatric femoral shaft fractures, treatment and results of 121 fractures. Eur J Trauma 26:25–32

Soft Tissue Injuries

4

4.1 Vascular Injuries

Causes, Mechanism of Injury

Vascular injuries in children occur in similar circumstances to those in adults, with penetrating trauma, e.g. from glass pieces (falls with a glass bottle), lacerations, and puncture wounds, or also with animal bites. When dealing with complex anatomical structures such as the hand, accompanying injuries to nerves and tendons must be taken into account. Puncture wounds especially can conceal serious injuries, as the injured and frightened child is often very difficult to examine. In case of doubt, and when there is suspicion for structural lesions, operative exploration should be carried out and adequate therapy given. In this way, partial or complete ischemia from vascular injuries and the resulting complications like growth disturbances or functional deficits can be prevented. Blunt vascular injuries are generally either direct arterial injuries in cases of contusion or compression, e.g. by haematoma or bony fragments, or indirect arterial injuries in cases of fracture or joint dislocation. Particular attention must be given to the risk of vascular injury in supracondylar humerus fractures, in which the brachial artery can be damaged by stretching, strain, or torsion. In the elbow region, around 2% of displaced fractures include vascular injuries requiring therapeutic intervention. However, approximately 10% of those with primary signs of vascular involvement will be basically clinically unremarkable after reduction.

Classification

- Sharp direct arterial injuries
- Blunt direct arterial injuries (Fig. 4.1)
- Indirect arterial injuries

Diagnostic Assessment

Initially, critical information is collected regarding mechanism of injury, time of injury, blood loss, and accompanying neurological complaints in particular. On examination, observations are made regarding the injury, bleeding, extent of haematoma, as well as swelling and other signs of compartment syndrome! The classical signs of ischemia such as pain, pallor, pulselessness, and paraesthesia are often not present, particularly with distal vascular injuries. In appropriate areas, an Allen test can be carried out to evaluate capillary refill, if necessary with a Doppler device. It

I. Marzi et al., *Pediatric Skeletal Trauma*, https://doi.org/10.1007/978-3-030-93685-3_4

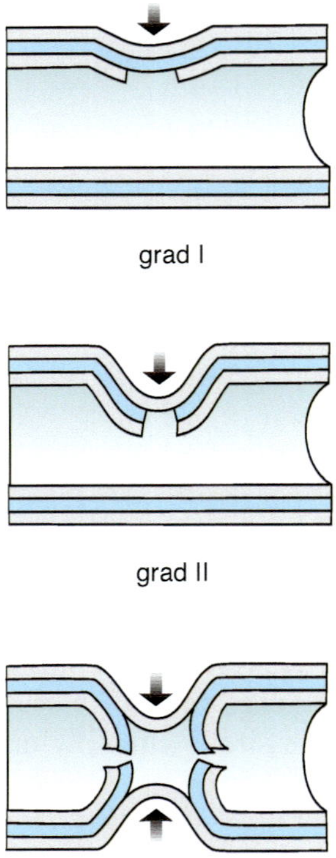

Fig. 4.1 Vascular wall injuries. Grade I: Intimal injury, Grade II: Intimal and muscular injury, Grade III: Lumen stenosis through curling of the intimal and muscular layers

is not uncommon that the actual extent of injury can be determined only at the time of surgical intervention. In cases of vascular injuries, when there is doubt, an x-ray examination should always be performed. Bony stability is essential for successful vascular reconstruction. Angiography is performed only in exceptional cases when the localization of injury is in question. In cases of dislocation and/or fracture, the location of the vascular injury is a given and thus, revascularization for complete ischemia should not be unnecessarily delayed.

Sharp Direct Vascular Injury

Incomplete arterial injuries are generally the consequence of stabbing or laceration wounds, or of iatrogenic aetiology. The vessel is damaged from the exterior to the interior, and bleeding can only be suspended by compression through haematoma or occlusion through curling of the intima/media. In addition to bleeding from the lesion, peripheral pulselessness is generated depending on localization.

Complete transection is identifiable, depending on the localization, as diffuse bleeding or haematoma. Smaller arteries can retract, and vascular spasm and tissue pressure can lead to haemostasis. However, this can also conceal the relevant vascular injury, so that the complete transection is only revealed during surgical exploration, unless angiography is performed.

Blunt Direct and Indirect Vascular Injury

Vascular contusion varies significantly from sharp injuries and can present very differently. Blunt injury leads initially to intimal lesions and only to medial lesions with more severe presentations and seldom to complete transections with adventitial injury. However, the lesion is often more extensive than in sharp injury, which must be taken into account during reconstruction to avoid post-operative thrombosis. The intimal lesion favours thrombosis formation and thus, vessel stenosis. Appropriate experience is required particularly to assess the extent of vascular damage. Bleeding into the vessel wall after vascular anastomosis, separation of the vessel wall layers, or areas with platelet aggregation or fibrin accumulation suggest more extensive intimal injury. The most important indirect vascular occlusions occur in joint dislocations around the femoral, popliteal, and axillary arteries or in deceleration trauma along the aorta.

Primary Treatment

Primary intervention, especially at the trauma scene, is focused on haemostasis, fighting shock, and avoiding further injury. Obvious bleeding must be treated with compression. A tourniquet should be applied as last resort. Extremity injuries and fractures in particular must be immobilized with a splint.

Therapy

Operative treatment ranges from direct vessel suture and venous patch to venous interposition, depending on the extent of injury. In cases of paediatric vessel injuries, exclusively autologous tissue must be used, since this is the only way to take further growth into account. Typical harvest areas for this are the underarm, cephalic, and basilar veins as well as the saphenous vein (Fig. 4.2). Continued growth must also be considered when choosing suture material and anastomosis technique. Especially when non-resorbable suture material is used, single-button techniques should be used to minimize the risk of secondary stenosis. Sutures should be applied without tension, so that rupture or secondary thrombosis can be avoided. When using venous interposition graft, the vessel must not kink, since this can also induce thrombosis. Once the vessel is reconstructed, the duration and magnitude of ischemia must be evaluated; with longer ischemia times, prophylactic fasciotomy for compartment syndrome must be performed when appropriate.

Short-term immobilization should be applied for approximately 2 weeks to protect the vessel repair. Close circulation control is needed within the first 48 h (beginning with every 2 h). This can be carried out with palpation of the pulses and inspection of capillary refill for extremity injuries. Pulse oximetry should supplement this monitoring. For vessel repairs in the microsurgical area or also the radial and ulnar arteries, postoperative thrombosis prevention can be improved with anticoagulants, e.g. heparin. This treatment can then be converted to short-term (3–4 weeks) therapy with low-dose ASA (acetylsalicylic acid).

Complications, Growth Disturbances

The major complications in the first 2 days are haemorrhage and immediate occlusion. Slower occlusion of reconstructed vessels can also occur. In such cases, when there is good circulation distal to the lesion without a detectable radial pulse, there is discussion whether to leave it under observation. In cases of relative ischemia after loading, however, revised reconstruction is needed. Other relevant complications are wound

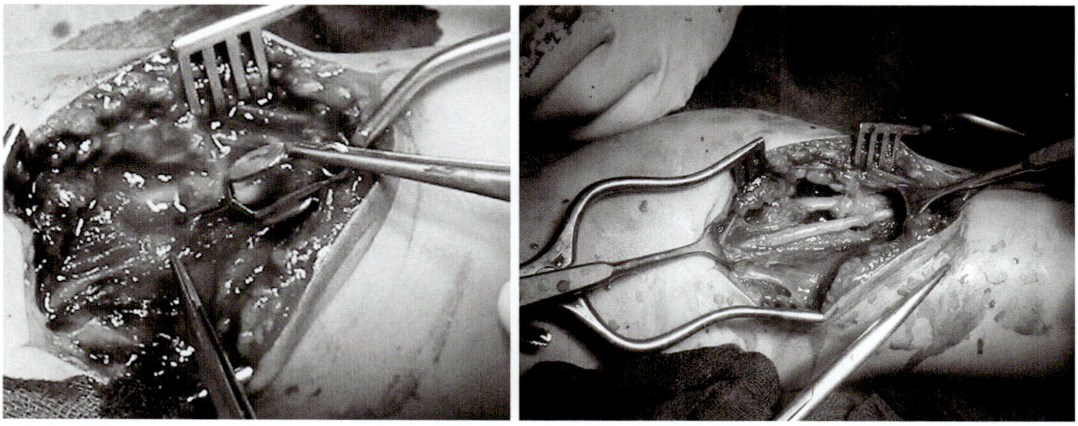

Fig. 4.2 Tear of the brachial artery with a supracondylar humerus fracture and vessel reconstruction with venous interposition graft

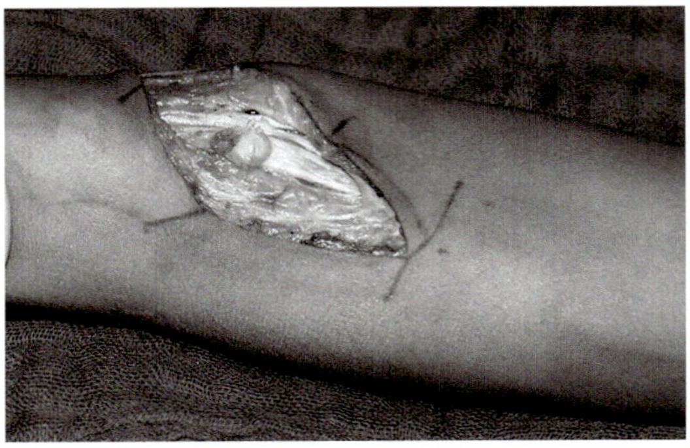

Fig. 4.3 Pseudoaneurysm and AV fistula after a stab wound

infections, compartment syndrome, and lymphatic fistulas or lymphoceles, especially in the groin area.

If an injury is overlooked, in addition to ischemic complications, a pseudoaneurysm requiring secondary surgical treatment, or arteriovenous fistula, especially in stab wounds, can develop (Fig. 4.3). Consequences of such AV fistulas include growth delay, tachycardia, increased blood volume, increased cardiac output, and increased venous pressure with the risk of congestive heart disease.

Investigations after subclavian artery ligation in Tetralogy of Fallot showed growth delay (radius) and reduced muscle mass. Thus, reconstruction of larger vessels is necessary. In cases of distal vessel injuries, such as of the wrist, palm, or finger, there is no uniform solution. Ligation of the ulnar artery yields a critical ischemia risk of 1.6%, and of the radial artery 5.1%. The risk can be minimized when the dominant vessel is known. In the wrist and finger regions, however, there is great variation and thus, when possible, microvascular surgery should be performed. Nerve injuries also recover better when there is combined neurovascular treatment.

Follow-Up

Follow-up is generally performed according to the concomitant injuries. After the initial phase of close circulatory monitoring for the first week after surgery, clinical checks should be made after 6 months and then annually for 2 years to identify any growth deficits. When findings are unclear during the course of follow up, colour duplex sonography or, in case of particular questions, magnetic resonance angiography can be performed.

4.2 Nerve Injuries

Causes, Mechanisms of Injury

The most common nerve injuries are lacerations of the distal forearm or hand, usually from glass. However, blunt injuries can also lead to full or partial nerve disruption through compression or tension. Sensory or motor nerve injuries are often identified especially in fractures of the elbow region, depending on displacement. Incomplete primary lesions generally have good prognoses after reduction and immobilization and recover after 2–4 months. Other common locations of injury include the extremities, shoulder and pelvic girdles, and the head/neck region. The most common causes of injury include:

- Ischaemia
- Mechanical causes (tension, compression, bending, cold, heat, electricity, toxic substances, radiation)
- Infection and inflammatory diseases
- Tumours
- Systemic diseases

In general, however, it's important to note that in cases of complete nerve disruption or even central plexus lesions, the developing nervous system displays more sensitive responses and relies on retrograde stimulation from the periphery. For example, in cases of plexus lesion from birth trauma, the cervical spinal canal shows marked atrophy.

Classification

The ultimate peripheral nerve conduction structure is the axon of the ganglion cell, located in the anterior horn of the spinal cord for motor nerves and in the spinal ganglion for sensory nerves. Several neurites are bound by connective tissue,

Table 4.1 Classification of nerve injuries according to Sunderland and Mackinnon

Severity	Tinel sign/distal progression	Recovery pattern	Recovery rate	Operative approach
I Neurapraxia	No T sign	Complete	Rapid (days to approx. 12 weeks)	None
II Axonotmesis	+/+	Complete	Slow (1 mm/day)	None
III Axonotmesis	+/+	Large variation	Slow (1 mm/day)	None/neurolysis
IV Continuity neuroma	+/–	None	No recovery	Nerve suture/nerve transplantation
V Neurotmesis	+/–	None	No recovery	Nerve suture/nerve transplantation
VI Combination injuries grades I–V	Varies according to fascicular injuries	Varies according to fascicle	Varies according to fascicle	Varies according to fascicle

and this perineurium forms the fascicle. A group of fascicles, in turn connected by interfascicular connective tissue, form a fascicular bundle. A group of these bundles ultimately forms the peripheral nerve, which is covered in a connective tissue sheath (epineurium). In cases when the axons have been disrupted, these will degenerate distal to the site of injury (Waller degeneration. However, since the nerve is not always completely disrupted, the possibility of regeneration depends on the degree of injury and the distance to the effector organ of the nerve and/or the anatomic location. The severity of nerve injuries was initially classified in 3 grades by Seddon:

- **Grade I**, Neurapraxia: conduction blockage at a particular point of the nerve not leading to axon degeneration.
- **Grade II**, Axonotmesis: axonal damage with degeneration distal to the lesion.
- **Grade III**, Neurotmesis: complete disruption of the nerve.

This classification, which is still somewhat commonly used in clinical practice, was expanded by Sunderland and later by Mackinnon (Table 4.1). It is aimed toward the axonal and connective tissue anatomy of the nerve.

Diagnostic Assessment

Children also show typical clinical presentations like drop hand or foot when motor function fails. During examination, attention must be given to identify dysesthesia, anaesthesia, weakness, paresis, and loss of function. However, this is a particular challenge for the examiner of children. For example, the child must be willing to spread the fingers (ulnar nerve) or bend the IP joint of the thumb or the DIP joint of the index finger (anterior interosseous nerve). It is also especially important to notice whether a child ignores part of an extremity and no longer uses it. This does not necessarily mean that there is a motor lesion; instead, it can be an isolated sensory deficit (e.g., spreading of the thumb and index finger with sensory loss of the median nerve). Children complain less often of pain, particularly in cases of complete disruption. It is found more commonly in cases of incomplete injuries and is then of varying duration and character. Sometimes there is warming and dry skin of the affected portion of the extremity. In cases of open wounds, the anatomic relationships to relevant nerve structures must be observed; in closed injuries, severity can be estimated based on hematoma formation, skin marks, and swelling.

During examination for paediatric spine injuries, it should be noted that the spinal cord fills the cervical canal and that spinal nerves emerge at almost right angles. Thus, separation is more likely than nerve root avulsion. Myelinisation is similarly not yet complete, and thus, nerve conduction is reduced by about 50% until around age 3. This must be particularly noted during the neurophysiological examination of paediatric nerve injuries. Increasing function or use (e.g., of the hand) often comes markedly later than the neurophysiological signs of re-innervation.

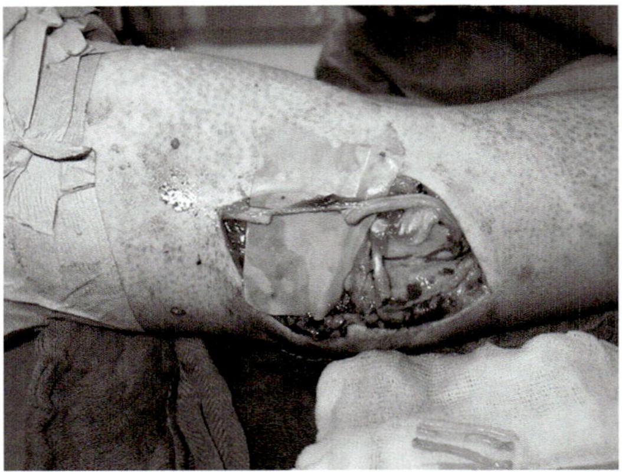

Fig. 4.4 Extensive tearing of the radial nerve

Primary Treatment

Treatment depends on the cause of injury. In cases of deep injuries (e.g. lacerations of the hand) and anatomic proximity to a nerve, nerve injury must be assumed, and local exploration must be performed—in children, generally under general anaesthesia (Fig. 4.4). In closed injuries, therapy is based on the cause of nerve injury. In cases of fracture (e.g. elbow with entrapment of a nerve), the focus is on reduction, exploration of the nerve, decompression and stabilization and immobilisation (Fig. 4.5). In cases of blunt nerve

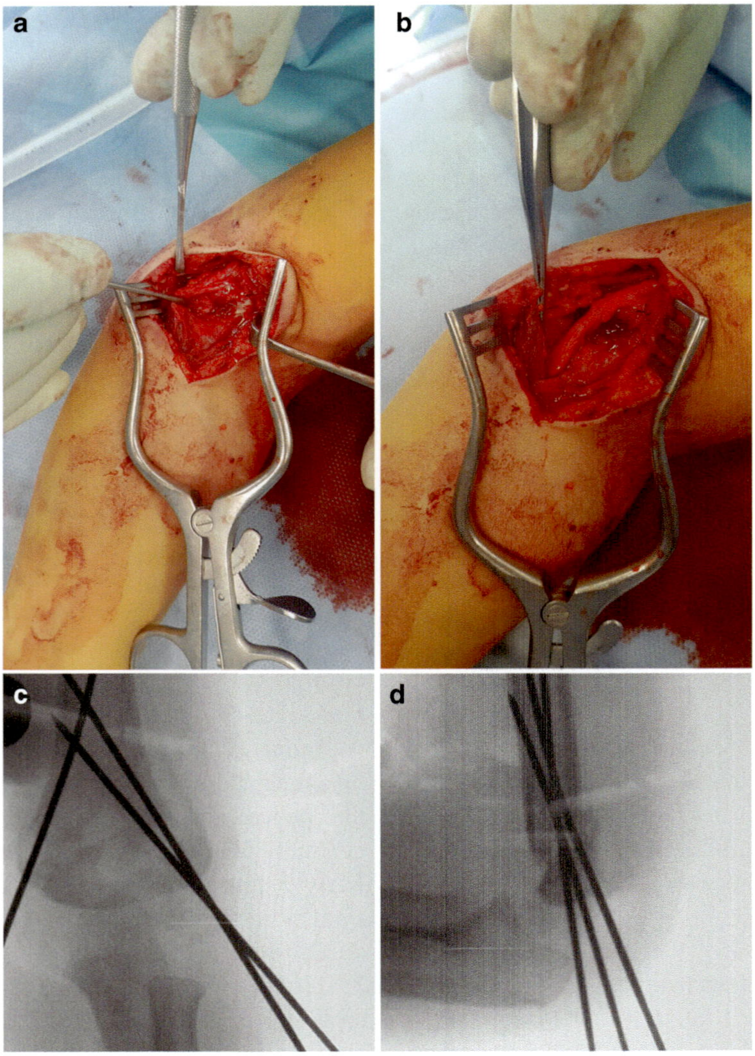

Fig. 4.5 Entrapment of the median nerve at a grade IV supracondylar humerus fracture. (**a**) Ventral approach to the elbow with entrapped median nerve. (**b**) Released median nerve, (**c, d**) Final reduction and K-wire osteosyntesis

injury from over-extension, there are high rates of spontaneous nerve regeneration after reduction (about 90%).

Treatment

Nerve transections must be treated operatively with microsurgical technique. Tension-free fascicular suture with additional epineural repair is carried out depending on the size of the nerve (Fig. 4.6). Non-resorbable suture is used, 10–0 for the finger and up to 7–0 for the large extremity nerves. In the case of nerve defects, nerve interponate graft must be used, e.g. with the sural nerve or the antebrachial cutaneous nerve.

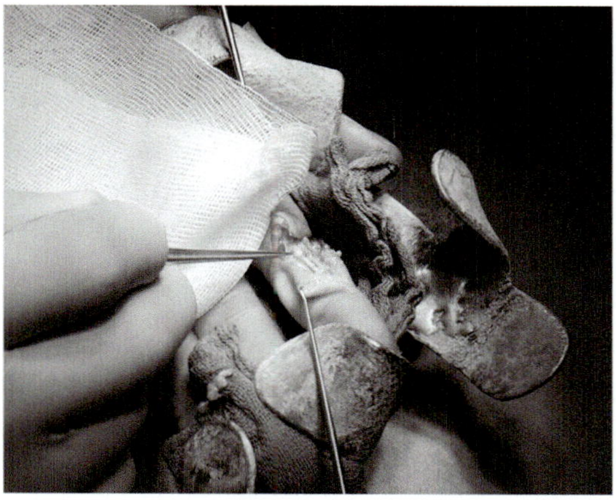

Fig. 4.6 Microsurgical nerve repair of the finger

Regeneration after complete nerve transection is only as good as the nerve suture or reconstruction. Nevertheless, it varies according to the amount of endoneural scarring and the degree of misdirection of sensory and motor axons within the injured nerve. This applies particularly for the spontaneous regeneration of Grade III, axonotmesis (Table 4.1). In this case, in addition to waiting, operative neurolysis can bring significant functional improvement, particularly when performed at a typical nerve compression site.

The regeneration rate is typically between 1 and maximal 3 mm per day. Remarkable in children is that pain is relatively rare.

Complications, Growth Disturbances

Incompletely released nerves from fractures or pronounced callus reactions can lead to compression or even complete nerve disruption. A secondary nerve lesion is the result, and it must be recognized early. In these cases, microsurgical neurolysis is required, which is often followed by rapid recovery of nerve function (Fig. 4.7). In some cases, however, the severely damaged nerve must be bridged with an interponate graft.

Denervation of an extremity leads to growth disruption; extensive birth-traumatic injuries to the plexus can create more than 20% differences. Even more important is the occurrence of muscular imbalance with the loss of particular muscle

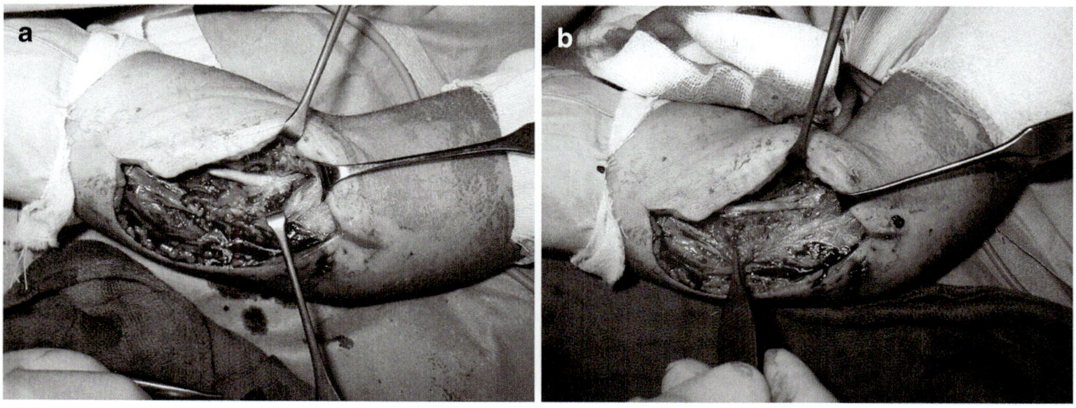

Fig. 4.7 (**a**, **b**) Radial nerve compression. (**a**) Secondary through callus, (**b**) Free course after neurolysis

groups. Such an imbalance must be eliminated in a timely manner to prevent a fixed deformity that can only be corrected by surgical intervention on the bony skeleton. Pain after nerve injuries has been reported for adults as following:

- CRPS (complex regional pain syndrome) Type 2
- Reflex Sympathetic Dystrophy (CRPS Type 1)
- Neuralgia
- Neurostenalgia (pain from compression, stretching or ischaemia)
- Central pain (e.g. due to spinal injury or chronic pain)
- Secondary gain

Most of these pain syndromes or aetiologies are not found in children and occur rarely even as neuralgia after plexus injuries. In contrast, pain as neurostenalgia is common in cases of nerve compression, e.g. in fractures, and can serve as an indication of the diagnosis. Postoperative pain pointing in a similar direction must also be noted. It could be an indication of nerve irritation along the bone or fracture fragments, compression from suture, or an increasing hematoma.

Follow Up

Follow up checks should occur every 2 weeks after an acute nerve injury; essentially this should be done to advise parents and to recognize signs of regeneration as soon as possible, which clearly decreases tension regarding the situation. After successful nerve repair, the Tinel sign can be used for clinical follow up. In cases of regeneration, this is stronger on the nerve regenerating from central to peripheral compared to the original location of repair. Neurophysiological examinations should be performed after 6 weeks, 3 and 6 months. If the axons are injured, there will be no motor stimulus response distal to the injury around 6 days post-injury.

The development or the appearance of a muscular imbalance should be checked every 6 months for the first 2 years. After that, annual follow up is needed. The functions that are ultimately regained can be classified according to the classification of the British Medical Research Council (1954, Table 4.2).

Table 4.2 Classification of nerve regeneration according to the British Medical Research Council

Motor	
M 0	No muscle contraction
M 1	Muscle contraction without movement
M 2	Minimal force generation, movement against gravity but not against resistance
M 3	Good movement, also against resistance
M 4	Active movement, also against resistance
M 5	Normal force
Sensory	
S 0	No sensation
S 1	Deep pain sensation
S 2	Tactile sensation
S 3	Partial two-point discrimination
S 4	Normal sensation

4.3 Tendon Injuries

Causes, Mechanism of Injury

Children and adolescents with open epiphysial junctures are more susceptible to avulsion or growth plate injuries than ligament, muscle, and tendon injuries. Biomechanically, the chondro-osseous tissue is the weakest link in the series when considering the musculotendinous or ligamentous units. Tendons and ligaments are not directly connected to the growing skeleton with Sharpey fibers as they are in adults. They are attached to the cartilage or the growth region via a fibro-cartilaginous connective tissue or the perichondrium or periosteum. This construct allows growth while bone size is increasing. The high elasticity and plastic deformability of the tendons and ligaments in children often lead to bony injuries and not to intra-ligamentous/intra-tendinous ruptures. Only at the end of the growth phase, in adolescents, does laxity decrease and the risk of intra-tendinous rupture increases. Thus, excessive strain in children is most likely to affect the nearby bone. This excessive strain can sometimes be seen as ossification and represents "failure" of the musculoskeletal system. These circumstances also appear to be the basis for pathologic changes in cases of avascular bone necrosis (e.g., Morbus Osgood-Schlatter).

Basically, it should be noted that muscles, tendons, and bones function together as a unit, and muscle injuries are common in sports medicine. These injuries are often misdiagnosed and inadequately treated. Thus, when there is suspicion for tendon injury, attention must be given to the entire muscle-tendon complex. Accordingly, injuries can be classified as lesions of the muscle, the musculotendinous transition, the tendon itself, and the insertion area.

Muscle contusions and strains are common in young adolescents with sports associated with that age, but uncommon in younger children. Acute tendon injuries are also rare in childhood, although sub-maximal strain can lead to an overload syndrome, e.g. to partial rupture of the biceps tendon in adolescent tennis players. Other contributing factors include suddenly increased load with overuse, walking on uneven terrain, hard or slick roads or on overly soft ground, sudden loads on untrained body regions without adequate adaptation of movement patterns or techniques, body growth, and insufficient rest after injury.

At rest, tendons have a wavy structure, and the collagen fibers are exposed to stress with stretching of 2%. The cross-linking of the collagen structures begins to fail at 4–8%. The Achilles tendon can bear maximal loads of some 12 times body weight. However, the cause for tissue damage is often recurrent strain in combination with pressure and shearing forces. Injuries are thus found in the following situations:

- rapid tension rise without warming up
- oblique tension lines
- tendon strain prior to trauma
- maximal contact surface to the attached muscle
- muscle stretching by external forces
- poor relation of the tendons to the muscles

Regarding open injuries, it must be remembered that children experience the world through sight, taste, and touch. Thus, they use their hands to touch dangerous objects that can lead to soft-tissue and tendon injuries. In children, such injuries can lead not only to loss of function, but also to reduced growth from accident-related damage. Tendon injuries of the hand are conspicuous in this regard.

Classification

Injuries to the muscles or muscle fibers of the muscle-tendon complex react quickly to changes, and lesions can heal within 3 weeks. There are several types of ruptures:

- **Strains:** lesions in the muscle-tendon transition caused by overstretching or eccentric overload.
  - **Grade I**, slight strain: less than 5% muscle fiber involvement; no reduced force or limitations in range of motion, but pain is present.
  - **Grade II**, moderate strain: significant but incomplete tearing of the muscle.
  - **Grade III**, severe strain: complete muscle tear.
- **Contusion** direct force when muscle is compressed against bone; problems are the muscle tearing and bleeding within the muscle.

The resulting hematomas can be differentiated into intra- and intermuscular hematomas. Intramuscular hematomas are within the muscle sheath and lead to increased pressure, which counteracts further bleeding. However, this can result in prolonged swelling over the first 48 h, marked tenderness and discomfort. Rarely, acute compartment syndrome can develop, in combination with additional osmosis-induced fluid overload. Intermuscular hematomas initially lead to increased pressure that rapidly drops, so that bleeding is distributed. Hematoma discoloration and swelling often occur distal to the injury. Because the pressure increase is small, muscle function returns rapidly.

Spontaneous tendon ruptures in particular are uncommon in children. There are 4 pathologic changes as signs of potential tendon failure, especially in adults:

- Peri-Tendinitis (inflammation of the tendon sheath)
- Peri-Tendinitis with tendinosis
- Tendinosis (tendon degeneration)
- Tendinitis (degeneration of the tendon with rupture and inflammatory repair processes)

Partial or complete tendon rupture/injury can be differentiated depending on the extent of damage. In contrast to bony injuries, tendons contribute less to the initial healing process. The majority of healing comes from tissue infiltration from the surrounding area. To ensure stability of the injured tendon, sufficient approximation of the ends is necessary. This can be attained easily with surgery, and there will be greater stability than with conservative treatment. However, since the tissue is still growing and has an enormous capacity for regeneration, especially in children, conservative therapy is still often indicated.

Extensor Tendons of the Hand

The extensor tendons run over the wrist under the broad extensor retinaculum and separated by tendon sheaths into 6 compartments. The long finger tendons are connected through cross-linking fibers (Juncturae tendineum). These cross-fibers can mask a tendon rupture, because they allow movement via the neighboring tendon (Fig. 4.8). At the level of the MCP joint, the tendons are centered over the metacarpal heads by the retinaculum and the extensor tendon hood. The extensor tendon divides at the distal end of the proximal phalanx, and the central slip bridges the PIP joint. At the same time, two side slips bypass this joint and unite with the intrinsic hand muscle tendons to attach at the base of the distal phalanx. The tendons of the intrinsic hand muscles are comprised of the 4 lumbrical, the 3 volar interosseous (finger adduction), and 4 dorsal interosseous (finger abduction) muscle tendons. Fine additional fibers complete the extensor apparatus in the long finger area. Similar to the intertendinous membrane of the proximal phalanx, the triangular ligament

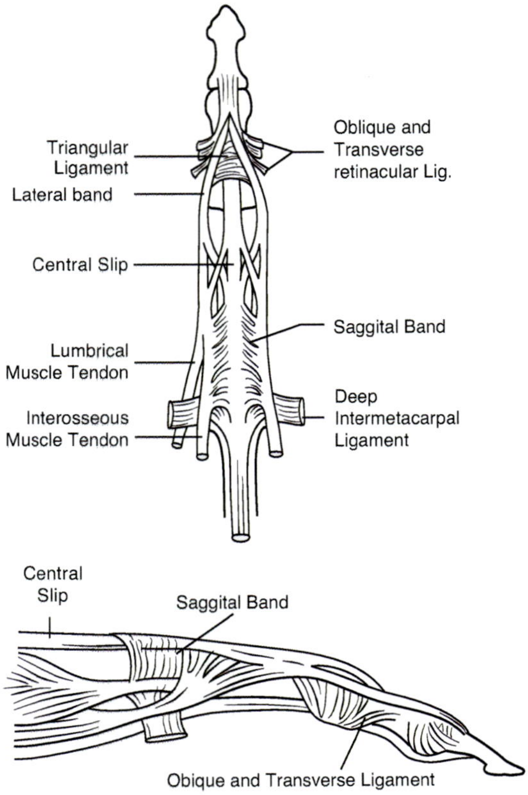

Fig. 4.8 Extensor tendons of the long fingers (needs to be labelled in English)

controls the lateral slips over the middle phalanx. Of particular importance are the Landsmeer ligaments (the transverse and oblique retinacular ligaments). Particularly the oblique band controls and coordinates flexion and extension between the two interphalangeal joints (Fig. 4.8).

Treatment of extensor tendon ruptures is carried out with various techniques and depends on localization, age of injury, and whether the injury is closed or open. The extensor apparatus is subdivided into extrinsic and intrinsic systems. The extrinsic extensor tendons extend from the forearm to the hand. The tendons of the lumbrical and interosseous muscles belong to the intrinsic extensor apparatus. Nine zones are distinguished in the hand and forearm, where zone 1 is at the level of the distal interphalangeal joint (DIP joint) or the interphalangeal (IP) joint of the thumb, and zone 8 is at the level of the distal half of the forearm.

Flexor Tendons of the Hand

The flexor tendons of the hand pass from the muscular origin of the forearm through the carpal tunnel into the deep palmar compartment, where they run towards the fingers. The four lumbrical muscles, which flex the fingers at the MCP joint and extend the middle and distal phalanges, also attach to the deep flexor tendons. The carpal tunnel and fiber separation provide a compact overview of the tendons on the bony skeleton. The tendons themselves are surrounded by the tendon sheaths, filled with synovial fluid, which also contribute to nutrition and optimize gliding function (Fig. 4.9). Special ring ligaments guide the tendons in the long finger regions. The ring ligaments over the proximal and middle phalanges are especially important and essential in cases of injury and reconstruction (A2 and A4). In addition, the deep flexor tendons pass through the superficial tendons at the level of the proximal phalanx (Chiasma tendinum). There are small slips on the side facing the bone, the Vinculae Tendineum, which also supply the tendons. The tendon of the flexor pollicis longus muscle runs to the thumb. In this case, the flexor pollicis brevis muscle, one of the thumb muscles that attaches to the sesamoid bones of the ulna and radius, is found instead of the superficial flexor tendon.

Because of the differences in the bearings of the flexor tendons, different zones have been established from the wrist to the fingertips (Fig. 4.10). This zone classification is essential to the choice of treatment and assessment of treatment outcomes. Zone II (Bunnell) is also called "no man's land," since prior to the development of dynamic flexor tendon treatment (Kleinert), no primary tendon repair was performed there. This zone extends from the insertion of the superficial flexor tendon to the proximal end of the A1 ring

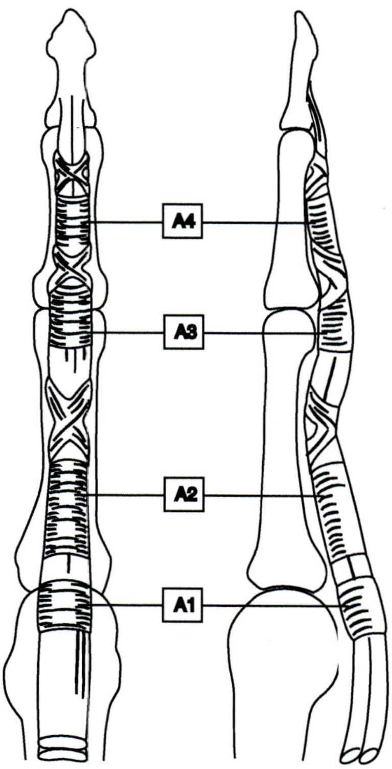

Fig. 4.9 Flexor tendons of the long fingers: ring ligaments A1 to A4

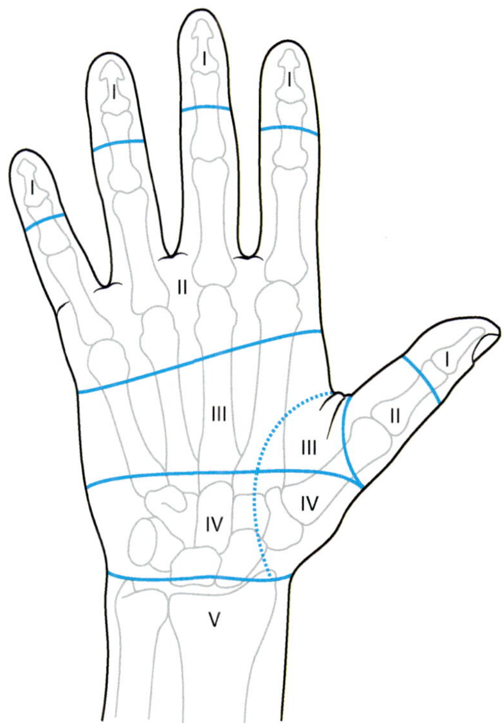

Fig. 4.10 Zones of the flexor tendon sheaths (IFSSH, International Federation of Surgeons for Surgery of the Hand)

ligament and thus, contains both flexor tendons in a tight, fibroosseous canal.

Diagnostic Assessment

In cases of muscle injury, the following characteristics should be observed:

- Sharp/stinging pain in cases of contracture
- Contraction limitations in cases of partial rupture, or total loss in complete rupture
- Palpation of the defect in cases of partial or complete rupture
- Tenderness and swelling
- Hematoma and discoloration after 24 h, possibly muscle spasms

Clinical examination with inspection and palpation as well as functional testing with and without resistance is essential. Ultrasound works well, particularly regarding delineation of an intramuscular hematoma.

Diagnostic assessment for tendon injuries is based essentially on analysis of the mechanism of injury, the clinical picture, and the examination with corresponding functional testing. In cases of complete tendon rupture, a sudden snap and pain is occasionally felt. Partial lesions often occur with sudden pain combined with certain events or movement patterns.

Conventional x-rays must be carried out for sport injuries in children or adolescents especially, to show growth plate and/or avulsion injuries. For certain tendon injuries, e.g. shoulder, wrist, quadriceps, patellar, or Achilles, ultrasound can be helpful. In certain clinical situations, magnetic resonance imaging is valuable. Certain problems such as osteochondritis, apophysiti, and chronic injuries of the growth region can be better analyzed; tendon injuries can be differentiated from tumor-related changes or infections.

Extensor Tendon Injuries of the Hand

Clinical diagnosis is difficult depending on the level of injury; in case of doubt, particularly in open wounds, exploration must be performed to exclude extensor tendon injury. For closed injuries, ultrasound can help. Initial assessment is difficult overall because of the lack of cooperation in small children, and must be repeated if necessary. Typical pitfalls should be noted using careful clinical examinations. For example, the cross-linking of the long finger tendons (Juncturae tendinum) can mask an extensor tendon rupture, because movement is still possible over the uninjured neighboring tendon.

Subcutaneous extensor tendon rupture in Zone I (mallet finger or baseball finger) occurs frequently after violent flexion of the distal joint, e.g. after moving a mattress, or after direct impact with a ball. In around a quarter of cases, a mallet fracture involves the epiphysis of the distal phalanx. It occurs with hyperextension of the PIP joint during flexion of the DIP joint.

With sudden violent flexion of the PIP joint (zone III) or in injuries of the PIP joint or volar dislocation of the PIP joint, rupture of the middle slip of the extensor tendon can occur. If initial findings are unclear due to swelling, the entire clinical picture might only become clear at a later time. Clinically, there is an extension deficit of the PIP joint with hyperextension of the DIP joint, also called a buttonhole deformity. This deformity arises from the loss of tension over the PIP joint by the extensor apparatus and the resulting volar slipping of the side slips below the PIP joint axis.

Extensor tendon injuries over the MCP joint and further proximal often occur in open injuries. In children, there are often problems associated with congenital anomalies first noticed at the time of injury. For example, injury of the long thumb extensor tendon can be confused with congenital trigger finger of the thumb, which prevents extension at the thumb IP joint through entrapment of the tendon.

Flexor Tendon Injuries of the Hand

Similar to extensor tendons, in the hand region, flexor tendons are subdivided into extrinsic and intrinsic. The extrinsic flexor tendons are comprised of the deep flexor tendons that pass through the superficial flexor tendons at the level of the proximal phalanx and insert onto the palmar base of the distal phalanx, as well as the superficial flexor tendons that insert onto the middle phalanx with the radial and ulnar slips. The lumbrical muscles as well as the dorsal and palmar interossei flex the MCP joints and form the intrinsic flexor system. Flexion of the distal phalanx of the thumb is performed by the flexor pollicis longus tendon, and that of the proximal phalanx by the flexor pollicis brevis.

Wound exploration should be performed in cases of transverse lateral, flexor side lacerations of the hand, since partial lesions cannot always be excluded clinically. With complete rupture of both flexor tendons, active flexion at the PIP and DIP joints is not possible, while isolated injury of the deep flexor tendon prevents active flexion at the DIP joint and injury to the superficial flexor tendon prevents flexion at the PIP joint.

Primary Treatment

For muscle injuries and bleeding, the following measures must be carried out in the acute phase

- Immobilization
- Bandaging of the affected muscle group without compression
- Cooling
- Elevation of the limb
- Unloading, e.g. crutches for the lower extremity; splinting of the upper extremity if needed
- Avoid additional injuries during the unstable phase (24–36 h).

The primary treatment for tendon injuries depends on the etiology. When it is a closed soft-tissue injury, the affected joint should be immobilized as much as possible. Position is selected so that the tendon is not further stressed. For example, flexor tendon injuries of the hand should be splinted in light flexion (approx. 20°) and moderate flexion of the finger, and Achilles injuries should be splinted with the foot in plantar flexion.

Sterile dressings should be applied to additional open injuries. If immediate treatment is not possible, antibiotics should be administered. If tendon injuries cannot be adequately treated and there is a significant time delay, e.g. prolonged transport to hospital/transfer hospital, treatment on the following day or in several days, the wounds should be surgically washed and initially closed. However, it should be noted that this will mean additional general anesthesia for children, since wound debridement can only be performed without excessive mental stress under local anesthesia when patients are older with greater understanding.

Therapy

After primary treatment of a muscle injury, depending on the clinical picture, the lesion should be initially considered serious and be observed for 2–3 days for circulation, swelling, and intramuscular pressure. Once this period is over, the clinical diagnosis should be differentiated between intramuscular and intermuscular hematoma. Milder ruptures/lesions can be treated with elastic bandages and heat or alternating heat/cold application if necessary. Compartment syndromes must be excluded in cases of painful swelling, exceptionally with pressure measurements of the compartments, and the assessment must be extended (ultrasound or MRI). With extensive bleeding, operative decompression might be necessary. During surgical intervention, the muscles should be adapted as far as possible with suture to minimize scarring. In cases of major findings, postoperative immobilization with a cast or brace is needed for 4–6 weeks.

Treatment of tendon injuries depends entirely on the anatomic localization. Various avulsion injuries, e.g. the hamstring muscles and the Achilles tendon, are generally treated conservatively. Rare lesions of the rotator cuff, the patellar and quadriceps tendons are treated surgically

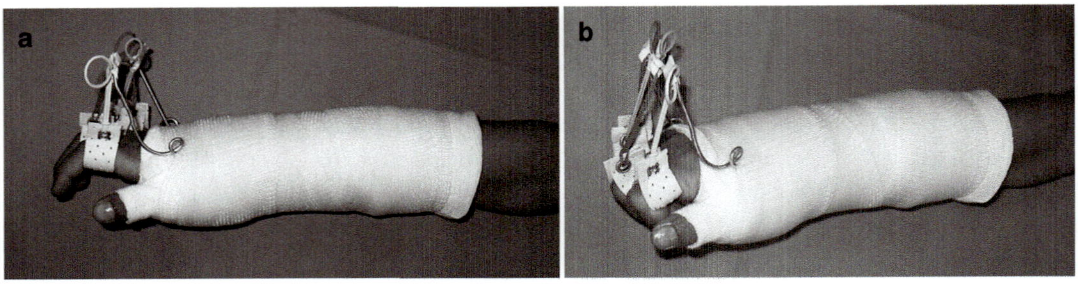

Fig. 4.11 (**a**, **b**) Dynamic extension splint for follow up care of reconstructed extensor tendons

according to the extent and degree of displacement.

In principle, after tendon injury, earliest possible mobilization should be sought, as this enables appropriate collagen alignment. This ensures good force transmission and recovery. Splints can limit the range of motion significantly enough that there is no overloading of the operative repair or disengagement of the tendon ends after conservative treatment.

Extensor Tendon Injuries of the Hand

Depending on the level (zone) of the injury, open injuries are generally treated with tendon reconstruction and adaptation of the extensor aponeurosis. In cases of closed subcutaneous extensor tendon ruptures (zone I), the distal joint is generally immobilized for 6–8 weeks with an aluminum finger splint, and then 2 weeks of hourly weaning, followed by 2 weeks of night splinting. In exceptional cases or in cases of mallet fractures, temporary Kirschner wire transfixation of the distal joint can be performed.

Injuries of zone III require immobilization of the PIP joint in extension for 6–8 weeks. Depending on age and understanding, this can be changed to a dynamic extension splint after 4 weeks.

Follow up care of extensor tendon injuries proximal to the proximal phalanx can proceed dynamically to rapid function optimization. To this end, the hand is immobilized postoperatively in extension with a plaster splint, and after several days, a forearm-based splint with a wrist extension of 30° is fitted. This splint is then combined with appropriate brackets to pull the finger(s) into extension with rubber loops (Fig. 4.11). Afterwards, there is progressive increase in finger flexion (e.g. 30° of MCP flexion in postoperative week 2, 60° in week 3, and then 90°). The splint generally remains in place for 5 weeks. Using this method, full hand function is often rapidly attained.

Acute Flexor Tendon Injuries of the Hand

Acute flexor tendon injuries are generally treated primarily. Once the tendon stumps are identified, they are fixed and smoothed with a canula. With many repair techniques, the principle is to create a core suture first, followed by continuous fine reconstruction of the tendon stumps (Fig. 4.12). If possible, the superficial flexor tendon should be treated as well, and uninjured ring ligaments should be protected as much as possible. In cases of heavily contaminated or bite wounds, an early secondary reconstruction can be performed up to 3 weeks after trauma.

Late tendon reconstruction generally requires a two-stage procedure. In the first step, a silicone rod is used as a placeholder to create a slide bearing. After 8–12 weeks, a tendon replacement graft reconstruction (usually with the palmaris longus or plantaris tendons) is performed when there is good passive motion. Tendon fixation is carried out with close observation of the epiphyses. The pull-out suture is placed on the fingernail along the bone of the fingertip (Fig. 4.13). The tendon graft is interlaced proximally to the corresponding muscle or tendon stump in the forearm, achieving very good primary fixation. In the case of the thumb

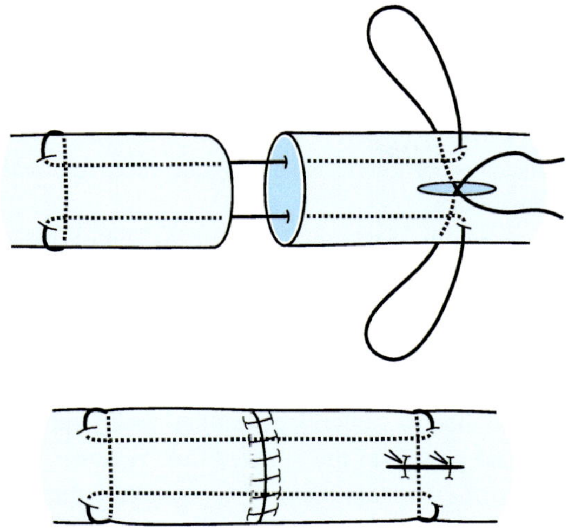

Fig. 4.12 Flexor tendon reconstruction: Core suture with fine adaptation

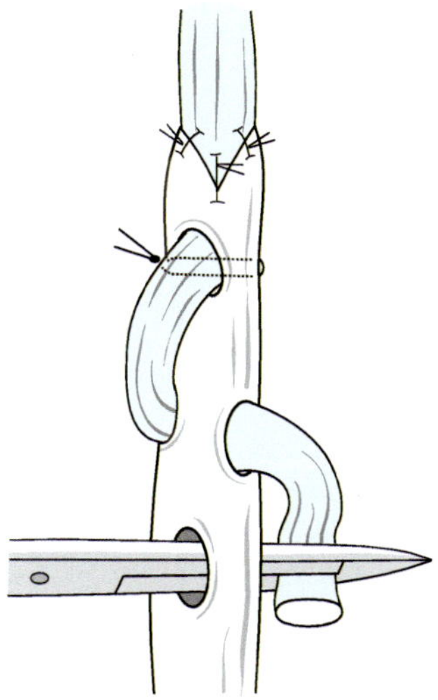

Fig. 4.14 Tendon interlace suture according to Pulvertaft

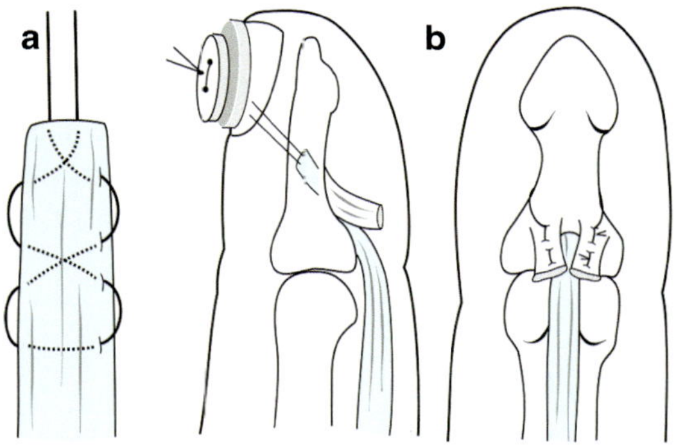

Fig. 4.13 (**a**, **b**) Flexor tendon reconstruction: (**a**) Paraosseous refixation of the deep flexor tendon, (**b**) stitching with the distal stump

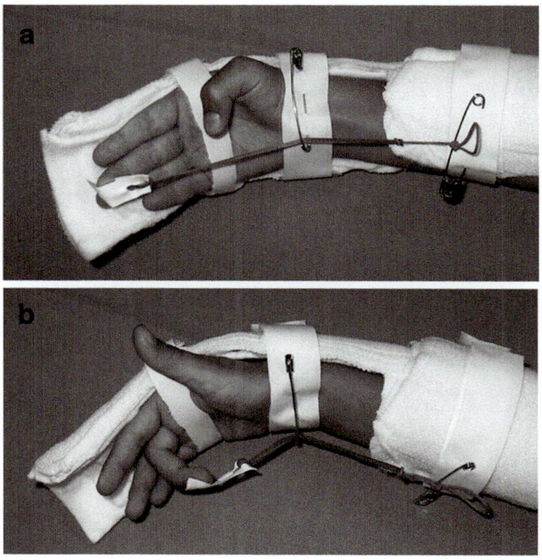

Fig. 4.15 Kleinert arrangement for the follow up of flexor tendon reconstruction. (**a**) extension block, (**b**) flexion with rubber gum

and the index finger flexor tendons, the original muscle tendon complex is used as much as possible; for the remaining long fingers, interweaving with the neighboring tendons can be carried out (Fig. 4.14).

After primary reconstruction of the flexor tendon in the fibro-osseous canal and at the level of the wrist, dynamic follow up treatment according to Kleinert is the method of choice, beginning on the first postoperative day (Fig. 4.15). Follow up treatment of these types of tendon injuries in children under 8 years can be problematic. Therapy must have the goal of protecting the tendon suture, since patient cooperation can't be assumed. A splint must be applied that prevents tension of the tendon suture and active access by the child, but also enables sufficient finger motion. These restrictions should be in

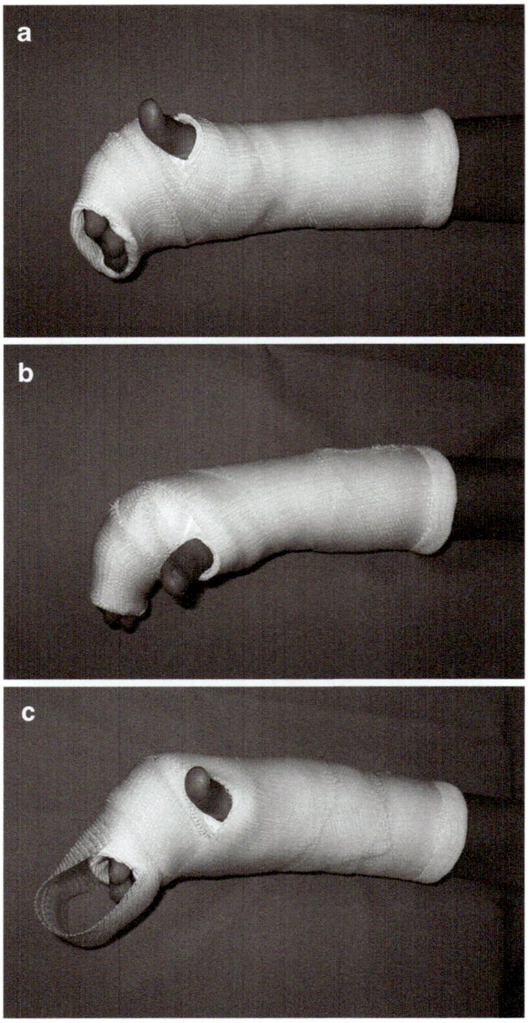

Fig. 4.16 (**a–c**) Plaster splint for children after flexor tendon reconstruction

place for a maximum of 4 weeks (Fig. 4.16). Children under 5 years must be immobilized over the elbow joint, since otherwise the splint or cast slips off.

Complications, Growth Disturbances

In principle, muscle and tendon injuries to be treated conservatively must be adequately unloaded. Sport activities in particular should be resumed only when the tendon has regained full strength and motion. Premature loading and re-injury can lead to more serious consequences, e.g. to myositis ossificans. However, depending on the extent, the formation of normal scar tissue can also leave areas of varying elasticity and thus, cause problems, so that in rare cases removal is necessary.

Although acute tendon injuries, apart from open hand injuries, are relatively rare, repetitive submaximal loading can lead to an overloading syndrome. Particularly in tendon injuries requiring operative reconstruction (e.g. flexor tendons of the hand), functional failure will lead to reduced growth of the affected limb region.

Insufficient treatment of an extensor tendon rupture in zone I can lead to a Swan Neck deformity with fixed hyperextension of the PIP joint and flexion of the DIP joint. In zone III, middle slip insufficiency leads to side slip sliding at the level of the PIP joint and to a fixed flexion deformity. The DIP joint is hyperextended. This is called a buttonhole deformity. Such fixed deformities are difficult to correct and generally must be treated with dynamic splints (Quengel splints) to achieve mostly free joint motion prior to surgery.

Follow Up

Complex tendon reconstructions need weekly follow up after initial parental instructions corresponding to patient age until the 6th or 12th postoperative week. Afterwards, monthly checkups should be performed until 6 months post-injury or until full function has been reached. In cases where growth disturbances might arise, annual clinical follow up should be performed.

Recommended Literature

Alves K, Spencer H, Barnewolt CE, Waters PM, Bae DS (2018) Early outcomes of vein grafting for reconstruction of brachial arterial injuries in children. YJHSU 43(3):287

Bertelli J, Soldado F, Ghizoni MF (2018) Outcomes of radial nerve grafting in children after distal humerus fracture. YJHSU 43(12):1140–1141

Birch R, Achan P (2000) Peripheral nerve repairs and their results in children. Hand Clin 16(4):579–595
Burnett MG, Zager EL (2004) Pathophysiology of peripheral nerve injury: a brief review. Neurosurg Focus 16(5):1–7
Costales JR, Socolovsky M, Lázaro JAS, García RÁ (2019a) Peripheral nerve injuries in the pediatric population: a review of the literature. Part I: traumatic nerve injuries. Child's Nerv Syst 35(1):29–35
Costales JR, Socolovsky M, Lázaro JAS, Costales DR (2019b) Peripheral nerve injuries in the pediatric population: a review of the literature. Part II: entrapment neuropathies. Child's Nerv Syst 35(1):37–45
Favetto JM, Rosenthal AI, Shatford RA, Kleinert HE (1999) Tendon injuries in children. In: Gupta A, Kay SPJ, Scheker LR (eds) The growing hand. Diagnosis and management of the upper extremity in children. Mosby, London, pp 609–627
Feliciano DV (2017) Pitfalls in the management of peripheral vascular injuries. Trauma Surg Acute Care Open 2(1):e000110
Fitoussi F, Lebellec Y, Frajman JM, Pennecot GF (1999) Flexor tendon injuries in children: factors influencing prognosis. J Pediatr Orthop 19(6):818–821
Friedrich H, Baumel D (2003) Die Behandlung von Beugesehnenverletzungen im Kindesalter. Handchir Mikrochir Plast Chir 35(6):347–352
Kleinert HE, Verdan C (1983) Report of the committee on tendon injuries. J Hand Surg 8A(5):794–798
Kleinert HE, Kutz JE, Atasoy E, Stormo A (1973) Primary repair of flexor tendons. Orthop Clin North Am 4(4):865–876
Kirchmayr L (1917) Zur Technik der Sehnennaht. Zentralbl Chir 40(44):906–907
Mackinnon SE, Dellon AL (1988) Surgery of the peripheral nerve. Thieme, New York
Matuszewski Ł (2014) Evaluation and management of pulseless pink/pale hand syndrome coexisting with supracondylar fractures of the humerus in children. Eur J Orthop Surg Traumatol 24(8):1401–1406
Millesi H (1985) Peripheral nerve repair: terminology, questions, and facts. J Reconstr Microsurg 2(1): 21–31
Missios S, Bekelis K, Spinner RJ (2014) Traumatic peripheral nerve injuries in children: epidemiology and socioeconomics. J Neurosurg Pediatr 14(6):688–694
Micheli LJ, Fehlandt AF (1992) Overuse injuries to tendons and apophyses in children and adolescents. Clin Sports Med 11(4):713–726
Prieto JM, Van Gent JM, Calvo RY, Checchi KD, Wessels LE, Sise CB et al (2020) Evaluating surgical outcomes in pediatric extremity vascular trauma. J Pediatr Surg 55(2):319–323
Sabharwal S, Tredwell SJ, Beauchamp RD, Mackenzie WG, Jakubec DM, Cairns R, Le Blanc JG (1997) Management of pulseless pink hand in pediatric supracondylar fractures of humerus. J Pediatr Orthop 17(3):303–310
Sebastin SJ, Chung KC (2011) A systematic review of the outcomes of replantation of distal digital amputation. Plast Reconstr Surg 128(3):723–773
Seigel DB, Gelberman RH (1991) Peripheral nerve injuries associated with fractures and dislocations. In: Gelberman RH (ed) Operative nerve repair and reconstruction. Lippincott, Philadelphia, pp 619–633
Shaw BA, Kasser JR, Emans JB, Rand FF (1990) Management of vascular injuries in displaced supracondylar humerus fractures without arteriography. J Orthop Trauma 4(1):25–29
Smith C, Green RM (1981) Pediatric vascular injuries. Surgery 90(1):20–31
Soh RCC, Tawng DK, Mahadev A (2013) Pulse oximetry for the diagnosis and prediction for surgical exploration in the pulseless perfused hand as a result of supracondylar fractures of the distal humerus. Clin Orthop Surg 5(1):74–81
Weller A, Garg S, Larson AN, Fletcher ND, Schiller JR, Kwon M et al (2013) Management of the pediatric pulseless supracondylar humeral fracture: is vascular exploration necessary? J Bone Joint Surg Am 95(21):1906–1912

Part II

Specific Injuries

5 Shoulder

5.1 Shoulder Girdle

Physiological Findings

The ossification centers of the shoulder girdle (Fig. 5.1) develop at various times during growth. When interpreting radiographic images, the possible presence of accessory bone in the shoulder joint area must be considered (Fig. 5.2a–c). In the shoulder girdle, growth plates close between the ages of 15 and 18 years; in the medial clavicle only, this can occur upto 25 years.

Most shoulder girdle injuries are straightforward and can be treated conservatively. However, grossly displaced injuries and fractures in adolescents also require open reduction and stabilization. Clavicle fractures occur frequently, while acromioclavicular joint injuries, sternoclavicular fractures or ligament injuries as well as scapular fractures are far less common. Traumatic shoulder dislocations increasingly occur in active, athletic adolescents and require thorough diagnostics including MRI and therapy.

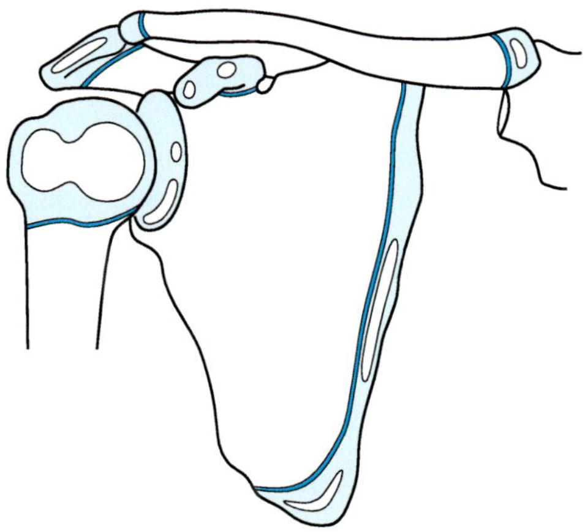

Fig. 5.1 Ossification centers of the scapula and humerus

Clavicle Fractures

Incidence, Mechanism of Injury and Clinical Picture

Clavicle fracture is the most common traumatic birth injury (1.7%) and is the fourth most common fracture in childhood, accounting for 5–15% of all fractures. However, clavicle fractures are also increasingly common among adolescents with the increase in high-intensity sports.

Traumatic birth fractures are often diagnosed only by early callus formation and the resulting swelling at the level of the fracture. Otherwise, a fall on the shoulder is the most common mechanism of injury along with a high proportion of athletic injuries. In babies and small children, fractures are generally non-displaced due to the thick periosteal sleeve, while displaced and comminuted fractures can also occur in adolescents. Shortening is relevant for adolescents, since it can begin affecting shoulder function if this exceeds 1.5 cm. Almost half of fractures occur in the first decade of life and are significantly more

I. Marzi et al., *Pediatric Skeletal Trauma*, https://doi.org/10.1007/978-3-030-93685-3_5

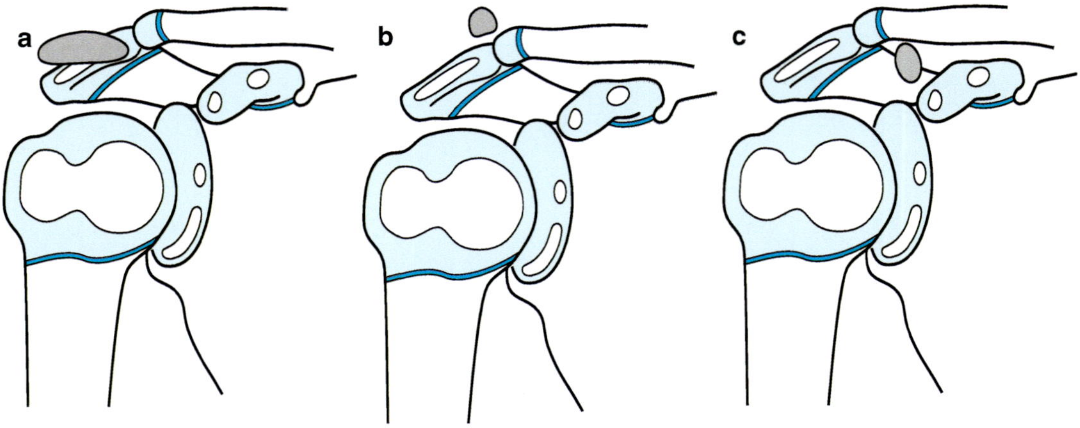

Fig. 5.2 Accessory ossification centers. (**a**) Acromion, (**b**) Capsular bones of the AC joint, (**c**) Large sesamoid bone in the coracoacromial ligament

common in boys. Clinical signs of fracture are obvious and clinical diagnosis is often possible. Soft-tissue involvement with skin tenting, pain and shortening should be evaluated and included in the decision making.

Classification

The Allman Classification is most commonly used for clavicle fractures.

Type I fractures are those of the middle third, Type II are those lateral to the coracoclavicular ligaments, and Type III are fractures of the medial third. The subtypes are:

- non-displaced (a),
- displaced (b) and
- comminuted (c) fractures.

The most common fractures of the middle third should be evaluated for soft-tissue injuries and shortening, as well as for extremely rare compression of the nerve plexus or the subclavian artery. In cases of 1.5 cm of shortening, the possible sequelae regarding shoulder function should be considered as an indication for surgery. In addition, pronounced pain, often from spearing of the soft-tissues, as well as athletic demands and more rapid recovery after surgery for either school or sports should be discussed with children and parents when considering treatment options.

Conservative treatment is equally effective with Desault or figure-of-eight slings. An advantage of the figure-of-eight bandage is freedom of both arms, but it should not be over-tightened as this can compress the axillary neurovascular structures. Lack of clavicular stabilization with a figure-of-eight bandage has been argued as a reason to use the Desault sling, but this doesn't achieve it either and the child has only one arm free.

In children, operative treatment with elastic intramedullary nail from medial or lateral is recommended over plate fixation. Both procedures are legitimate and can be adapted to the size of the child. The ESIN procedure, however, often also requires open reduction after closed attempts are unsuccessful. In addition, there is a scar from the medial approach in the visible area. On the other hand, the lateral approach is complicated by proximity to the AC joint and open reduction is relatively often required. If a plate osteosynthesis is required, a 4-hole plate is sufficient for fixation in small children, while in adolescents a six-hole or longer plate should be used, according to the fracture.

At the medial end, three types of injury occur. The most common is a fracture through the growth plate. True shaft fractures of the medial third, i.e. fractures between the medial attachment of the sternocleidomastoid muscle and the medial epiphysis, which is responsible for 80% of growth, are much less common. Sternoclavicular dislocations continue to be reported, but in children, MRI often reveals that these are misdiagnosed joint injuries. Fractures of the medial epiphysis are classified with the Salter and Harris system. These are usually Salter-Harris I and II type fractures. The epiphyseal fragment—with or without a small metaphyseal wedge--remains in the (not directly injured) sternoclavicular joint, while the medial shaft end can be markedly displaced. Further classification of this injury indicates the direction of shaft displacement. Anterior displacement is most common. Posterior displacement, with potential injury to mediastinal structures, is more critical and requires definitive diagnosis with MRI and CT 3D reconstruction. Here, operative reduction is recommended, if necessary, with vascular surgery backup, and in most cases a fixation with stable suture or cerclage can be achieved. Fixation with wires must be avoided as these can migrate into the mediastinum.

The adult Rockwood Classification is used to evaluate the less common AC joint injuries on the lateral third of the clavicle. Fractures of the lateral third are classified according to the Dameron and Rockwood system (Fig. 5.3). Injuries in this region are generally lateral clavicle fractures and not true AC joint ruptures. The forces of trauma and the attaching muscles cause the medial fragment to displace, sometimes markedly superiorly but also horizontally towards posterior, after piercing and rupturing the thick periosteal sleeve. The periosteal sleeve remains in contact with the peripheral fragment, and the coracoclavicular ligaments stay intact on the inferior aspect of the periosteal tube!

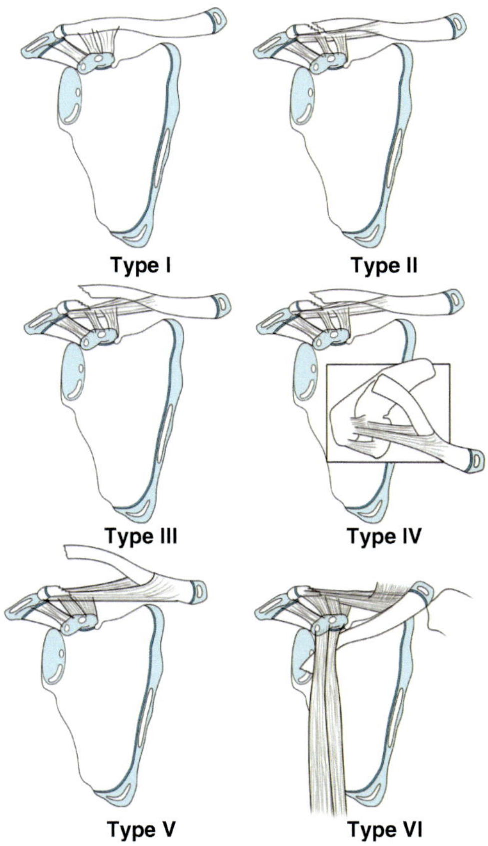

Fig. 5.3 Dameron and Rockwood classification of lateral clavicle fractures

According to Dameron and Rockwood, the following types are described:

- Type I: Strain of the acromioclavicular ligament or fissure of the lateral clavicle without periosteal tube disruption. No radiological evidence of displacement.
- Type II: Partial perforation and tear of the periosteal tube, mild instability with widening of the AC joint/fracture line without significant widening of the acromioclavicular space on radiographs.
- Type III: Extended tear of the periosteal tube with marked instability and elevation of the medial fragment. Coracoclavicular distance is increased by 25–100%.
- Type IV: Corresponds to Type III, but with posterior displacement of the medial fragment. The fragment can also create a buttonhole perforation of the trapezius muscle, preventing closed reduction. This injury can be underestimated on AP radiographs. The posteriorly-displaced fragment is only recognizable on axial projection.
- Type V: Complete disruption of the periosteal tube, proximal subcutaneous displacement of the medial fragment. The coracoclavicular distance is widened by more than 100%.
- Type VI: Medial fragment displaced distally with entrapment beneath the coracoid process.

Lateral clavicle injuries are thus created by displacement of the medial fragment. Differentiation between joint injuries and shaft fractures is not clinically relevant as both has to be treated similarly.

The therapeutic options of the different localizations are indicated in Tables 5.1, 5.2, and 5.3.

Technical aspects of the treatment of clavicular fractures are shown in Table 5.4.

Table 5.1 Fractures of the middle third—Allman classification Type I (Fig. 5.4)

Special features	Most common type of clavicle fracture
Diagnostic assessment	Radiology AP is generally sufficient, ultrasound can be used over the course in individual cases
Goals of treatment/limits of correction	In adolescents only, shortening should be avoided as much as possible (<1.5 cm) There is good potential for correction through remodeling
Primary treatment	Immobilization with Desault splint Figure-of-eight bandage offers pain relief by putting traction on the painful bony ends and must be regularly tightened. Customized bandages are practical.
Conservative treatment	
Indication	The usual conservative approach is a figure-of-eight or Gilchrist sling or a Desault bandage for 3–4 weeks (Fig. 5.5).
Follow up	Functional follow up once pain-free
X-ray controls	Consolidation control after about 4 weeks, in small children clinical findings also using ultrasound if applicable.
Return to sports	Approximately 4 weeks after consolidation
Operative therapy	
Indication	Open fracture, neurovascular injury, risk of tissue spearing In cases of shortening more than 1.5 cm, with pronounced pain, with soft tissue puncture or skewering, after extensive consultation for adolescents to expedite return to school or sports activities.
Procedure	Case-by-case selection of ESIN (Fig. 5.6) or plate fixation (Fig. 5.7)
Follow up	Functional follow up once pain-free
X-ray controls	Consolidation control about 4 weeks post-operatively.
Hardware removal	Plate or ESIN after 3–6 months
Return to sports	Approximately 4 weeks after consolidation
Complications	Occasional irritation of the plexus from ball callus, which sometimes needs to be reduced in order to decompress the plexus Re-fracture of Clavicula possible (Fig. 5.8)
Growth disturbances	Not generally expected
Follow up controls	Not required

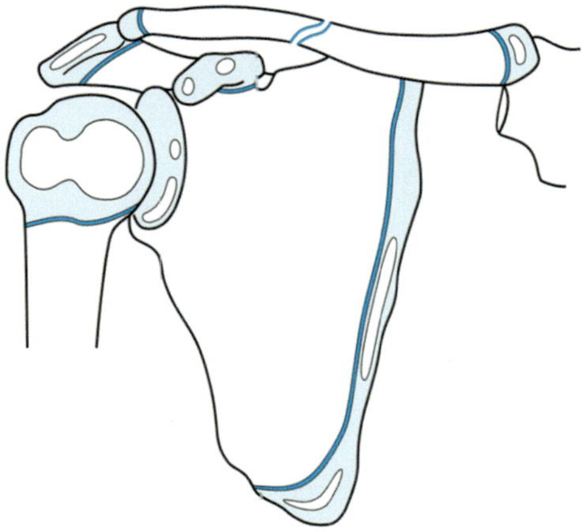

Fig. 5.4 Medial fracture of the clavicula type Allmann I

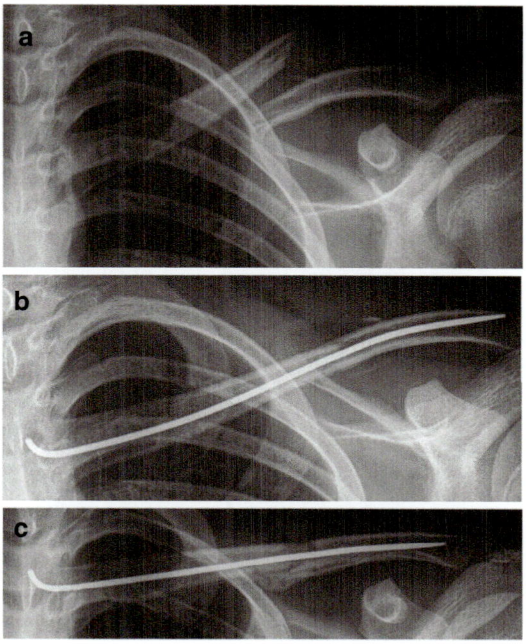

Fig. 5.6 Fracture of the clavicula shaft of a 14 year old boy. Stabilization with ESIN from medial due to strong dislocation and shortening. (**a**) Trauma image, (**b**) Postoperative x-ray with ESIN, (**c**) Healing after 10 weeks, before metal removal

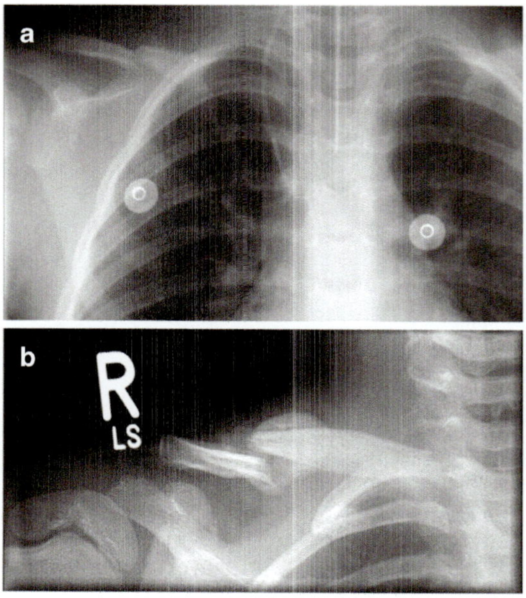

Fig. 5.5 Clavicle shaft fracture, Allman type I. (**a**) Trauma image. (**b**) Conservative treatment with callus cloud

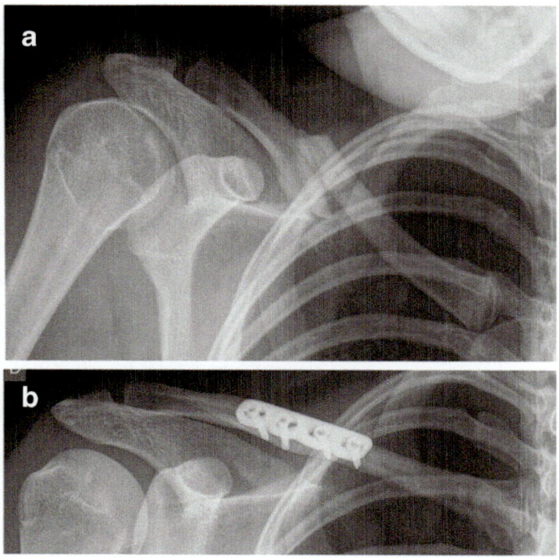

Fig. 5.7 Fracture of the clavicula in the middle third. Plate Osteosynthesis due to closed meduallary canal. (**a**) Trauma image, (**b**) Plate osteosynthesis, 18 weeks post operative prior to metal removal

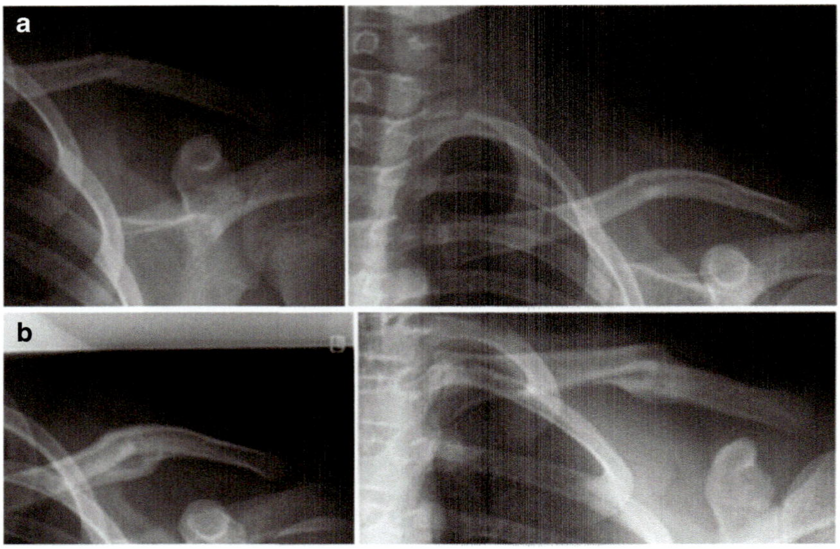

Fig. 5.8 Fracture of the clavicula in the middle third of a 11 year old boy. (**a**) Conservative treatment, (**b**) Pre-fracture after new fall

Table 5.2 Lateral third fractures—Allman classification Type II (Fig. 5.9)

Special features	Periosteal sleeve remains intact as do the coracoclavicular ligaments Consolidation through periosteal bone formation
Diagnostic assessment	Radiology AP and axial shoulder views to check for direction and magnitude of displacement
Goals of therapy/ limits of correction	Dameron and Rockwood Types IV, V and VI require reduction Good potential for correction through remodeling Formation of a new clavicle within the periosteal sleeve is possible
Primary treatment	Immobilization with Gilchrist sling Figure-of-eight bandage is an alternative
Conservative treatment	
Indication	All Dameron and Rockwood Type I, II and III injuries
Procedure	Gilchrist sling for 2 weeks, 3–4 weeks in adolescents (Fig. 5.10)
Follow up	Functional follow up once pain-free
X-ray controls	Consolidation control at approximately 4 weeks
Return to sports	Approximately 4 weeks after consolidation
Operative therapy	
Indication	Dameron and Rockwood Type IV, V and VI injuries Open fracture, neurovascular injury, risk of tissue skewering occurs occasionally in adolescents with severe shortening
Procedure	In cases of children in whom the periosteal sleeve is still robust, periosteal sleeve suture In adolescents, tension banding fixation (Fig. 5.11), with drilled wires and cord if needed (Fig. 5.12a–c) alternative is fixation with resorbable suture to the coracoid
Follow up	Functional follow up once pain-free
X-ray controls	Consolidation control at approximately 4 weeks
Hardware removal	In cases of tension banding through the AC joint, at 5–6 weeks
Return to sports	Approximately 4 weeks after consolidation or hardware removal
Complications	Seroma formation after tension banding, infection
Growth disturbances	Not generally expected
Follow up	Not required

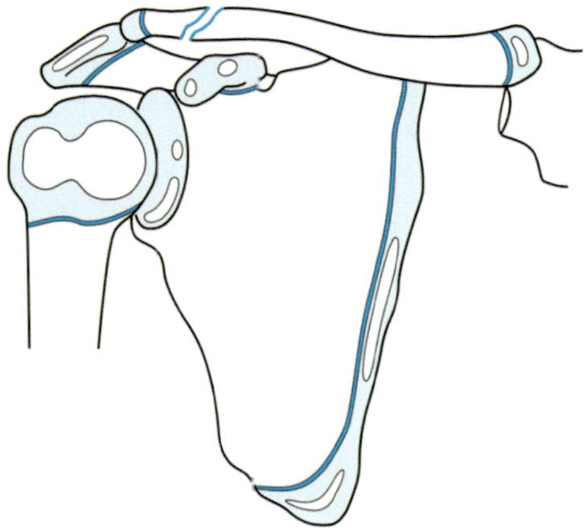

Fig. 5.9 Lateral fracture of the clavicula type Allmann II

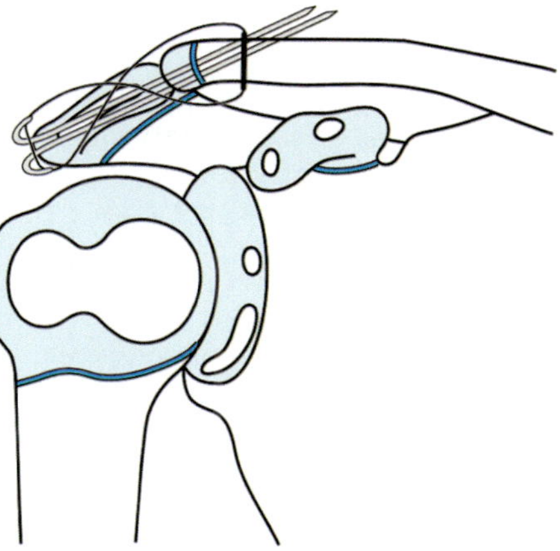

Fig. 5.11 Scheme tension band wiring of lateral. Clavicula fractures using 2 K-wires and a resorbable band

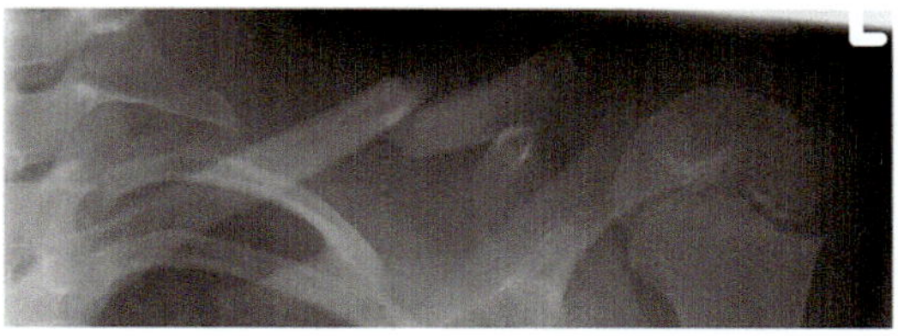

Fig. 5.10 Lateral clavicula fracture, 5 years girl; indication for conservative treatment

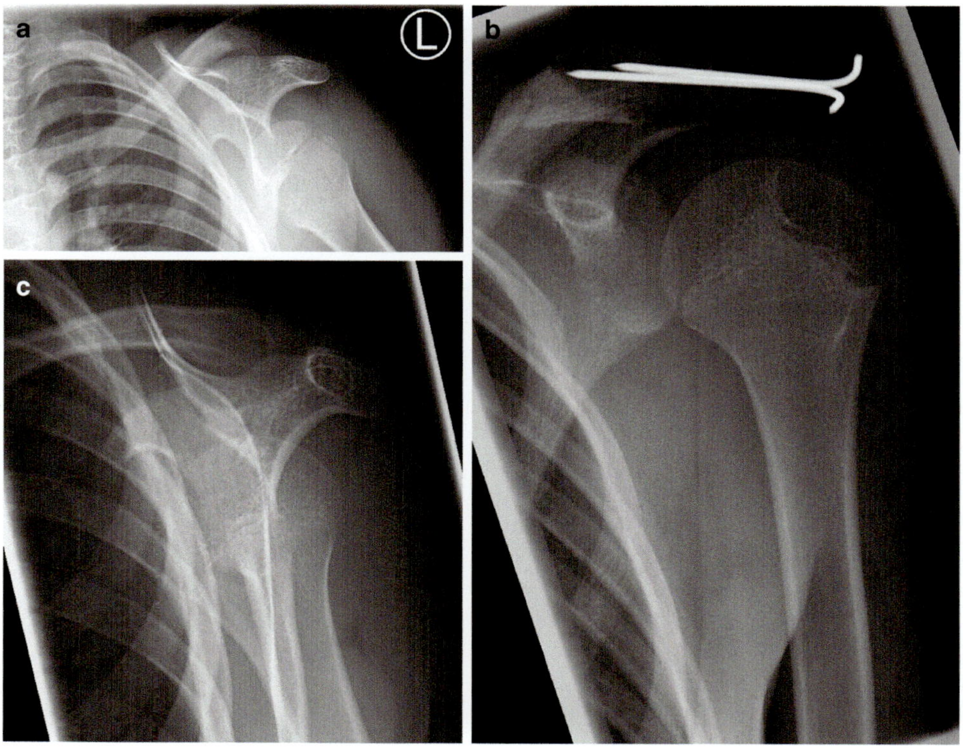

Fig. 5.12 Lateral fracture of the clavicula, 8 years boy (**a**) Dislocated lateral fracture, (**b**) Tension band wiring with 2 K-wires and resorbable band. (**c**) Consolidation and implant removal

Table 5.3 Fractures of the Medial Third—Allman classification Type III (Fig. 5.13)

Special features	Very rare Most fractures are through the growth plate as an epiphysiolysis (salter-Harris II). Displacement of the shaft fragment towards the mediastinum, can compress mediastinal structures.
Diagnostic assessment	Radiology AP x-ray, CT with reconstructions (!), also MRI with reconstructions is possible, showing the joint injury
Goals of therapy/ limits of correction	Pain relief Reduction of the displacement and shortening and decompression of the mediastinal structures Good potential for correction through remodeling
Primary treatment	Reduction is rarely required Only in cases of displacement toward the mediastinum with compression of the mediastinal structures may closed or open reduction be required Immobilization with Gilchrist sling
Conservative treatment	
Indication	Almost always (see primary treatment)
Procedure	Gilchrist sling for 2–4 weeks
Follow up	Functional follow up once pain-free
X-ray controls	Consolidation control at approximately 4 weeks
Return to sports	Approximately 4 weeks after consolidation
Operative therapy	
Indication	Reduction of mediastinal displacement is most important, but also anterior dislocations causing symptoms. Tendency to re-displace; observe during follow up!
Procedure	Fixation with resorbable suture after reduction K-wire fixation alone can't be performed because of the tendency for wire migration! Fixation with PDS suture along the sternum plus capsule suture. Optional plate Osteosynthesis (Fig. 5.14)
Follow up	Gilchrist sling for 4 weeks
X-ray controls	Consolidation control at approximately 4 weeks
Hardware removal	No metal implants
Return to sports	After confirmed consolidation
Complications	Wire migration with K-wire fixation alone, thus not to be performed! Rupture of the tension banding (resorbable material, also theoretically possible for the suture knot to loosen)
Growth disturbances	Not generally expected
Follow up	For a few years to exclude retrosternal growth

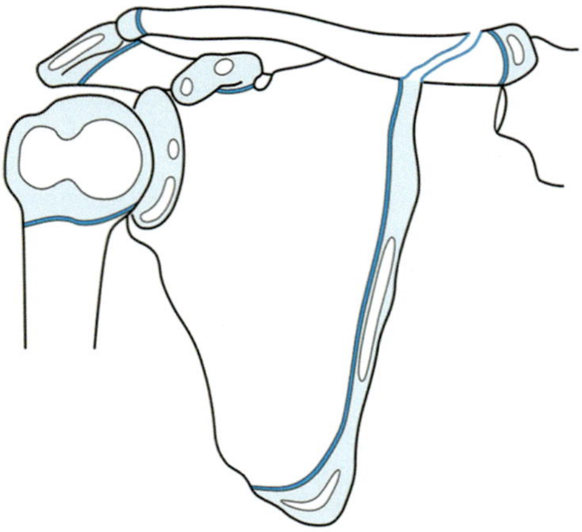

Fig. 5.13 Medial fracture of the clavicula type Allmann III

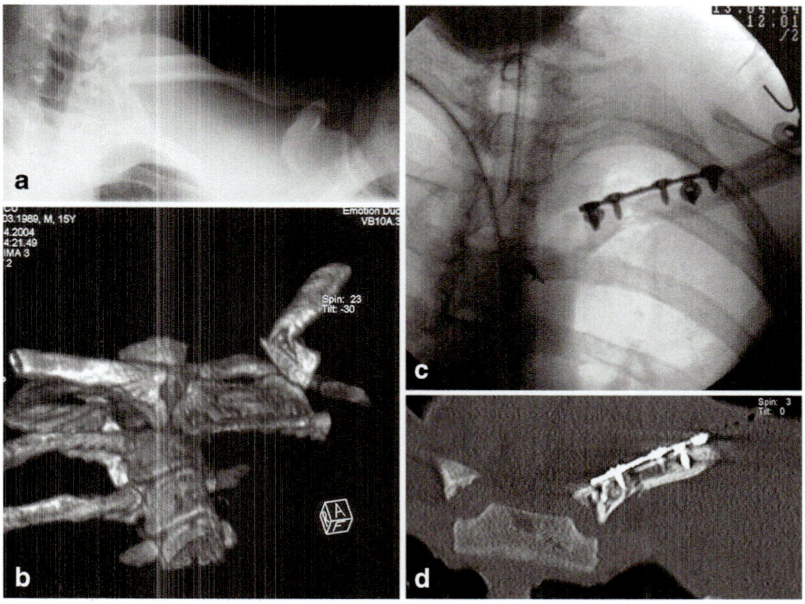

Fig. 5.14 Medial clavicula shaft fracture Typ III acc. to Allmann with dislocation in the sternoclavicular joint. 14 Year old girl. (**a**) Trauma image, (**b**) CT control with 3 D reconstruction, (**c**, **d**) Reconstruction with plate and bone anchor

Table 5.4 Technical aspects of the treatment of clavicular fractures

Material	Vicryl (3.0) for periosteal suture K-wires (1.4 or 1.6 mm), cerclage wire (1.25 for tension banding) Small fragment reconstruction plate (3.5 mm) for plate fixation Titanium elastic nail (2.0) for ESIN
Positioning	Supine positioning, freely movable arm, shoulder table or fluoroscopic capability Beach chair positioning is less favorable for small children
Approach	Incision along the clavicular axis at fracture level, alternatively a saber-cut incision
Special explanation	Conservative alternatives must be discussed, and this should be documented. Seroma formation, risk of infection, scar formation Less risk of neurovascular injuries
Surgical principle	Periosteal suture Closure of the thick periosteal sleeve after reduction of the clavicle. Tension banding: Classic tension banding, also resorbable suture around the coracoid with possible plate fixation with comminuted fractures—biological osteosynthesis, no denuding of the free fragments; ESIN as alternative: Threading of the fracture from lateral or medial, if necessary with percutaneous or open reduction (Figs. 5.15 and 5.16).
Hardware removal	ESIN, plate or tension banding fixation

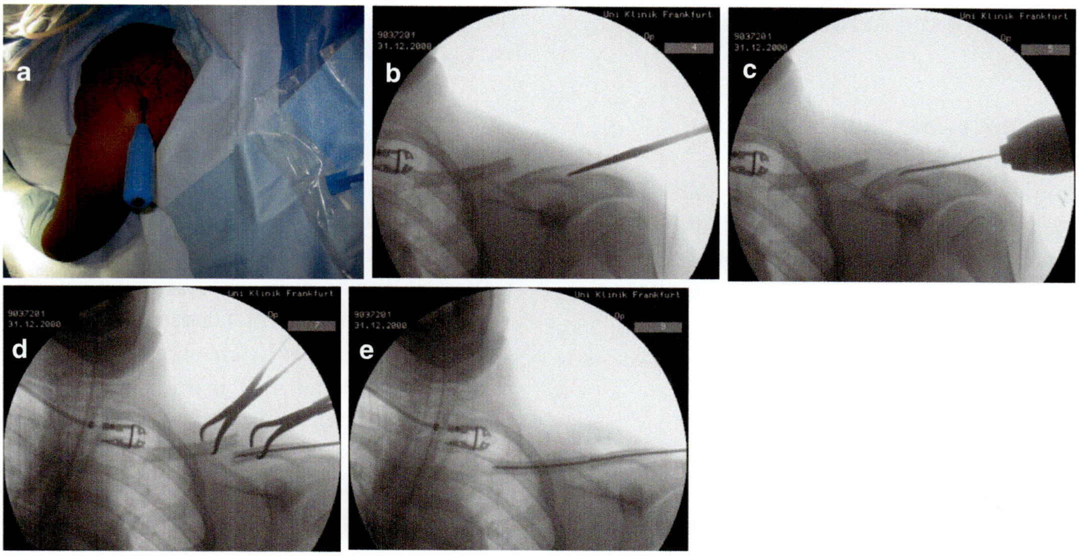

Fig. 5.15 Clavicula fracture treatment with ESIN from latero-dorsal in a 13 years old boy. (**a**) Entry point clinically. (**b**) Opening of medullary canal, (**c**) Introduction of elastic wire, (**d**) Indirect percutaneous reduction with forceps. (**e**) Final reduction and stabilization

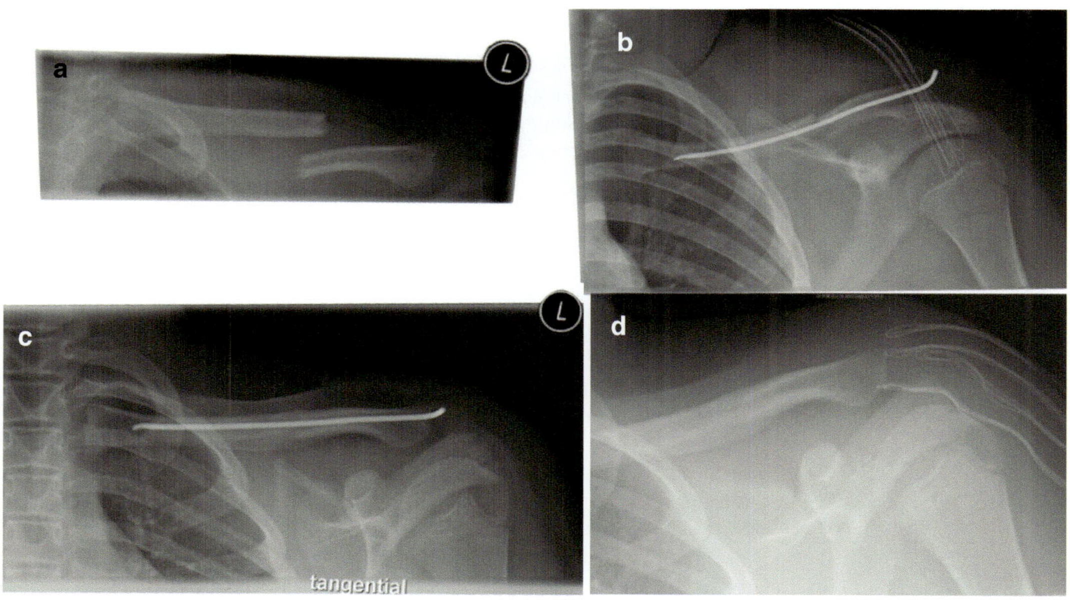

Fig. 5.16 Clavicula fracture, 14 years boy; (**a**) Fracture, (**b**) Post-operative ESIN form dorsolateral, (**c**) Healing, (**d**) After ESIN removal

Injuries of the Acromioclavicular Joint

Incidence, Mechanism of Injury and Clinical Picture

Injuries of the acromioclavicular joint are rarely seen during growth. Possible causes is direct shoulder trauma, for example in adolescent wrestlers. The mechanism of injury is more likely to cause a metaphyseal fracture. The clinical picture correlates with the injury in adults (piano-key sign).

Classification

The Rockwood Classification differentiates six types. Type 3–6 injuries require specific treatment (see also lateral clavicle fractures), while type 1,2,and 3 corresponds to the well known Tossy classification.

Treatment

Rockwood or Tossy Type 1–2 injuries are generally treated conservatively in children. For Tossy Type 3 or Rockwood Type 3 and on (till 6), operative treatment must at least be considered. Healing of considerable shoulder step injuries with tearing of the acromioclavicular in addition to the coracoclavicular ligaments, without repercussions, is also the goal in treating children. Horizontal instability in particular should be repaired and stabilized to avoid sequelae (Table 5.5).

Technical Aspects of acromio-clavicular joint disruptions are shown in Table 5.6.

Table 5.5 Acromioclavicular joint injuries (AC joint injuries) (Fig. 5.17)

Special features	During growth, it's important to differentiate this from epiphyseal rupture of the lateral clavicle
Diagnostic assessment	Loading images for analysis of shoulder joint instability are better avoided. Ultrasound or MRI imaging is most accurate for choice of therapy as well as for clinical diagnosis, but mostly standard x-ray is sufficient (Fig. 5.18)
Goals of therapy/limits of correction	The goal of treatment is maintenance of shoulder joint stability and prevention of factors that might lead to long-term deformity, pain and/or arthritis
Primary treatment	Figure-of-eight bandage or Gilchrist sling
Conservative treatment	
Indication	Most of the cases
Procedure	Immobilization bandage for approximately 3–4 weeks
Follow up	Early functional treatment, no sports for 8 weeks
X-ray controls	Generally not necessary
Return to sports	At 8 weeks
Operative therapy	
Indication	In exceptional cases with complete joint disruption (Types 3–6)
Procedure	Tension banding with drilled wires and resorbable suture material (PDS) as needed. Alternatively arthroscopic tight-rope procedure (clavicle to coracoid) or hooked plate in mature adolescents.
Follow up	Early functional follow up avoiding overhead movements for 6 weeks
X-ray controls	Prior to removal of the transfixing drilled wires
Hardware removal	At 6 weeks
Return to sports	At 8–12 weeks
Complications	Persistent instability
Growth disturbance	Unknown

Table 5.6 Technical aspects of acromio-clavicular joint disruptions

Material	Resorbable suture (PDS) Drilled wires 1.8 mm
Positioning	Beach chair positioning
Approach	Lateral incision over the AC joint
Special explanation	Secondary hemorrhage, nerve injury, infection
Surgical principle	Protection of re-inserted ligament tears and temporary holding with tension banding (see Fig. 5.12a–c)
Hardware removal	In intervals after 6 weeks, outpatient

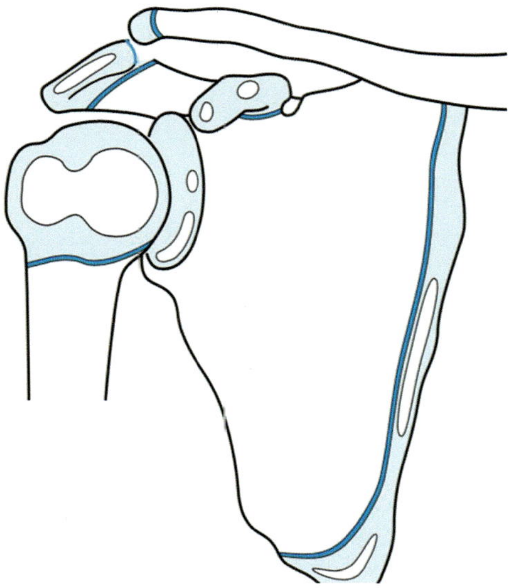

Fig. 5.17 Acromioclavicular joint injuries

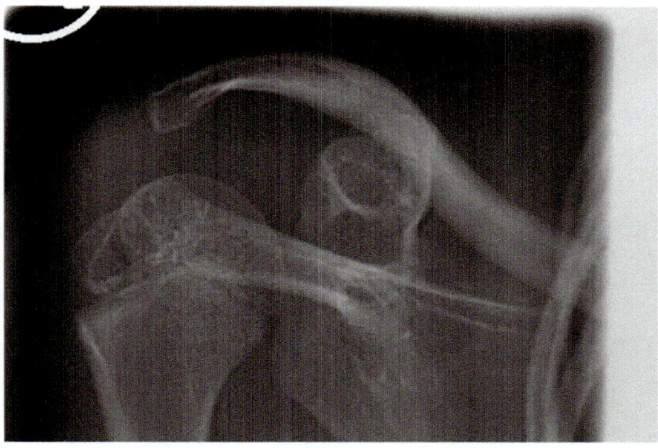

Fig. 5.18 Acromio-clavicular joint disruption, type Tossy 3, 13 years old boy

Injuries of the Sternoclavicular Joint

Incidence, Mechanism of Injury and Clinical Picture

Typical SC joint disruption as occurs in adults is extremely rare in children (Fig. 5.19a); differential diagnosis is to rule out more common traumatic epiphysiolysis (Fig. 5.19b).

Cause of injury to the sternoclavicular joint can be a fall onto the outstretched arm. Sports like wrestling and gymnastics are likely to lead to these types of trauma. The clinical picture shows impressive swelling and pain. Differential diagnosis should include rheumatic changes (Sjögren's syndrome).

Classification

Injuries are differentiated according to the direction of displacement (anterior, posterior). The clinical features and the diagnostic and therapeutic algorithms are shown in Table 5.7. Technical aspects are mentioned in Table 5.8.

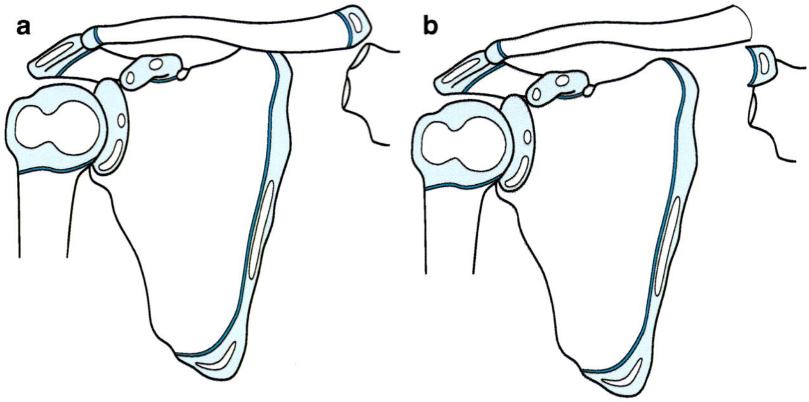

Fig. 5.19 Sternoclavicular joint disloaction (**a**) Complete joint luxation. (**b**) Epiphyseolysis

Table 5.7 Sternoclavicular joint injuries (SC joint injuries)

Special features	Concomitant injuries to the thoracic organs (pneumothorax) are reported, especially in cases of posterior dislocation (Fig. 5.20)
Diagnostic assessment	Conventional AP radiographs often don't enable diagnosis; in cases of suspicion of dislocation, cross-sectional imaging should be considered the method of choice. CT offers better reconstructions and MRI better visualization of the soft-tissues, vessels and affected joints
Goals of therapy/limits of correction	The goal of treatment is the restoration of stability
Primary treatment	Immobilization in Gilchrist sling
Conservative treatment	
Indication	In cases of partial instability, good secondary remodeling can be expected
Procedure	Closed reduction maneuvers are not promising, findings check with MRI; no reduction maneuvers are indicated, since they aren't successful without fixation
Follow up	Rest for 3 weeks; explanation regarding residual swelling.
X-ray controls	Only with unclear findings.
Return to sports	At 6 weeks
Operative therapy	
Indication	In cases of instability, marked anterior or posterior dislocation, secondary in cases of complaints
Procedure	Open reduction; 8–0 wire suture or PDS suture, trans-osseous drill canal, with additional periosteal flap and capsular reconstruction (Fig. 5.21)
Follow up	Rest and avoidance of external rotation movements of the shoulder joint for 4–6 weeks
X-ray controls	Prior to resuming full activities
Hardware removal	Optional for wire suture after about 3 months
Return to sports	3 months
Complications	Intraoperative injuries of neighboring structures (lungs, large vessels), thus no drilled wires! Residual swelling, prominence and scar formation
Growth disturbance	Not expected
Follow up	Functional checks over the course of treatment

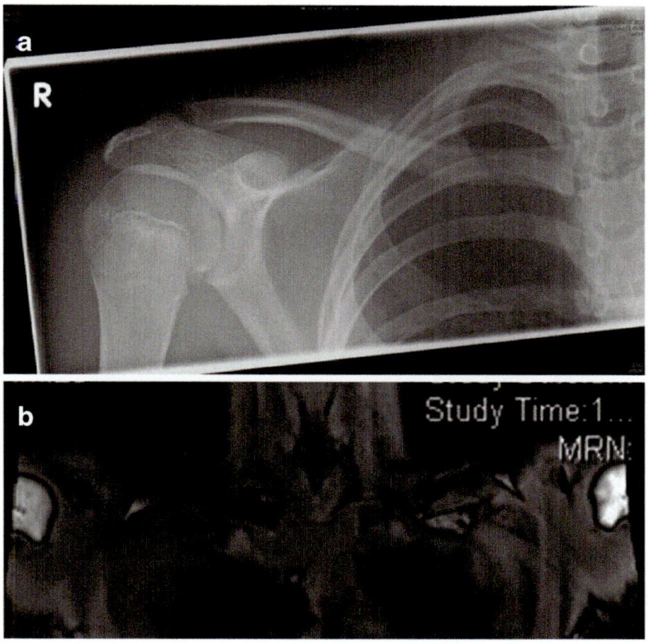

Fig. 5.20 Epiphyseolysis type Salter-Harris II of the sterno-clavicular joint right side in a child. (**a**) X-ray, (**b**) MRI. Tension band wiring was performed with fiber wire and bone anchor

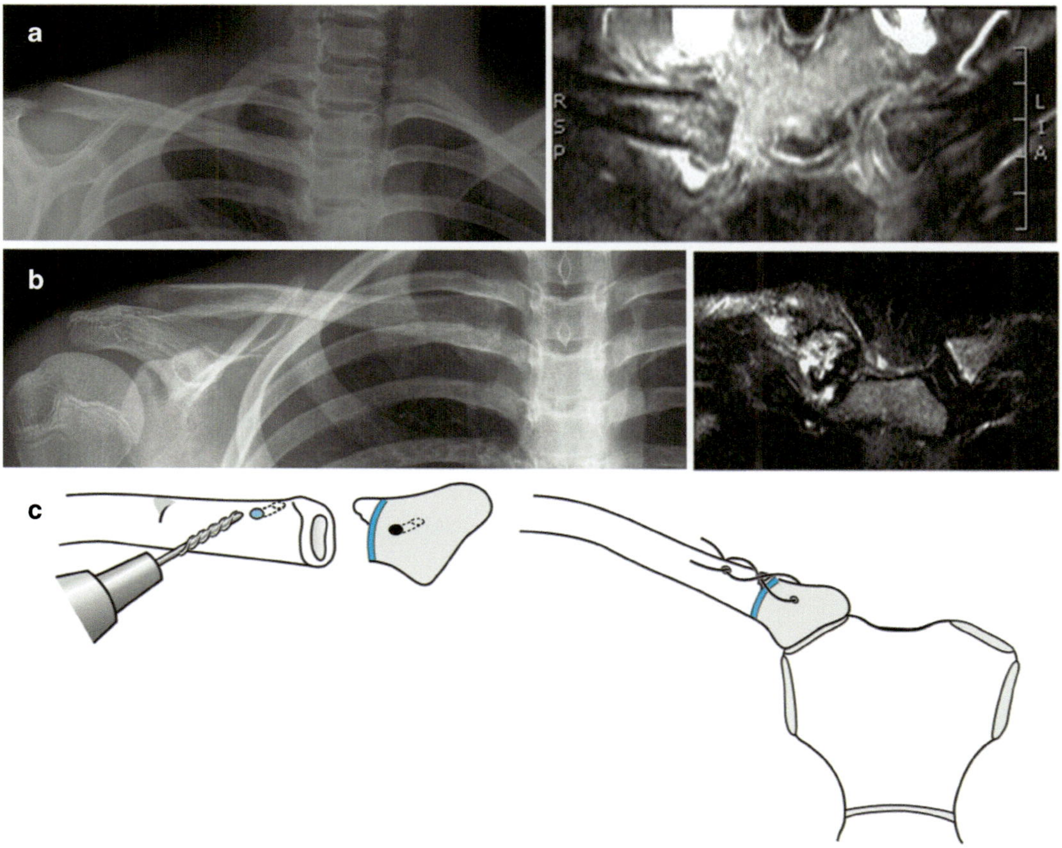

Fig. 5.21 Medial luxation of the clavicula (Salter-Harris II) in a 13 year old girl. (**a**) Trauma images x-ray and MRI; (**b**) Postoperative x-ray and MRI of correct healing. (**c**) Operative principle with trans-osseous sutures

Table 5.8 Technical aspects of SC joint

Material	Wire 8–0 suture through drilled canals, alternatively PDS if necessary
Positioning	Beach chair positioning
Approach	Bow-shaped incision over the SC joint
Special explanation	Injury to neighboring structures, remarkable scar formation
Surgical principle	Tension banding
Hardware removal	Optional after about 3 months when wire suture is used

Scapular Fractures

Incidence, Mechanism of Injury and Clinical Picture

Scapular Fractures are rare and make up fewer than 1% of fractures.

Shearing injuries along the glenoid occur during shoulder dislocations (including bony Bankart Lesions, see there). Coracoid avulsion fractures can occur together with lateral clavicular fractures and AC joint injuries. The remaining scapular fractures are consequences of high-speed trauma with traffic accidents and falls from a great height with direct force. Concomitant rib or vertebral fractures dominate the clinical picture, so that scapular fractures are often initially seen only on the polytrauma CT scan. Targeted assessment of clinical and radiological signs of fracture is necessary when there is clinical suspicion of shoulder injury.

Classification

There is no specialized classification for pediatric scapular fractures. Generally they are classified according to fracture localization (Fig. 5.22):

- Body Fractures (1),
- Spine Fractures (2),
- Acromial fractures (3),
  - with narrowing of the subacromial space,
  - without narrowing of subacromial space,
- Coracoid fracture (4),
- Scapular neck fractures (5),
- Glenoid fractures (6),
- Thoracoscapular dissociation (Fig. 5.23).

Table 5.9 shows the clinical signs and options and Table 5.10 the technical approaches.

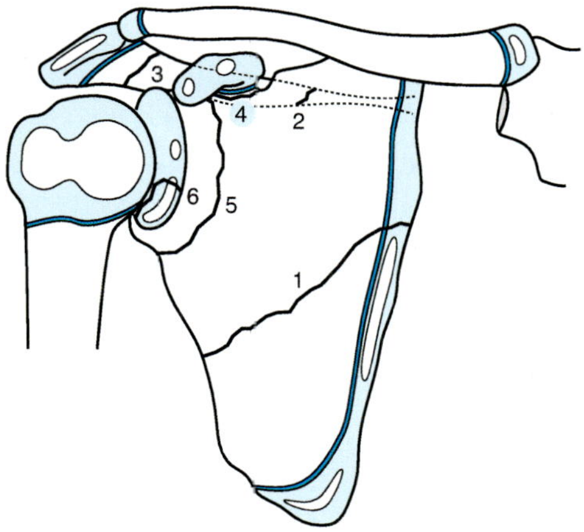

Fig. 5.22 Types of scapula-fractures (1) Body (2) Spine (3) Acromial (4) Coracoid (5) neck (6) Glenoid

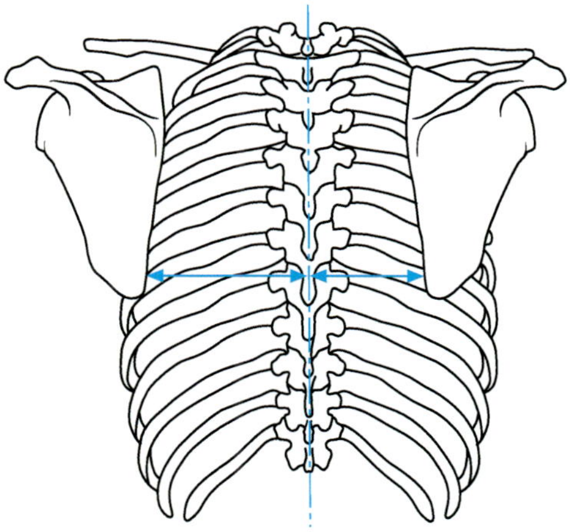

Fig. 5.23 Thoraco-scapular dissociation

Table 5.9 Scapular fracture

Special features	Very rare
Diagnostic assessment	Radiology: AP and axial shoulder X-ray tangential scapula Over the course of healing, the fractures and magnitude of displacement cannot always be assessed on conventional radiographs; in these cases, CT
Goals of therapy/limits of correction	Pain relief Glenoid reconstruction in cases of increased displacement and instability
Primary treatment	Immobilization in Gilchrist sling
Conservative treatment	
Indication	Usually conservative (Fig. 5.24)
Procedure	Gilchrist sling for 2–3 weeks
Follow up	Early functional spontaneous exercises
X-ray controls	Consolidation control at approximately 4 weeks
Return to sports	Approximately 4 weeks after consolidation
Operative therapy	
Indication	In cases of floating shoulder, treatment of the clavicle or scapula as needed, treatment of the scapula only when there is gross displacement; plate support of the scapular neck in floating shoulder through a posterior approach to the lateral margin. Grossly displaced glenoid fractures supported arthroscopically if needed.
Procedure	Plate and screw fixation (Fig. 5.25)
Follow up	Functional follow up once pain-free
X-ray controls	Consolidation control at approximately 4 weeks
Hardware removal	At 8–12 weeks (only clavicle, scapular plates can be left)
Return to sports	Approximately 3 weeks after hardware removal
Complications	Morbidity from approach, scars
Growth disturbances	Not generally expected
Follow up	Not required

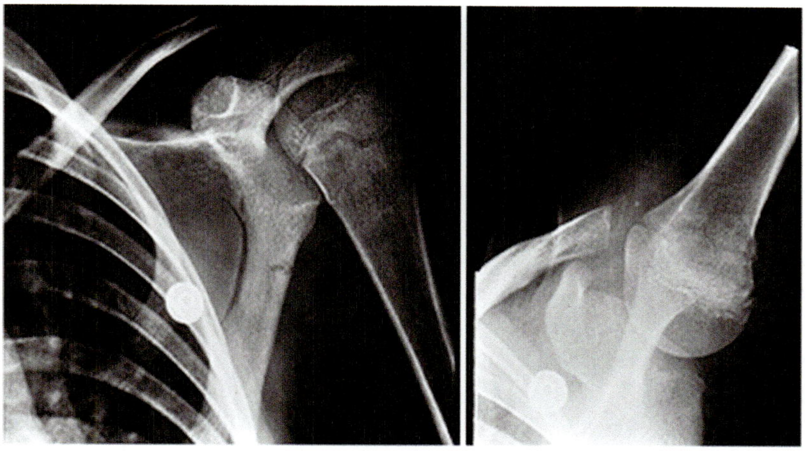

Fig. 5.24 Scapula fracture, undisplazed

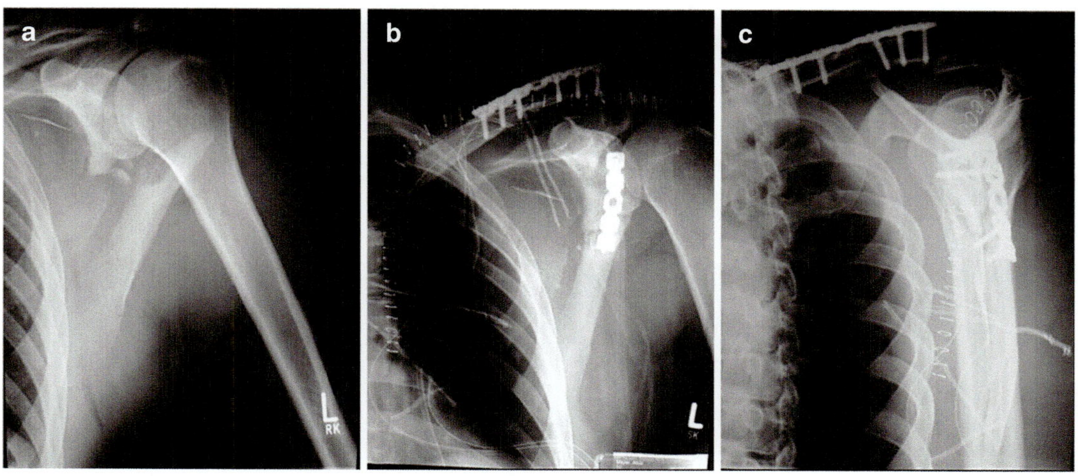

Fig. 5.25 (**a**–**c**) Floating shoulder with clavicule fracture type Allman I and concomitant scapular neck and body fractures. Treatment with plate fixation of the clavicule and lateral scapula

Table 5.10 Scapula—technical aspects of surgery

Material	Screws (2.0–3.5 mm) Plate fixation (2.0–3.5 mm)
Positioning	Beach chair positioning, arm freely movable for the anterior approach (glenoid) Prone positioning, arm free movable in posterior approach In cases of combined approach, use lateral positioning on the opposite side with fluoroscopic capability, arm mobile and with sterile cover.
Approach	Anterior Deltopectoral approach or arthroscopic (glenoid) Posterior Generally sufficient to stabilize the lateral margin along the lateral scapular border and under and over the Teres major muscle (two window approach), rarely a second plate over the spine
Special explanation	Risk of injury to the suprascapular and axillary nerves
Surgical principle	Plate fixation posterior Classic plate fixation Screw plate fixation Classic screw plate fixation (posterior glenoid)
Hardware removal	At 8–12 weeks; posterior scapular plate stays

5.2 Shoulder Joint

The shoulder joint is a ball joint that is not primarily stable since the glenoid is flat compared to the spherical humeral head; it is maintained only by the labrum, the joint capsule, the glenohumeral ligaments and the rotator cuff. On the one hand, this predominantly soft-tissue stabilization enables the greatest range of motion of all the joints; on the other hand, the lack of bony stabilization makes it particularly susceptible to joint capsule injuries, subluxations and dislocations.

Glenohumeral Shoulder Dislocation and Rotator Cuff Injuries

Incidence

The incidence of glenohumeral dislocation is about 2% in children and adolescents. In children, because of the strength of the ligaments and soft tissues, the proximal humeral growth plate is the weakest mechanical part of the shoulder joint complex. Thus, a Salter-Harris II can take place, but are difficult to show. When the growth plates ossify during puberty, there is a marked increase in capsule and rotator cuff injuries, subluxations and dislocations. Shoulder dislocations with Bankart lesions occur most frequently after 10–12 years and the number has increased in recent years with the surge in intensive sport participation (Fig. 5.26a–d). The majority of shoulder dislocations recur and show relevant labral injuries on MRI (Fig. 5.27a). More than half of dislocation injuries are not the initial event. Therefore, even in adolescents, separated labral injuries should also be fixed arthroscopically to avoid recurrent shoulder dislocations (Fig. 5.27b, c). But even rotator cuff injuries or rupture of the subscapular tendon (Fig. 5.28) can be observed. In addition, regularly recurrent shoulder dislocation should be identified as well as unusual situations in cases of congenital condition (Ehlers-Danlos or Marfan syndrome) or plexus palsy.

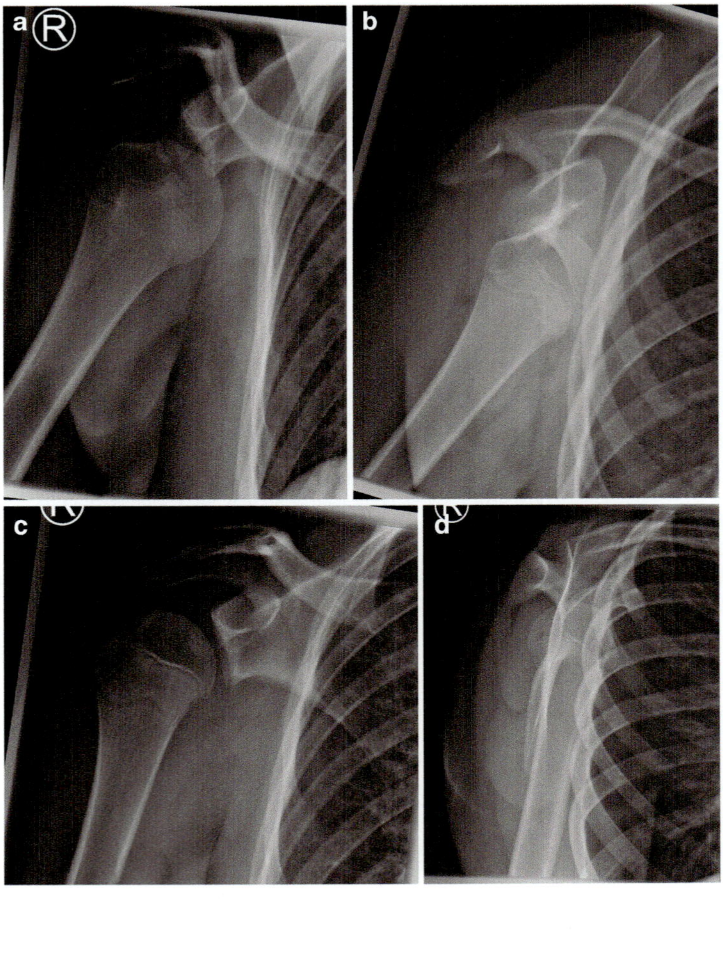

Fig. 5.26 (**a**, **b**) Gleno-humeral dislocation in a 13 years old boy; (**c**, **d**) After reduction

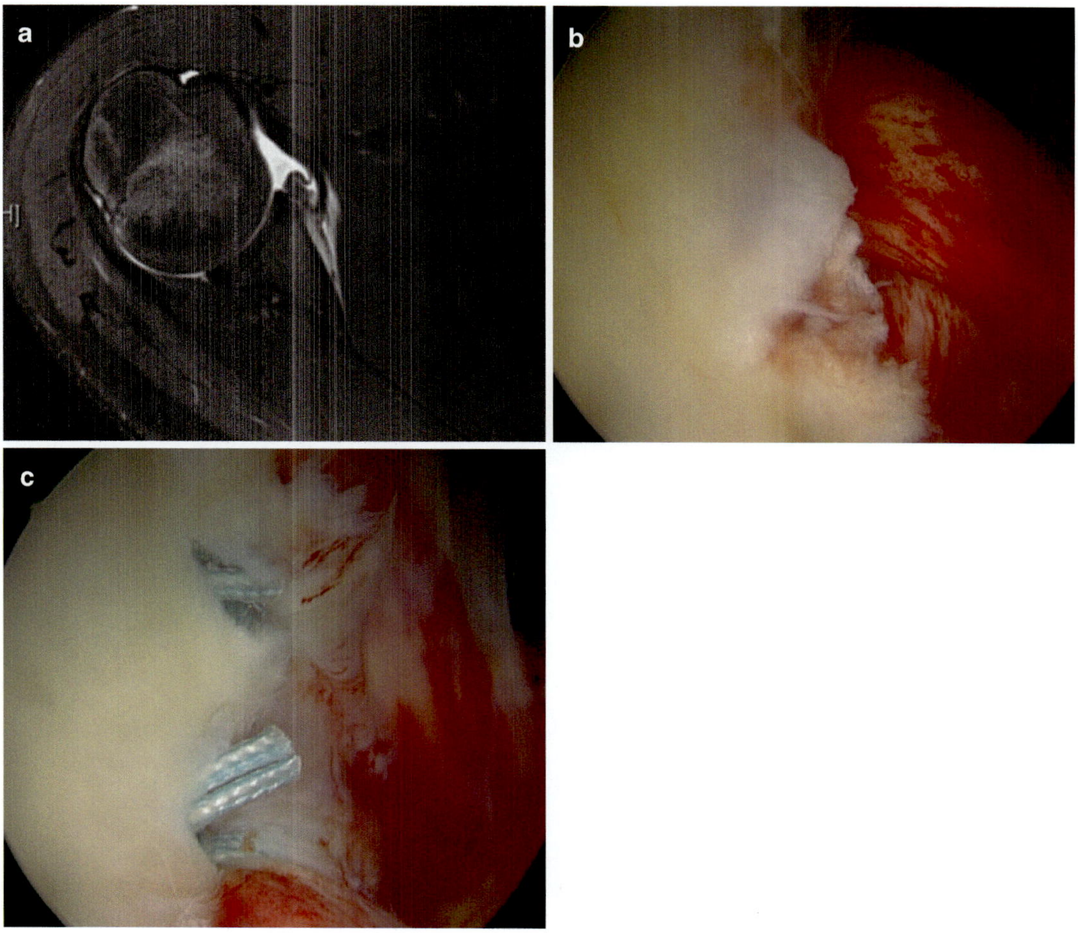

Fig. 5.27 Lesion of the anterior gleno-humerus labrum in a 13 years old boy (**a**) MRI, (**b**) Corresponding arthroscopic view of labrum lesion, (**c**) Refixation with arthroscopic suture anchor

Mechanism of Injury and Clinical Picture

Anterior shoulder dislocation is caused by a fall on the arm that is extended, externally rotated and abducted. The position of the humeral head creates anterior leverage, overextending the anterior and inferior capsule or even tearing it from the glenoid neck. Anterior labral tears, with or without bony avulsion, are of paramount importance regarding long-term shoulder stability (Bankart lesion Fig. 5.29).

Posterior shoulder dislocation is caused either by a fall on the anterior shoulder with the adducted arm in internal rotation or during epileptic seizures because of imbalanced muscle contraction with internal rotator predominance. The humeral head is levered posteriorly, the capsule stretched or torn. Indirect trauma is the most common mechanism of injury. While in children these injuries lead to growth-plate lesions, more common in adolescents and adults are metaphyseal fractures and soft-tissue injuries, for example rotator cuff injuries, subluxations or dislocations.

Shoulder dislocations have also been reported as birth traumas. An epiphysiolysis of the proximal humeral growth plate can actually occur as a consequence of difficulty delivering the shoulder during birth. The humeral epiphysis is within the joint, and the metaphysis slips as a result of the trauma and epiphysiolysis. Because the core of the head is not yet ossified and is invisible on x-ray, this is misinterpreted as shoulder dislocation and ultrasound might help to differentiate.

Another form of shoulder dislocation is the so-called "atraumatic" or habitual dislocation, in which children can arbitrarily sublux or dislocate the shoulder. It is not clear whether this phenom-

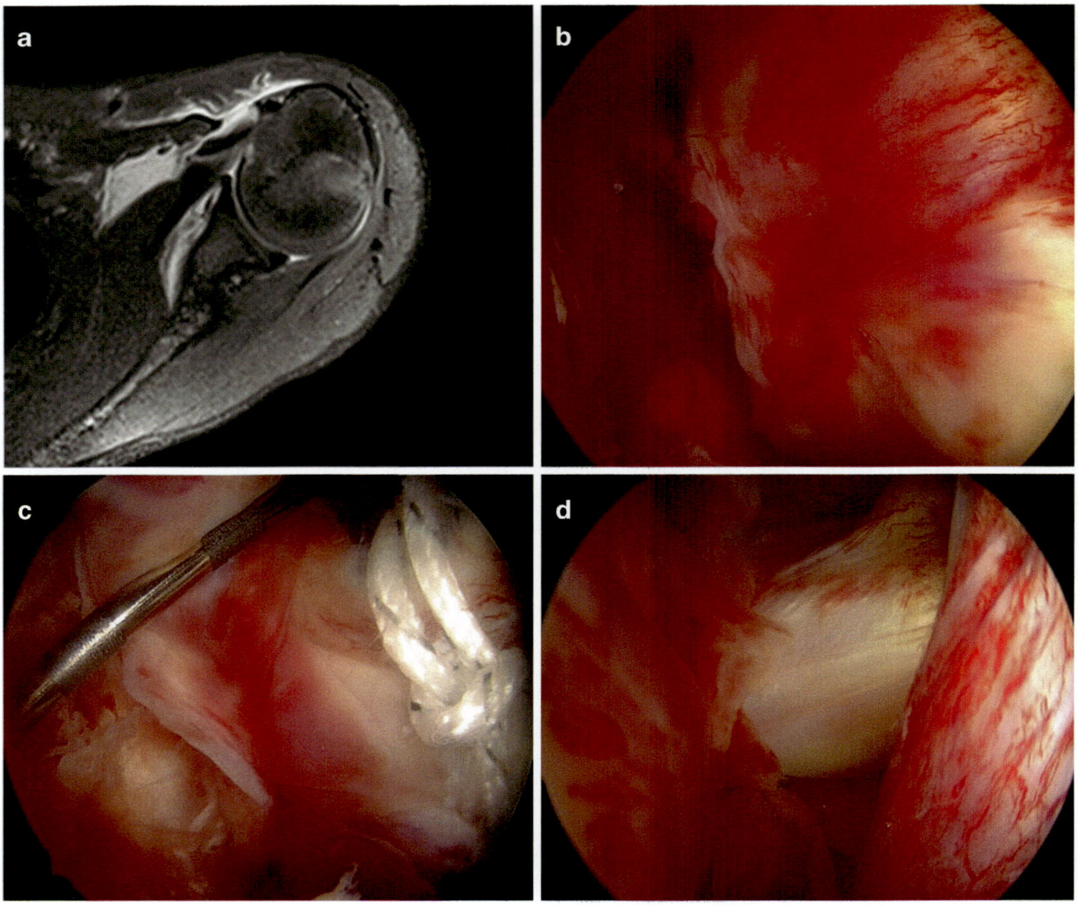

Fig. 5.28 Rupture of the subscapular tendon in an 10 years old boy after fall. (**a**) MRI with complete rupture from the humerus, (**b**) Corresponding arthroscopic view, (**c**) Suture of the tendon with push-loc anchor, (**d**) Stable refixation of the tendon

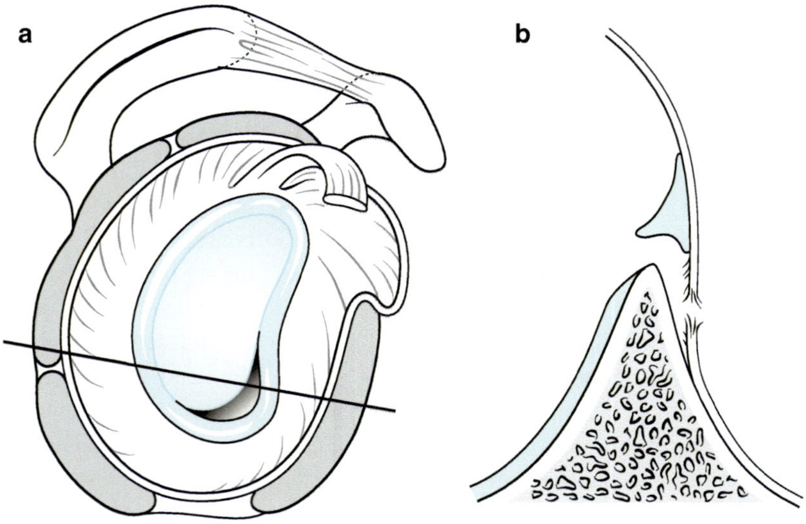

Fig. 5.29 Bankart lesion (**a**) Horizontal view, (**b**) Transversal view

enon occurs spontaneously or as a consequence of minor trauma. In this form of dislocation, psychological factors also play a role. On the other hand, causes such as glenoid dysplasia or habitual shoulder dislocation-even after a traumatic primary dislocation with persistent instability—must be ruled out in these cases.

Traumatic dislocation causes pain, swelling and functional impairment of the shoulder region. The position of the arm depends on the direction of dislocation. In anterior dislocation, the arm is held in mild abduction and external rotation, and the empty glenoid is clinically detectable (Fig. 5.30). A posterior dislocation presents in adduction and internal rotation. Inferior dislocation also presents with the arm in abduction, although the arm is behind or over the patient's head luxatio erecta). Arbitrary subluxation or dislocation causes mild to no pain and swelling.

Classification

Shoulder dislocations are classified according to direction as anterior, posterior, inferior or multidirectional dislocations. By far the most common is the anterior dislocation. Another system classifies according to the cause as traumatic, atraumatic, arbitrary, habitual, congenital (Table 5.11).

The specific clinical signs are shown in Table 5.12 and technical aspects are shown Table 5.13.

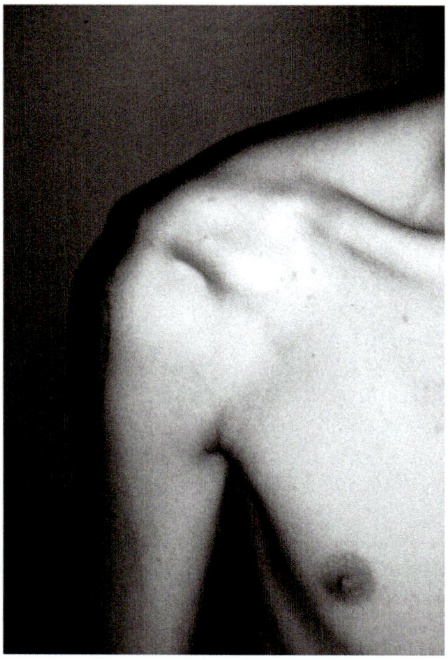

Fig. 5.30 Clinical picture of an anterior shoulder dislocation; empty glenoid

Table 5.11 Mechanism-oriented classification of shoulder dislocation

Traumatic etiology	No trauma
Primary dislocation: Traumatic dislocation with capsule tear, Bankart lesion etc.	Congenital dislocation: Laxity, connective tissue diseases
Recurrent dislocation: Dislocation in post-traumatic capsule insufficiency, Bankart dislocation, Hill-Sachs deformity	Acquired dislocation: Plexus palsy, neurological disorders Arbitrary dislocation: Laxity, psychological factors

Table 5.12 Shoulder dislocation

Special features	Primary traumatic shoulder dislocation during growth is rare, but seen in adolescents during sports (Fig. 5.26) Congenital skeletal anomalies (glenoid dysplasia and congenital neurological disorders) can favor dislocation; children with arbitrarily elicited subluxations and dislocations should be worked up for behavioral disorders and need special muscle-building exercises
Diagnostic assessment	Clinical: Anterior dislocation (common): position in non-fixed abduction and empty glenoid; Posterior dislocation: adduction and internal rotation; Inferior dislocation: arm over or behind the head (luxatio erecta). Exclude injury to the axillary nerve or the brachial plexus. Control arm circulation before and after reduction. Radiographs of the shoulder AP (second plane usually unnecessary). MRI for clarification of the injury and assessment of the labrum, cartilage and any other abnormalities and/or additional injuries; Generally, MRI is required to assess the extent of injury including the labrum, the rotator cuff and/or other injuries, such as an apophyseal cartilage rupture in adolescents. Non-invasive ultrasound examination is also useful in newborns and infants as well as in cases of soft tissue injury.
Goals of therapy/limits of correction	Reduction with restoration of the articular surface contact; prevention of joint instability, functional impairment, neurovascular injury; prevention of re-dislocation
Primary treatment	Radiographs required prior to reduction maneuvers to verify diagnosis and rule out proximal humerus fracture (Fig. 5.31) In children, closed reduction with similar to technique to that used in adults is performed under short general anesthesia with short-term muscle relaxation to prevent secondary damage; Emergency indication of reduction procedure and control x-ray
Conservative treatment	
Indication	First dislocation without morphological damage on MRI, or well-fitting labrum
Procedure	After successful reduction, immobilization in Gilchrist sling for 2–3 weeks, rule out injury requiring surgery with MRI
Follow up	4 weeks of progressive physical therapy while avoiding external rotation for anterior dislocations
X-ray controls	Reduction control with radiographs; MRI to exclude labral lesion
Return to sports	No sooner than 6 weeks, contact sports and overhead sports (tennis) at 10–12 weeks
Operative therapy	
Indication	Cases of clear undisplaced and displaced lesions of the anterior labrum and recurrent dislocation
Procedure	Arthroscopic labrum refixation with suture anchor (resorbable or titanium and capsule tightening, occasionally open refixation is needed (glenoid fracture)
Follow up	Immobilization in a shoulder vest for 4 weeks, avoiding external rotation for at least 6 weeks
X-ray controls	Not usually required
Return to sports	No sooner than 6 weeks, contact sports and overhead sports (tennis) at 10–12 weeks
Complications	Re-dislocation; education regarding risk of re-dislocation
Growth disturbances	Not expected, except with concomitant injuries to the proximal humeral epiphysis
Follow up	None

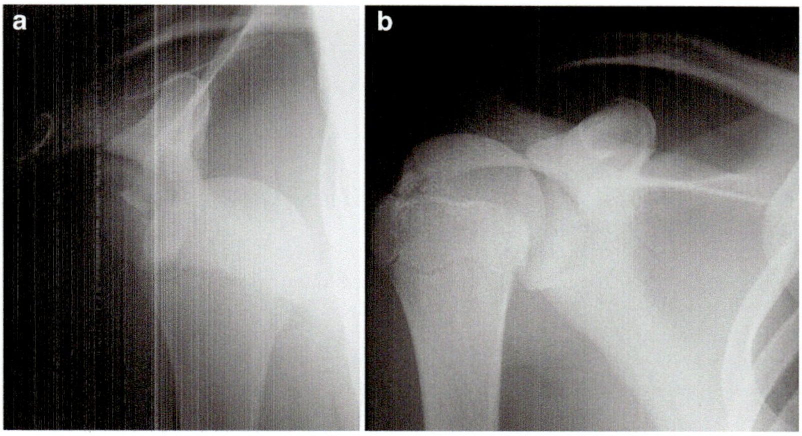

Fig. 5.31 Anterior luxation of the gleno-humeral joint. (**a**) Luxation, (**b**) After reduction

Table 5.13 Technical aspects shoulder dislocation

Material	Anchor suture, resorbable (Fig. 5.32)
Positioning	Beach chair positioning or extended shoulder (lateral)
Approach	Arthroscopic, mini-open if needed
Special explanation	Risk of recurrence
Surgical principle	Stabilization of the injured capsule structures, labrum refixation with suture anchor debridement of the rupture and zone of insertion Exclude additional intra-articular injuries during arthroscopy
Other special features	Usually a primary arthroscopic procedure, also useful for repeat procedures. Difficult stabilization in habitual dislocation, in these cases a capsular arthroscopic shift in addition to the labrum refixation is mostly successful. In cases of glenoid dysplasia and persistent dislocation a bony glenoid rim reconstruction, J-span, or Latarjet procedure might be necessary. Conservative operative indication in cases of multidirectional instability, due to high risk of recurrence

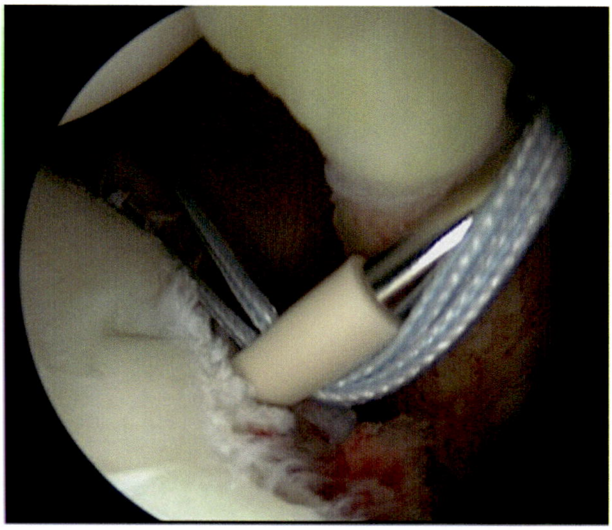

Fig. 5.32 Refixation of the anterior labrum in an adolescent with a suture anchor

Recommended Literature

Faust KC, Lark RK, Leversedge FJ (2018) Pediatric clavicle injuries. In: Gordon I (ed) Undefined. Springer, Cham, pp 205–214

Gao B, Dwivedi S, Patel SA, Nwizu C, Cruz AI (2019) Operative versus nonoperative management of displaced midshaft clavicle fractures in pediatric and adolescent patients: a systematic review and meta-analysis. J Orthop Trauma 33:e439–e446

Gottlieb M (2018) Current approach to the diagnosis and management of shoulder dislocation in children. Pediatr Emerg Care 34:357–362

Janicki JA (2020) Adolescent clavicle fractures. In: Christopher A, Frick SL (eds) Undefined. Springer, Cham, pp 19–22

Kraus R, Zwingmann J, Jablonski M, Bakir MS (2020) Dislocations of the acromioclavicular and sternoclavicular joint in children and adolescents: a retrospective clinical study and big data analysis of routine data. PLoS One 15:e0244209

Labronici PJ, da Silva RR, Franco MVV, Labronici GJ, Pires RES, Franco JS (2016) Distal clavicle fractures in children. Rev Bras Ortop 51:24–28

Lampert C, Baumgartner G, Slongo T, Kohler G, Horst M (2003) Traumatic shoulder dislocation in children and adolescents. Eur J Trauma 29:375–378

Milewski MD, Nissen CW (2013) Pediatric and adolescent shoulder instability. Clin Sport Med 32:761–779

Nawar K, Eliya Y, Burrow S, Peterson D, Ayeni O, de Sa D (2020) Operative versus non-operative management of mid-diaphyseal clavicle fractures in the skeletally immature population: a systematic review and meta-analysis. Curr Rev Musculoskelet Med 13:38–49

Pandya NK, Namdari S, Hosalkar HS (2012) Displaced clavicle fractures in adolescents: facts, controversies, and current trends. J Am Acad Orthop Surg 20(8):498–505

Rapp M, Prinz K, Kaiser MM (2013) Elastic stable intramedullary nailing for displaced pediatric clavicle midshaft fractures: a prospective study of the results and patient satisfaction in 24 children and adolescents aged 10 to 15 years. J Pediatr Orthop 33:608–613

Rockwood CW, Wilkins K, King R (1984) Fractures and dislocations of the elbow region. Fract Children

Swarup I, Maheshwer B, Orr S, Kehoe C, Zhang Y, Dodwell E (2021) Intermediate-term outcomes following operative and nonoperative management of midshaft clavicle fractures in children and adolescents: internal fixation may improve outcomes. JB JS Open 6(e20):00036

6 Humerus

6.1 Physiological Findings

The growth plate of the proximal humerus is tent-shaped in the anterior-posterior view of an x-ray (Fig. 6.1a, b). It is convex (proximally) on lateral projection; the vertex is posteromedial. A narrow margin of proximal metaphysis (posteromedial) is intracapsular and not covered by cartilage. The strong joint capsule attachment begins precisely under this strip. Because of this, and because the periosteum is thicker posteromedially and thinner anterolaterally, the metaphyseal fragment tears the periosteum anterolaterally in proximal humerus fractures. In these cases, a strip of metaphyseal fragment often remains along the epiphysis (Fig. 6.2).

Ossification Centers and Growth Plate Fusion

The primary ossification center of the humerus appears around the sixth embryonic week. The secondary ossification center of the humeral head arises between 6 and 12 months after birth, and that of the greater tuberosity between 7 months and 2 years. Two years later, i.e., between 2.5 and 4 years, the ossification center appears in the lesser tuberosity. Fusion of these proximal secondary ossification centers occurs between the ages of 4 and 6 years. The proximal humeral growth plate closes between 14 and 17 years in girls and 16 and 18 years in boys (Fig. 6.3). An age-dependent, radiological representation of the proximal humerus is depicted in Figs. 6.4, 6.5, 6.6, and 6.7.

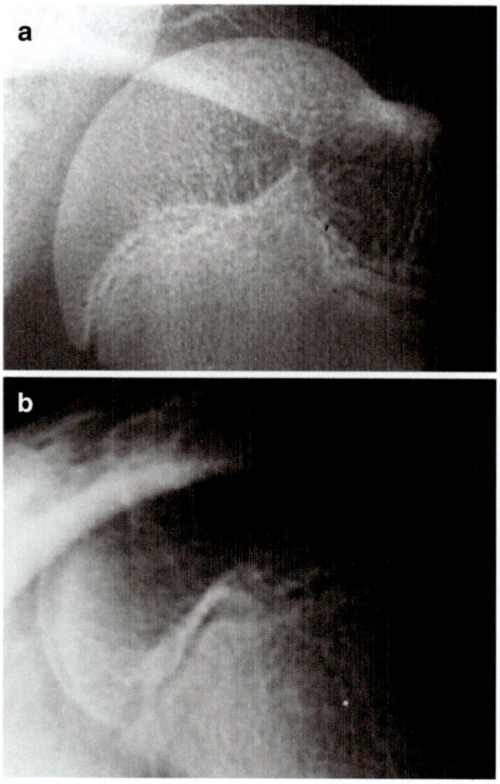

Fig. 6.1 (**a**) A.P. view X-ray image of the juvenile humerus head with tent-shaped growth plate, (**b**) Lateral view with convex growth plate

80% of longitudinal growth of the humerus occurs at the proximal growth plate. Thus, even adolescents have good potential for spontaneous correction after fractures, and significant deformity can be tolerated in young children.

I. Marzi et al., *Pediatric Skeletal Trauma*, https://doi.org/10.1007/978-3-030-93685-3_6

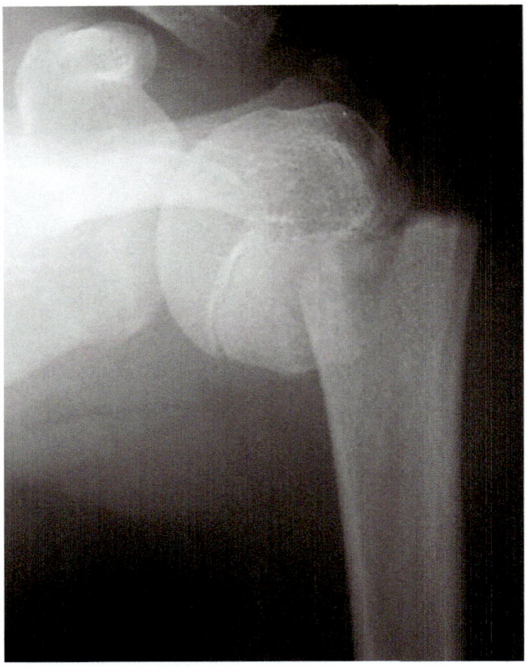

Fig. 6.2 Typical Salter-Harris II injury: epiphysiolysis with a posteromedial metaphyseal fragment. The metaphysis is displaced anterolaterally and the humeral head is tilted posteriorly within the socket

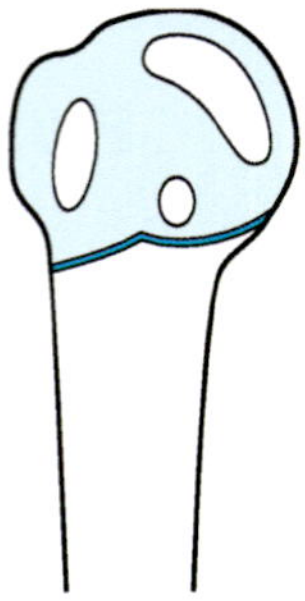

Fig. 6.3 Ossification centers of the proximal humerus

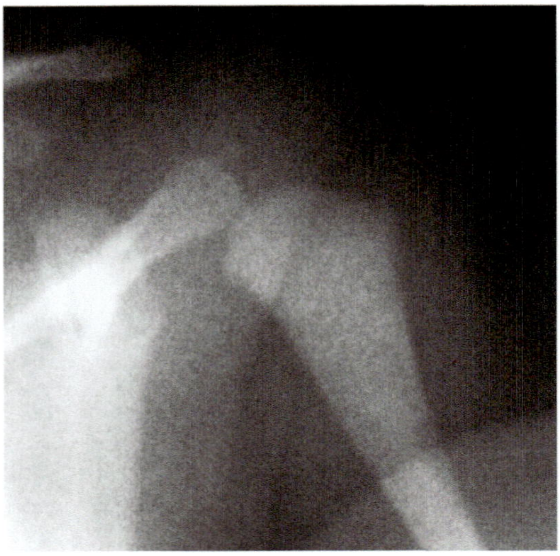

Fig. 6.4 X-ray of a newborn humeral head

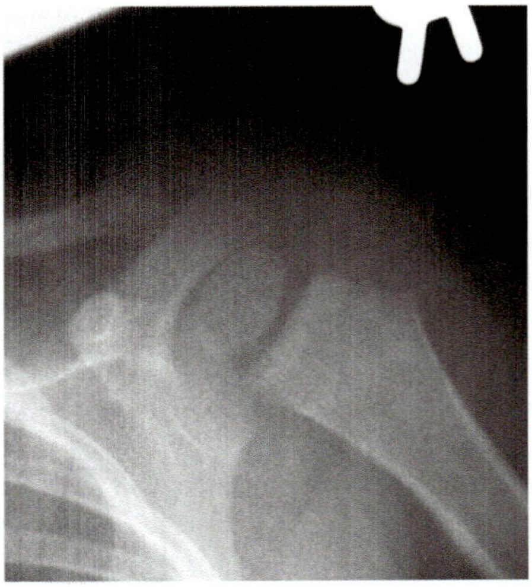

Fig. 6.5 X-ray of a one year old child of the humeral head

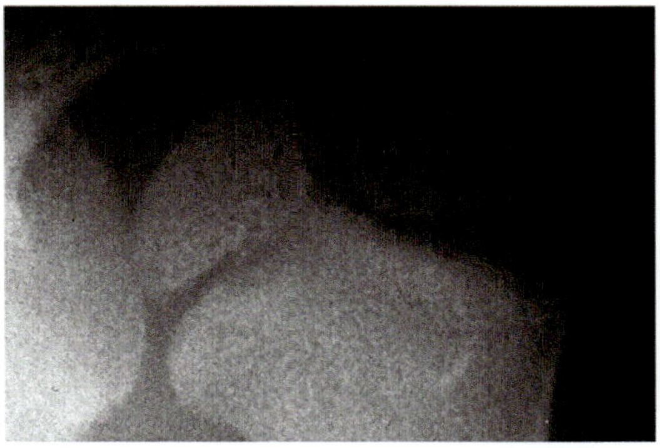

Fig. 6.6 X-ray of a 2 year old child, of the greater tuberosity

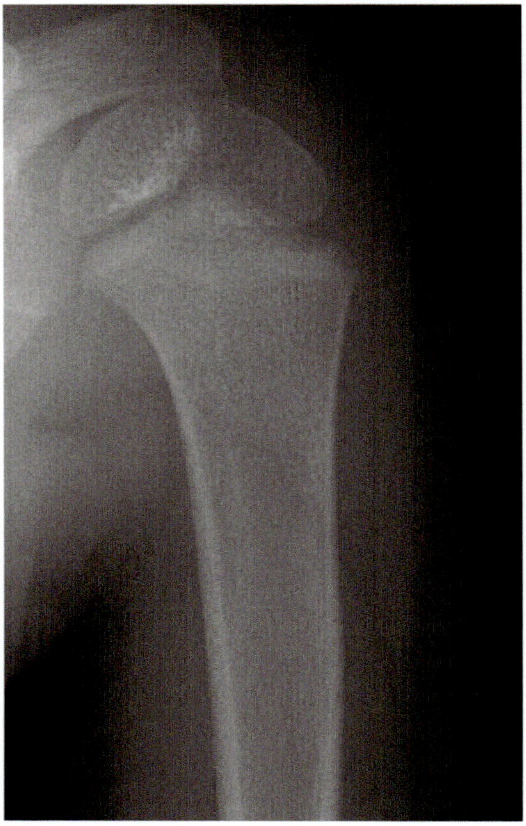

Fig. 6.7 X-ray of a four year old child at the humeral head

6.2 Proximal Humerus Fractures

Incidence, Mechanism of Injury and Clinical Picture

Approximately 40% of all bony upper arm injuries occur proximally (Fig. 6.8). A third of cases are epiphysiolysis, some do not have a metaphyseal wedge (Salter-Harris I), but most do (Salter-Harris II). Two-thirds of cases involve subcapital humerus fractures in children aged 5–14 years. Epiphyseal and epi-metaphyseal fractures are extremely rare.

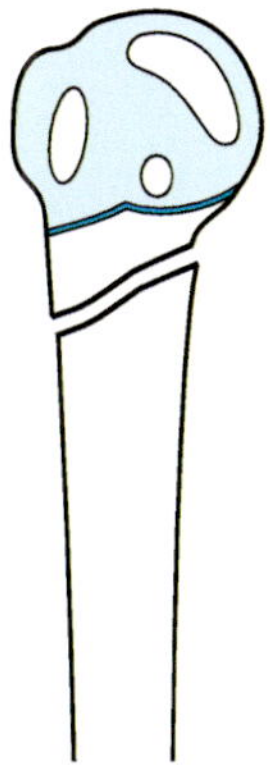

Fig. 6.8 Fractures of the proximal humerus

Proximal humerus fractures result from direct trauma, such as a fall on the shoulder, and indirect trauma after falling backward onto an outstretched arm (Fig. 6.9). In newborns, there are birth trauma injuries. Child abuse must be considered in infants and toddlers (Fig. 6.10a, b). Pathological fractures from juvenile bone cysts are prevalent in the upper arm (Fig. 6.11).

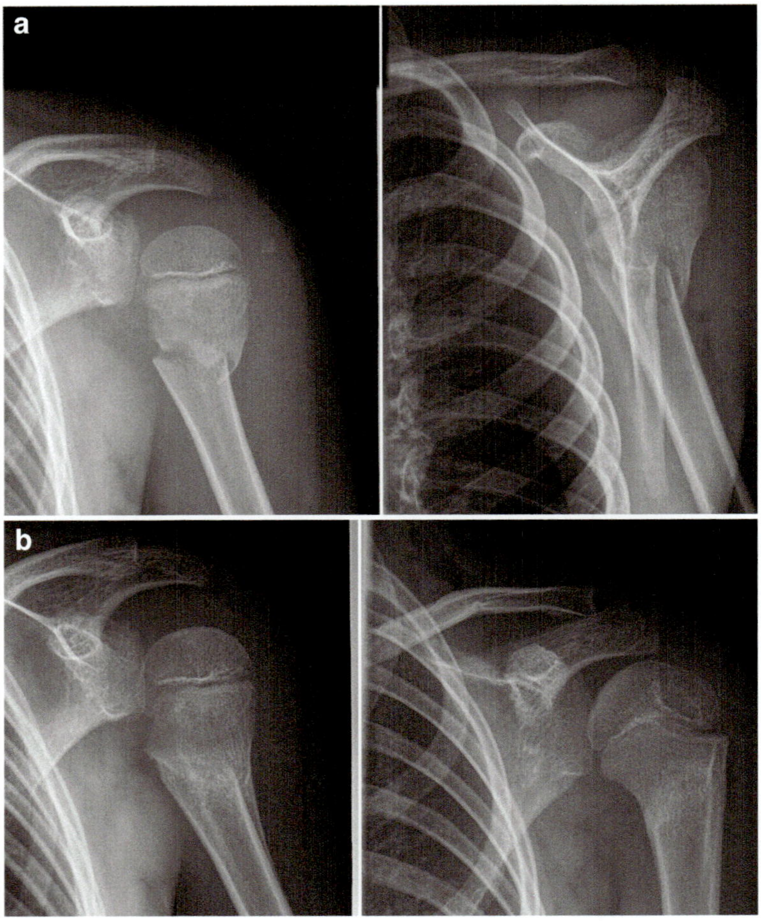

Fig. 6.9 Subkapital humerus fracture of a 7 year old boy, conservative treatment with Desault bandage. (**a**) Trauma image. (**b**) Healing with good callus after 6 weeks

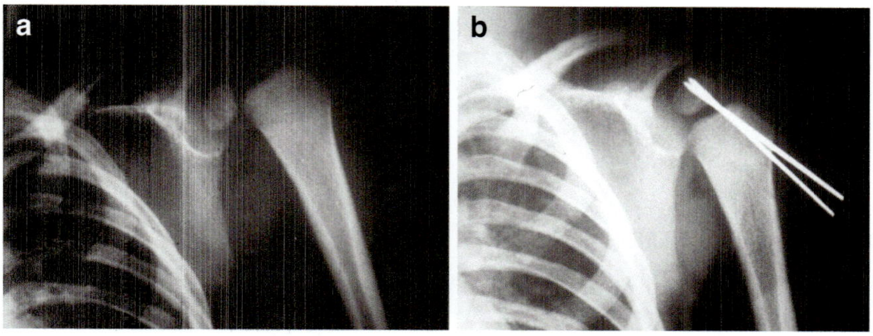

Fig. 6.10 (**a**, **b**) Epiphyseal disruption on the proximal humerus from child abuse. Boy, 2 years. (**a**) X-ray findings on admission. (**b**) Fixation after closed reduction with 2 K-wires

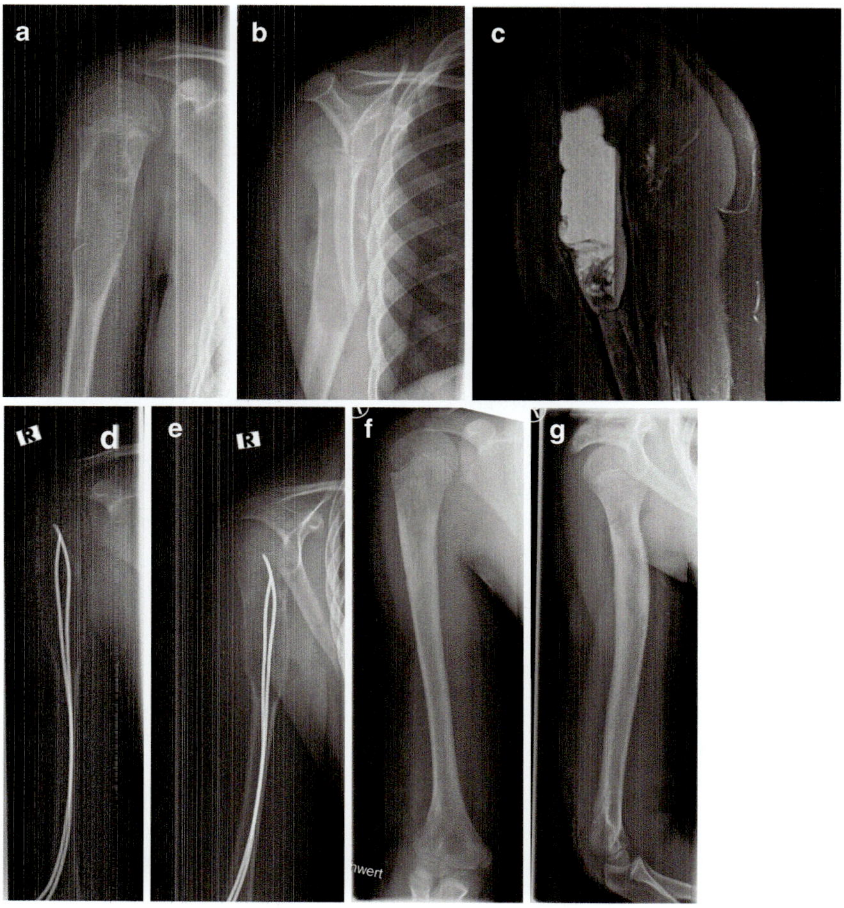

Fig. 6.11 Typical pathological fracture of a juvenile cystic lesion of the proximal humerus. (**a**, **b**) X-ray of Pathological fracture with cyst without adequate trauma, (**c**) MRI showing typical fluid, (**d**, **e**) Primary stabilization with retrograde ESIN, (**f**, **g**) Healing after metal removal

The clinical presentation varies according to age. Diagnosis can be challenging in newborns, infants, and toddlers, due to the incomplete imaging in x-ray. The clinical picture can range from pain on movement to complete loss of function. In any case, osteomyelitis, brachial plexus injury, and clavicle fracture must be excluded. In older children and adolescents, localized swelling occurs with pain and corresponding movement limitations (Table 6.1).

Table 6.1 Proximal humerus fractures

Special Features	Because there are three and then two unique ossification centers of the humeral head, it can be challenging to diagnose nondisplaced fractures. An oblique joint projection can simulate a fracture; pathological fractures from juvenile bone cysts can occur (Fig. 6.12).
Diagnostic techniques	AP and lateral radiographs; on the AP image, the growth plate appears "tent-shaped," it is convex on the lateral image.
Goals of treatment/ correction limits	Rapid pain resolution, Unlimited shoulder mobility and symmetrical shoulder contours (cosmetic). There is much potential for spontaneous correction of deformities, especially side-to-side translation and frontal/sagittal angulation. When considering operative treatment, the following correction limits are relevant: <5 years: 70–90° angulation in the frontal plane and bone contact with translation up to one shaft width; 5–12 years: 20–70° angulation in the frontal plane, translation up to 2/3 shaft width; >12 years: < 20°, translation less than 1/2 shaft width.
Primary treatment	Medical analgesia as needed, immobilization in Gilchrist bandage (Fig. 6.12).
Conservative treatment	
Indications	Displacement within correction limits
Approach	Immobilization in Gilchrist or Desault bandage for 3–4 weeks (Fig. 6.12)
Follow up	Mobilization and physical therapy are generally not necessary
X-ray controls	Trauma radiographs and controls
Return to sports	3–4 weeks after fracture consolidation
Operative treatment	
Indications	Displacement outside of correction limits Functional indication for early mobilization after consultation with parents Severe pain due to fragment dislocation
Approach	Closed reduction usually possible; occasionally, open reduction is necessary when there is soft-tissue interposition (biceps tendon) Percutaneous K-wire fixation; supplemental Gilchrist bandage (Figs. 6.13 and 6.14) Retrograde ESIN (more for older children), stable for mobilization (double S-technique see Fig. 6.15)
Follow up	K-wire fixation: Gilchrist/Desault bandage for 3–4 weeks ESIN: functional
X-ray controls	Trauma radiographs, intraoperative position check, consolidation checks at 3–4 weeks
Hardware removal	K-wires: at 3–4 weeks (after consolidation x-rays) ESIN: at 12–16 weeks
Return to sports	2–4 weeks post-consolidation
Complications	Partial, premature growth plate fusion, misalignment after conservative and operative treatment due to inadequate reduction or fixation, infections after operative treatment and restricted mobility after excessive immobilization
Growth disturbance	Occurs rarely as a result of premature, partial, or complete growth plate fusion; according to age, stimulative (clinically irrelevant) and inhibitory growth disorders are possible (birth trauma)
Follow up	Functional checks until unhindered mobility, annual clinical checks in cases of angulation until deformity resolves
Classification	AO: 11-E/1-9.1-3 11-M/1-9.1-3 LiLa: 1.1.a.5.0-2. 1.1.s.1-5.0-2.

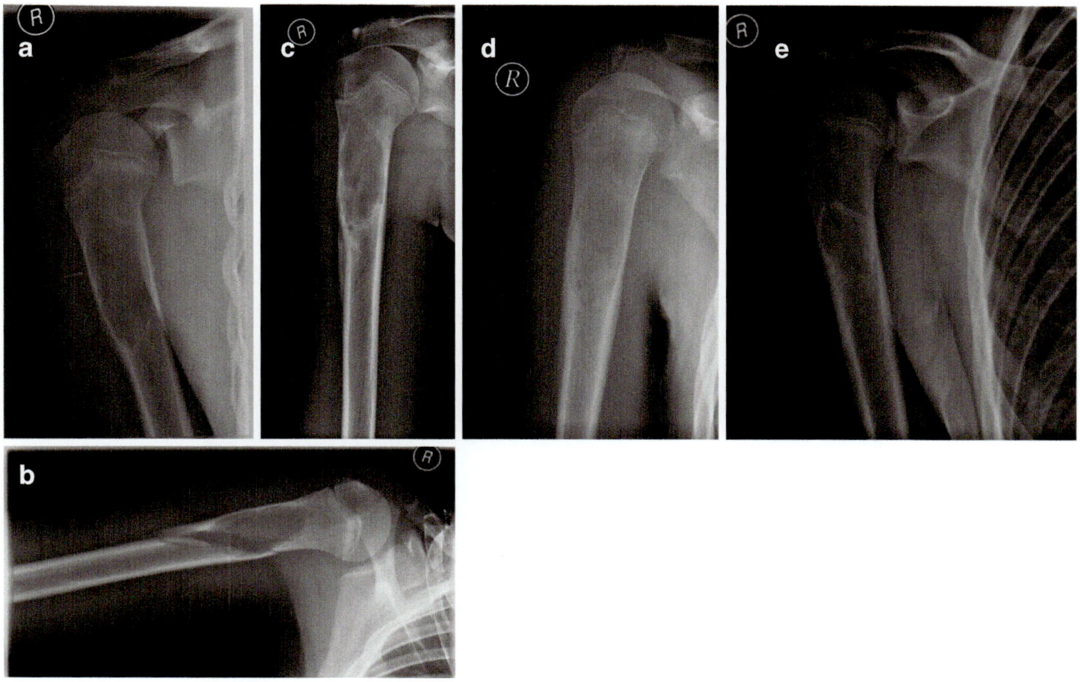

Fig. 6.12 Pathological oblique fracture of humerus with juvenile bone cyst. (**a**, **b**) Trauma image, (**c**) Healing after 4 weeks, (**d**) X-ray after 4 months, (**e**) Complete healing after 9 months

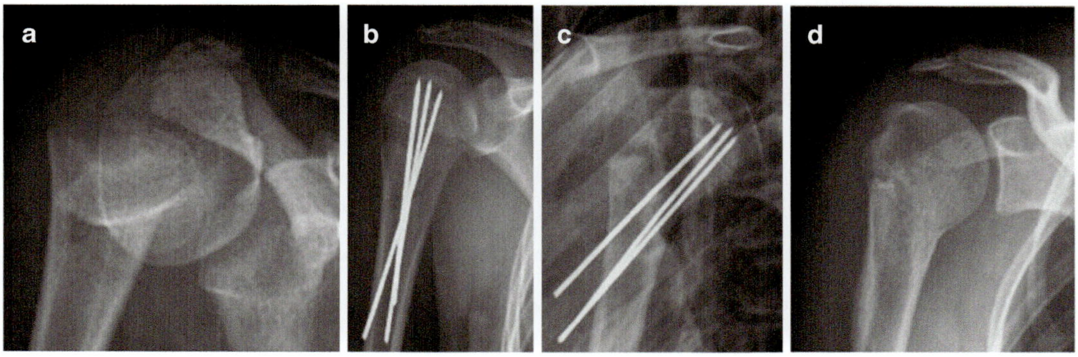

Fig. 6.13 Completely dislocated Salter-Harris-II fracture of a 13 years old girl. (**a**) Injury, (**b**, **c**) Postoperative reduction and K-wires crossing the growth plate, (**d**) Healing after 14 weeks and metal removal

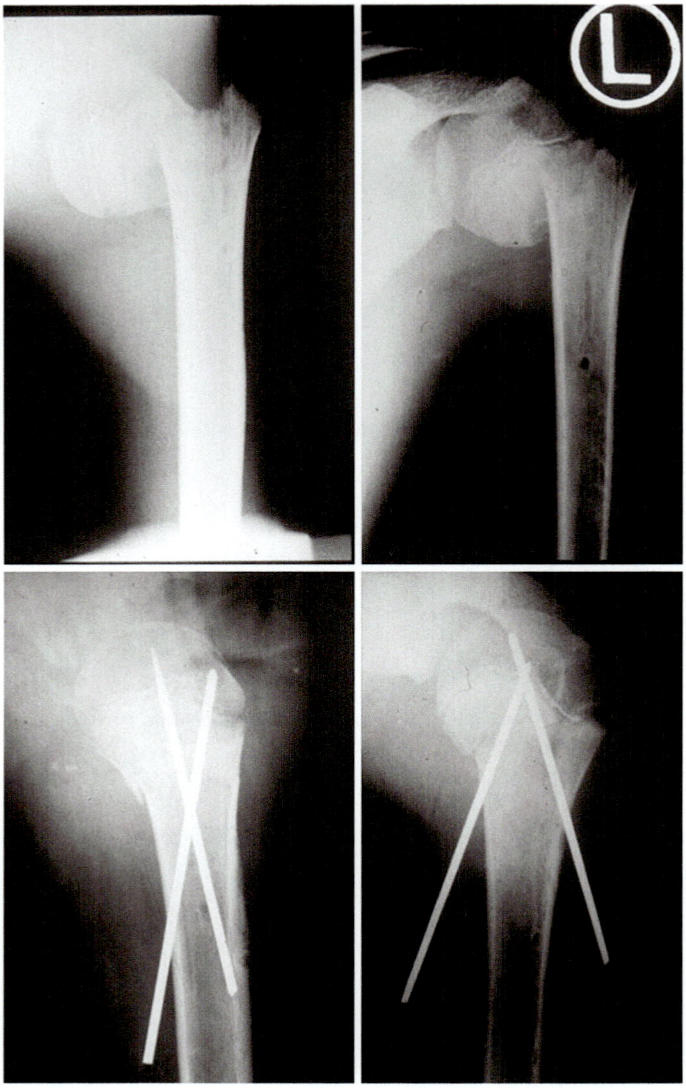

Fig. 6.14 Salter-Harris-II fracture of a 14 years old boy. (**a**) Injury and complete dislocation, (**b**) Reduction and fixation with 2 k-wires, crossing the growth plate

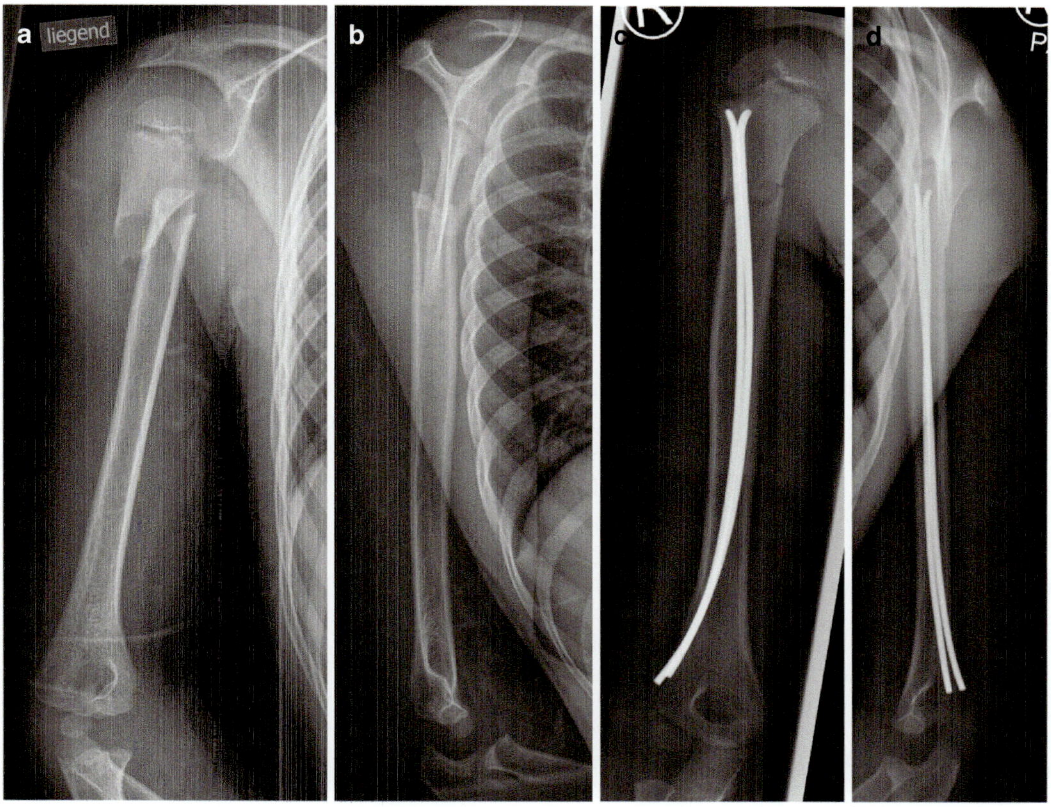

Fig. 6.15 Subcapital humerus fracture, completely displaced. (**a**, **b**) Trauma image, (**c**, **d**) Closed reduction and stabilization with retrograde ESIN

Classification

The Aitken and Salter and Harris Classifications are most commonly used for growth plate injuries. Salter III and IV injuries are extremely rare in the proximal humerus. There are also subcapital humerus fractures not involving the growth plate and apophyseal avulsion injuries affecting the greater and lesser tuberosities.

6.3 Diaphyseal Humeral Fractures

Incidence, Mechanism of Injury and Clinical Picture

Diaphyseal fractures are usually the result of direct forces and occur in just 10–20% of all bony humeral injuries.

The clinical presentation is localized swelling and pain in the area of the humeral shaft. Crepitation of the bone and pain intensity depending on fracture instability.

Transverse and short oblique fractures are typically the result of direct trauma, which is the most common mechanism of injury. Indirect forces cause long oblique or spiral fractures, a fracture type also seen in child abuse. Minor trauma can lead to pathological fractures when juvenile bone cysts are present. This is the most common localization for this clinical entity. Fractures at the transition from the mid to distal humeral thirds can be associated with radial nerve irritation or damage. Although direct nerve tears are rare, callus encroachment is possible when the fracture line is angled. An isolated post-traumatic radial nerve lesion is generally not a sufficient indication for primary surgical nerve revision since there is a high probability for spontaneous regeneration (motor function of the brachioradialis muscle returns first). In most cases, residual sensitivity can still be detected. The exception is a nerve lesion that appears after reduction, worsens, or shows no improvement during the initial 6–8 weeks. In these cases and cases of long, oblique fracture lines in the direction of the radial nerve, early nerve revision might be necessary (Tables 6.2 and 6.3).

Table 6.2 Diaphyseal humerus fracture (Fig. 6.16)

Special Features	Newborns sometimes show what is known as pseudoparalysis of the arm. The goal here is to exclude osteomyelitis/septic joint, brachial plexus injury, clavicular fracture, or rupture of the proximal humeral growth plate; in cases of primary radial palsy, conservative treatment with neurological follow-up examinations is tried initially, with secondary release only in special cases	
Diagnostic techniques	Radiographs in two planes Ultrasound	
Goals of treatment/ correction limits	Analgesia; no angulation (varus, valgus, anteversion, or retroversion over 10°), side-to-side translation to just under a shaft width; only minor rotational deformity is tolerated; cosmetic symmetry	
Primary treatment	Analgesia, immobilization in Gilchrist bandage	
Conservative treatment		
Indications	Nondisplaced oblique or spiral fractures to limits of correction (Fig. 6.17)	
Approach	Gilchrist bandage for 3–4 weeks	
Follow up	Mobilization of the arm after immobilization, no primary physical therapy necessary	
X-ray controls	Consolidation radiographs	
Return to sports	Approximately 4 weeks post-consolidation	
Operative treatment		
Indications	In open fracture grades 2 and 3; in painful, unstable shaft fractures (fracture end crepitus); in fractures where correction limits are not retained conservatively; in polytrauma; relative surgical indication in transverse and short oblique fractures of adolescents when early functional treatment is desired	
Approach	ESIN (Fig. 6.18) alternatively external fixateur (Fig. 6.19)	
Follow up	Functional with stable bony fixation	
X-ray controls	Intraoperative reduction check, consolidation radiographs	
Hardware removal	ESIN at 3 months, fixator at 6–8 weeks	
Return to sports	Approximately 4 weeks after the conclusion of treatment	
Complications	Secondary angulation, infection, neurovascular injury, fracture healing disorder	
Growth disturbance	No clinical relevance	
Follow up	Functional checks until unhindered mobility, annual clinical checks in cases of angulation	
Classification	AO: 12-D/1-9.1-3	LiLa: 1.2.s.2-5.0-2.

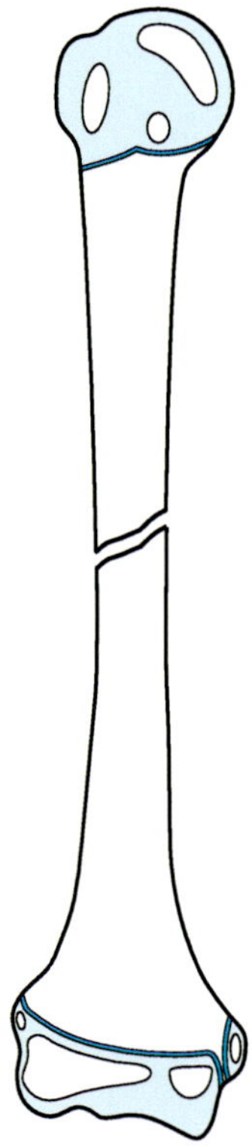

Fig. 6.16 Diaphyseal fracture of the humerus

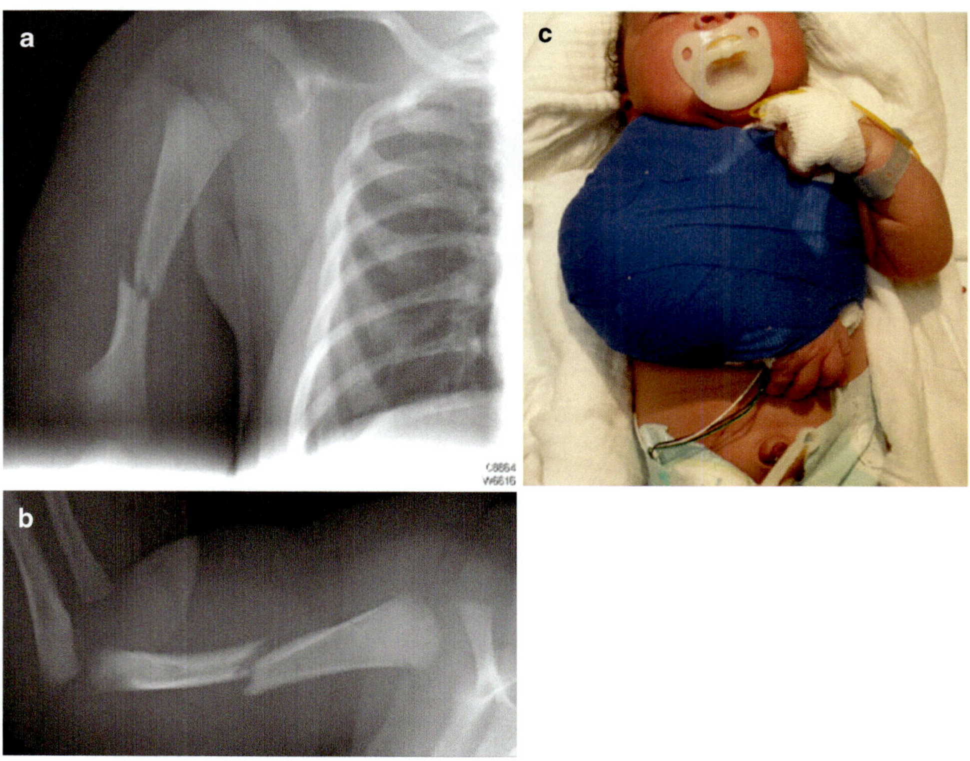

Fig. 6.17 Conservatively treated oblique shaft fracture of the humerus. (**a**) Injury, (**b**) Healing after 6 weeks. (**c**) In additional cast after 2 weeks

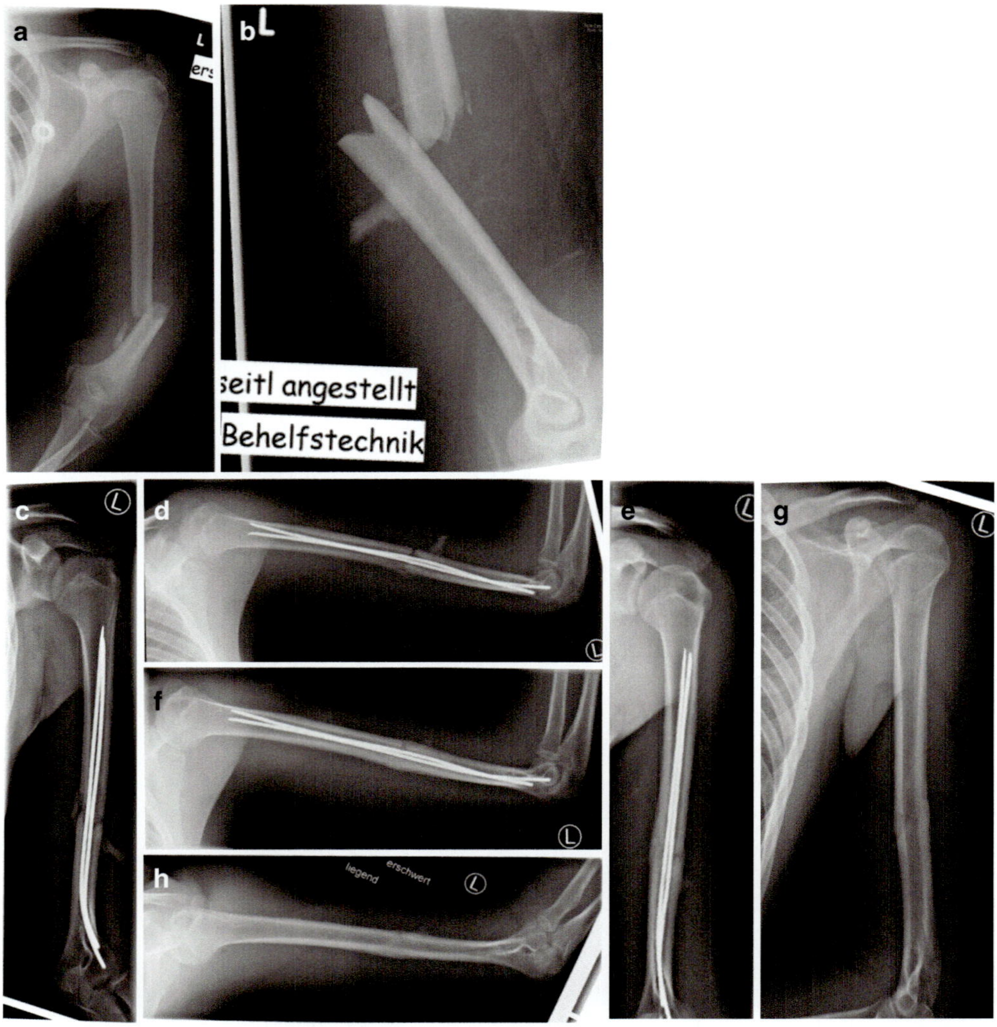

Fig. 6.18 Shaft fracture of the humerus, 14 year old boy. (**a**, **b**) Trauma image, (**c**, **d**) Postoperative with retrograde ESIN, (**e**, **f**) Bony healing with ESIN, (**g**, **h**) Healed bone after removal of ESIN

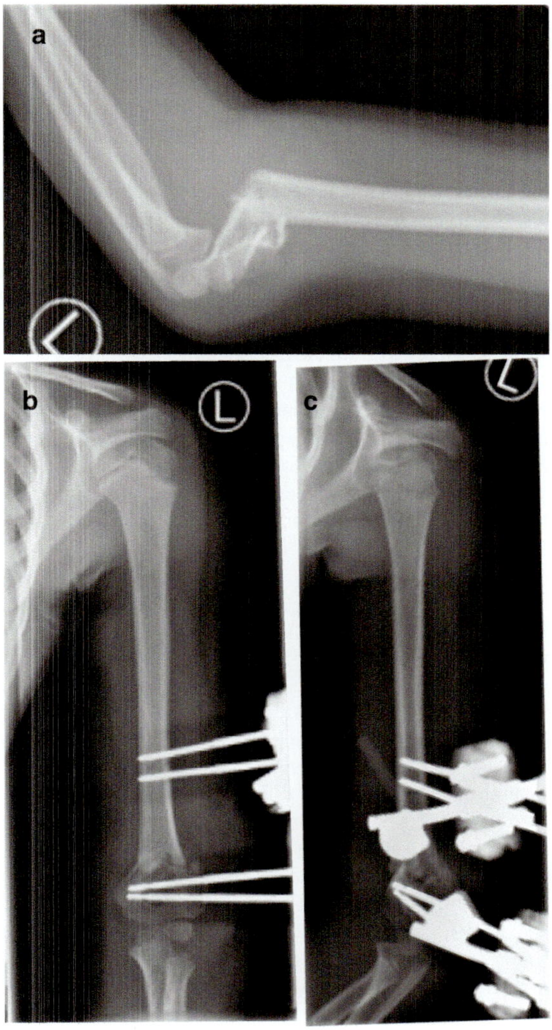

Fig. 6.19 Severely dislocated fracture of the distal humerus in a 5 year old girl. (**a**) Trauma image with dislocation, (**b**, **c**) Stabilization with external fixateur

Table 6.3 Technical aspects humerus fractures

Retrograde ESIN in proximal humerus and humeral shaft fractures	
Material	Titanium or steel nails, 2–3.5 mm diameter according to child age; titanium has a similar elasticity coefficient as bone and produces less foreign body reaction than steel nails External fixator from various manufacturers; minor additional soft-tissue irritation; pin positioning under visualization, risk of nerve lesion (radial nerve!) very high
Positioning	Supine position, no tourniquet (image intensification), drape to the elbow, rotation checks
Approach	Lateral incision over the lateral epicondyle or combined medial and lateral approaches (with ulnar nerve exposure) over both epicondyles Insertion of the two nails via lateral and medial or two lateral oblique cortical perforations Advance the nails across the fracture and anchor in the proximal humeral metaphysis Depending on the fracture line, the nails can be crossed retrograde or anterograde (deltoid tuberosity) or inserted from the exterior alone. Open reduction in primary radialis nerve lesion and retrograde ESIN (Fig. 6.20)
Closed reduction and K-wire fixation for very proximal humerus fractures or epiphysiolysis	
Closed reduction and percutaneous introduction of K-wires is technically demanding because of the steep angle and physiological retroversion of the humeral head. Post-reduction introduction of two 1.6–2 mm K-wires under image intensification in two planes, ascending from the metaphysis into the humeral head and crossing the growth plate. This is unstable fixation; thus, additional immobilization in a Gilchrist bandage or something similar is necessary.	
External fixator on the humerus (in special cases only, as there is a high risk for radial nerve injury)	
Approach and operative principle (external fixator)	The proximal pins of the external fixator are inserted in the area of the deltoid tuberosity, the distal pins proximal to the distal humeral growth plate Care must be given to avoid the radial nerve along the humerus at the middle to distal third transition The pins must be visualized during positioning!
Approach and operative principle (open reduction)	A skin incision is made over the humerus to expose the shaft and explore the radial nerve between the brachialis and brachioradialis muscles While protecting the nerve, the soft tissues are released from the fracture line, and the fracture stabilized with ESIN or an external fixator
Complications	Radial nerve injury as a result of reduction, infection Ulnar nerve injury through a medial approach No potential for stimulative growth disturbance
Operative principle	Closed reduction and fixation with ESIN or external fixator through 2 or 4 stab incisions, without growth plate contact Open reduction can only be justified in cases of hindered reduction and open fractures grades 2 or 3
Hardware removal	ESIN at 12 weeks, external fixator at 6–8 weeks
Special features	

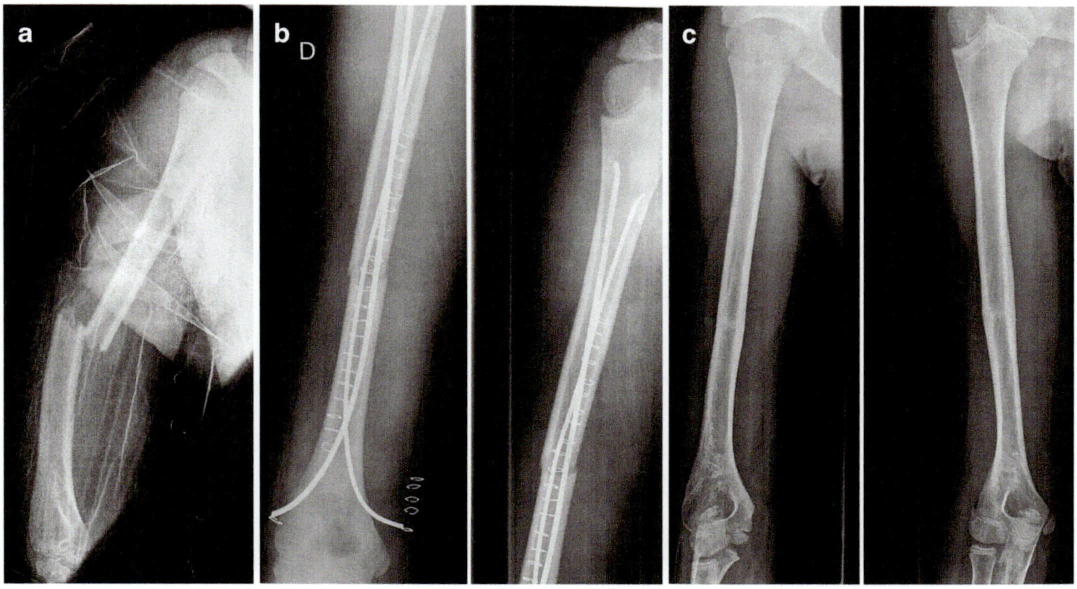

Fig. 6.20 Oblique fractures in a 5 year old boy fall during football with primary radialis nerve injury. (**a**) Oblique humerus mid shaft fracture with complete primary sensomotoric palsy of radial nerve. (**b**) Primary open reduction and nerve release from periostal fixation in the fracture. Retrograde elastic nail fixation. (**c**) Complete remission of nerve function and consolidated fracture after 6 months

Recommended Literature

Dietz HG, Schmittenbecher PP, Illing P (1997) Intramedulläre Osteosynthese im Wachstumsalter. Urban & Schwarzenberg, Munich

Dietz HG, Schmittenbecher PP, Slongo T, Wilkins KE (2006) Elastic stable intramedullary nailing (ESIN) in children. Thieme, Stuttgart

Dietz HG, Illing P, Schmittenbecher PP, Slongo T, Sommerfeldt DW (2011) Praxis der Kinder- und Jugendtraumatologie, 1st edn. Springer, Berlin

Khan A, Athlani L, Rousset M, Samba A, Canavese F (2014 Jan 1) Functional results of displaced proximal humerus fractures in children treated by elastic stable intramedullary nail. Eur J Orthop Surg Traumatol 24(2):165–172

Knorr P, Joeris A, Lieber J, Schalamon J, Dietz HG (2005 Jan 1) The use of ESIN in humerus fractures. Eur J Trauma 31(1):12–18

Marzi I (2016) Kindertraumatologie, 3rd edn. Springer, Berlin

Ogden JA (2006) Skeletal injury in the child. Springer, New York

Rang M, Pring ME, Wenger DR (2005) Rang's children's fractures. Lippincott Williams & Wilkins, Philadelphia

Rockwood CA (2010) Rockwood and Wilkins' fractures in children, vol 3. Lippincott Williams & Wilkins, Philadelphia

Roposch A, Saraph V, Linhart WE (2000 Jan 1) Flexible intramedullary nailing for the treatment of unicameral bone cysts in long bones. JBJS 82(10):1447

Sommerfeldt DW, Dietz HG (2011 Apr) Pediatric and adolescent traumatology - upper extremity. Der Unfallchirurg 114(4):284–284

von Laer L, Kraus R, Linhart WE (2012) Frakturen und Luxationen im Wachstumsalter 6., überarbeitete und erweiterte Auflage. Thieme Verlag, Stuttgart

7 Elbow

7.1 Physiological Findings

The ossification center (OC) of the humeral capitellum is already present at birth; it arises in the 5th–6th month of gestation. In the proximal radius, the OC develops around age 2. Around age 4, the OC of the medial humeral epicondyle appears. The medial condyle OC arises between 6 and 8 years. It's frequently irregular and asymmetrical compared to the other side. The OC for the olecranon develops between 9 and 11 years. Finally, the OC for the lateral humeral condyle develops between the ages of 12 and 14 years. The distal humeral growth plate closes functionally between ages 8 and 10, sometimes even up to age 12. The ossification centers of the epicondyles unite with the distal humerus at 14–18 years. The growth plate of the radial head fuses with the radius between ages 10 and 18, and the ossification center of the olecranon connects with the proximal ulna between 14 and 16 years (Fig. 7.1).

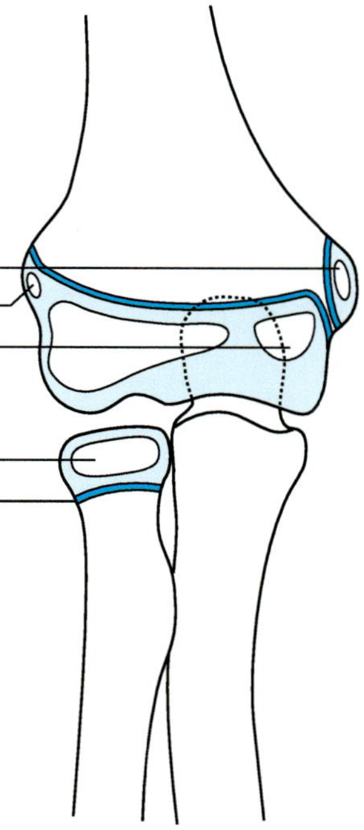

Fig. 7.1 Ossification centers growth plate fusion in the elbow (y=years)

Age-Dependent X-ray Findings

The growth plate of the distal humerus can hardly be seen at birth because most of the epiphysis is cartilaginous. In the lateral plane, it can appear quite oblique and irregular, with an aspect toward the epiphysis that can mimic epiphysiolysis. In any case, the lateral x-ray does not show the "fat pad" sign as an indication of an intra-articular effusion (Fig. 7.2a). This fat pad sign can be visualized even better with ultrasound and is a strong indication for a fracture (Fig. 7.2b–d).

Prior to the closure of the distal humeral growth plate, a number of ossification centers may have developed in the trochlea. These should not be confused with fractures or aseptic bone necrosis. Because ossification centers appear successively, the exact course of the distal humeral joint surface can only be imagined through familiarity with the anatomy, as shown in illustrations and radiologi-

I. Marzi et al., *Pediatric Skeletal Trauma*, https://doi.org/10.1007/978-3-030-93685-3_7

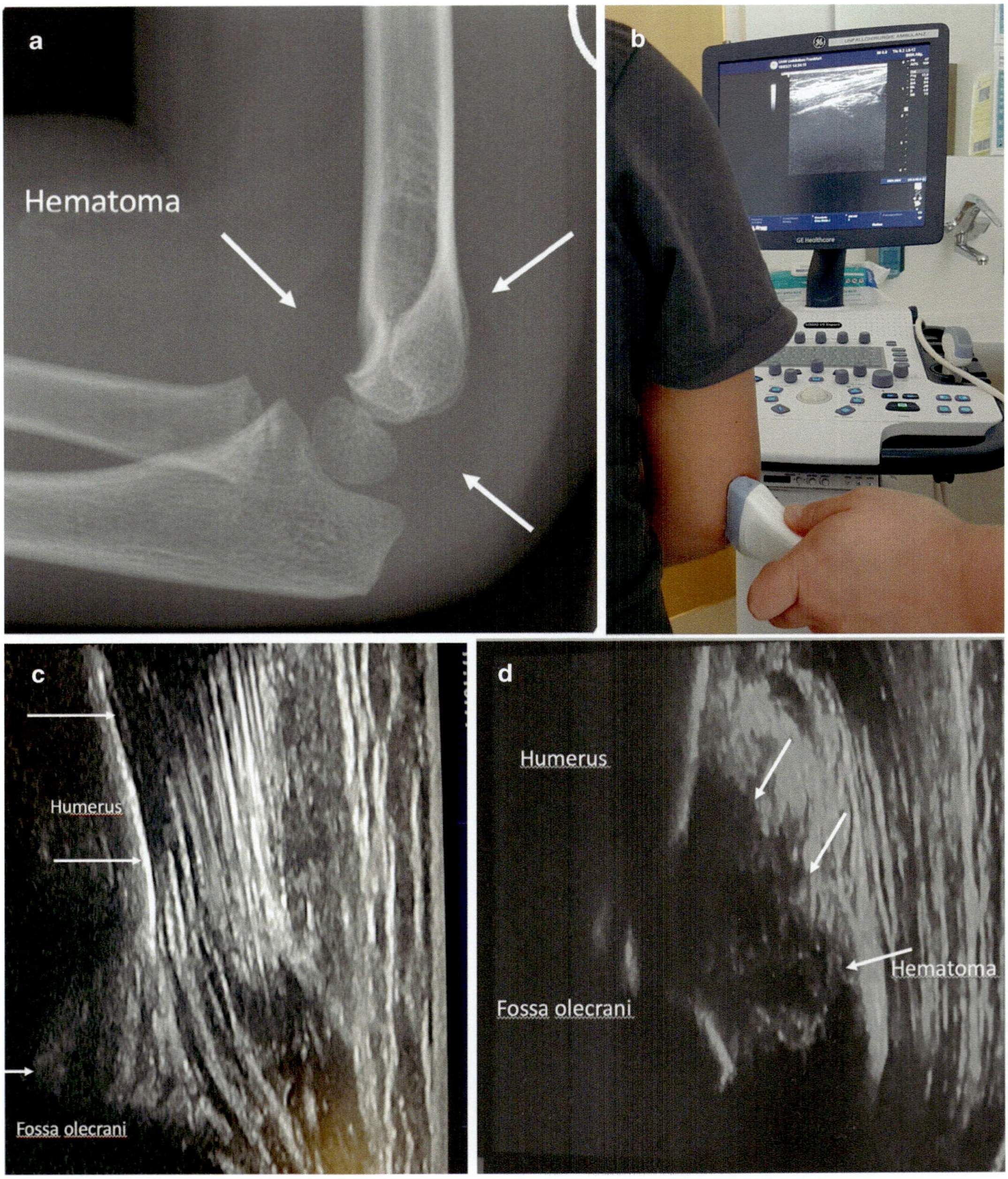

Fig. 7.2 Anterior and posterior fat-pad sign in a supracondylar humerus fracture type I

cally here in Figs. 7.3, 7.4, 7.5, and 7.6. Extra-articular supracondylar and epicondylar fractures should be distinguished from intra-articular fractures. Extra-articular entities include the common lateral condyle fracture and less prevalent medial condyle fractures. Sometimes, the supracondylar fracture line extends directly within the joint; this is referred to as a T-fracture of the distal humerus.

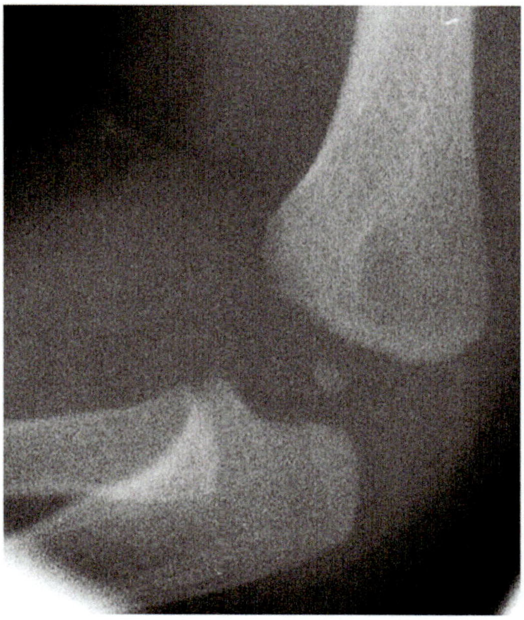

Fig. 7.3 6 Months: ossification center humeral capitellum

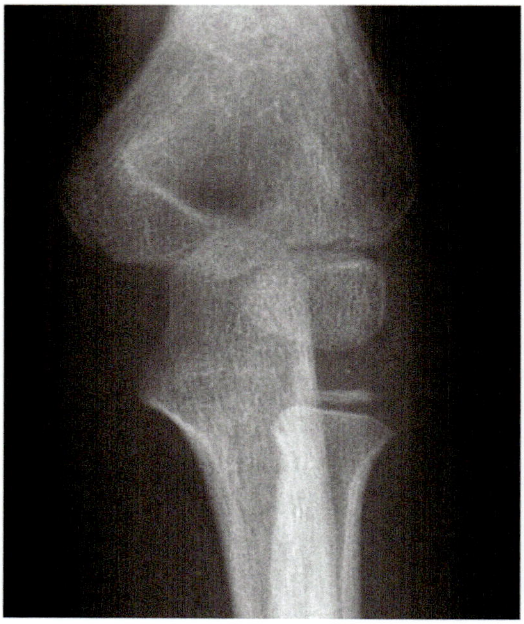

Fig. 7.4 3 Years: ossification center radial head

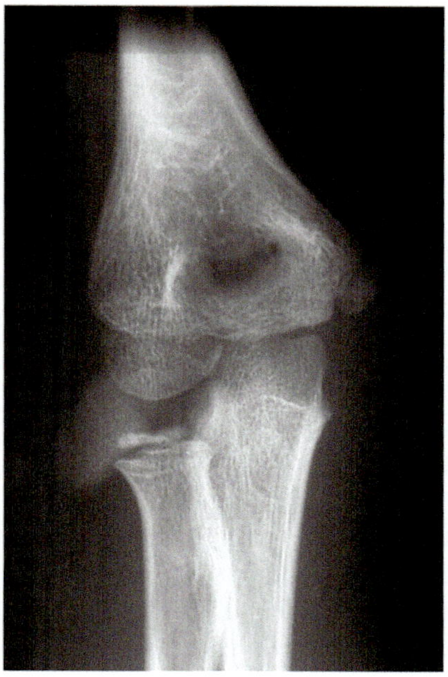

Fig. 7.5 8 Years: Ossification center medial epicondyle

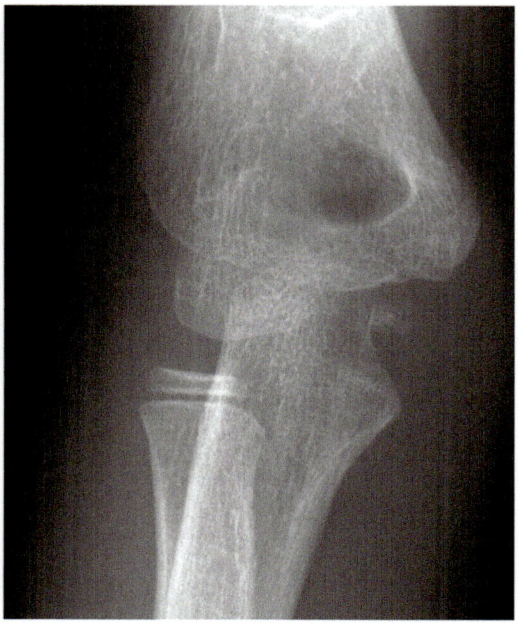

Fig. 7.6 12 Years: ossification center trochlea

7.2 Supracondylar Humerus Fractures

Incidence, Mechanism of Injury, and Clinical Presentation

Elbow lesions have an overall incidence of 7–9% of all fractures, of which 86.4% involve the distal humerus. Further breakdown shows 69.8% supracondylar fractures, 16.9% lateral condyle fractures, 12.5% avulsions of the medial epicondyle, and fewer than 1% medial condyle or T-fractures. Thus, the total incidence of supracondylar fractures is about 5–6%.

Supracondylar humerus fracture is a characteristic pediatric injury; shortly before the growth plate closes, its frequency diminishes, replaced by elbow dislocations. The classic peak age of injury is around 5 years. The etiology is generally a fall on the outstretched, hyperextended arm. Usually, they are bracing themselves during a fall. The olecranon is levered into the olecranon fossa, and a fracture occurs in the metaphysis of the distal humerus. Thus, in most cases, it is an extension injury; only occasionally (approx. 2%) are flexion injuries caused by a direct fall onto a partially flexed elbow. Injuries can be seen best on lateral x-ray using the anterior humeral line, the so called Roger's line (Fig. 7.7).

The history includes an injury consistent with this pattern, usually a fall. The clinical picture depends on the amount of displacement and is characterized by significant hematoma and elbow swelling. When there is displacement, deformity of the joint is unmistakable. Circulation must be assessed by palpating peripheral pulses. Peripheral nerves must be evaluated for both sensory and motor function, although this can be difficult. The radial nerve is assessed by extending the wrist and fingers, the median nerve by flexing the distal phalanx of the index finger, and the ulnar nerve by splaying the fingers. This confirmation is crucial for differentiating intra and postoperative nerve lesions.

Classification and Treatment Concept

The Von Laer classification with 4 types of fractures often used, but the classifications of Gartland and Baumann and others are also common used. These systems distinguish three to four different fracture types (Fig. 7.8).

Type I is a non-displaced fracture. Type II is displaced in the sagittal plane. 98% of these cases show deviation towards anterior (antecurvation), with only occasional posterior deviation (recurvation). Stable injuries (maximum 30° antecurvation) should be distinguished from impending instability (antecurvation >30° with lateral translation). Type III injuries are displaced in two planes with malrotation. Type IV is a completely displaced fracture. Some classifications do not differentiate Types III and IV. The epiphyseal disruption (Salter-Harris I injury) and occurs only in newborns and up to 1 year of age (Table 7.1, Figs 7.9, 7.10, and 7.11).

While Type I injuries are always treated conservatively (Table 7.2). Type II injuries (Table 7.3) can be treated with reduction, cast immobilization, and a collar and cuff sling, but also with operative reduction and wire fixation. Type III and IV injuries (Table 7.4) are always reduced and retained with drilled wires.

The technical aspects of the treatment of distal humerus fractures are indicated in Table 7.5.

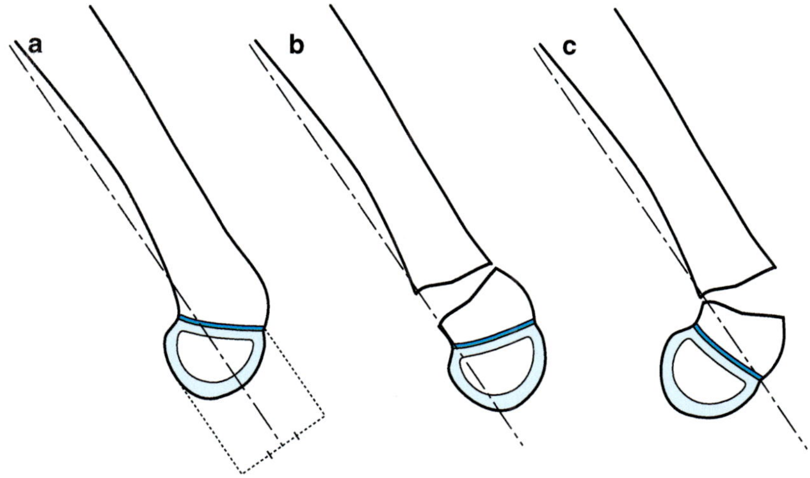

Fig. 7.7 Anterior humeral line to diagnose a supracondylar humerus fracture on lateral x-ray. (**a**) Physiological finding: lengthening of the anterior humeral cortex cuts the capitellum at the transition from mid to posterior third. (**b**) Extension fracture: the intersection lies further anterior. (**c**) Flexion fracture: the intersection lies further posterior

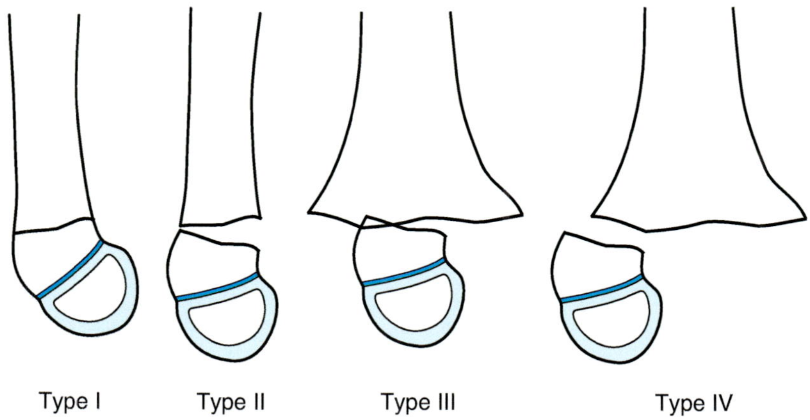

Fig. 7.8 Classification of supracondylar humerus fractures acc. Von Laer

Table 7.1 Salter-Harris I injury—epiphyseal disruption (Fig. 7.9)

Special features	Extremely rare, occurs in newborns and up to 1 year of age, possible birth trauma, Exclude child abuse Epiphysis is not visible in newborns; secondary fracture signs such as fat-pad are unreliable; thus, diagnosis is not simple	
Diagnostic approach	AP and lateral x-ray (Fig 7.10a, b); initially sometimes not visible Alternatively ultrasound to demonstrate fracture MRI in exceptional cases (Fig. 7.11a, b) x-ray control in cases of persistent complaints; pronounced callus formation and metaphyseal consolidation during healing course	
Treatment goal/ limits of correction	No malrotation, no varus or valgus >10° Theoretically, spontaneous correction is only possible in the plane of motion (sagittal up to 20° ante/recurvation) up to age 5 or 6 years	
Primary treatment	Medical analgesia; upper arm plaster splint	
Conservative treatment		
Indication	Almost always, except in non-reducible fractures	
Approach	2–3 weeks upper arm cast	
Follow up	Once cast is removed, release for independent movements; in the first year of life, physical therapy is impractical	
Radiology controls	Day 4–5: position check in cases of impending instability, e.g. by ultrasound, otherwise no clinical consolidation check, indolent callus	
Return to sports	Not applicable	
Operative treatment		
Indication	In cases of malrotation or complete displacement	
Approach	Closed reduction with clinical control; reduction result not visible on x-ray; ultrasound controls Percutaneous K-wire fixation if needed Open reduction and percutaneous K-wire fixation for clinical signs of complete displacement	
Follow up	2–3 weeks upper arm plaster splint	
Radiology controls	Postoperative position check, before hardware removal, cast-free for consolidation check (at 3–4 weeks)	
Hardware removal	At 3 weeks; consolidation check before hardware removal	
Return to sports	Not applicable	
Complications	Overlooked injury in mostly young babies Deviation of the elbow axis (mostly due to malrotation; occasionally because of radial overgrowth) Nerve lesions, also difficult to determine (avoid iatrogenic damage to the ulnar nerve, traumatic damage to radial and median nerves, then always motor and sensory deficits) Vascular injury Rare compartment syndrome	
Growth disturbance	Cubitus varus/valgus are theoretically possible from asymmetrical growth, incidental, rare, not pronounced with malrotation not addressed, combined deformity with clinical Cubitus varus is possible	
Follow up	Elbows should be examined for axial asymmetry and growth irregularities until there is unlimited function and comparable axes	
Classification	AO: 13-E/1.1-3	LiLa: 1.3.s.1.0-2.

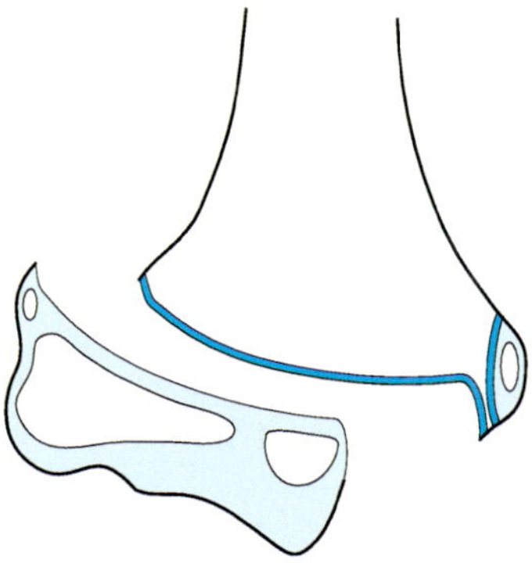

Fig. 7.9 Epiphysiolysis of distal humerus, type Salter-Harris I

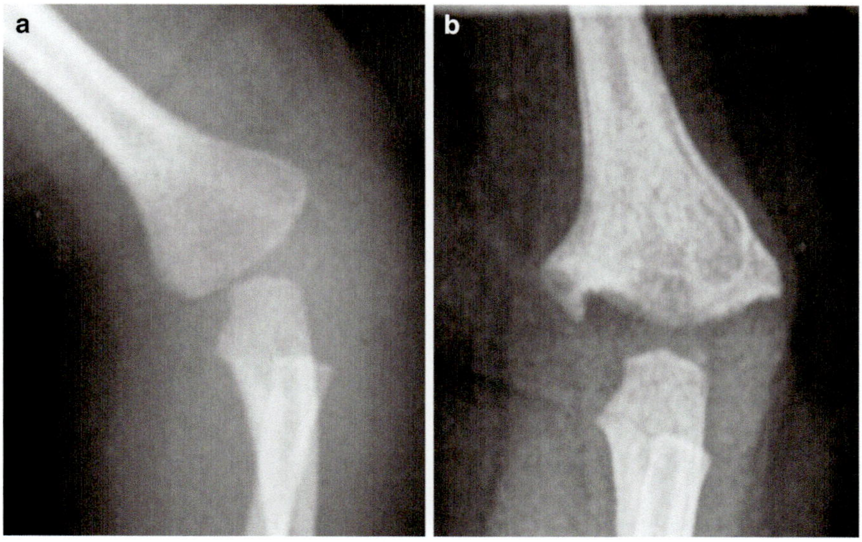

Fig. 7.10 Epiphysiolysis of distal humerus, infant, 4 months, child abuse. (**a**) Trauma image. (**b**) After cast immobilization, metaphyseal consolidation visible

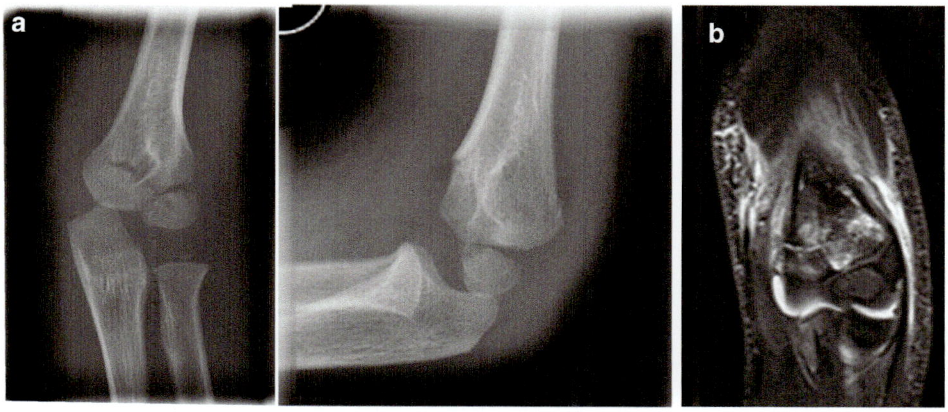

Fig. 7.11 Salter-Harris-I injury. Epiphysiolysis with metaphyseal fracture of the distal humerus; conservative treatment. (**a**) Trauma image, (**b**) MRI

Table 7.2 Supracondylar Humerus Fracture Type I without displacement (Fig. 7.12)

Special features	Always preceded by commensurate trauma Minimal swelling and pain-limited movement These are non-displaced, stable fractures	
Diagnostic approach	AP and lateral x-ray; fat-pad sign (!), anterior humeral line normal (Figs. 7.13 and 7.14) Sometimes not evident initially, only during secondary diagnosis at 10–14 days there is a periosteal reaction	
Treatment goal/limits of correction	Analgesia Since there is no displacement, healing is uncomplicated	
Primary treatment	Pain control, upper-arm plaster splint or collar and cuff sling	
Conservative treatment		
Indication	Always, because no displacement or complications are expected	
Approach	2–3 weeks upper-arm plaster splint or collar and cuff sling (Fig. 7.15)	
Follow up	After cast-removal, independent movements, physical therapy not necessary	
Radiology controls	No controls necessary	
Return to sports	2–4 weeks after consolidation	
Operative treatment		
Indication	None	
Approach	Not applicable	
Follow up	See above	
Radiology controls	Not necessary	
Hardware removal	Not applicable	
Return to sports	See above	
Complications	Asymmetrical growth is theoretically possible, but there have been only poorly documented individual cases and rather unlikely	
Growth disturbance	See above	
Follow up	Not necessary	
Classification	AO: 13-M/3.1-3.I	LiLa: 1.3.s.3.0-2.

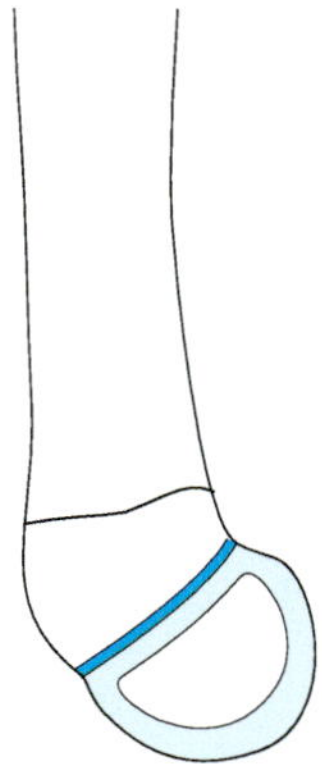

Fig. 7.12 Supracondylar humerus fracture Type I

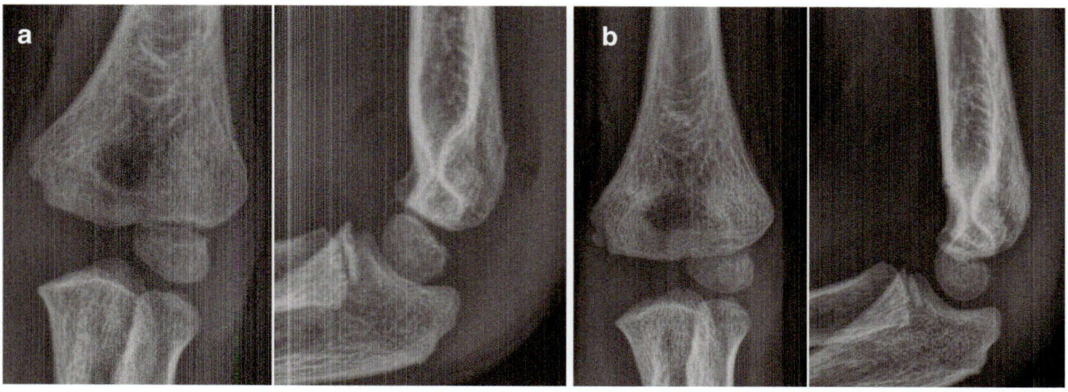

Fig. 7.13 Supracondylar fracture Type I in an 8 year old boy; conservative treatment. (**a**) Trauma image, fat-pad sign (**b**) Consolidation after 3 weeks

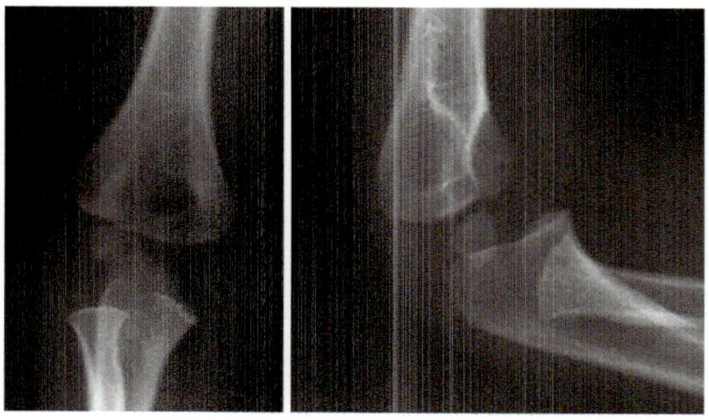

Fig. 7.14 Supracondylar fracture Type I in an 5 year old boy; indication for conservative treatment

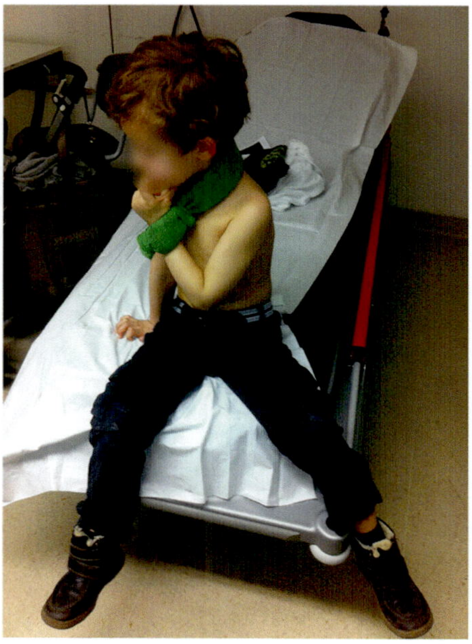

Fig. 7.15 Individually adapted Blount sling for treatment of Type I supracondylar fracture

Table 7.3 Supracondylar humerus fracture Type II (displaced in the sagittal plane) (Fig. 7.16)

Special features	Common injury; in >95% of cases, there is antecurvation; recurvation deformity is rare (approx. 2%) Differentiation between stable (only antecurvation to a maximum 20°) and impending unstable fractures (antecurvation at least 30°, recurvation; evidence for translation in the frontal plane) Certain combinations of deformity are possible, which can be aggravated by anterior rotation of the lateral condyle; the consequence is Cubitus varus	
Diagnostic approach	AP and lateral x-ray; fat-pad sign, anterior humeral line runs too far to the flexor side	
Treatment goal/limits of correction	No malrotation, no varus or valgus Theoretically, spontaneous correction is only possible in the plane of motion (sagittal up to 20° ante/recurvation) up to age around 6 years.	
Primary treatment	Medical analgesia Upper-arm plaster splint	
Conservative treatment		
Indication	In stable fractures; conditional in impending unstable fractures in the age below 6 years; healing with cuff and collar in good position is possible (Fig. 7.17a, b)	
Approach	In good position: upper-arm plaster splint Compensation of persisting antecurvation deformity by reduction in hyperflexion under analgesia; immobilization with collar and cuff sling possible	
Follow up	3 weeks after removal of upper-arm plaster splint or collar and cuff sling	
Radiology controls	At 3–5 days to exclude malrotation At 4 weeks for consolidation check	
Return to sports	With almost unlimited mobility of the elbow joint	
Operative treatment		
Indication	In older children, when Roger's line does not meet the capitulum anymore; in impending unstable fractures if reduction is unsuccessful or when malrotation occurs or stabile fixation is safer for after-treatment (compliance)	
Approach	Closed reduction under general anesthesia, supine with arm bench Exclude evidence of rotation Percutaneous crossed K-wire transfixion radial and ulnar with open localisation of ulnar nerve!) Open reduction is only required when closed reduction is impossible Percutaneous lateral parallel or crossed K-wire fixation Alternatively, descending ESIN or lateral external fixator (with localization of radial nerve) Stable fixation and intraoperative control of mobility (pay attention to ipsilateral forearm axis and free extension/flexion to 120°, detailed description in technical section!) Figures 7.18 and 7.19	
Follow up	With percutaneous K-wire fixation, wire ends can protrude above the skin; 3–4 weeks upper-arm plaster splint With external fixator or ESIN, cast-free follow up is possible	
Radiology controls	At 3–4 weeks for consolidation check	
Hardware removal	At 3–4 weeks	
Return to sports	When there is free mobility of the elbow joint	
Complications	Growth irregularities with development of cubitus varus/valgus very rare and incidental; Fluoroscopy and radiological controls can only give approximate assessments; thus, clinical controls are necessary The ulnar nerve can be injured in up to 15% of closed K-wire fixation procedures; thus, the nerve should be exposed through a small incision if it is not readily palpable and easily protected	
Growth disturbance	Cubitus varus/valgus are theoretically possible from asymmetrical growth, incidental, less pronounced version happens very rarely Cubitus varus mostly due to overlooked malalignment during initial treatment	
Follow up	Until free function and axial symmetry Controls of axial asymmetry or growth irregularity	
Classification	AO: 13-M/3.1-3.II	LiLa: 1.3.s.3.0-2.

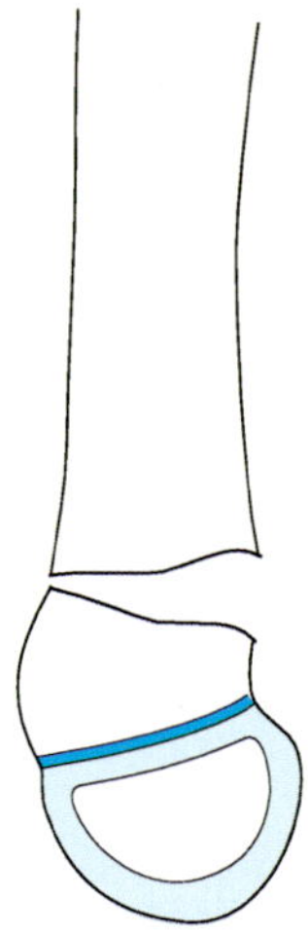

Fig. 7.16 Supracondylar humerus fracture Type II (Scheme)

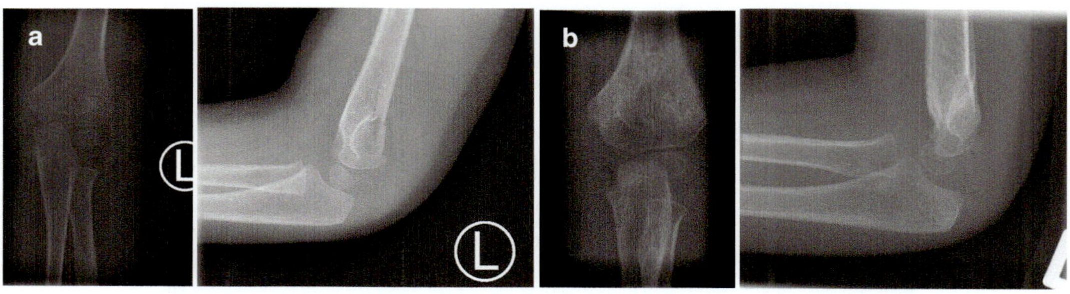

Fig. 7.17 Supracondylar fracture Type II in a 2.5 year old girl. (**a**) Trauma image, (**b**) Consolidation after 4 weeks

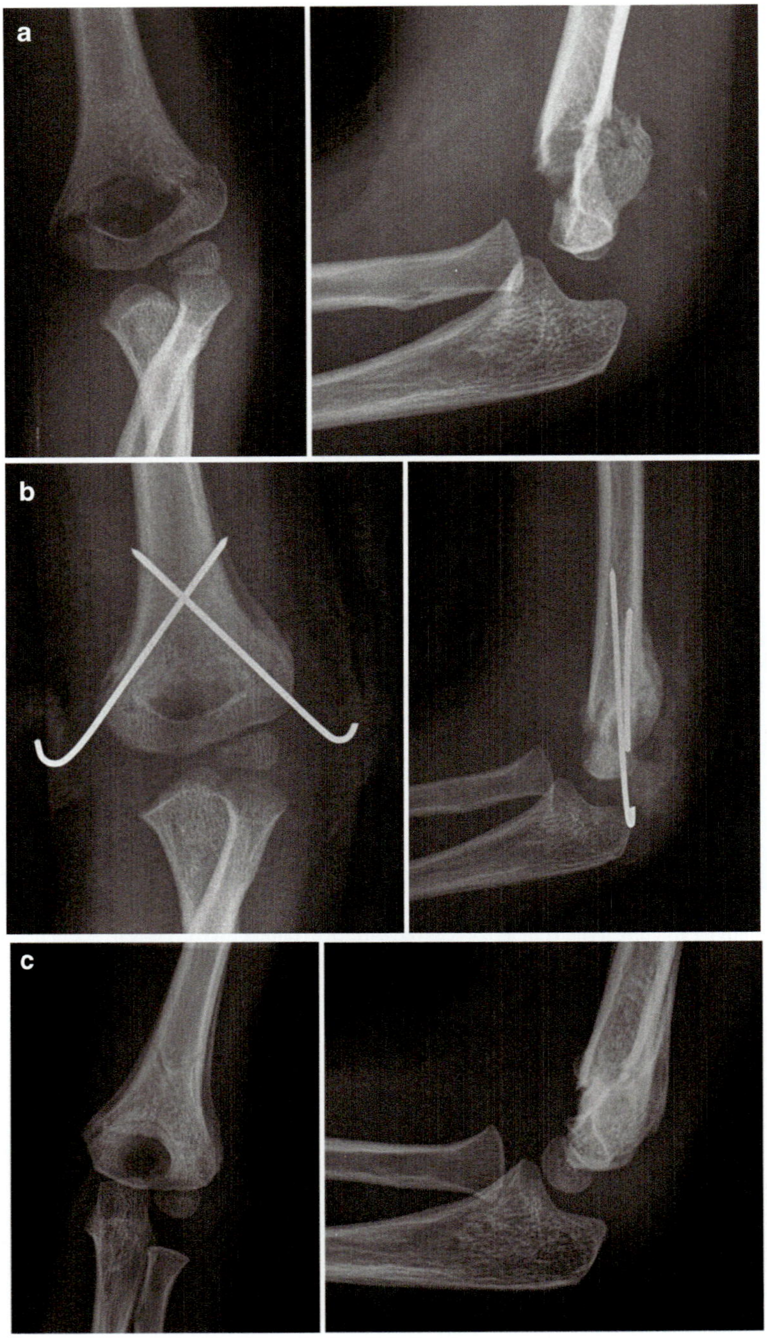

Fig. 7.18 Supracondylar humerus fracture Type II in a 4 year old girl. (**a**) Trauma image, (**b**) Indication for reduction and stabilization in instable situation with 2 crossed K-wires after closed reduction and upper arm plaster. After 4 weeks metal removal. (**c**) Consolidation and callus formation after 8 weeks

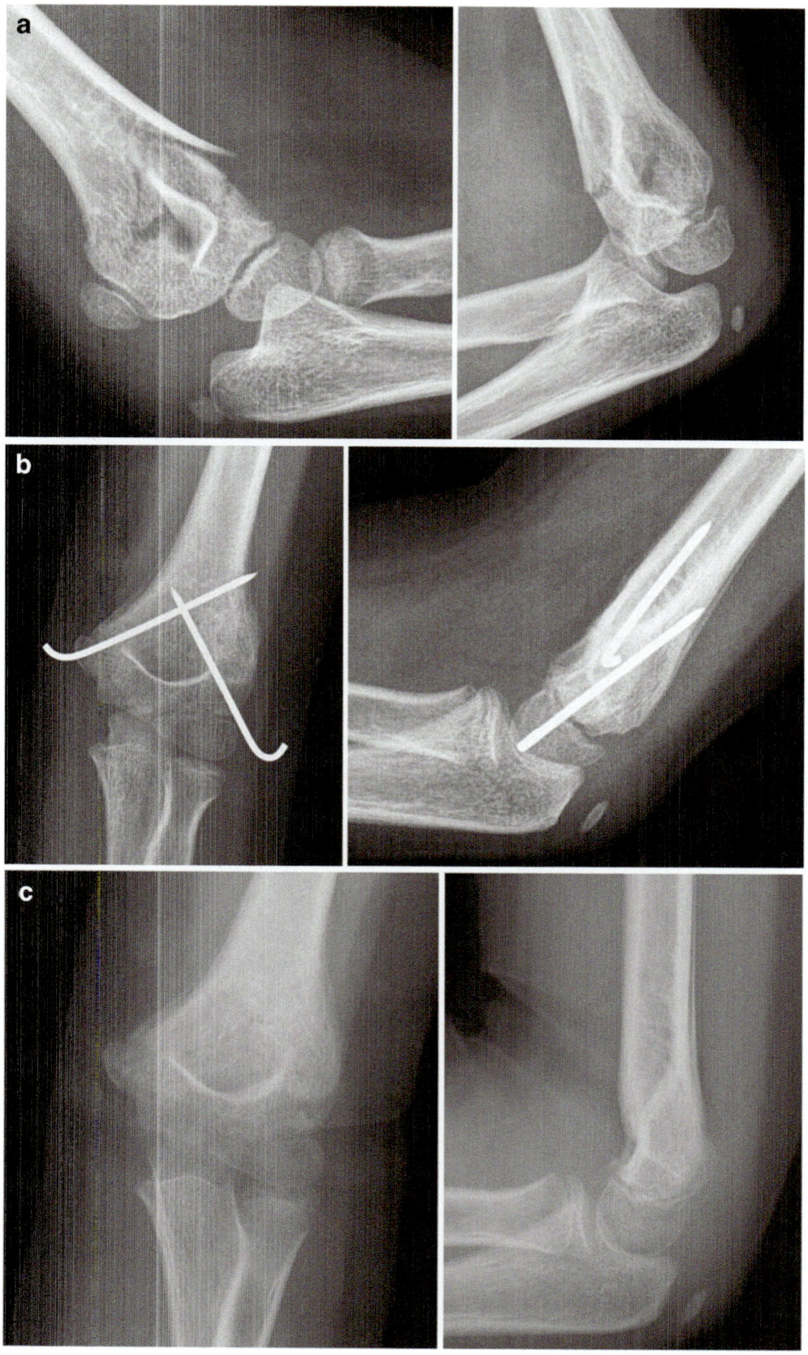

Fig. 7.19 Supracondylar humerus fracture Type II in a 8 year old boy. (**a**) Trauma image, (**b**) 4 Weeks after closed reduction and crossed K-wire osteosynthesis, (**c**) Consolidation image after 6 weeks

Table 7.4 Supracondylar humerus fracture Type III and IV. Supracondylar humerus fracture Type III (displaced in three planes with malrotation). Supracondylar humerus fracture Type IV (displaced in all planes; no contact between fragments) (Fig. 7.20)

Special features	Common injury; deformity is clearly visible on presentation; once reduced, assessment is always approximate (risk of overlooked malalignment!); marks can indicate malrotation, which can lead to complex deformity over time; anesthesia is always necessary to treat these fractures, and definitive treatment should always be attempted under anesthesia; clear indication for surgery!	
Diagnostic approach	x-ray elbow in two planes (in pronounced deformity, one plane is sufficient to indicate the need for surgery); assess peripheral circulation (Pulse or and Doppler sonography if needed) and nervous function (sensory and motor) as thoroughly as possible	
Treatment goal/limits of correction	No malrotation, no varus or valgus deformity accepted; theoretically, corrective compensation can only be expected in the plane of motion (sagittal up to 20° ante-/recurvation) until age 5 or 6 years	
Primary treatment	Medical analgesia; upper-arm plaster splint, rapid surgical organization	
Conservative treatment		
Indication	Not indicated because secondary displacement with complex malalignment occurs in 30–50%, with frequent need for repeat reduction	
Operative treatment		
Indication	For all displaced fractures; because they are unstable and most with axial deviation and malrotation as well as considerable pain; additional risk of neurovascular injury because of displacement	
Approach	Closed (two attempts) or open reduction under general anesthesia Fixation with K-wire (Figs. 7.21 and 7.22), ESIN, external fixator (more details in technical section below)	
Follow up	In percutaneous K-wire fixation, ends do not need to be below the skin because protrusion makes removal possible as an outpatient without anesthesia; 3–4 weeks upper-arm plaster splint With external fixator or ESIN, cast-free follow up is possible	
Radiology controls	Definitive intraoperative or postoperative controls; At 3–4 weeks for consolidation check (before hardware removal) (note: usually no strict AP films are present because the arm is bent in plaster!)	
Hardware removal	At 3–4 weeks	
Return to sports	When there is free mobility of the elbow joint	
Complications	Growth irregularities with development of cubitus varus/valgus rare and incidental; fluoroscopy and radiological controls can only give approximate assessments; thus, clinical controls are necessary; comparison with uninjured arm is clinically recommended in cases of closed percutaneous K-wire fixation Ulnar nerve injury in up to 15% of cases, thus exposure (open) or protection (mini-incision, guarding with finger) of the nerve during the procedure	
Growth disturbance	Growth irregularities with the development of cubitus varus/valgus through uneven growth is very rare and incidental; Cubitus varus mostly due to overlooked malalignment during initial treatment (see Chap. 19).	
Follow up	Until free function and axial symmetry Controls of axial asymmetry or growth irregularities	
Classification	AO: 13-M/3.1-3.III (IV)	LiLa: 1.3.s.3.0-2.

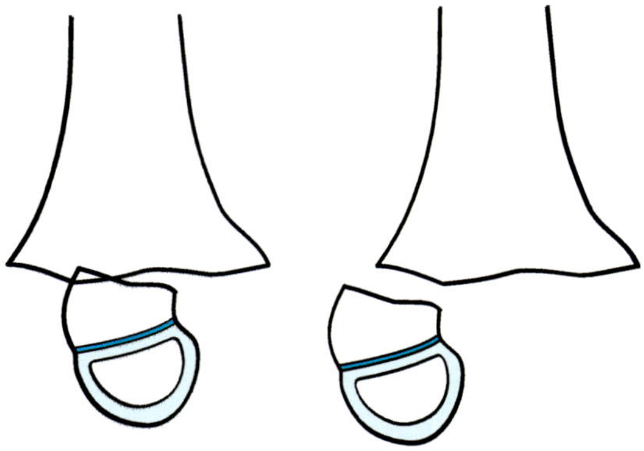

Fig. 7.20 Supracondylar humerus fracture Type III and IV (scheme)

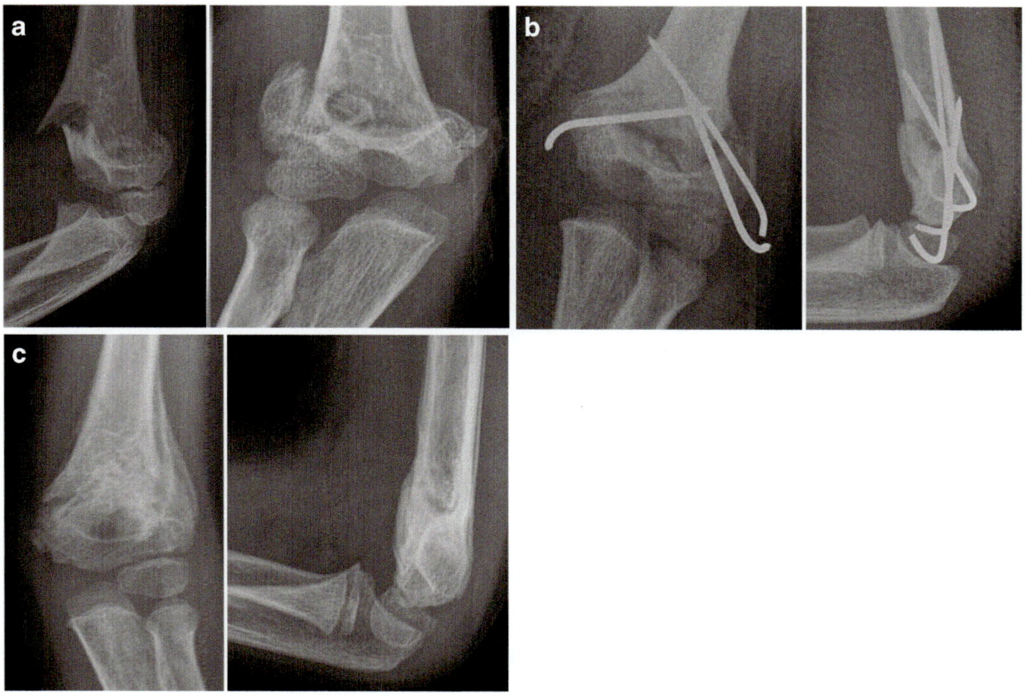

Fig. 7.21 Supracondylar humerus fracture Type III. (**a**) Trauma image, (**b**) 2 Weeks after closed reduction and K-wire fixation and upper arm plaster, (**c**) Correct healing with new callus after 3 months

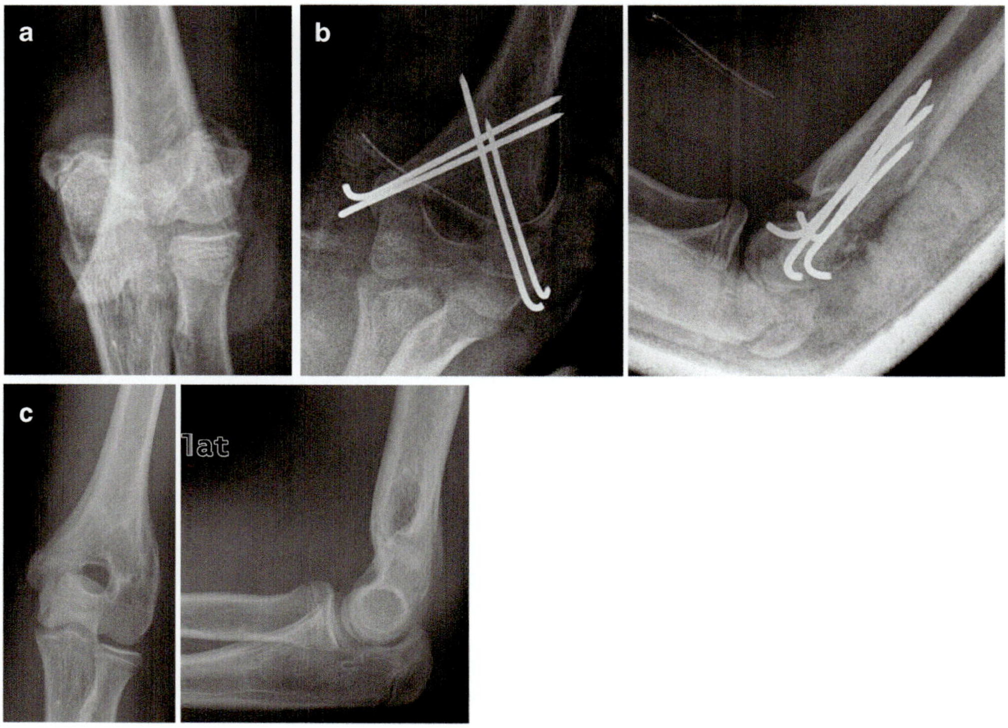

Fig. 7.22 Supracondylar humerus fracture Type IV of a 13.5 year old boy after fall; open fracture with median nerve elongation and brachial artery disrupture. (**a**) Trauma image, (**b**) Reduction and K-wire stabilization and vein graft. (**c**) Healing after 1 year with correction of antecurvation with free function and remission of median nerve function

Table 7.5 Technical aspects distal humerus

Material	K-wires thickness 1.4–1.8 mm External fixator (to 2.5 mm) ESIN (size 1/3 shaft diameter)
Positioning	Supine, arm on armrest; Optional tourniquet for the open approach
Approach	Medial approach to protect the ulnar nerve, possibly combined with a lateral approach, an alternative is posterior approach in prone position
Special considerations	During crossed percutaneous K-wire fixation, there is a risk of ulnar nerve injury with troublesome but generally reversible paresis (Fig. 7.23) With lateral external fixator placement, radial nerve injury, varus malalignment due to incidental growth irregularities are possible but extremely rare (Fig. 7.24) After surgical treatment, especially with the posterior approach, persistent range of motion limitations are possible
Operative principle	Reduction under general anesthesia with relaxation (important!), as if shaking hands with the patient under constant tension and the elbow joint flexes slowly with proximal to distal dorsal manipulation. Varus and valgus malalignments are compensated for with pronation and supination, respectively, followed by maximum flexion (caution: hyperflexion can over-reduce the fracture into the flexion type), the lateral view is especially useful to detect malrotation. **K-wires:** the radial wire is inserted first, visualized under lateral beam at approx. 30° to the longitudinal axis of the upper arm in the humeral center, the wires must lie entirely in the lateral and medial pillars With crossed K-wire fixation, the medial wire is inserted from the anteriorly palpable tip at the same angle (secure palpation but much safer is open exposure of the ulnar nerve!); the crossing point of the wires always proximal to the fracture; otherwise, fracture rotation is possible! For the alternative, somewhat less stable parallel fixation, two wires are inserted parallel through the lateral condyle with a separating distance of 1 cm At the end of the surgery, a clinical control of the axis and movement has to be performed (Fig. 7.25).
	Lateral external fixator, 2 stable wires (2–2.5 mm) are inserted from lateral into the epiphysis and the metaphysis (caution radial nerve!). Then, reduction of the fracture is possible and temporary fixation with the rod; control by x-ray in lateral and AP view. Fine correction possible with loosening and fixation of the ext. fixator. This procedure is in particular useful, of reduction and fixation with K-wires fails and needs to many approaches. In largely dislocated fractures, also 4 pins can be used (Fig. 7.26 new) Additionally, 2 K-wires can be introduced thereafter to stabilize the reduced situation (Fig. 7.27). **ESIN**: incision below the insertion of the deltoid muscle on the proximal upper arm and 2 windows; after advancing two ESIN, final reduction and divergent (S-type) insertion of the two intramedullary nails is performed under fluoroscopy (challenging because of the narrow, column-shaped medullary canal) (Figs. 7.28 and 7.29)
Hardware removal	K-wire fixation at 3–4 weeks External fixator: at 3–4 weeks ESIN: elective at 3–4 months
Special features	Assessment of sagittal malalignment using the anterior humeral line (Fig. 7.7); normally, this intersects the middle of the lateral condyle's ossification center; when there is antecurvation, the line is anterior to the capitellum, and in recurvation posterior to the capitellum. Correction in small childs is possible (Fig. 7.30), but not sure. For ESIN, conspicuous scar formation on the proximal upper-arm should be discussed

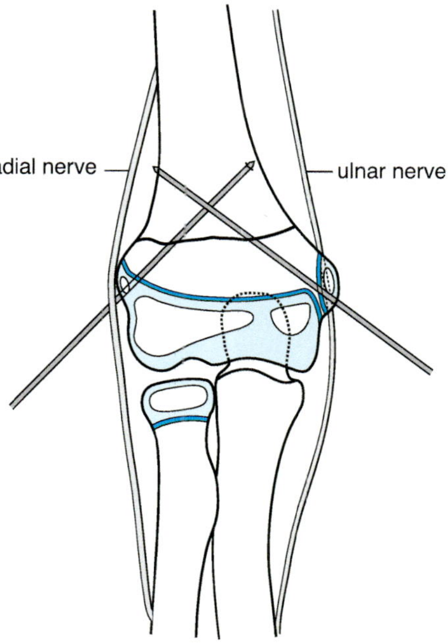

Fig. 7.23 Crossed K-wire transfixion in supracondylar humerus fracture, scheme, The K-wires can be left above the skin in order to remove them easier after 4 weeks. Steril dressing under the upper arm plaster is necessary and a weekly control

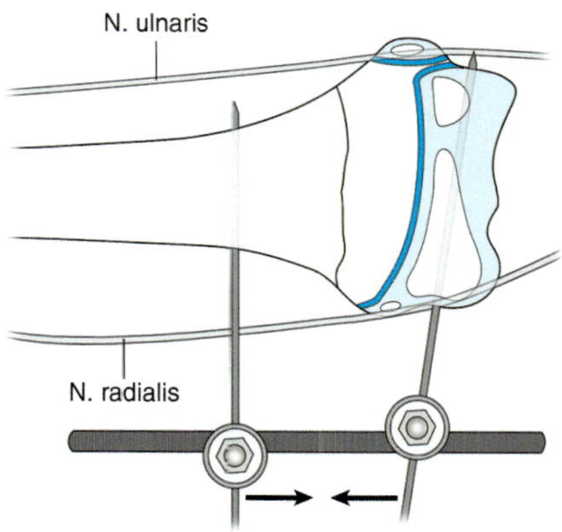

Fig. 7.24 Lateral external fixator for supracondylar humerus fracture. This is particular useful in difficult reduction

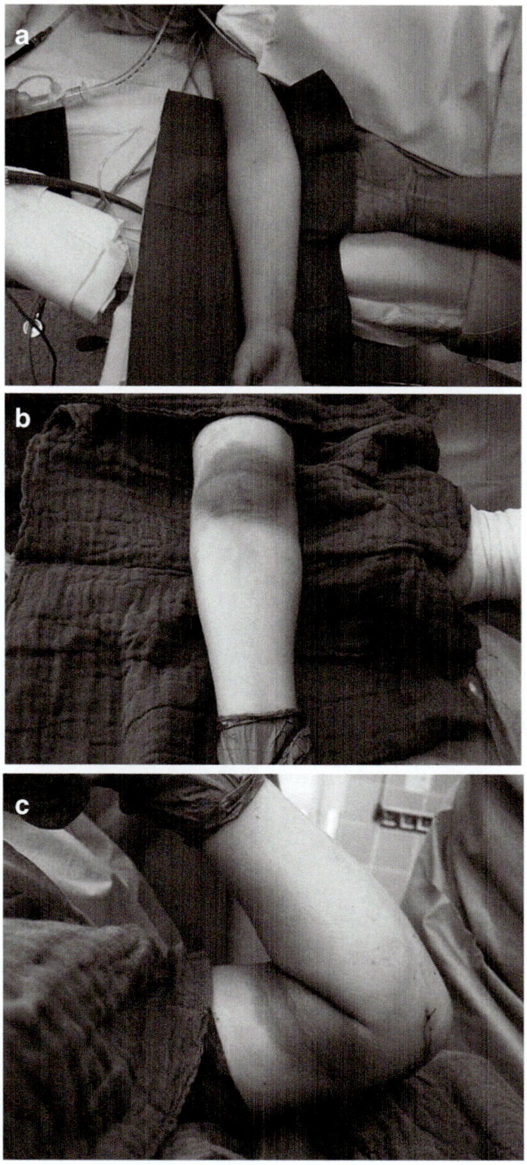

Fig. 7.25 Reduction of supercondylar Elbow fracture (**a**–**b**) Intraoperatively, the slightly valgus elbow axis must be assessed for symmetry to the contralateral side. (**c**) If there is full extension, flexion is possible up to at least 120°, so a relevant deformity is excluded

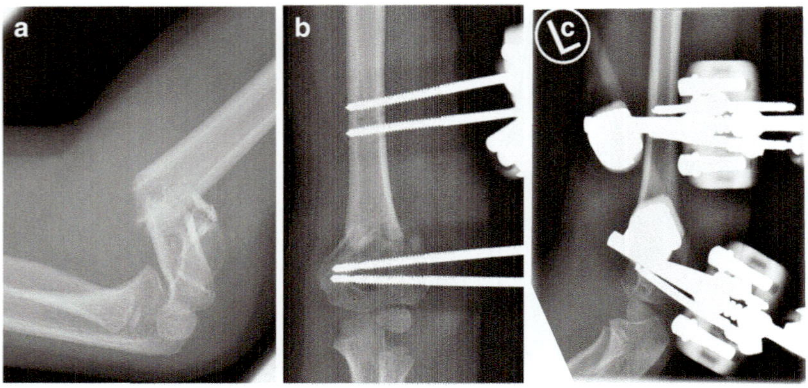

Fig. 7.26 Largely dislocated distal humerus fracture in an 8 year old boy. (**a**) Trauma image, (**b**, **c**) Reduction and stabilization with an external fixateur above the growth plate

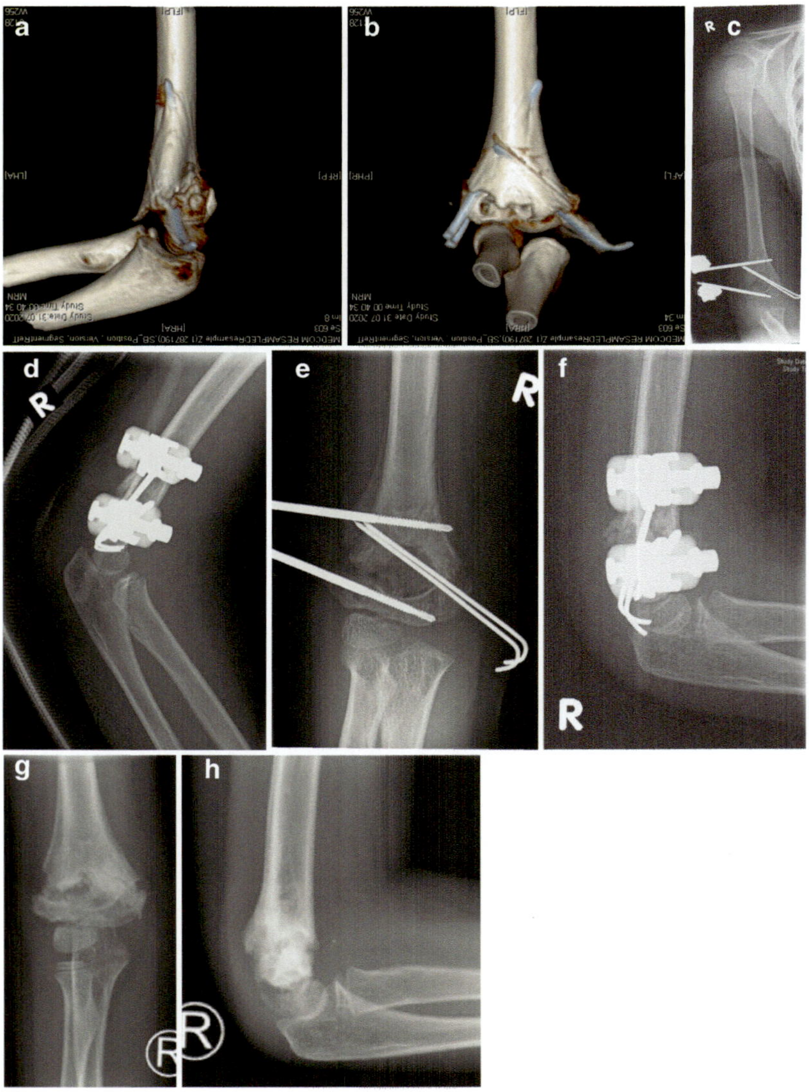

Fig. 7.27 Insufficient reduction of a supracondylar humerus fracture, type 4. (**a**, **b**) CT scan of insufficiently reduced fracture with K-wires; (**c**, **d**) Postoperative image after metal removal, reduction with external fixateur and additional 2 K wires; (**e**, **f**) Healing after 4 weeks; (**g**, **h**) Consolidation after metal removal in good axis with good function

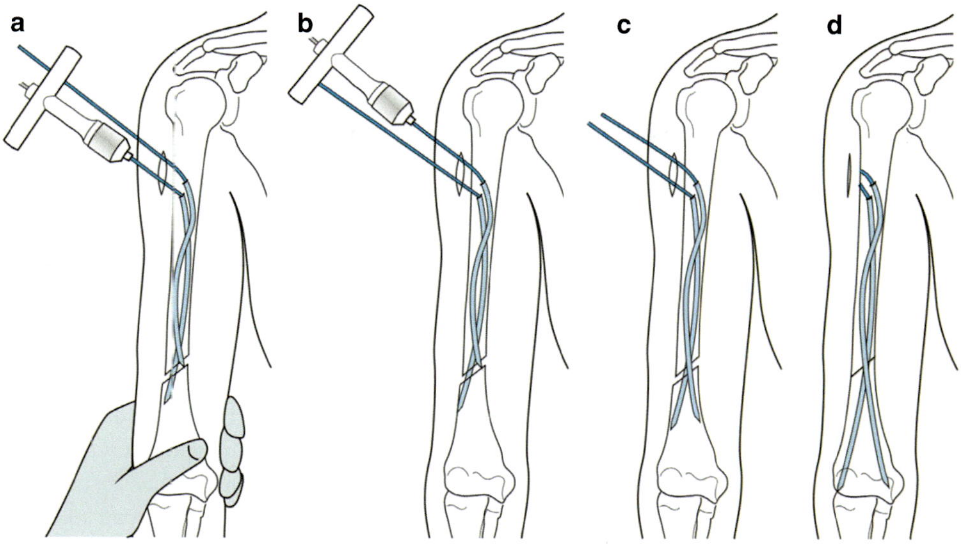

Fig. 7.28 Descending elastic stable intramedullary nailing (ESIN). Entry point proximal upper arm; 1 nail is inserted in C-form, a second nail needs to be twisted by 180° and is inserted in S-form. Stabilization with the tips of the 2 nails in the distal fragment

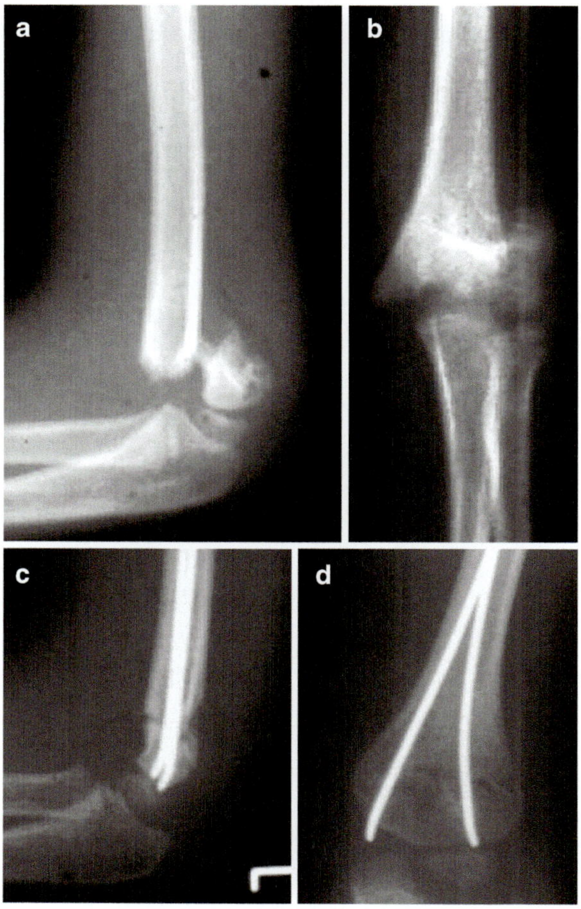

Fig. 7.29 (**a**, **b**) Supracondylar humerus fracture type IV, in which there is no contact between fracture surfaces. (**c**, **d**) The fracture was treated with two descending ESIN in axial-appropriate positions after closed reduction

7.3 Distal Humerus Transcondylar Fractures

Incidence, Mechanism of Injury, and Clinical Presentation

Transcondylar humerus fractures—fractures of the lateral and medial condyles and T-fractures—are the second most common pediatric elbow injuries, with 1.8% of all extremity fractures (Fig. 7.30). The most common fracture is the lateral condyle (90%) (Fig. 7.30), followed by the medial condyle and T-fractures (each about 5%). The peak age incidence of lateral condyle fractures is 4–5 years, just under supracondylar humerus fractures. The peak age for medial condyle fractures is around the age of 12 years (Table 7.6).

The trauma mechanism is usually a fall onto the outstretched hand, and occasionally, it is a direct trauma. The extent of transcondylar fractures is often challenging to evaluate because the visible ossification center does not show the joint surface. Thus, assessment of the joint space is only possible indirectly by the displacement of the radial condyle and metaphysal fracture. Only with MRI it may be visualized, but MRI is generally not indicated and necessary in children, requiring sedation or anesthesia.

Thus, it is essential to differentiate displaced from non-displaced lateral condyle fractures (Fig. 7.30a, b) from the x-ray images. The non-displaced variant is called a "hanging fracture" because it is still fixed by the invisible cartilage (see Fig. 7.31a, b). The dorso-lateral displacement shows only the metaphyseal part but not the joint itself. If the joint surface is fractured and thereby the fracture instable, can only be estimated by the fracture fragment's dislocation. This can be judged by a lateral dislocation of the capitulum humeri and a 'gap' in the joint line (Fig. 7.32), by a further dislocation of the metaphyseal part to the dorsal side (Fig. 7.33) or an additional antecurvation of the distal humerus.

In consequence, and since this cartilaginous portion is not visible on x-ray, conservative primary treatment must be followed up every time (!) with a radiological control cast-free (!) after a few days to confirm the initial assessment of stability (Fig. 7.34). If the lateral condyle fragment has further displaced in the x-ray control after 4 days, it is clearly an unstable fracture situation with dislocation of the joint surface that must undergo open surgery (Fig. 7.35). On the other hand, in primarily-displaced fractures, there can be a considerable step formation and malrotation with the joint injury that must be reduced and stabilized surgically (Fig. 7.36).

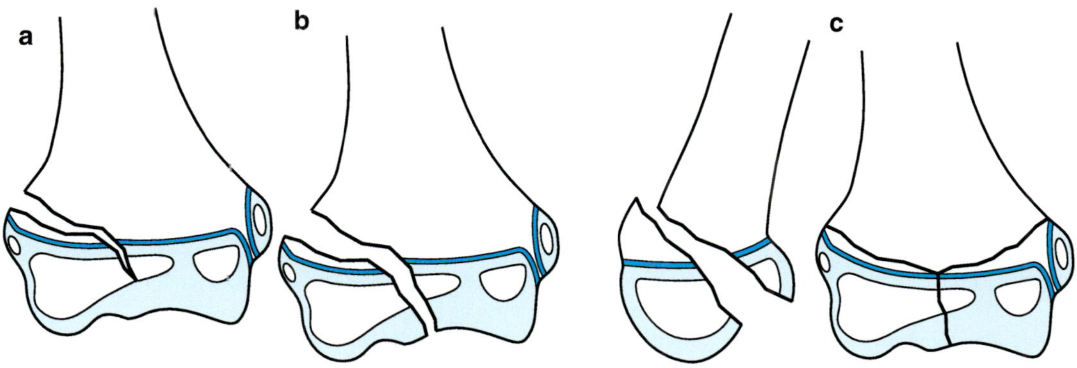

Fig. 7.30 Lateral condyle fracture of the distal humerus. (**a**) Complete, instable fracture A.P. view and lateral view, (**b**) Stable lateral condyle fracture (hanging fracture), (**c**) Y-fracture of the distal humerus

Table 7.6 Distal humerus transcondylar fracture. Fracture of the lateral condyle, the medial condyle, and T-fracture of the distal humerus (Fig. 7.30)

Special features	Risk of non-union and joint malalignment after lateral condyle fractures
Diagnostic approach	AP and lateral x-rays. Indirect signs: lateral soft-tissue swelling and cortical disruption on the AP image; on lateral: fracture line running posterior (proximal) to anterior (distal). Fractured cartilage is not visible radiologically: if it is an incomplete, "hanging" fracture, in which the cartilaginous portion of the joint is stable, there is no risk of secondary displacement; if it is a complete articular fracture, it will progressively displace even with plaster immobilization. This can be differentiated theoretically with MRI Clinical practice, however, is that secondary displacement has to be excluded with a second, cast-free x-ray control on the 4th–6th post-traumatic day
Treatment goal/limits of correction	Stabilization of unstable complete articular fractures to prevent secondary displacement and consequent non-union and to keep growth irregularities to a minimum Because it is an articular fracture, no spontaneous correction can be expected and the dislocation is usually larger than expected from the x-ray; the first principle is anatomical joint reconstruction and secure stabilization
Primary treatment	Upper-arm plaster splint
Conservative treatment	
Indication	Non-displaced stable (incomplete articular, "hanging") fractures (Figs. 7.31 and 7.34)
Approach	Upper-arm cast in 90° position
Follow up	3–4 weeks; spontaneous movements and physical therapy as needed during follow up after cast-removal or immediately postop when there is stable fixation
Radiology controls	4–6 days: x-ray control to exclude secondary displacement without cast Consolidation x-ray at 4 weeks
Return to sports	With free function
Operative treatment	
Indication	Operative treatment of lateral/medial condyle fractures: primary and secondary displaced fractures Operative treatment of T-fractures: primary and secondary displaced fractures
Approach	Operative treatment of lateral/medial condyle fractures: open reduction with visualization of the joint surface, anatomical adjustment, screw fixation of metaphysis and K-wire or screw fixation for the epiphysis if needed; alternatively, 2 divergent K-wires for small children with additional plaster immobilization (Fig. 7.41) (see also Figs. 7.32, 7.33, and 7.35) Operative treatment of T-fractures: open reduction with screw fixation both transverse to the joint line and the metaphyseal are, not crossing the growth plate (Fig. 7.42) (see also Fig. 7.40); when growth plate fusion has begun, a supplemental plate is indicated for mobility-stable fixation
Follow up	Functional as tolerated according to pain
Radiology controls	Postoperative (either during surgery or within the first week), Consolidation check after 4 weeks
Hardware removal	At 12–16 weeks
Return to sports	With free function, movement can be begun immediately with stable fixation
Complications	Most serious problem in fractures of the lateral condyle Overestimation of stability and missing a secondary displacement
Growth disturbance	Risk of partial growth plate fusion and avascular necrosis. However, the typical growth irregularity is a temporary stimulation of the growth plate, which leads to varus alignment after lateral and T-fractures and valgus alignment after medial fractures. The extent of varus after lateral and T-fractures depends on the duration of consolidation and, thus, on fracture stability and fixation method
Follow up	6–12 month checks at least 2 years post-surgery
Classification	AO: 13-E/4.1-3 LiLa: 1.3.a.1-5.0-2.

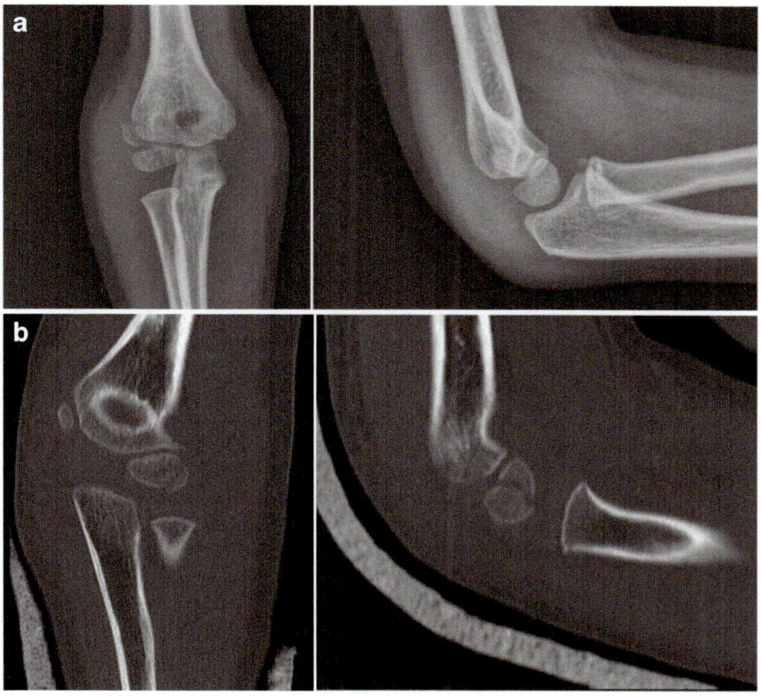

Fig. 7.31 Incomplete articular hanging fracture of the distal radial condyle. Indication for primary conservative therapy. (**a**) X-ray, (**b**) CT scan

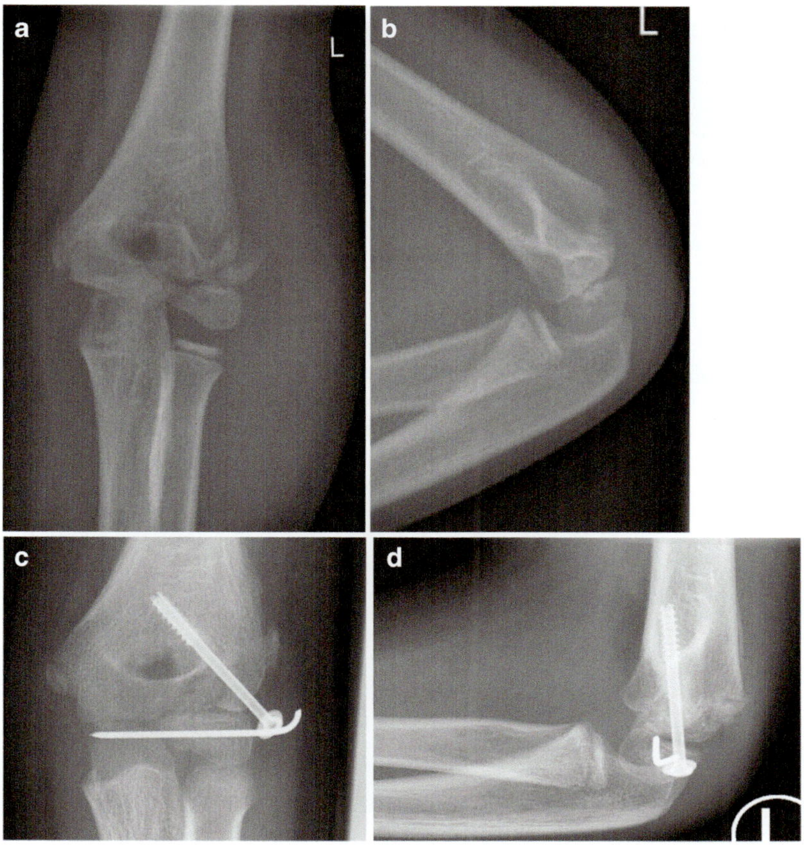

Fig. 7.32 Instable condylus radialis fracture with visible dislocation. (**a**, **b**) Trauma image, (**c**, **d**) After reduction, K-wire in the epiphysis and metaphyseal lag screw 4 mm

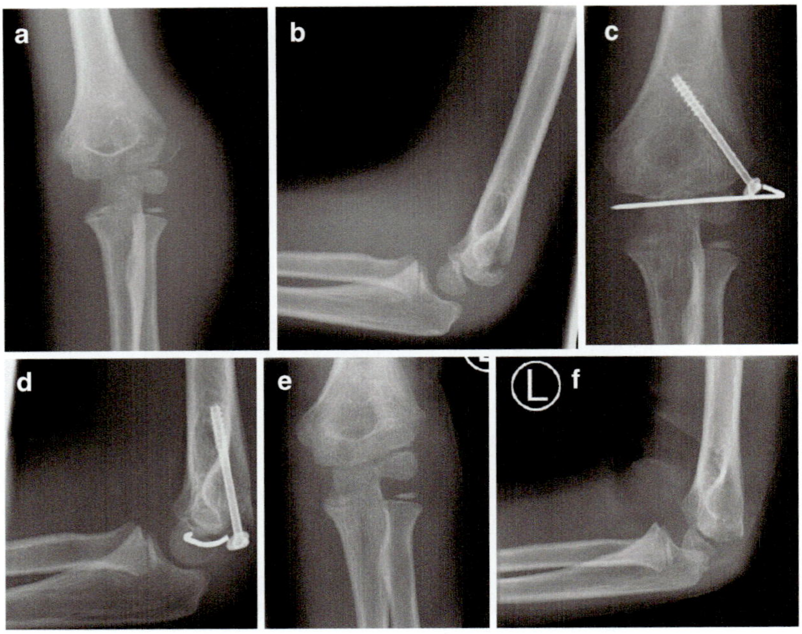

Fig. 7.33 Instable condylus radialis fracture with visible dislocation in A.P. view and lateral view. (**a**, **b**) Trauma image, (**c**, **d**) After reduction, K-wire in the epiphysis and metaphyseal lag screw 4 mm, (**e**, **f**) After metal removal complete healing

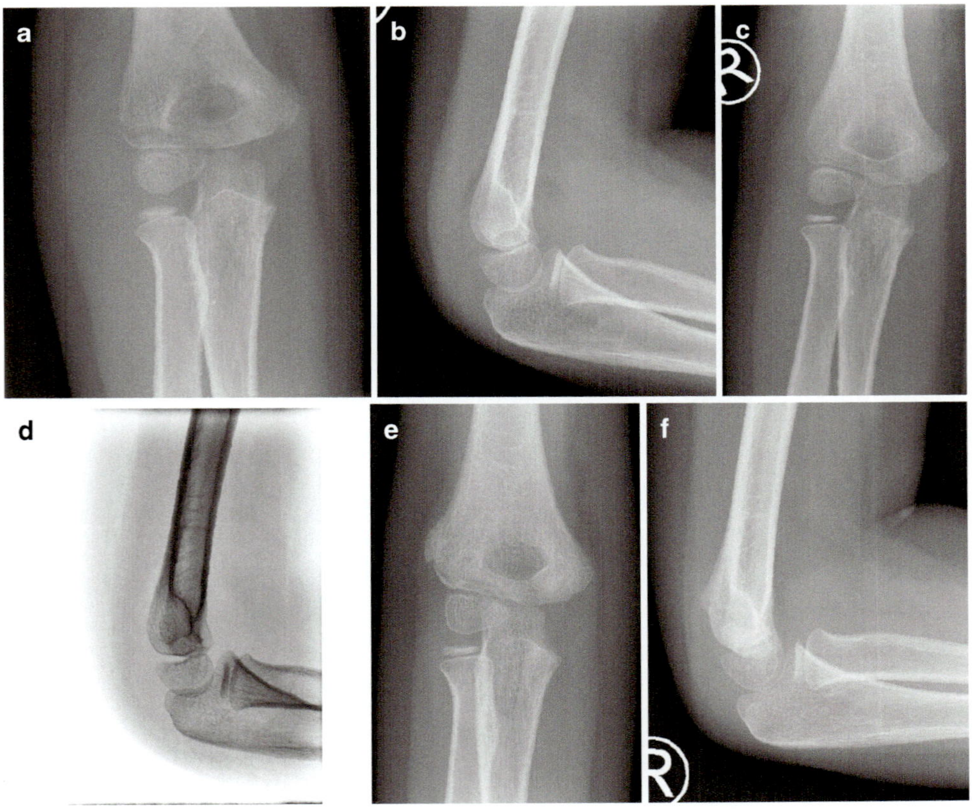

Fig. 7.34 Hanging fracture of the radial condyle in a 6 year old girl. (**a**, **b**) Trauma image, (**c**, **d**) X-ray control after 4 days showing no further dislocation; (**e**, **f**) Healing after 4 weeks in a upper arm plaster

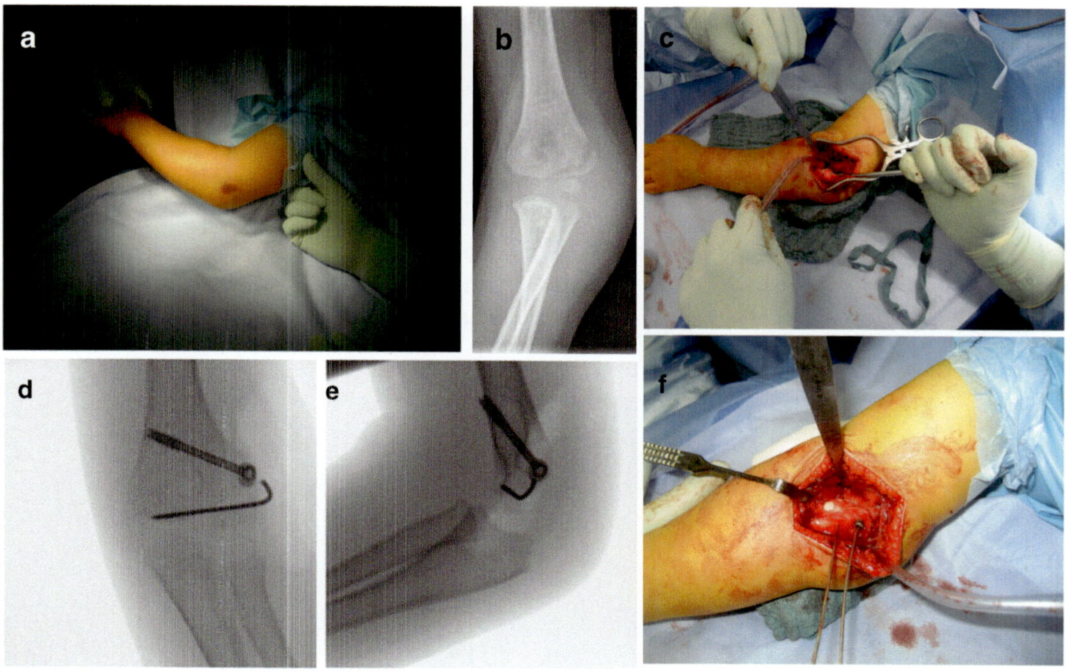

Fig. 7.35 Instable radial condyle fracture (**a**) Swelling and hematoma, (**b**) Trauma image, (**c**) Intraoperative view of displaced radial condyle with fracture gap, (**d**, **e**) Intraoperative x-rays after fixation with K-wire and screw, (**f**) Intraoperative image of reduced radial condyle

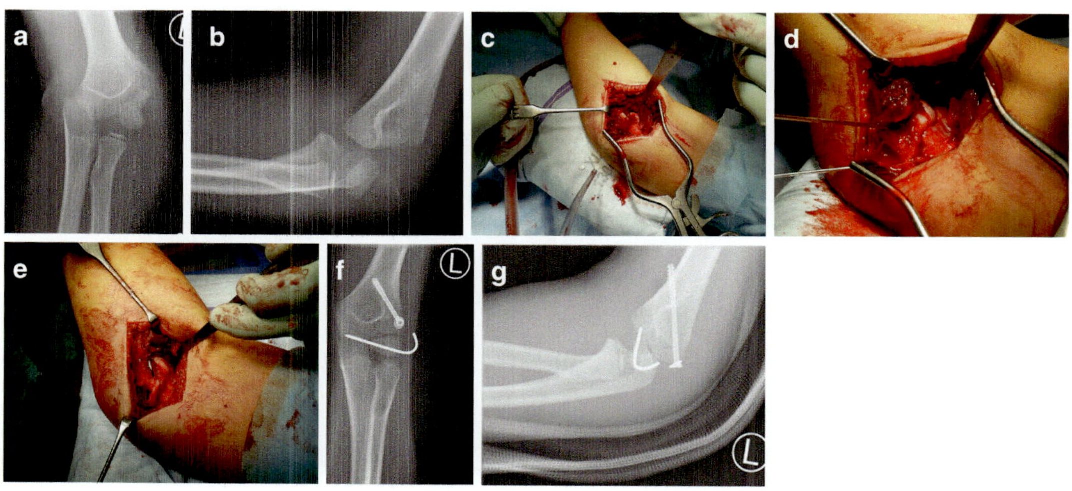

Fig. 7.36 8 years old boy with large radial condyle fracture and subluxation of elbow. (**a**, **b**) Trauma image, (**c**) Intraoperatively completely displaced joint surface, (**d**) Reduction and K-wire fixation, (**e**) After screw and K-wire osteoynsthesis, (**f**, **g**) Postoperative image

Lateral condyle injuries that are missed (Fig. 7.37) instable fractures and not reduced or sufficiently fixed operatively (Fig. 7.38) can lead to significant functional deficits, deformity, non-union, and growth plate closure such as fishtail deformity or cubitus valgus. The instable situation will lead to a subsequent dislocation in a valgus deformity and to non-union with pain and impaired movement. Valgus deformity furthermore may lead to an ulnar nerve irritation. Early secondary reconstruction is the best and most successful treatment option (see Figs. 7.37 and 7.38). Injury of the central growth plate leads to a central fusion and pathological growth of the distal humerus with a fish-tail deformity, usually without large movement restrictions. Closure of the radial part of the growth plate may lead to a valgus deformity and ulnar nerve irritation. Further details see also the chapter on upper extremity reconstruction (Chap. 19).

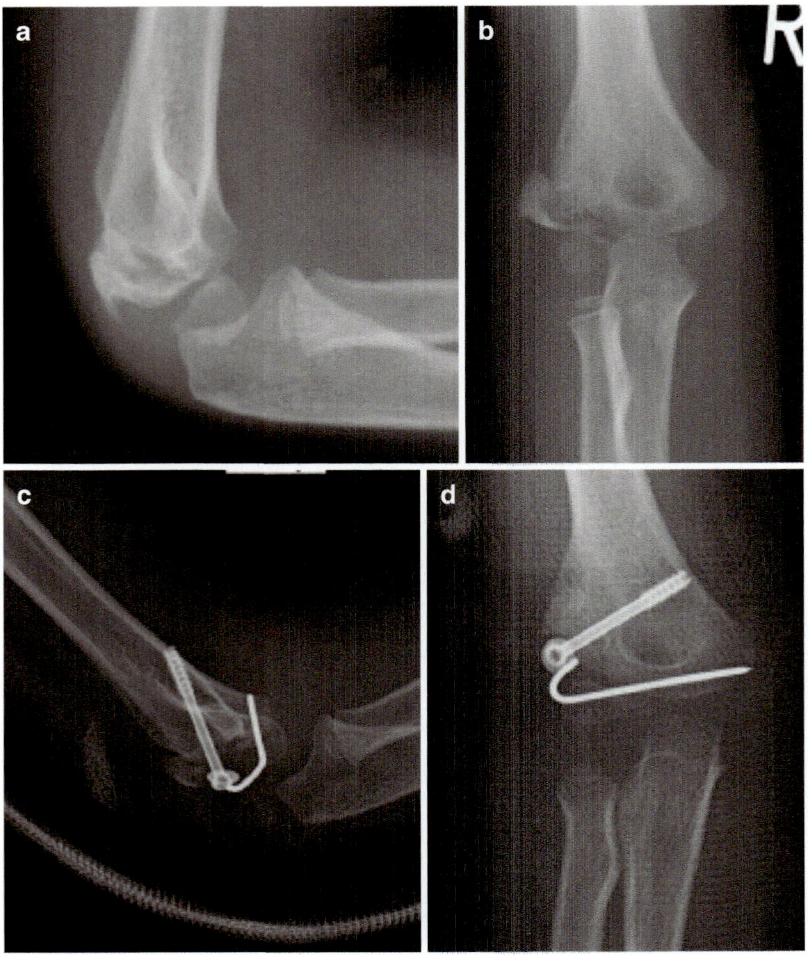

Fig. 7.37 Conservatively treated radial condyle fracture. (**a, b**) Image after 3 months with impaired range of movement and pain. (**c, d**) Postoperative image after open reduction, reduction of insufficient callus formation and fixation with K-wire and screw

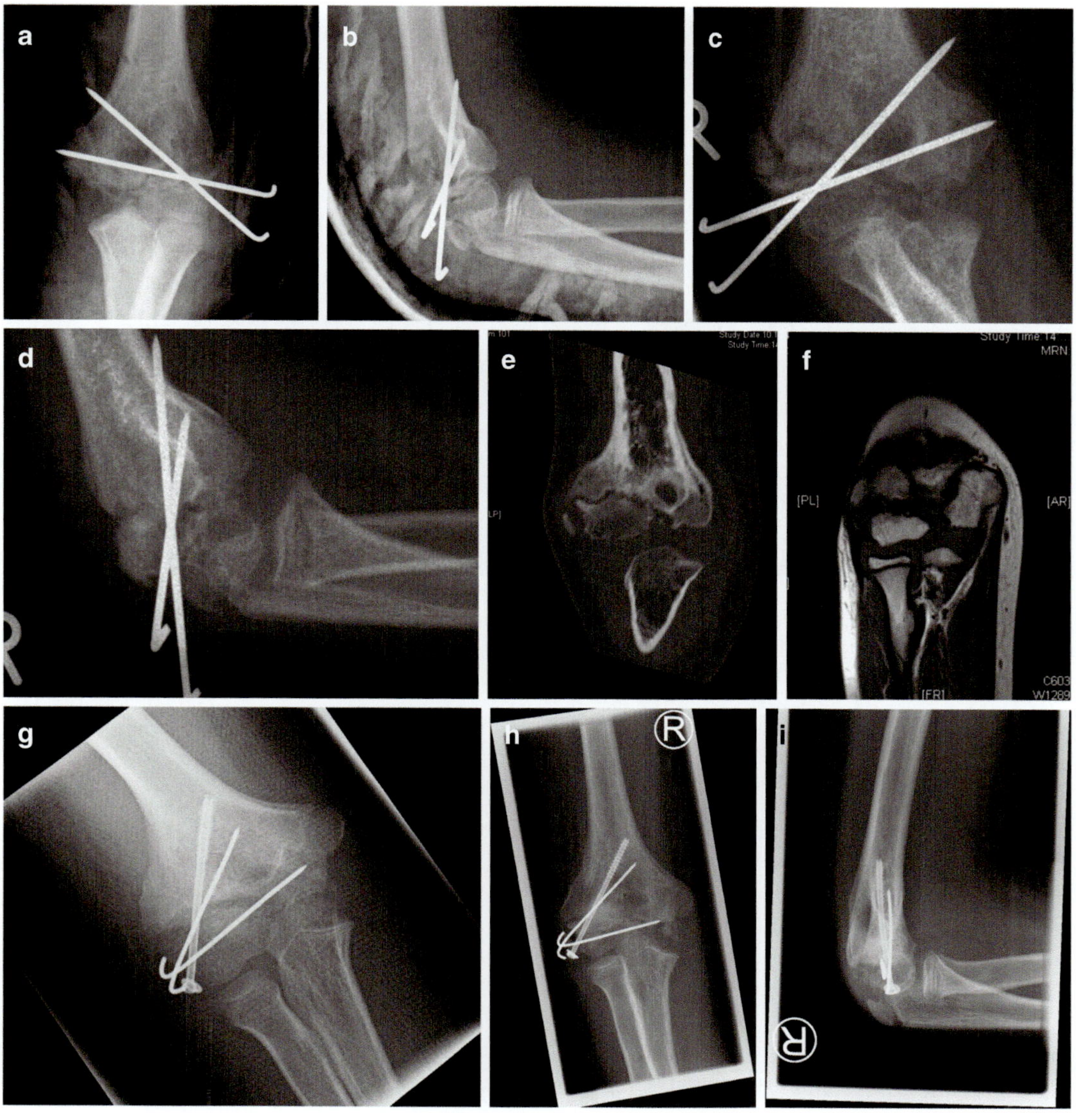

Fig. 7.38 Insufficiently fixed radial condyle fracture in a 10 year old boy. (**a**, **b**) Postoperative images with instable K-wire fixation, (**c**, **d**) Development of nonunion visible, (**e**, **f**) CT and MRI after 6 months showing nonunion, (**g**) Postoperative x-ray after open clearing of nonunion, reduction and interposition of bone graft from the iliac crest and stabilization with screw and K-wires. (**h**, **i**) Complete healing after 4 months

Fractures of the ulnar condyle with dislocation are very rare. Since these fractures are joint fractures, the degree of dislocation is important for the definition of the treatment. Undisplaced fractures can be treated conservatively in a cast (Fig. 7.39), while displaced joint fractures need operative reduction and screw fixation without crossing the growth plate.

T-fractures are rare. In children around the age of 6–7, a central line of the supracondylar fracture is formally a joint fracture (Fig. 7.40) but treated with crossed K-wires like the supracondylar fractures. Dislocated T-fractures of older childs and adolescents might need open reduction and plate ostesynthesis, like in adults.

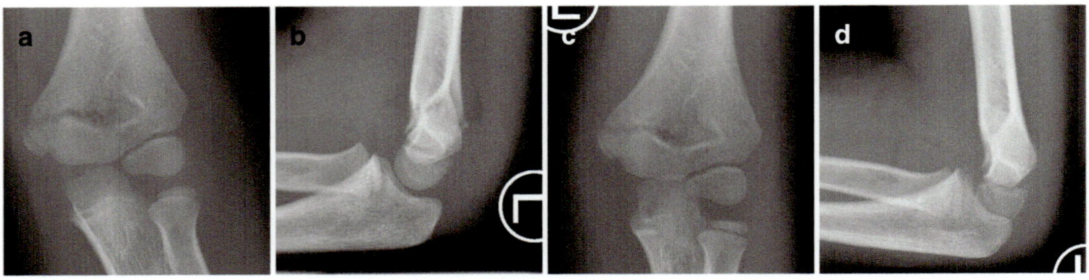

Fig. 7.39 Ulnar condyle fracture in a 8 year old boy. (**a**, **b**) Trauma image; (**c**) X-ray control after 4 days without further displacement, (**d**) Complete healing after 4 weeks in a cast

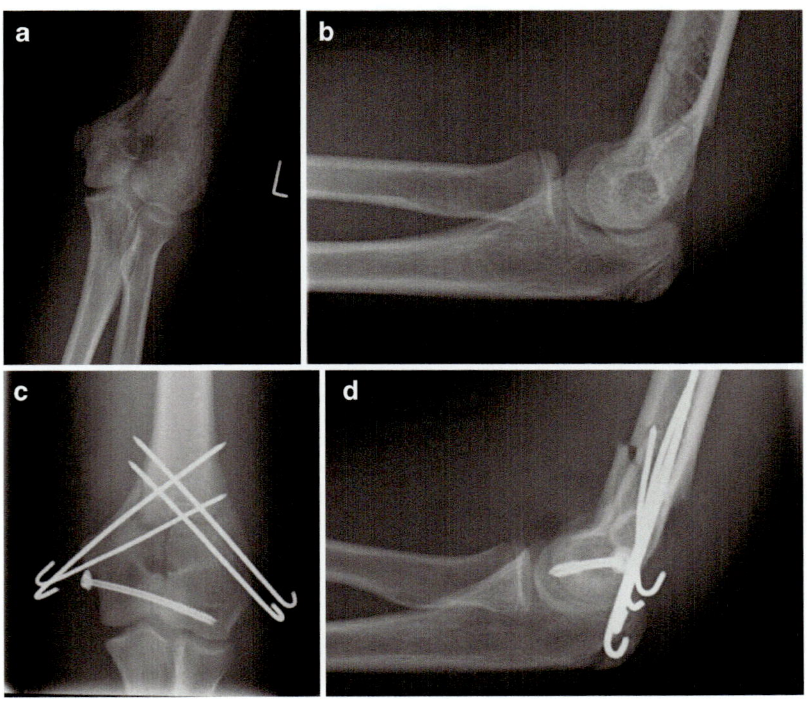

Fig. 7.40 Y-fracture of the distal humerus in a 14 year old boy. (**a**, **b**) Trauma image, (**c**, **d**) Postoperative x-ray after reduction and fixation with lag screw of the distal joint surface and K-wires

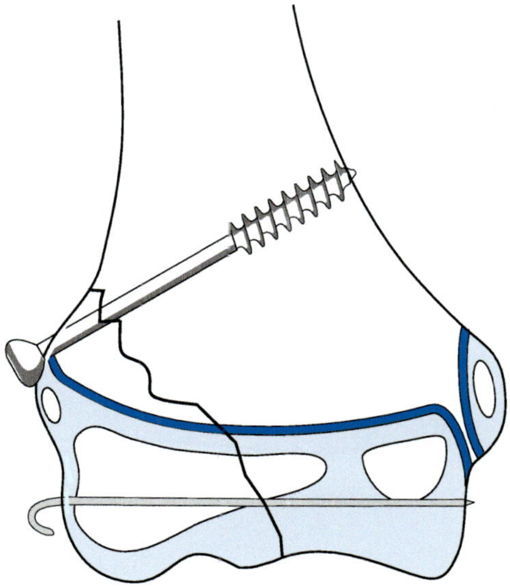

Fig. 7.41 Principle of osteosynthesis of a condylar humerus fracture. After reduction a lag screw superior to the growth plate is inserted via a K-wire (cannulated screw) from dorso-lateral in order not to injure the growth plate. Often a K-wire parallel to the growth plate helps to anatomical fix the joint surface after reduction

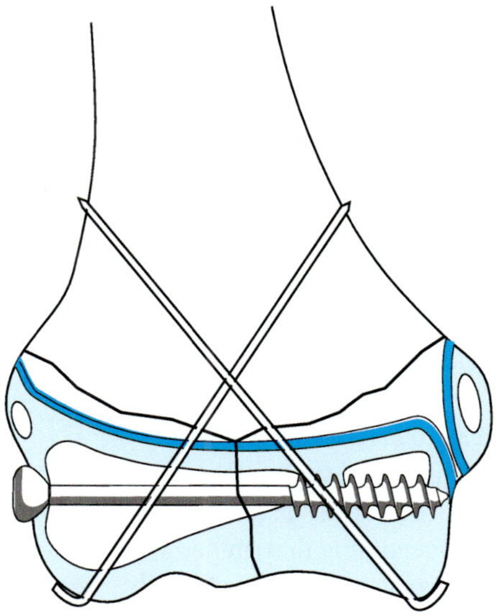

Fig. 7.42 Options for the osteosynthesis of a T-fracture of the distal humerus

Clinically, the elbow joint injuries are characterized by considerable swelling with hematoma formation and pain, combined with severely restricted motion and deformity. It is of outmost importance to judge the peripheral circulation and the neurological sensible and motoric nerve functions, even it might be challenging in small children. However, for the post-operative evaluation this information might be of great importance.

7.4 Elbow Dislocation

Incidence, Mechanism of Injury, and Clinical Presentation

Elbow dislocations are more prevalent after age 10 and appear not infrequently together with medial epicondyle fractures (Fig. 7.43).

This injury usually occurs when a fall on the outstretched hand leads to posterolateral dislocation; rarely, a direct fall on the posterior elbow will lead to anterior dislocation.

Because only the apophyses are injured, no growth irregularities are expected. The prognosis after dislocation is determined by the associated injuries and treatment. Usually, the elbow remains stable after reduction (Fig. 7.44). In instable situation after reduction and testing in anesthesia an MRI for further evaluation might be indicated. Occasionally, avulsions of the radial head might occur (Fig. 7.45).

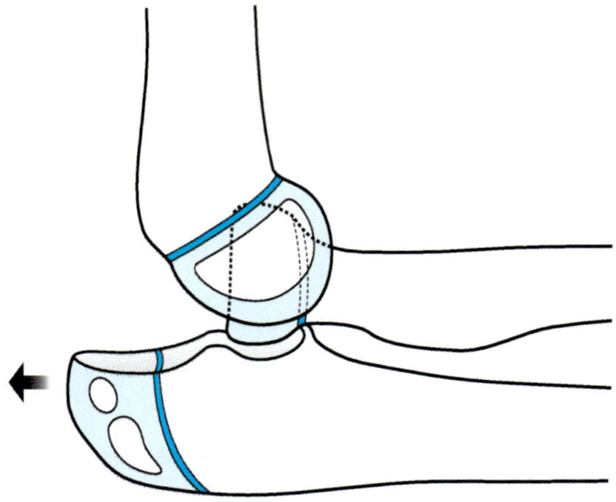

Fig. 7.43 Elbow luxation

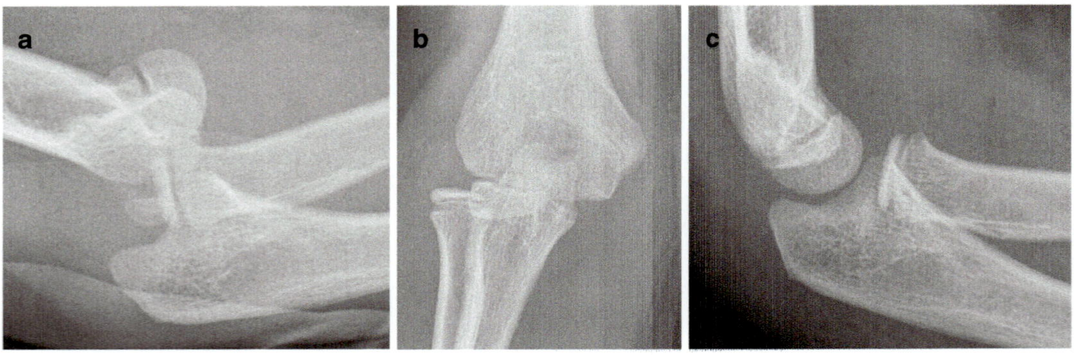

Fig. 7.44 Elbow dislocation after fall of a 9 year old girl. (**a**, **b**) Trauma image, (**c**) Reduction in anesthesia, control of stability and upper arm plaster for 1 week

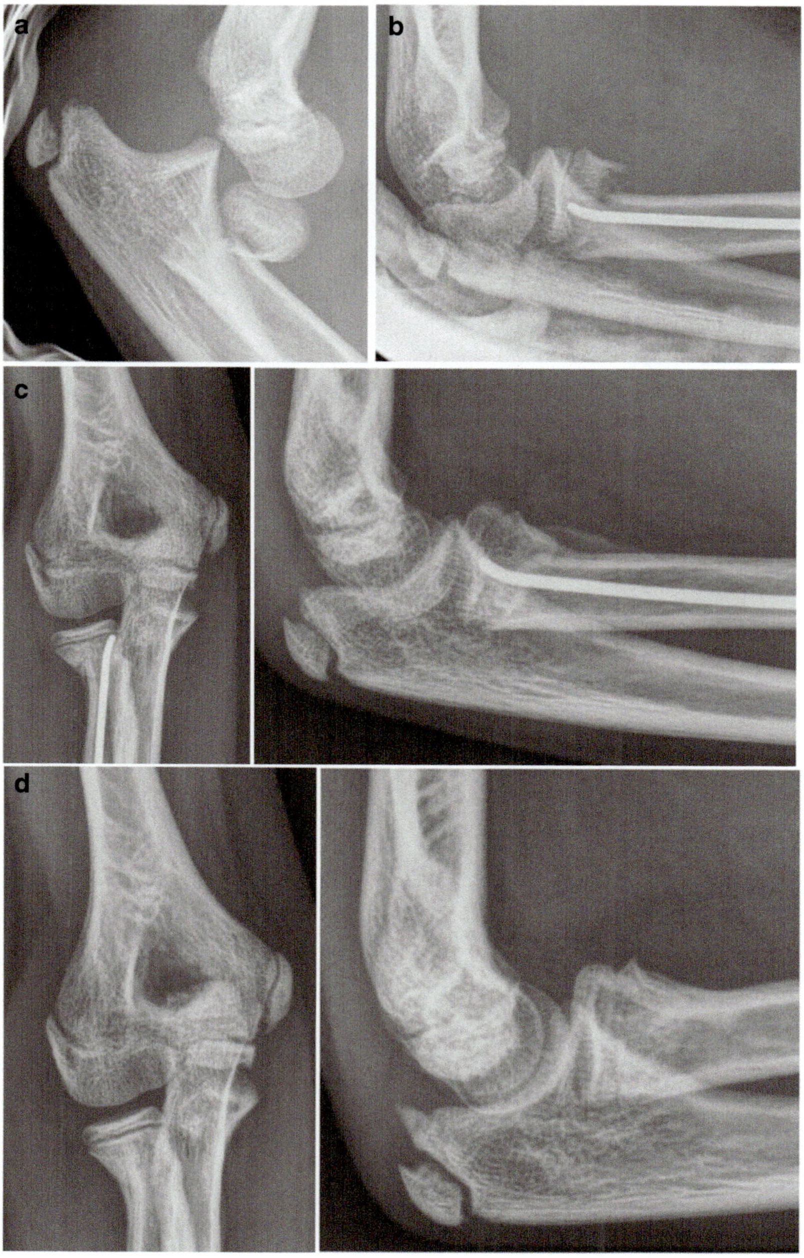

Fig. 7.45 Elbow dislocation with radial head fracture after fall from horse in a 11 year old girl. (**a**) Trauma image, (**b**) 10 Days later, after reduction and retrograde fixation of radial head fracture, (**c**) Healing after 2 months, (**d**) After metal removal at 4 months free function

Avulsion of the medial epicondyle is the most common injury that occurs in 2/3 of all elbow dislocations (Fig. 7.46). The medial epicondyle is usually shifted distally but can occasionally also lie within the joint (Fig. 7.47). In such cases, it is often unrecognizable. Even in small children, when the epicondyle is not yet visible, it can be avulsed with the ligament. Thus, elbow dislocation is often recognizable after-the-fact from the disrupted medial epicondyle. In cases of displacement, these should be re-fixed operatively, if possible, with wire or preferably cannulated screws, with the ulnar nerve under visualization and being protected. Stabilization enables functional follow up with better outcomes. Only small children should be treated conservatively; otherwise, range of motion limitations may occur from immobilization.

Lateral collateral ligament or medial intraligament tears are rare (Fig. 7.48). Occasionally, children suffer avulsion injuries of the lateral epicondyle or the coronoid process, but both are usually treated conservatively.

An overlooked lateral collateral ligament tear can lead to recurrent dislocations. Persistent ulnar instability is uncommon and can lead to a distressing sensation of instability (Table 7.7).

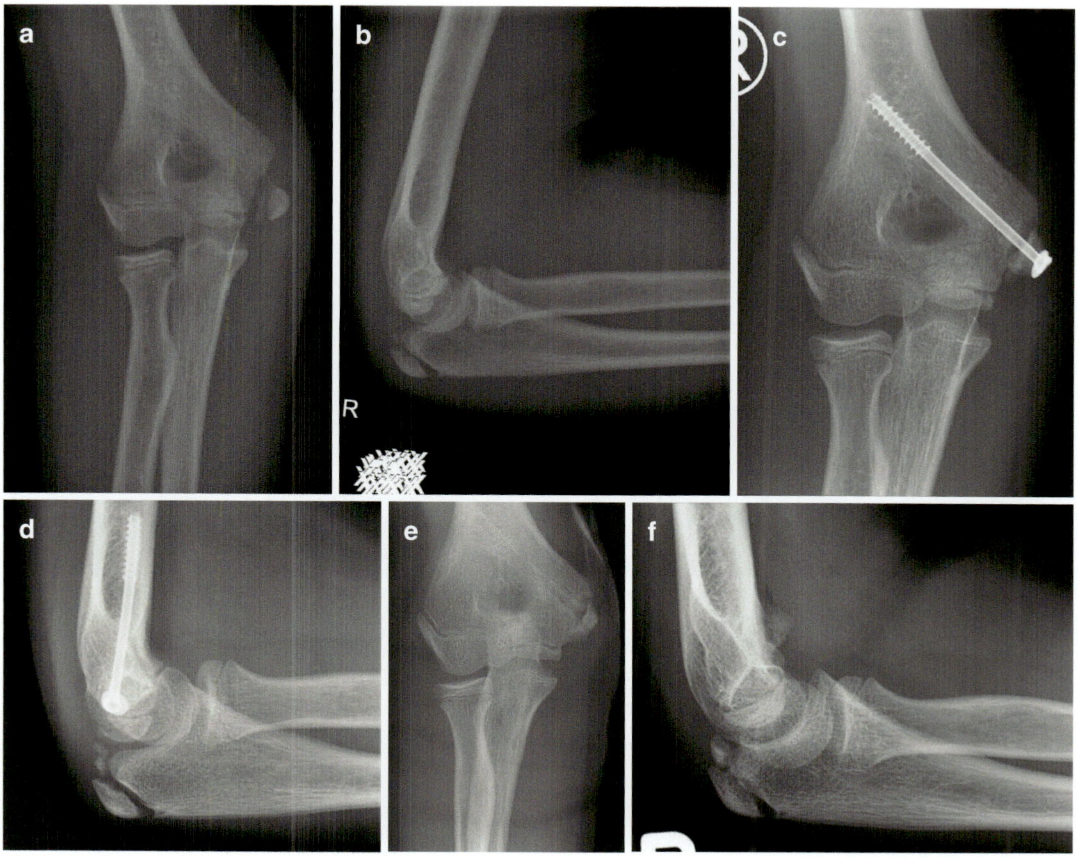

Fig. 7.46 Elbow luxation with ulnar epicondyle dislocation in a 7 year old girl. (**a**, **b**) Trauma image, (**c**, **d**) After open reduction and screw osteosynthesis, (**e**, **f**) After metal removal 3 months later

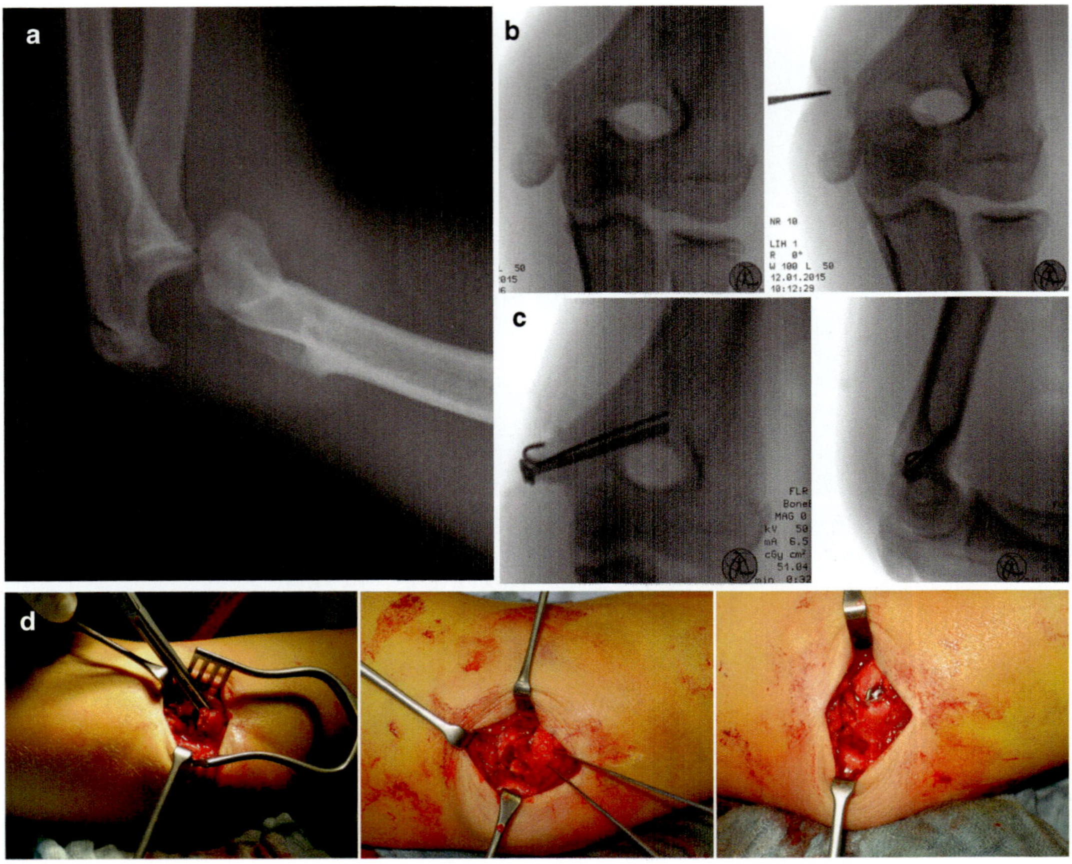

Fig. 7.47 Elbow luxation with substantial dislocation of ulnar epicondyle in a 13 year old boy. (**a**) Trauma image with luxation, (**b**) Dislocation in functional testing in OR, (**c**) Reduction and stabilization of ulnar epicondyle with screw and K-wire. (**d**) Operative situation of dislocated epicondyle, reduction and control of ulnar nerve (bottom) and final image with screw, washer and K-wire

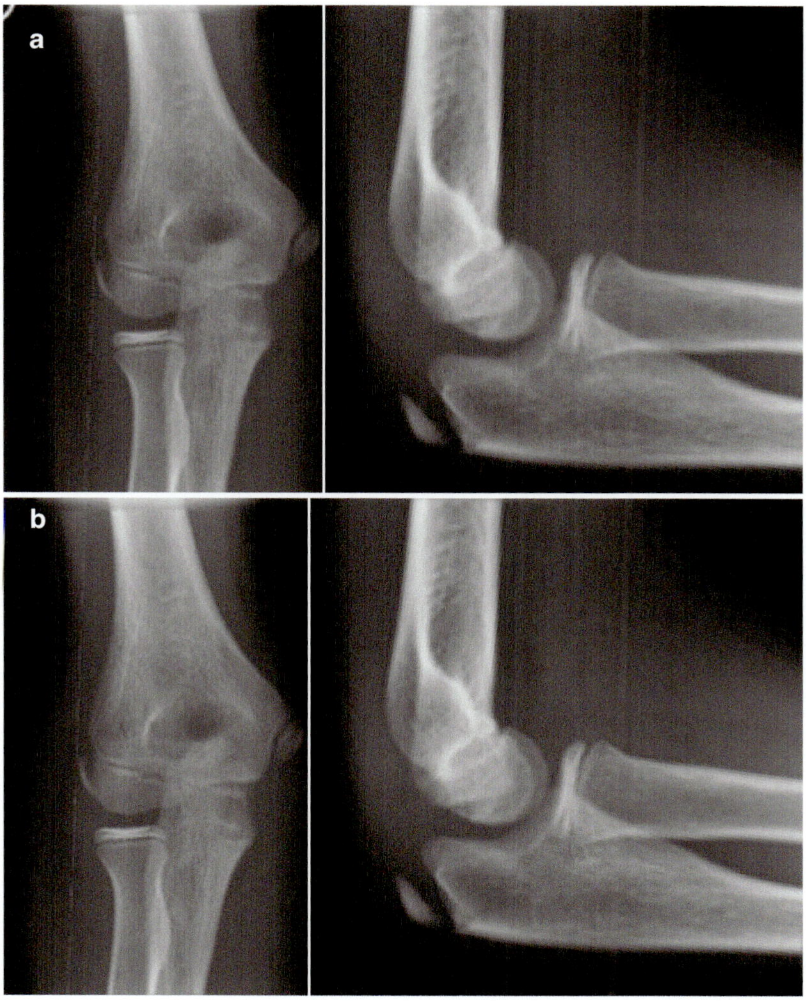

Fig. 7.48 Rare radial epicondyle fracture. Conservative treatment, (a) Trauma Image, (b) Healing after conservative treatment

Table 7.7 Elbow dislocation

Special features	Particularly in adolescents
Diagnostic approach	x-ray overview films with evidence of dislocation or fracture-dislocation, associated bony injuries are often only radiographically evident on post-reduction AP and lateral images; clinical assessment of lateral and medial ligament stability on the extended elbow after reduction under anesthesia or sedation.
Treatment goal/limits of correction	Articular reduction, prevention of instability, treatment and healing of associated injuries, rapid recovery of full function
Primary treatment	Emergency closed reduction, ideally under short anesthesia, along with assessment for instability or associated bony injuries that can be treated at the same time
Conservative treatment	
Indication	Stable elbow joint post-reduction, lack of or anatomically-positioned concomitant bony injuries
Approach	Immobilization in upper-arm cast for 2–3 weeks, initially as plaster splint
Follow up	Functional treatment after cast-removal
Radiology controls	7 days: x-ray control in upper-arm cast to exclude secondary displacement
Return to sports	3 weeks after cast-removal
Operative treatment	
Indication	Lack of stability after primary reduction with tendency to re-dislocate; ligament instability which might be further evaluated with MRI. With bony apophyseal avulsions, especially of the medial epicondyle, the operative fixation of the epicondyle with the medial ligament is a good indication
Approach	Open reduction of the bony avulsion (medial or lateral epicondyle) and fixation with small fragment tension screw; exposure of the ulnar nerve in medial epicondyle avulsions; In lateral instability, direct suture, re-fixation of bony avulsion fragments with mini-screw or K-wires or band fixation with tendon anchor (2.4 mm) Follow up with 2–3 week upper-arm cast, except for stable re-fixation with screws; in these cases, upper-arm plaster splint to allow swelling reduction
Follow up	Plaster immobilization for 2 to maximum 3 weeks, then independent exercises and physical therapy if needed
Radiology controls	Post-reduction; consolidation check
Hardware removal	K-wire at 3 weeks, screws at 12–16 weeks
Return to sports	With free function
Complications	Secondary irritation of the ulnar nerve after medial approach; limitations in elbow range of motion, non-union, re-dislocation rare in pure ligament instability
Growth disturbance	Rare, since growth plates are not directly involved
Follow up	6–12 month checks at least 2 years post-surgery, discharged with free function

7.5 Distal Humerus Epicondylar Fractures

Incidence, Mechanism of Injury, and Clinical Presentation

Overall, the incidence of epicondylar fractures including elbow dislocations, is 1.3% of all extremity injuries. Fractures of the medial epicondyle are much more common (over 90%) than those of the lateral epicondyle. Mostly the medial epicondyle fracture is the result of an elbow dislocation; thus refixation of the epicondyle stabilizes the elbow dislocation as well. Isolated medial epicondyle injuries can occasionally occur through direct trauma. Injuries of the lateral epicondyle are rare and ligamental tears of the lateral ligament and capsule (Fig. 7.49). It must clearly be differentiated from the intra-articular lateral condyle fractures (see Fig. 7.3).

These are extra-articular fractures (Table 7.8). The affected growth plate is an apophysis that functions mainly as an attachment for ligaments and for bone shape and does not contribute to the arm's longitudinal growth. Rapid refixation and return to movement has the best functional results (Table 7.9).

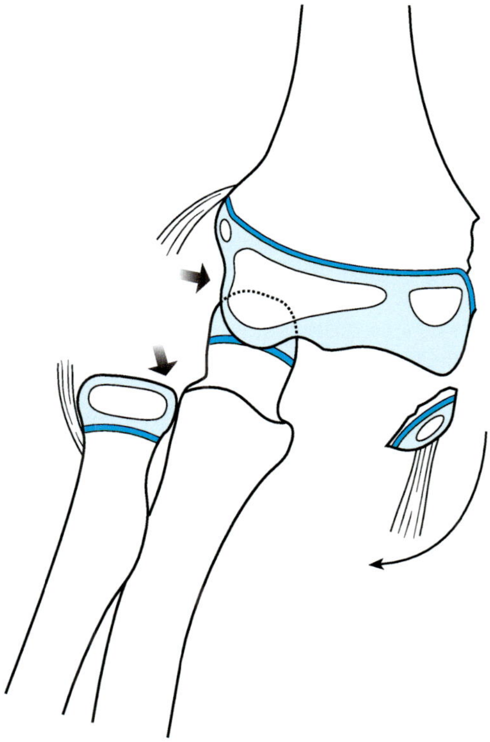

Fig. 7.49 Additional injuries of an elbow dislocation. Mostly associated with an ulnar condyle avulsion, but sometimes with ligamentous injuries of the radial collateral ligament and the anterior capsula

Table 7.8 Distal humerus epicondyle fracture (Fig. 7.50)

Special features	Extra-articular fracture; the affected growth plate is an apophysis that contributes mainly to bone shape and not to longitudinal growth of the arm	
Diagnostic approach	AP and lateral x-ray; in children under 5 years, in whom the ossification center of the epicondyle is not yet visible, diagnosis must be made clinically: direct trauma, swelling, and evident pain medially; in this age, the degree of displacement is less critical because it has no sequelae	
Treatment goal/limits of correction	Unlimited elbow function without instability; The associated growth plates are apophyseal plates; thus, spontaneous correction is not expected	
Primary treatment	Immobilization in upper-arm plaster splint; controls of neurovascular status (sensory and motor)	
Conservative treatment		
Indication	All non-displaced fractures: non-displaced includes displacement up to 0.5 cm (Fig. 7.51)	
Approach	Upper-arm cast in neutral position with 90° elbow flexion	
Follow up	Physical therapy is not necessary initially; only when range of motion limitations do not improve for 6–8 weeks	
Radiology controls	At 3–5 weeks consolidation check	
Return to sports	With free function	
Operative treatment		
Indication	All displaced fractures, especially when they are driven into the joint; displacement of 0.5 cm or more, for some authors greater than 0.2 cm is an operative indication; When there is concomitant elbow dislocation, surgery should proceed urgently; with epiphyseal avulsion alone, immediately or after a few days to decrease swelling (Fig. 7.52)	
Approach	Screw fixation with cannulated, self-tapping screws, with a washer if necessary (approx. 3.5 mm), K-wire transfixion or tension banding only in exceptional cases; intraoperative visualization of the ulnar nerve that can be displaced due to instability (Figs. 7.53 and 7.54).	
Follow up	In screw fixation, as early functional as possible; in K-wire fixation for small children, 3 weeks immobilization in upper-arm cast; After stable fixation, spontaneous movement can be started immediately Physical therapy is not necessary initially; only when range of motion limitations do not improve for 6–8 weeks	
Radiology controls	Postoperative: either during surgery or within the first week; consolidation check	
Hardware removal	Screws after 3–4 months; K-wires at the time of consolidation if they are protruding, otherwise at 8–12 weeks	
Return to sports	With free function	
Complications	Non-union of the medial epicondyle occurs in up to 40% of cases treated conservatively and in around 10% treated surgically; symptoms are only present in 10% of all non-unions; occasional irritation of the ulnar nerve	
Growth disturbance	Because this is an apophysis, resulting growth irregularities are not expected	
Follow up	Treatment can be concluded with full function since there is no risk of growth disturbance	
Classification	AO: 13-M/7.1-3	LiLa: 1.3.s.5.0-2.

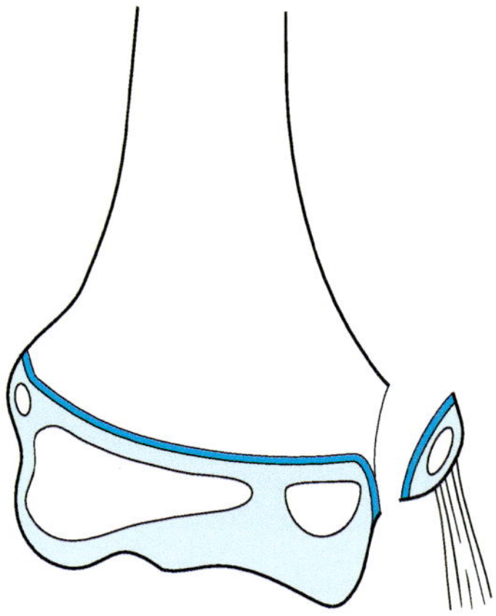

Fig. 7.50 Avulsion fracture with dislocation of the attached medial collateral ligament of the ulnar condyle

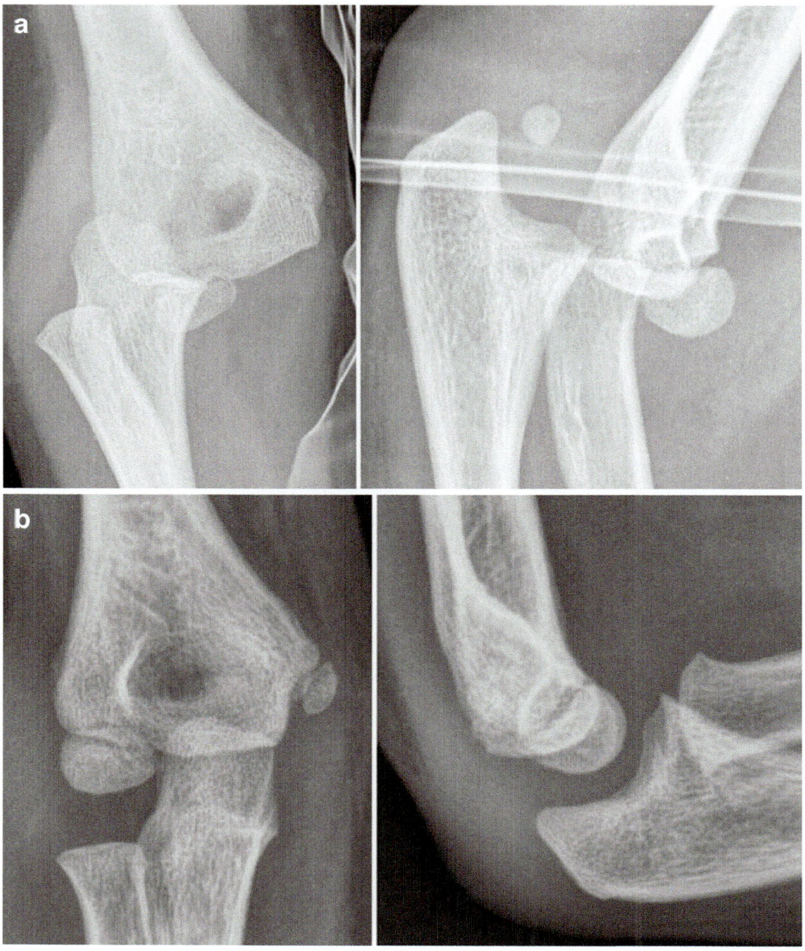

Fig. 7.51 Epicondyle avulsion fracture after elbow luxation. Since it was not recognized initially, a conservative treatment was successfully achieved, due to the anatomic reduction of the ulnar epicondyle. (**a**) Trauma images, (**b**) conservative treatment with healing after 6 weeks in correct position

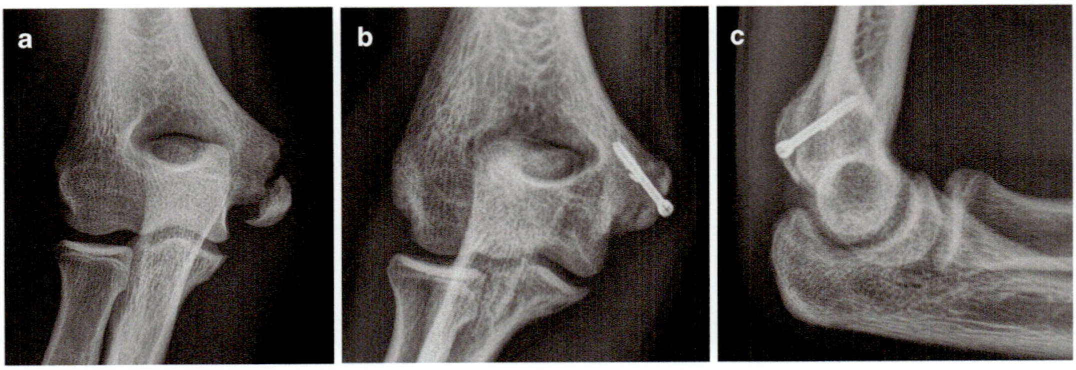

Fig. 7.52 Isolated epicondyle fracture of a 15 year old boy. (**a**) Trauma image, (**b**, **c**) Open reduction and Cannulated lag screws osteosynthesis

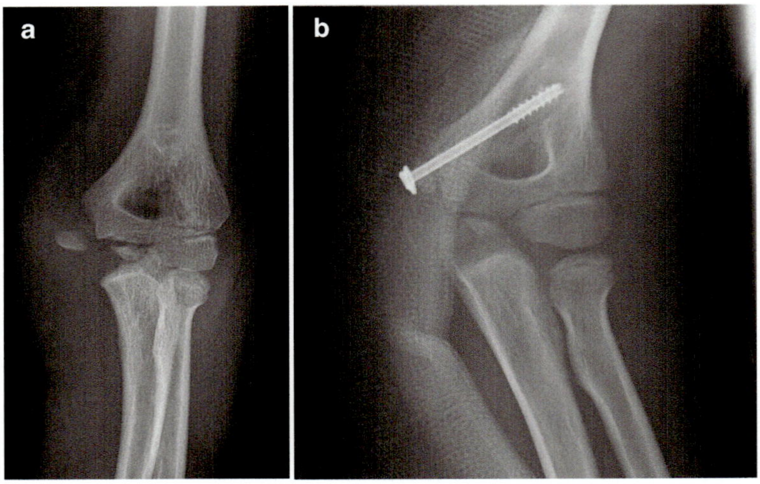

Fig. 7.53 Largely displaced ulnar epicondyle avulsion fracture. (**a**) Trauma image, (**b**) Fixation with cannulated lag screw after open reduction

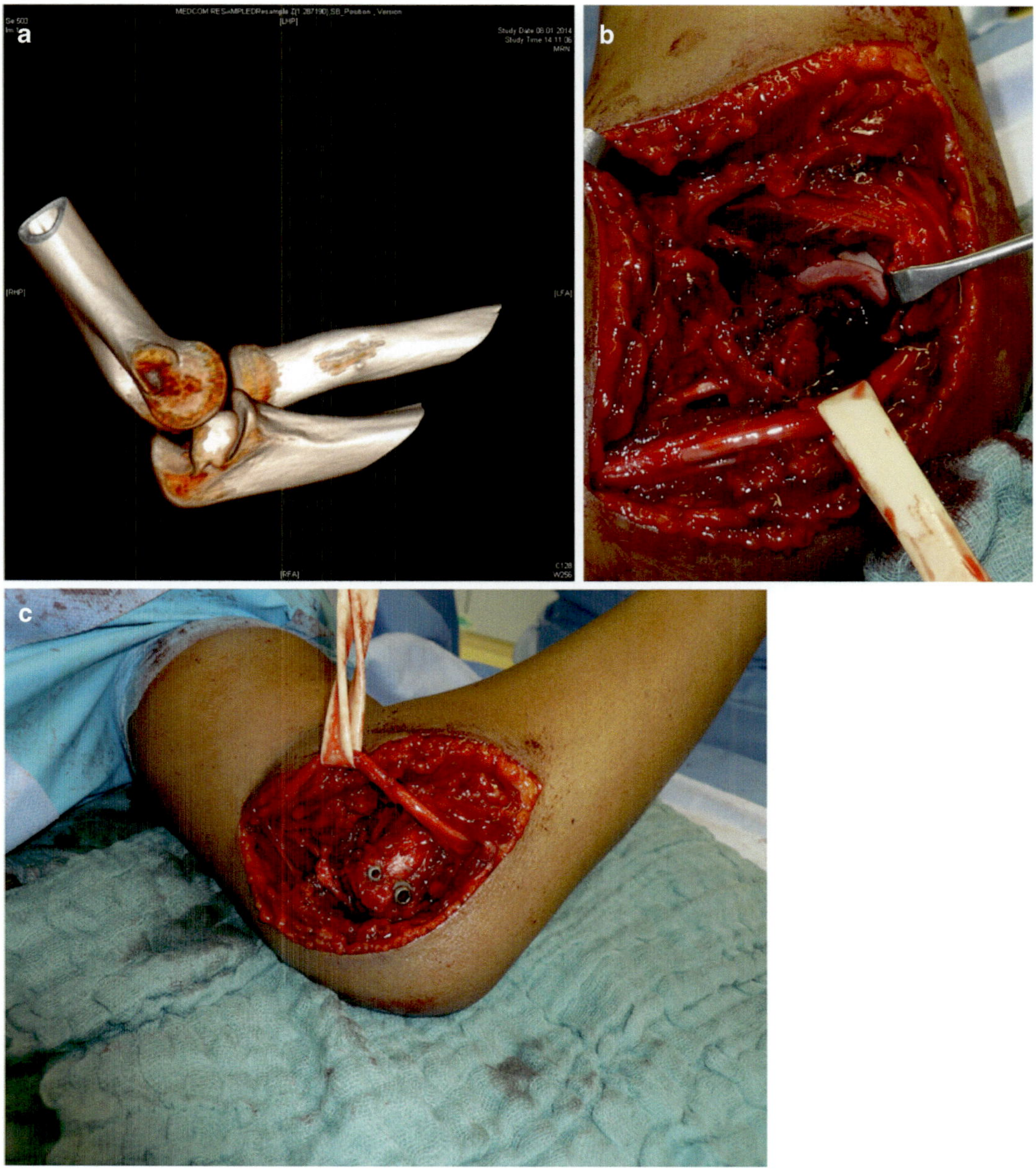

Fig. 7.54 Ulnar nerve is mostly fixed to the epicondyle avulsion fracture and needs to be controlled during operation. (**a**) Entrapment of the displaced epicondyle ulnaris into the elbow joint, (**b**) Neurolysis of ulnar nerve, distally visible wide dislocation of ulnar epicondyle; (**c**) Refixation of ulnar epicondyle ulnaris and ulnar nerve prior to reposition dorsally

Table 7.9 Technical aspects—condylar fractures

Distal Humerus epicondyle fracture	
Material	Screws (cannulated self-tapping screws, mostly 3.5 mm)
Positioning	Supine, prone also possible
Approach	Medial approach to the elbow. The avulsed fragment is easily visualized with hematoma. The ulnar nerve must be exposed. At the tip of the fragment, a hole is drilled from oblique posterior to anterior at 30° to the humeral shaft. A small fragment cancellous screw with short threads or a cannulated self-tapping screw can be used. The latter has the advantage that the fragment can be temporarily fixed with a K-wire, over which the screw can be inserted. K-wire fixation alone with 1–2 K-wires is only appropriate when other options are not feasible, e.g., for small fragments.
Special considerations	Ulnar nerve lesions, non-union, restricted mobility, joint stiffening (heterotopic ossification, soft-tissue scarring)
Distal Humerus Transcondylar fracture (fracture of the lateral condyle, the medial condyle, and T-fracture)	
Positioning	Prone or supine position: prone is somewhat easier for reduction of lateral condyle fractures; T-fractures should only be treated operatively in the prone position
Approach	Lateral approach for lateral condyle fractures Medial approach for medial condyle fractures Posterior approach with/without olecranon osteotomy in transcondylar fractures (in adolescents as in adults)
Special considerations	Nerve lesions according to approach Non-union with lack of healing, restricted ROM Post-traumatic arthritis
Approach	Operative treatment of lateral condyle fractures Lateral approach Exposure of the displaced fracture, opening of the capsula, removal of hematoma and exposure of the joint surface without exception; the lateral joint and metaphysal fragment is usually largely dislocated and twisted: then: anatomical reduction of articular congruity under full view and temporary fixation with a K-wire parallel to the joint and perpendicular to the fracture surface above the growth plate. Stabilization with cannulated, over-drilled screws and/or K-wires, these can be inserted parallel to the oblique tension screws (3–3.5 mm) for rotational safeguarding; this screw has start above the growth plate from dorsally to anterior-medial; the K-wires (1.4–1.6 mm) inserted into the trochlea parallel to the joint surface increase fixation stability and prevent secondary displacement. Controrl by intraoperative x-ray. Alternatively, divergent insertion of two K-wires in small children; these will need additional plaster immobilization Operative treatment of medial condyle fractures Medial approach Visualization of the ulnar nerve for mobilization Exposure of the joint surface and anatomical reduction of joint incongruity Temporary fixation with K-wires parallel to the joint and perpendicular to the fracture surface Stabilization with cannulated, over-drilled screws and/or K-wire, these can be inserted parallel to the oblique tension screws (3–3.5 mm) for rotational safeguarding; the K-wires (1.4–1.6 mm) inserted into the trochlea parallel to the joint surface increase fixation stability Reposition of the ulnar nerve, anterior shift is generally not necessary

	Operative treatment of T-fractures Prone position Incision parallel to the triceps tendon Exposure and mobilization of the ulnar nerve Reduction of the T-fracture beneath the triceps tendon, temporary fixation with K-wires parallel to the joint line and the metaphysis, intraoperative x-ray controls When anatomic reduction is achieved, stabilization with cannulated tension screws over the K-wires In adolescents with high tensile forces, one or both pillars can be fixed with small fragment plates (3.5 mm reconstruction plate, rarely low contact plate); since the epiphyses are placed under compression here, it should not be performed before growth plate fusion Olecranon osteotomy if the above approach does not yield a secure anatomical reduction; if this is performed, then anatomical mobilization-stable reduction and fixation with plates, closure of the osteotomy with tension banding, and functional follow up
Hardware removal	Tension screws at 3–4 months, olecranon osteotomy at 3 months, plates at 5–6 months
Special features	Anatomical reconstruction of the joint is the first priority to avoid post-traumatic arthritis

Recommended Literature

Slongo T (2014 Feb) Radial external fixator for closed treatment of type III and IV supracondylar humerus fractures in children. A new surgical technique. Oper Orthop Traumatol 26(1):75–96

Ulrich D, Voth M, Frank J, Marzi I (2015 Mar 25) Dislocation fractures of the elbow in childhood. Trauma Berufskrankheit 17(S2):253–259

Fernandez PDFF (2015 Mar 11) Ellenbogenverletzungen im Kindesalter. Trauma Berufskrankheit 17(1):48–54

Müller LP, Hollinger B, Burghart K (2016) Expertise Orthopädie und Unfallchirurgie – Ellenbogen, 1st edn. Thieme, Stuttgart

Chirurg PSD (2017) Frakturen der oberen Extremität im Kindes-/Wachstumsalter. Orthopäde. Springer, New York

von Laer L, Kraus R, Linhart WE (2012) Frakturen und Luxationen im Wachstumsalter 6., überarbeitete und erweiterte Auflage 2012 512 S., 1380 Abb. Thieme, Stuttgart

Green DP, Hotchkiss MDRN, Pederson MDWC, Wolfe MDSW (2005) Green's operative hand surgery. Churchill Livingstone, Edinburgh

Marzi I (2016) Kindertraumatologie, 3rd edn. Springer, New York

Thielemann F, Biewener A, Schaser KD (2017 Mar) Korrekturosteotomien bei posttraumatischen Fehlstellungen des Ellenbogengelenks. Oper Orthop Traumatol 30:1–11

Frank J, Sander AL, Voth M, Marzi I (2016) Sekundäre Rekonstruktionen am Ellenbogengelenk im Kindesalter. Trauma Berufskrankheit. 19:126–134

Linhart WE, Kraus T (2008 Nov 16) Reconstruction of humeroradial joint. Oper Orthop Traumatol 20(4–5):396–408

Rang M, Pring ME, Wenger DR (2005) Rang's children's fractures. Lippincott Williams & Wilkins, Philadelphia

Dietz HG, Illing P, Schmittenbecher PP, Slongo T, Sommerfeldt DW (2011) Praxis der Kinder- und Jugendtraumatologie, 1st edn. Springer, Heidelberg

Pathy R, Dodwell ER (2015 Jan 1) Medial epicondyle fractures in children. Curr Opin Pediatr 27(1):58–66

Green NE, Swiontkowski MF (1998) Skeletal trauma in children, 2nd edn. W.B. Saunders, Philadelphia

Müller LP, Hollinger B, Burkhart K (2018 May 3) Expertise Orthopädie und Unfallchirurgie. Ellenbogen. Thieme, Stuttgart, pp 1–64

8 Proximal Radius and Olecranon

8.1 Physiological and Radiological Findings

The anatomy of the elbow joint is depicted in Fig. 8.1 demonstrating the collateral ligaments and bony structures in AP view and lateral view and the close anatomic relationship to the radial nerve. The ossification centers of the proximal olecranon and the radial head occur at different time points: at first of the radial head, then of the olecranon (Fig. 8.2). The vascular situation of the radial head is very critical (Fig. 8.3) and is to be considered for any surgical exploration. In small and school children, therefor, a direct surgical exposure of the radial head and neck should be only intended if absolutely necessary and most of the treatment can be done indirectly.

The joint function depends absolutely on the correct position of the radius in respect to the capitellum humuri. Regardless of age and developmental stage of the ossification center, the radial neck axis must always meet the capitellum in any position. The radiocapitellar line of the center of the radius enables a reliable assessment of proximal radius position (Fig. 8.4a, b).

If epiphyseal ossification is largely or entirely absent in small children, injuries to the proximal radial metaphysis can be underestimated; epiphysiolysis or compression may appear only as minimal metaphyseal plate loosening (Fig. 8.5).

The olecranon apophysis might still be absent in small children, or it could have one or several separate tiny ossification centers. Its course distinguishes it from a fracture. The proximal radial epiphysis might be absent, very small, or occasionally divided in two (Fig. 8.5).

I. Marzi et al., *Pediatric Skeletal Trauma*, https://doi.org/10.1007/978-3-030-93685-3_8

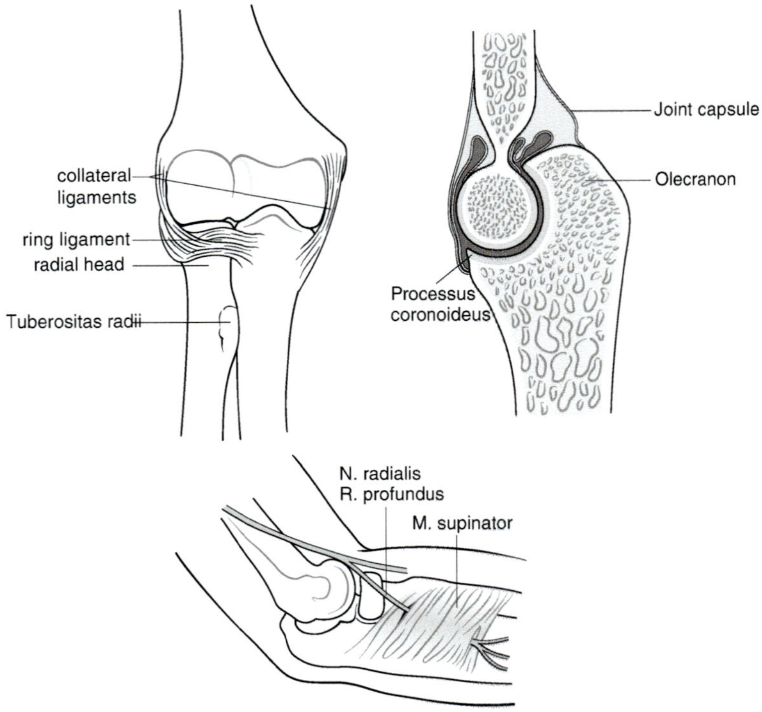

Fig. 8.1 Anatomy of the proximal forearm

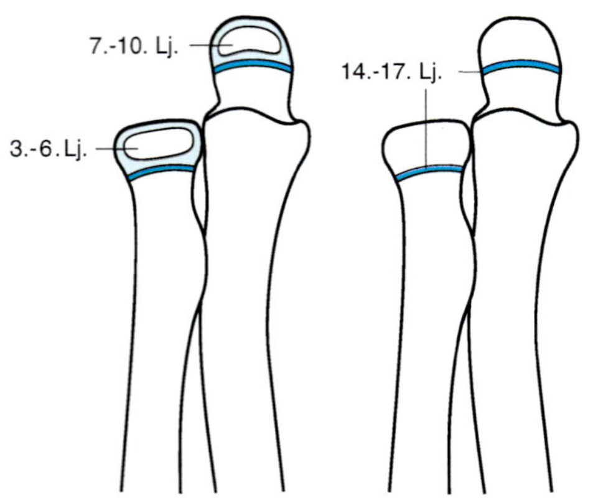

Fig. 8.2 Ossification centers and growth plate fusion. (*Lj*) life year

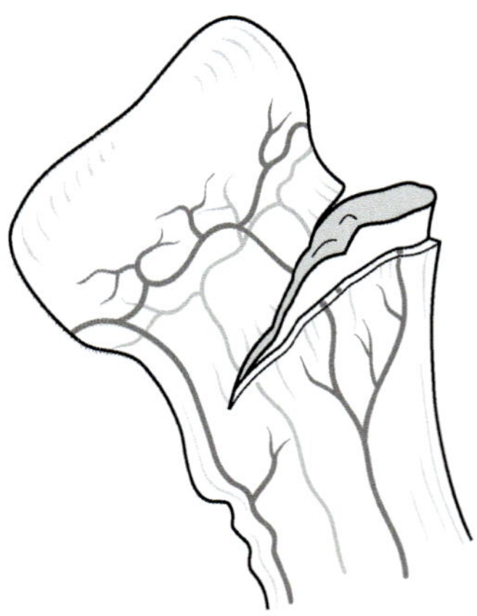

Fig. 8.3 Blood circulation of the proximal radius

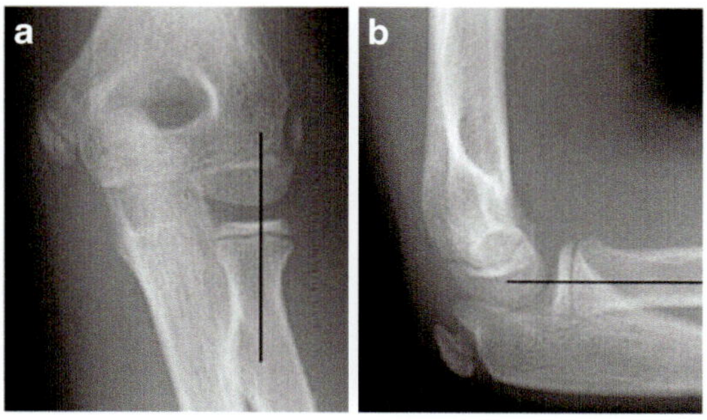

Fig. 8.4 (**a**, **b**) Elbow jcint with correct position of the radial head to the capitellum. For all movements and in each x-ray projection, the extended radial axis intersects the capitellum

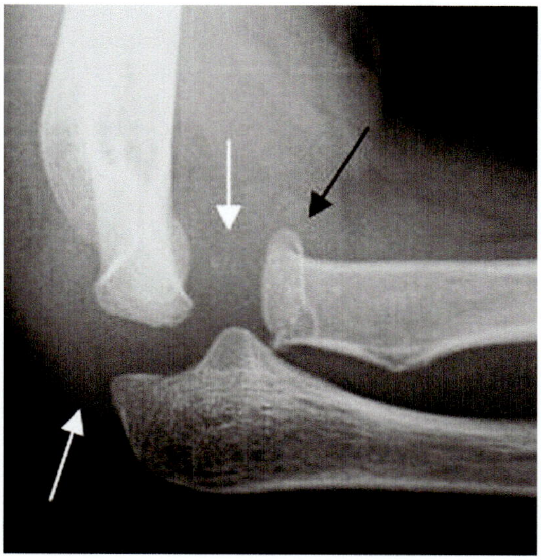

Fig. 8.5 Toddler with racial neck fracture (black arrow); centers of the proximal radial epiphysis and the olecranon apophysis are still lacking (white arrows)

8.2 Fractures and Dislocations of the Proximal Radius

Radial Head Dislocation (Table 8.1) Temporary subluxation is the most common injury in the proximal radius region. It is also called "nursemaid's elbow," with an incidence of 3.4–5.6% of all skeletal injuries and 27% of elbow traumas. The diagnosis is usually made based on clinical history in children up to 4 years of age. It results from the abrupt force exerted when an adult catches a stumbling child by the extended arm or when the extended arm is twisted. Occasionally, an arm is caught between crib slats and subsequently twisted. The child presents holding the injured elbow in moderate extension and pronation. The proximal radius slips out of the annular ligament when the muscles cannot counter-stabilize the joint. The trauma is often not witnessed, and the parents are unaware of the reason for the sudden onset of pain. The radial head has reached its final size by the age of four, and the injury is markedly less common.

If several reduction attempts are unsuccessful despite the typical history and presentation, the arm should be immobilized in a splint for a couple of days. Once the splint is removed, the arm usually moves freely, or another injury, e.g., a non-displaced supracondylar humerus or radial neck fracture, becomes evident, which might be found by a control x-ray at that time (Fig. 8.6).

Table 8.1 Radial head subluxation

Special features	Synonyms: pulled elbow, nursemaid's elbow Incidence: 3.4–5.6%
Diagnostic approach	Typical history: abrupt pull on the arm, sudden favoring of the entire arm Clinical: guarding of the elbow in moderate extension and pronation ("painful pronation") AP and lateral x-ray only after unsuccessful reduction attempt
Treatment goal/limits of correction	Reduction, immediate unlimited mobility
Primary treatment	Immediate reduction, if possible
Conservative treatment	
Indication	Always indicated
Approach	Manual reduction without anesthesia: shake hands with the child while lightly grasping the elbow with the other hand; traction of the forearm, then supination, and finally complete elbow flexion until the radial head snaps into position. The first attempt should succeed; otherwise, it becomes more challenging and is only possible if the child is distracted. Before a second attempt, an elbow x-ray should be performed to exclude fracture. If 1–3 initial reduction attempts are unsuccessful (not resulting in free mobility), a posterior plaster splint can be placed for 2–4 days; function is often restored afterward (spontaneous reduction or "relaxation"), or another reduction should be attempted.
Follow up	None; check for unlimited function during play minutes after reduction
Radiological controls	None, only in persistent pain and dysfunction, a x-ray control might be indicated in these cases.
Return to sports	Immediately
Operative treatment	
Indication	None
Complications	Recurrence rate: 40%; caution after multiple reduction attempts; misdiagnosis: supracondylar humerus fracture or occult elbow injury (conservative treatment for several days in cast); conditioning questionable with ligament laxity; permanent damage not observed
Growth disturbances	Not applicable
Follow up	Not necessary

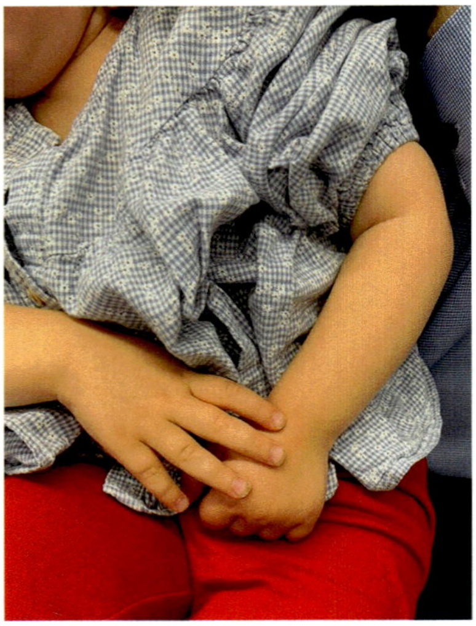

Fig. 8.6 Chassaignac luxation. Prone position of the forearm (pronation doloreuse)

Isolated Radial Head Dislocation This is an infrequent injury, and there is usually an overlooked ulnar fracture (Monteggia fracture with a slight, barely noticeable bowing of the ulna or plastic deformation: an "occult ulnar fracture") (Fig. 8.7 and Table 8.2).

The mechanism of injury is the same as a Monteggia fracture. Under strong forearm traction, the radial head slips under the annular ligament, or the ligament tears when there is pronounced elbow stress (sports injury) (Fig. 8.8). Immediate reduction is usually achieved with closed maneuvers (Fig. 8.9). If the radius has pierced the capsule or the injury is missed and reduction is delayed, an open approach might be necessary.

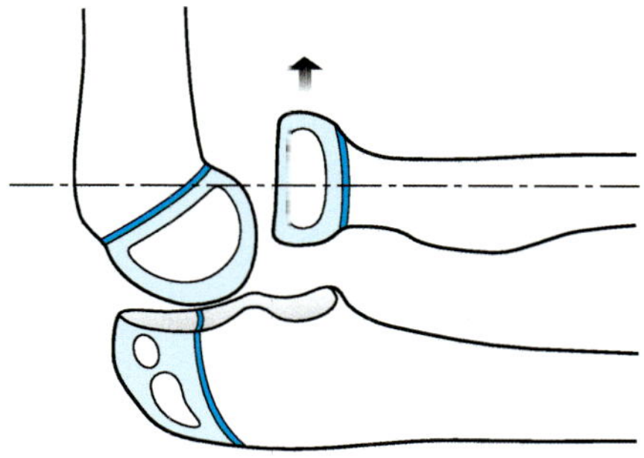

Fig. 8.7 Isolated proximal radial head luxation

Table 8.2 Isolated proximal radius dislocation

Special features	Rare; mostly misdiagnosis in cases of missed ulnar fracture (Monteggia injury) Differential diagnosis: congenital dislocation
Diagnostic approach:	AP and lateral x-rays of the forearm, drawing in the radial axis Clinical: swelling, painful pro/supination
Treatment goal/limits of correction	Stable reduction of the dislocation
Primary treatment	Positioning in long-arm splint
Conservative treatment	
Indication	Closed reduction attempt is strictly indicated
Approach	Traction on the forearm with alternating pronation and supination, with direct pressure on the proximal radius, if needed; Check stable reduction (flexion/extension and pro/supination) under fluoroscopy
Follow up	Posterior long-arm plaster splint in elbow flexion and neutral forearm position for 2–3 weeks, then mobilization as tolerated, no physical therapy until 6 weeks after splint removal
Radiological controls	At 1 week: Articular check in splint
Return to sports	When there is generally free mobility, usually 2–3 weeks after splint removal
Operative treatment	
Indication	Usually dislocations that have occurred more than 3 weeks previous and cannot be reduced closed
Approach	Open reduction, if needed tension suture, no ligament reconstruction In absolute exceptions, percutaneous trans-ulnar K-wire fixation, no trans-articular fixation
Follow up	As with conservative treatment
Radiological controls	At 1 week: articular check in splint
Hardware removal	3 weeks post-surgery
Return to sports	When there is generally free mobility, usually 2–3 weeks after splint removal
Complications	Unstable reduction and re-dislocation (search for other causes: Monteggia injury, ulnar bowing) Calcification of the joint capsule or the torn ligament Permanent mobility deficits (pro/supination)
Growth disturbances	None
Follow up	Until there is full mobility

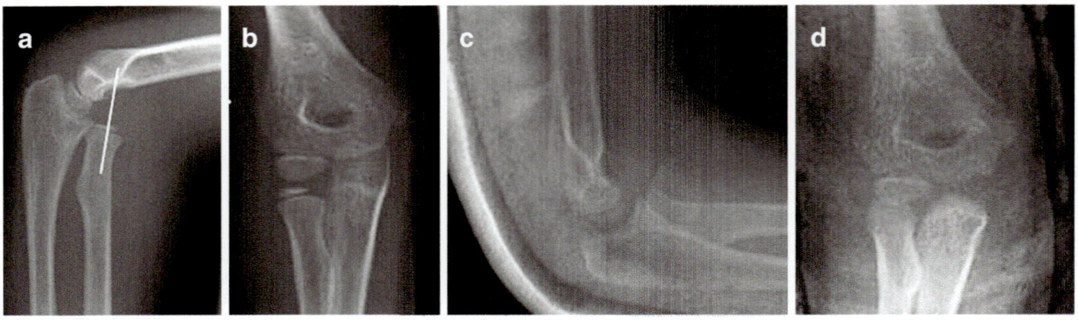

Fig. 8.8 Isolated proximal radial head dislocation, girl, 7 years, unclear fall. (**a**, **b**) Trauma images, with auxiliary line. (**c**, **d**) Immediate reduction, cast immobilization

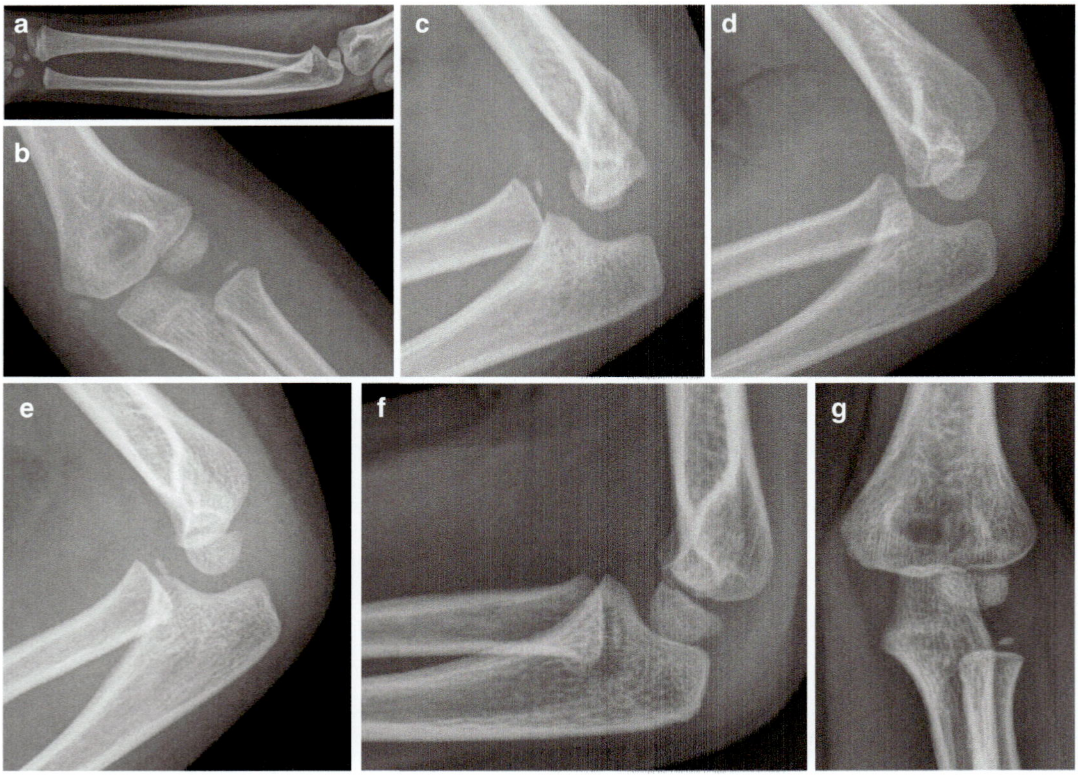

Fig. 8.9 Isolated radial head luxation after fall. (**a**) X-ray of the elbow and forearm with unclear clinical signs. (**b**–**d**) Specific x-rays for further clarification of radial head luxation, (**e**) X-ray of contralateral elbow, (**f**, **g**) After intraoperative pressure on radial head and snapping 2 weeks cast and then regular x-ray at free function

Congenital dislocation must always be included in the differential diagnosis! In such a case, the deformed epiphysis appears rounded and convex, often with posterior deviation. The radius is also too long, the capitellum is hypoplastic, and there is "no place" for the radial head on the AP image. The deformity is usually bilateral (see also Chap. 19).

Epiphyseal Fractures of the Radial Head This is an absolute exception in childhood; it is possible with premature growth plates. The cause is usually valgus elbow stress, which can shear off a lateral epiphyseal fragment. Another possible cause is severe axial compression trauma, e.g., from falling on the outstretched hand with a pronated forearm. The injury can occur as part of a dislocation. Thus, the collateral ligaments, coronoid process, and medial epicondyle must also be checked (Table 8.3).

Table 8.3 Epiphyseal radial head fracture

Special features	Absolute exception in childhood, possible in rare cases with premature growth plate The cause is generally valgus stress or severe axial compression trauma Associated with elbow dislocation: check the collateral ligaments, coronoid process, medial epicondyle	
Diagnostic approach:	AP and lateral x-rays of the elbow	
Treatment goal/ limits of correction	Exact restoration of the articular surface No spontaneous correction is expected	
Primary treatment	Immobilization in a long-arm splint	
Conservative treatment		
Indication	Non-displaced fractures	
Approach	Cast immobilization for 3 weeks	
Follow up	Mobilize as tolerated, (usually) no physical therapy	
Radiological controls	Position check at 1 week (secondary displacement?); Consolidation check at 3 weeks	
Return to sports	When there is generally free mobility, usually 3 weeks after cast removal	
Operative treatment		
Indication	Fractures with a step or dehiscence of the articular surface (can only be diagnosed with x-rays in adolescents)	
Approach	Open reduction and fixation with K-wire, mini-screw, or resorbable pin	
Follow up	Immobilization for 7–10 days, then early functional follow up	
Radiological controls	Day 0 (intraoperative), day 21/28 (consolidation), before hardware removal	
Hardware removal	K-wire: 3–4 weeks post-surgery Screws: 4–6 weeks post-surgery	
Return to sports	When there is generally free mobility, usually about 6 weeks	
Complications	Injuries to the deep branch of the radial nerve during open reduction Forearm rotation deficits because of post-traumatic radial head shape changes	
Growth disturbances	Irrelevant regarding epiphyseal growth impairment	
Follow up	Until free mobility is reached	
Classification	AO: 21-E/3(4).1-3	LiLa: 2.1.a.5.0-2.

Classification This is descriptively called a chisel fracture (Fig. 8.10). When the growth plates are (still) open, epiphyseal fractures are classified according to Salter-Harris; this injury is a Salter-Harris III or IV fracture or a transitional fracture. It is very rare and in children due to the high regeneration potential of the proximal radius usually a conservative approach (Figs. 8.11 and 8.12).

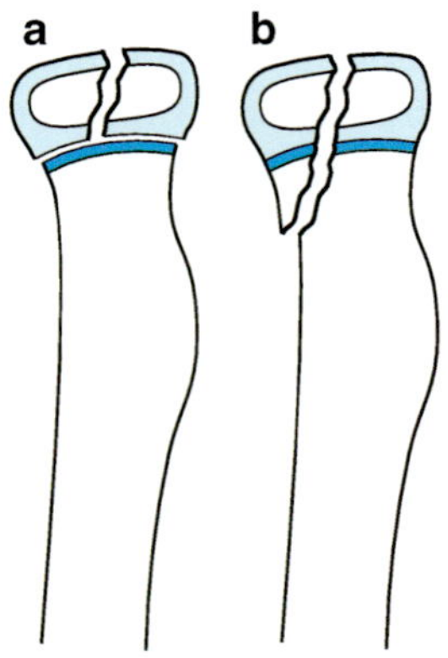

Fig. 8.10 Radial head fracture of the epiphysis. (**a**) Salter-Harris II, (**b**) Salter-Harris IV

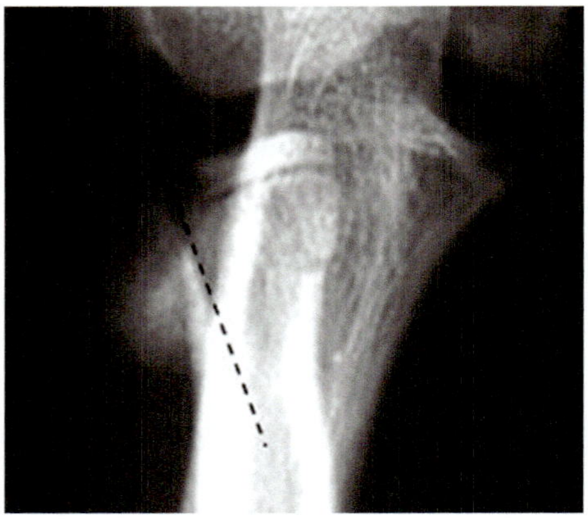

Fig. 8.11 Dislocated epiphyseal radial head fracture

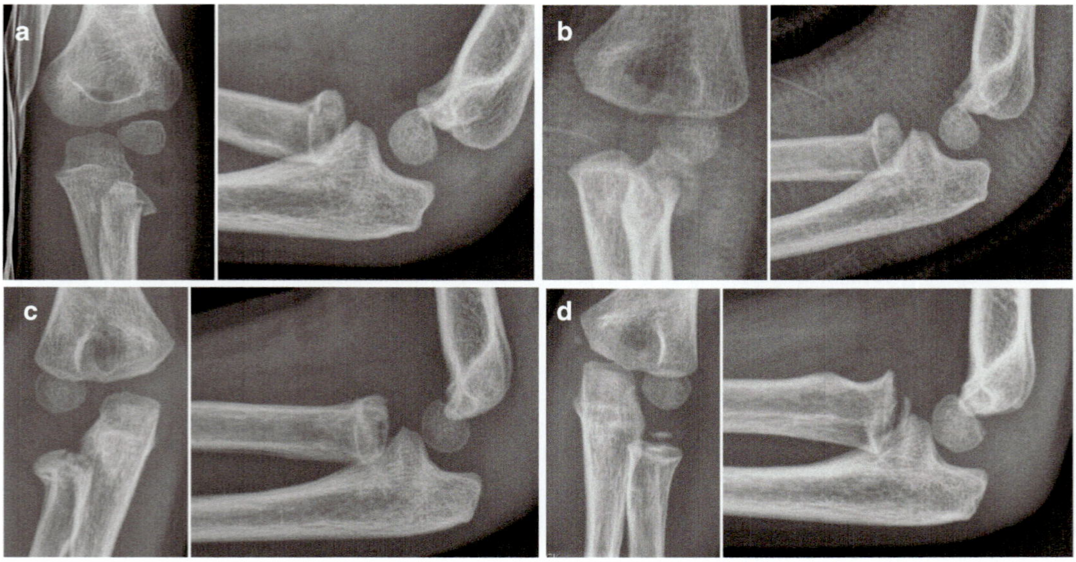

Fig. 8.12 (**a**–**d**) Epiphyseal radial head fracture, 5 years old boy. (**a**) Trauma image. (**b**) (**c**) after 7 months, (**d**) 13 months later

Metaphyseal Radial Neck Fracture This is a common pediatric elbow injury, with 1–1.3% of all fractures (Fig. 8.13). It can be associated with elbow dislocation but is more often caused by a fall on the pronated arm with an extended elbow or along with an ulnar shaft "parry" fracture as a Monteggia equivalent. Valgus stress shears off the head of the radius. Two-thirds to three-quarters of fractures are subcapital and metaphyseal, and a third to a quarter are tepiphyseal disruptions; most fractures are extracapsular with the proximal fragment displaced within the joint capsule. The classification is indicated in Table 8.4.

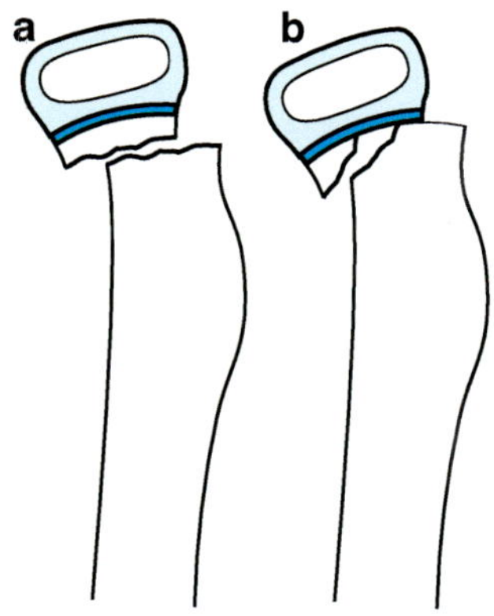

Fig. 8.13 (**a**) Radial neck fracture, (**b**) Salter-Harris II fracture

Table 8.4 Radial neck fracture classification

Judet classification	Metaizeau classification	AO classification
Type I Minimal translation	Type I <3 mm translation, tilt <20°	Type I Non-displaced
Type II Tilt <30°	Type II Tilt 20°–45°	Type II < 50% offset
Type III Tilt 30°–60°	Type III Tilt 45°–80°	Type III > 50% offset
Type IV Tilt >60°	Type IV Tilt >80°	
Type V Complete tilt		

Special Features The metaphyseal periosteal vessels are exclusively responsible for the blood supply to the proximal epiphysis (see Fig. 8.3). When there is severe tilt, there is a risk of ischemia with consequent changes to the shape of the proximal radius and mobility deficits. The proximal radial growth plate accounts for only a small proportion of radial growth; relevant growth irregularities are thus uncommon, and most are minimal. Partial growth plate fusion is possible when there is ischemia. Metaphyseal radial neck fracture information is given in Table 8.5.

The treatment of radial neck fractures in the metaphysis as well as Salter-Harris I and II fractures depend strongly on the age of the children. The remodeling capacity ranges from 60° in small childs to 10° around 10–12 years. Thus, conservative treatment is the first choice in most small children (Fig. 8.14). With increasing dislocation and age, an operative treatment should be performed, but without exposure of the radial neck, due to the critical vascularization. Indirect reduction and retrograde ESIN is the method of choice in these cases (Figs. 8.15 and 8.16).

Table 8.5 Metaphyseal radial neck fracture

Special features	Common; incidence 1–1.3% of all pediatric fractures Typically associated with elbow dislocation; Concomitant ulnar parry fracture (Monteggia equivalent), Fall on a pronated arm with extended elbow
Diagnostic approach:	AP and lateral x-rays, drawing the epiphyseal axis angle Clinical: Swelling, painful limited rotation
Treatment goal/limits of correction	Straightening of the proximal radius protecting head circulation as much as possible <10 years: Tilt to 45° can correct itself, intervention only for >45° >10 years: Tilt to 20° can self-correct, intervention for >20°, translation will not self-correct
Primary treatment	Positioning in long-arm splint
Conservative treatment	
Indication	Up to 45° tilt in patients <10 years, up to 20° tilt >10 years
Approach	<10 years: long-arm cast immobilization for 3 weeks >10 years: closed reduction with direct pressure on the proximal fragment under varus stress and elbow extension, to reach <20° of angulation
Follow up	Long-arm cast, remove at 3 weeks to mobilize as tolerated
Radiological controls	Day 1 (post-reduction only), day 7 (position check), day 21 (consolidation check)
Return to sports	When there is generally free mobility, usually 3–4 weeks after cast removal
Operative treatment	
Indication	Tilt >45° or > 20° (depending on age) or translation >½ shaft width
Approach	Closed reduction and fixation by retrograde ESIN Indirect reduction with K-wire joystick from posterolateral; direct open reduction rarely necessary and only indicated in exceptional cases because of circulation risk
Follow up	Functional with ESIN; possibly with long-arm splint for 1–2 weeks; Loading with full mobility at 4–6 weeks
Radiological controls	Day 0 (intraoperative), day 28 (consolidation check)
Hardware removal	At 4–6 weeks
Return to sports	After hardware removal with good mobility
Complications	Radial head shape changes, bulging, mobility deficits (pro/supination), non-union, head necrosis, radioulnar synostosis
Growth disturbances	Minimal, partial growth inhibition is possible
Follow up	Until free function From time of complication until growth is completed
Classification	AO:21-E/1(2).1-3.I–III I 21-M/2(3).1-3.I–III I LiLa: 2.1.s.1-5.0-2.

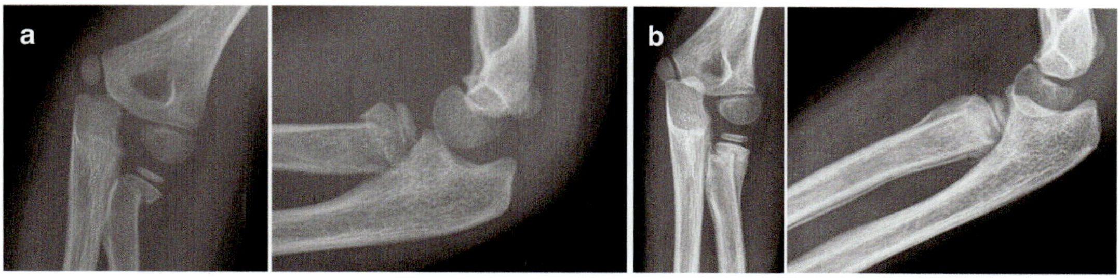

Fig. 8.14 Metaphyseal fracture of radial neck in a 5 year old boy. (**a**) Trauma Image. (**b**) 2 Months after conservative treatment with complete healing

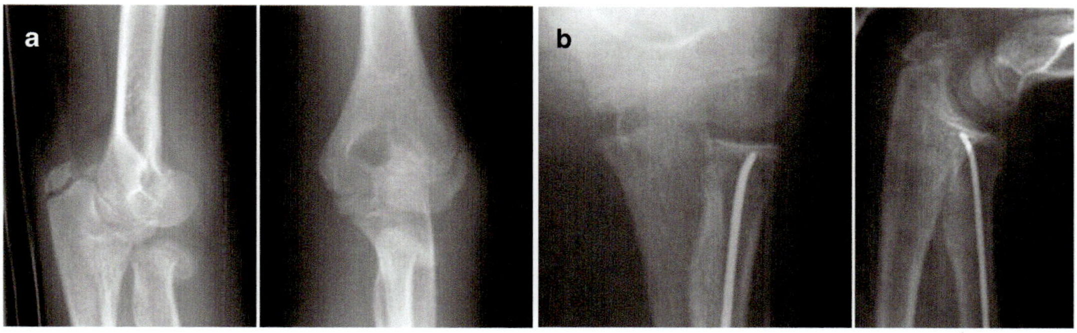

Fig. 8.15 Metaphyseal radial neck fracture of a 12 year old girl, Judo. (**a**) Trauma image, (**b**) Operative treatment with indirect reduction and retrograde intramedullary nailing, ESIN

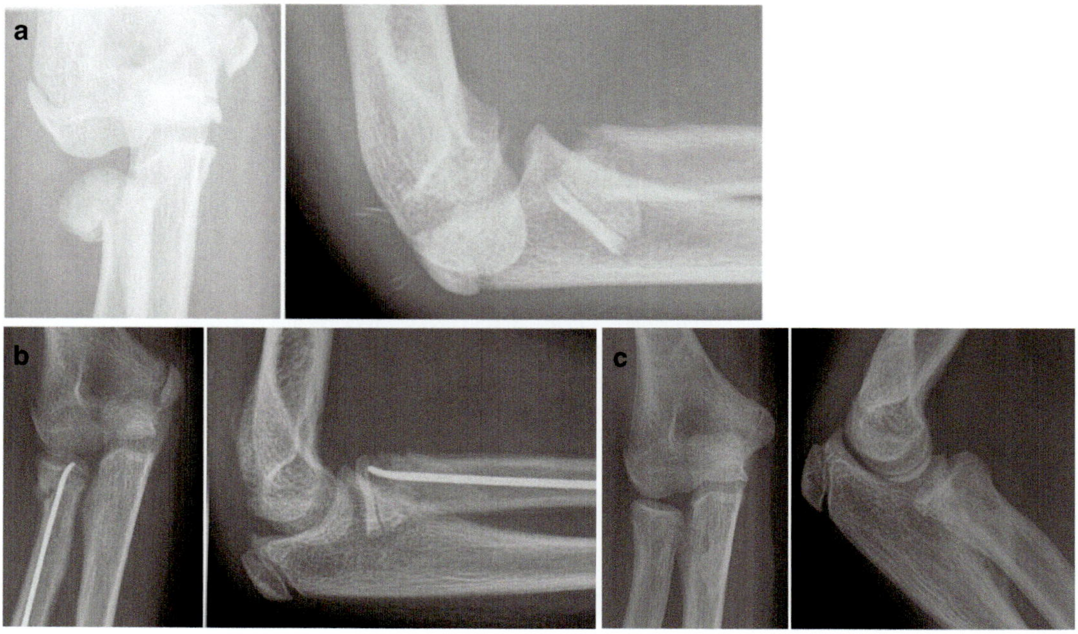

Fig. 8.16 Strongly dislocated radial neck fracture (70°) of a 11 year old girl. (**a**) Trauma image, (**b**) 4 Weeks after closed reduction and retrograde ESIN. (**c**) After metal removal at 4 months

8.3 Fractures of the Proximal Ulna

Intraarticular Olecranon Fracture (Fig. 8.17)
Together with extraarticular fractures, these make up <1% of all pediatric bony injuries and almost 5% of elbow injuries. The fracture results from the tensile forces of the brachialis and triceps muscles after a direct fall on the flexed elbow or a fall on the outstretched hand with varus or valgus stress. This type of oblique articular fracture also occurs with humeral lateral condyle fractures (Table 8.6).

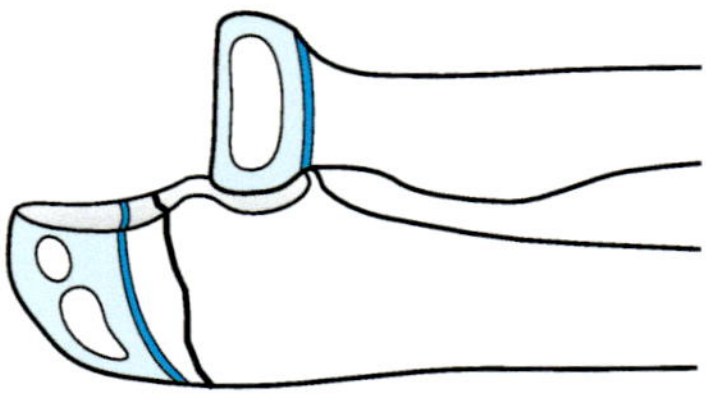

Fig. 8.17 Intraarticular metaphyseal fracture of the olecranon

Table 8.6 Intraarticular olecranon fracture

Special features	Incidence <1% of all fractures	
Diagnostic approach:	AP and lateral x-rays of the elbow Clinical: swelling especially posterior elbow, painful limited extension	
Treatment goal/limits of correction	Healing without an articular step No spontaneous correction	
Primary treatment	Immobilization in a long-arm splint	
Conservative treatment		
Indication	Non-displaced fractures (no articular step, max 2 mm dehiscence)	
Approach	Long-arm cast for 3 weeks	
Follow up	Mobilization as tolerated	
Radiological controls	Day 7 (secondary displacement), day 21 (consolidation check)	
Return to sports	When there is generally free mobility, usually 2–3 weeks after cast/splint removal	
Operative treatment		
Indication	Displaced fractures (articular step or dehiscence >2 mm)	
Approach	Open reduction and fixation Transverse fracture: tension band Alternative: (only) 2 K-wires (<5 years) or tension screw (for longitudinal or oblique fractures)	
Follow up	Tension band: immobilization until the wound is healed, then free mobility K-wires, screws: long-arm cast (splint) for 3 weeks	
Radiological controls	Day 0 (intraoperative), day 21–28 (consolidation check)	
Hardware removal	At 6–8 weeks (tension band, screw), K-wires at 4 weeks	
Return to sports	When there is generally free mobility, usually 2–3 weeks after cast/splint removal	
Complications	Residual articular step	
Growth disturbances	Not applicable as there is no proximal ulnar growth plate	
Follow up	Until free mobility	
Classification	AO: 21-M/3.1-3	LiLa: 2.1.a.5.0-2.U.

Special Features The fragment can appear tiny in younger children because a large part of the olecranon metaphysis remains cartilaginous (Fig. 8.18). The apophysis can show multiple ossification centers. Triceps muscle forces can increase secondary displacement of the olecranon (Figs. 8.19 and 8.20). The goal of treatment is anatomical joint reconstruction, because the apophyseal growth plate does not contribute to ulnar growth and thus, no spontaneous correction is expected. However, due to the ongoing growth and compression of the growth plate, an early removal of the tension bend wiring is recommended.

In undisplaced fractures, a conservative treatment is possible with a upper arm plaster for 3 weeks. Fractures can be transverse (Fig. 8.21) or oblique (Fig. 8.22).

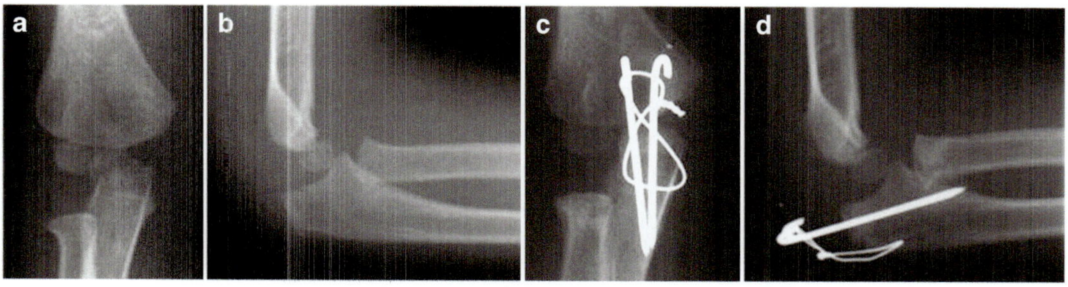

Fig. 8.18 Intraarticular olecranon fracture in toddler, girl, 2 years, fall on elbow at home. (**a**, **b**) Trauma images; dislocation due to ossification status better visible in A.P. view. (**c**, **d**) Tension band wiring after open reduction

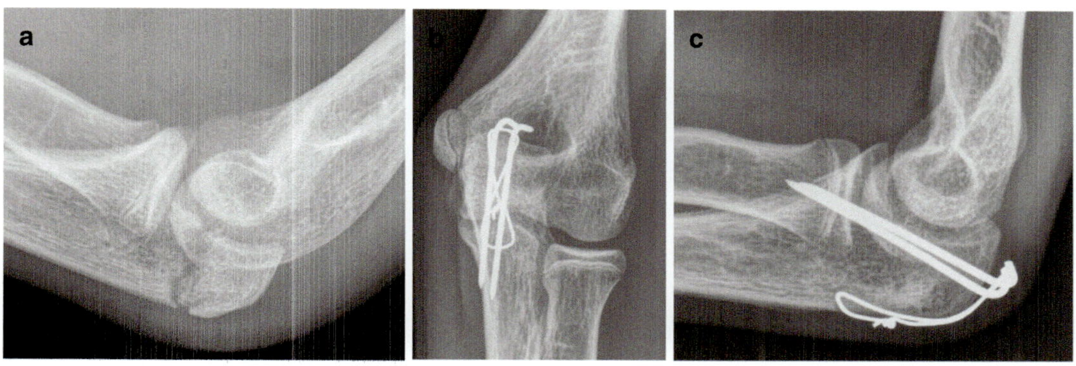

Fig. 8.19 Intraarticular olecranon fracture of a 14 year old boy after bicycle fall (with splenic rupture). (**a**) Trauma image, (**b**, **c**) 3 Months after tension band wiring with complete healing; prior to metal removal

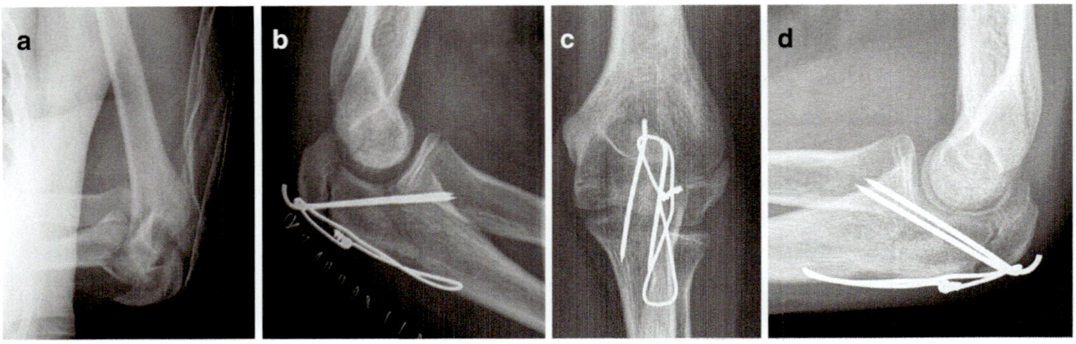

Fig. 8.20 Intraarticular olecranon fracture of a 13 year old boy. (**a**) Trauma image, (**b**) 2 Weeks postoperatively, (**c**, **d**) 2 Months later healing and prior to metal removal

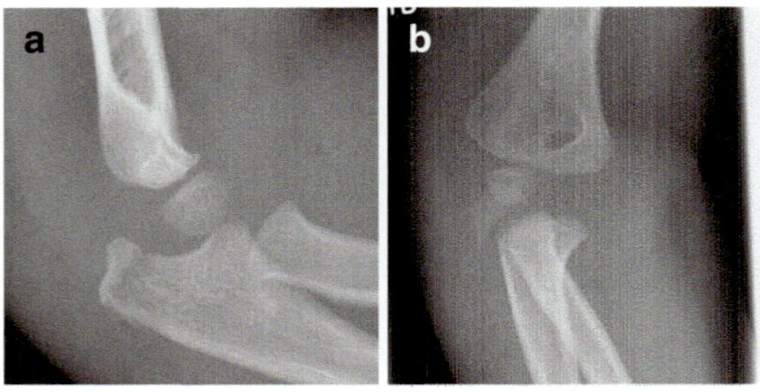

Fig. 8.21 (**a**, **b**) Undisplaced intraarticular olecranon fracture with indication for conservative treatment 4 year old girl

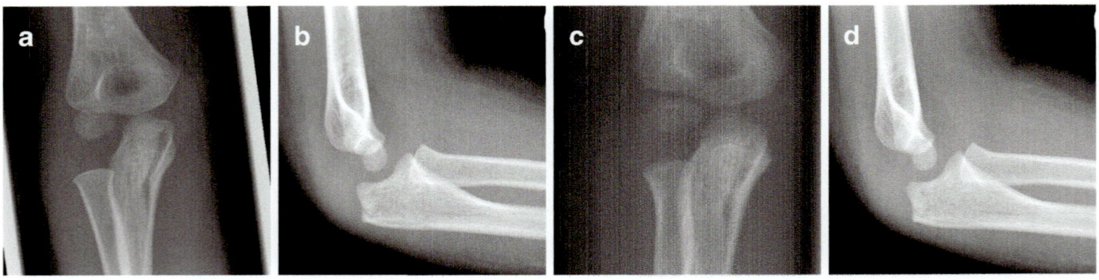

Fig. 8.22 (**a**, **b**) Undisplaced longitudinal olecranon fracture 5 year old boy, (**c**, **d**) Healing after conservative treatment

Extra-Articular Proximal Ulnar Fracture This usually arises from direct trauma, e.g., a fall on the elbow or the proximal ulna, and possibly along with a proximal radius dislocation (Monteggia fracture) or proximal radius fracture. Healing with even a minor axial deviation (especially varus) can lead to deficits in pronation/supination. Thus, operative reduction and tension band wiring is the method of choice. The possible concomitant injuries need to be treated as well. Undisplaced fractures might be treated conservatively (Table 8.7).

The technical consideration for the treatment of the proximal radius and ulna are shown in Tables 8.8 and 8.9.

Table 8.7 Extraarticular proximal ulnar fracture

Special features	Mostly direct trauma Can be associated with proximal radial dislocation (Monteggia fracture) or proximal radius fracture	
Diagnostic approach:	AP and lateral x-rays of the elbow, with forearm shaft if necessary, drawing of the radial axis	
Treatment goal/limits of correction	Healing without angulation; no spontaneous correction	
Primary treatment	Immobilization in a long-arm splint	
Conservative treatment		
Indication	Generally, a conservative attempt is indicated	
Approach	Non-displaced fractures: immobilization	
Follow up	Immobilization in a upper arm plaster for 3–4 weeks, then mobilization as tolerated	
Radiological controls	Day 0 and day 7 (control of secondary displacement), day 21/28 (consolidation check)	
Return to sports	When there is generally free mobility, usually 2–3 weeks after cast removal	
Operative treatment		
Indication	For insufficient reduction or retention	
Approach	Open reduction and screw fixation (Fig. 8.23) Tension band wiring after open reduction	
Follow up	With tension screw, immobilization in a long-arm cast for 3 weeks, then release; With tension band wiring 2 weeks upper arm cast	
Radiological controls	Day 0 (intraoperative), day 28 (consolidation check)	
Hardware removal	At 6–8 weeks	
Return to sports	When there is generally free mobility, after hardware removal	
Complications	Residual deformity in the AP plane, often underestimated and resulting in mobility deficits (pronation/supination)	
Growth disturbances	None	
Follow up	Until free function	
Classification	AO: 21-M/2(3).1-3	LiLa: 2.1.s.5.0-2.U.

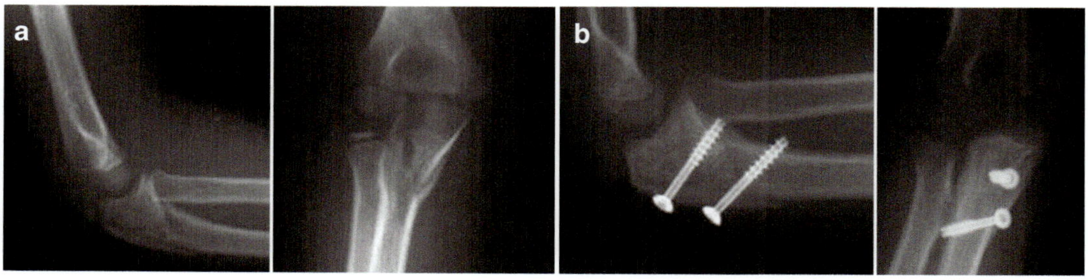

Fig. 8.23 Extraarticular fracture of the olecranon of a 6 year old girl after fall from a high bed. (**a**) Trauma image, (**b**) Lag screw osteosynthesis after open reduction

Table 8.8 Technical aspects: proximal radius

	Rarely open reduction via a posterolateral approach in pronation (caution: deep branch of the radial nerve) (Fig. 8.24) if possible, without opening the joint capsule and using trans-capsular reduction (protection of the periosteal vessels), intramedullary fixation regardless!
Material	Mini screws for proximal epiphyseal radial fractures ESIN diameter 2.0–2.5 mm, retrograde from distal radius metaphysis
Positioning	Supine positioning, arm table, tourniquet, draping above the elbow, hand wrapped
Access/approach (Figs. 8.25 and 8.26)	Posterolateral approach to the proximal radius in pronation Radial head dislocation or non-reducible radial neck fracture: removal of intraarticular obstacles to reduction (ligament structures), if necessary, with ligament repair, no ligament reconstruction Caution: deep branch of the radial nerve; the joint capsule must not necessarily be opened to reduce a radial neck fracture Metaphyseal radial neck fracture Reduction and fixation with intramedullary nail (2.0–2.5 mm), inserted from the distal radius In high-grade tilt, thumb pressure or percutaneously-placed K-wire can be used to assist reduction (Fig. 8.27) Hold, reduce, and fix the head with the sharpened nail tip, which is anchored in the epiphysis (Fig. 8.28)
Special clarification	Nerve injuries, joint infections In proximal radial dislocation: redislocation In proximal radial fracture: radial head necrosis, bulging of the radial head For all proximal forearm fractures: mobility deficits, especially pronation/supination
Hardware removal	ESIN at 6–8 weeks
Special features	None

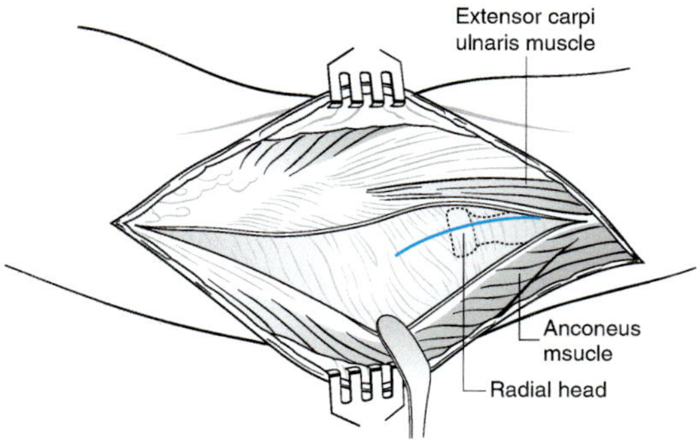

Fig. 8.24 Deep dorso-radial approach to the proximal radius in pronation of the forearm. Cave: deep branch of the radial nerve. Mostly, the opening of the joint capsula necessary Fig. 8.25

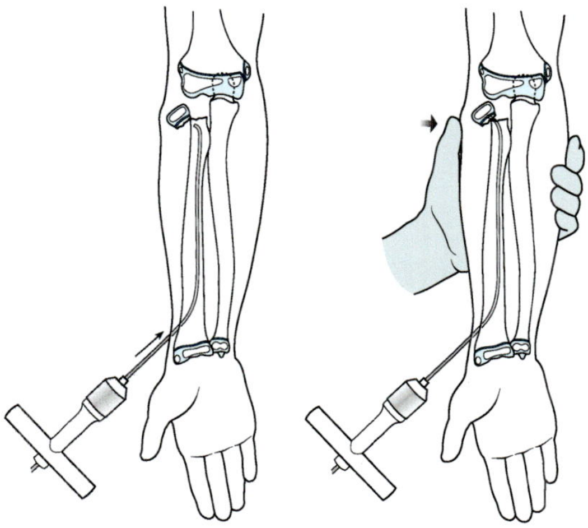

Fig. 8.25 (**a**, **b**) Retrograde elastic-stable intramedullary nailing of a radial neck fracture. (**a**) Insertion of the nail (2–2.5 mm), (**b**) Manual reduction with the thumb of the radial head. If this is not successful, a K-wire can be used percutaneously as a joy-stick

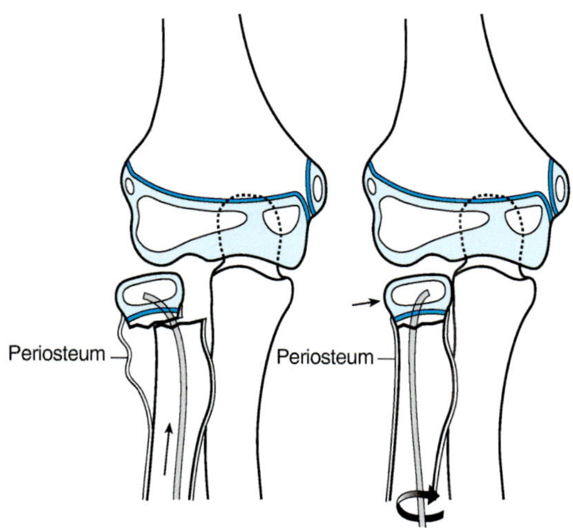

Fig. 8.26 (**a**) Retrograde protrusion of the nail into the largely reduced radial heads. (**b**) By turning of the nail, a better reduction and final position can be achieved. Occasionally, the perforation of the growth plate is necessary for this procedure

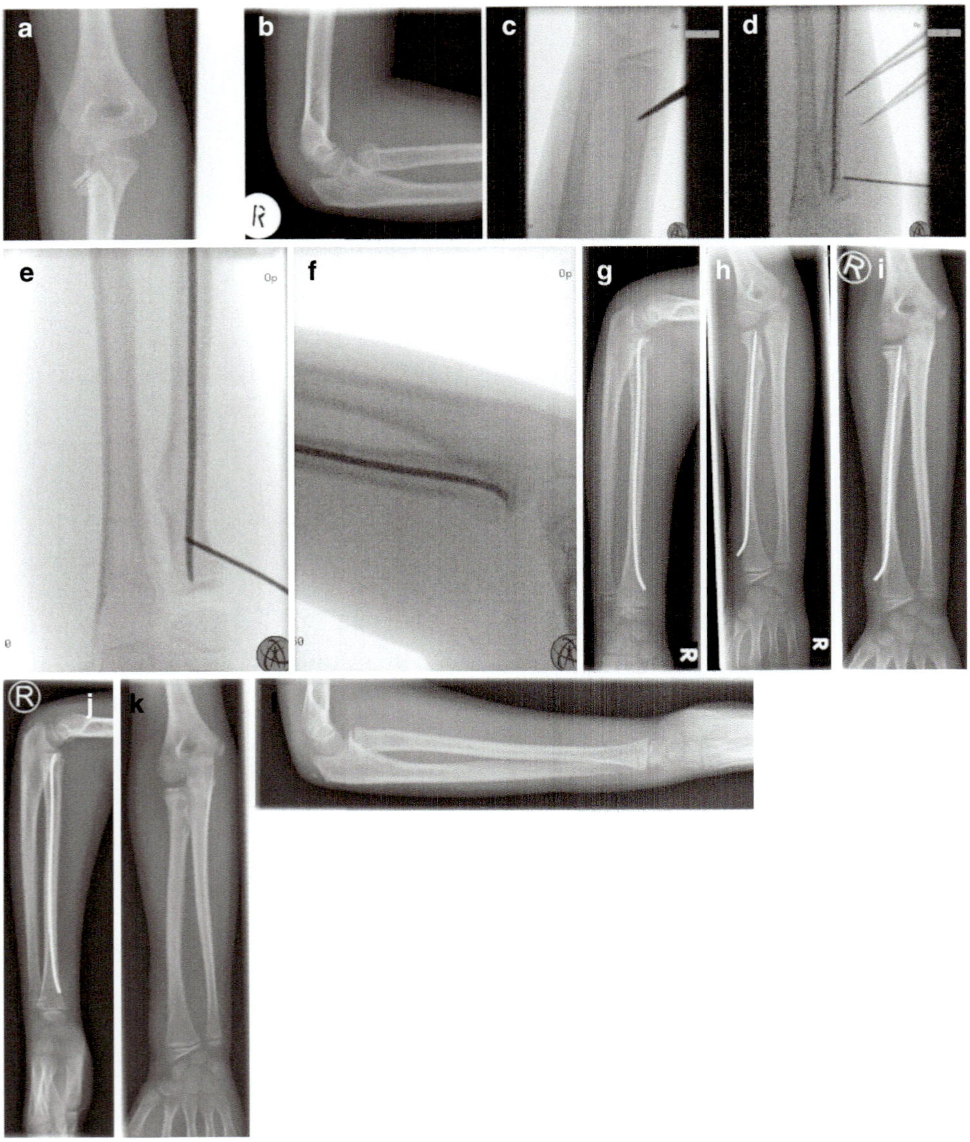

Fig. 8.27 Displaced radial head fracture in a 10 year old girl. (**a**, **b**) Trauma image, (**c**) Insertion of retrograde ESIN from distal radius, (**d**) Percutaneous K-wire in Kapandji technique for difficult reduction, (**e**) Successful reduction, (**f**) Advancement of ESIN into epiphysis to fix the reduction, (**g**, **h**) Postoperative x-ray; (**i**, **j**) Healing after 4 weeks, (**k**, **l**) After metal removal 4 months

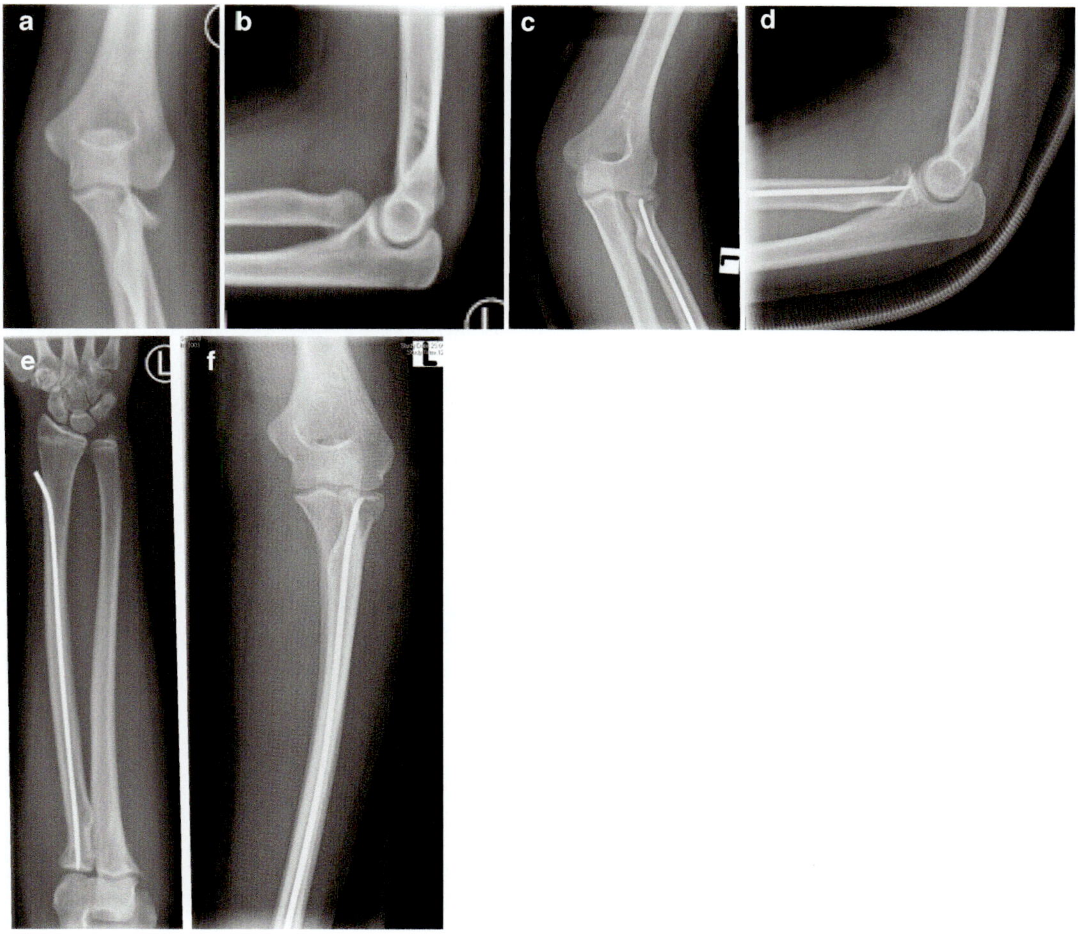

Fig. 8.28 12 year old girl with wide dislocation of proximal radial head. (**a**, **b**) Trauma image, (**c**, **d**) Postoperative x-ray after closed reduction and retrograde ESIN, (**e**, **f**) Healing after 4 month

Table 8.9 Technical aspects: proximal ulna

Material	K-wires 1.4–1.8 mm and cerclage wire 0.8–1.2 mm for olecranon fractures Small fragment screws for extraarticular proximal ulnar fractures ESIN diameter 2.0–2.5 mm
Positioning	Prone position with the forearm hanging over an arm table is helpful for olecranon fractures; supine position for ESIN
Access/approach	Posterior approach to the olecranon with lateral dissection Intraarticular olecranon fracture Open reduction from posterior with lateral dissection of the olecranon (Fig. 8.29) If needed, visualization of the ulnar nerve and tension band, especially for transverse fractures Tension band: placement of two parallel K-wires over the olecranon apophysis, drilled through the anterior cortex of the ulnar metaphysis Wire cerclage around the K-wire ends and through a transverse-drilled ulnar canal Alternative: (only) 2 K-wires (<5 years) or tension screw (for oblique fractures) Extraarticular olecranon fracture: open reduction and screw fixation tension band wiring or plate osteosynthesis in proximal fractures
Special clarification	Nerve injuries, joint infections For all proximal forearm fractures: mobility deficits, especially pronation/supination
Hardware removal	Tension band at 2–3 months
Special features	None
	Deeper posterolateral approach to the proximal radius in pronation. Caution: Deep branch of the radial nerve; the joint capsule must not necessarily be opened to reduce a radial neck fracture.

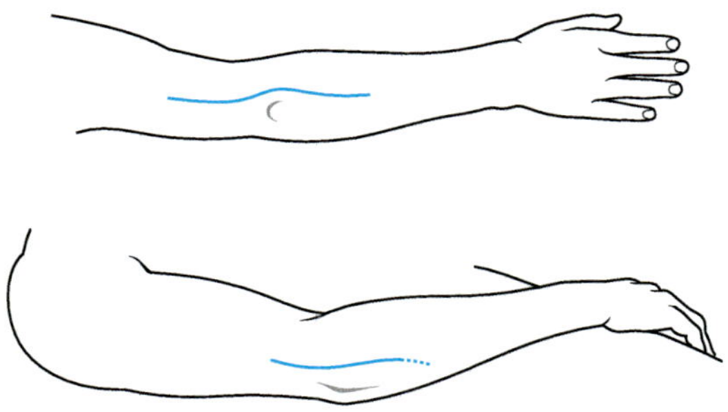

Fig. 8.29 Above: posterior approach to the olecranon with lateral dissection, visualization of the ulnar nerve; below: posterolateral approach to the radial head

Recommended Literature

Çevik N, Cansabuncu G, Akalın Y, Otuzbir A, Öztürk A, Özkan Y (2018) Functional and radiological results of percutaneous K-wire aided Métaizeau technique in the treatment of displaced radial neck fractures in children. Acta Orthop Traumatol 52:428–434

Chirurg PSD (2017) Frakturen der oberen Extremität im Kindes-/Wachstumsalter. Orthopäde. Thieme, Stuttgart. https://doi.org/10.1007/s00104-017-0420-5

Dietz HG, Illing P, Schmittenbecher PP, Slongo T, Sommerfeldt DW (2011) Praxis der Kinder- und Jugendtraumatologie, 1st edn. Springer, New York

Gortzak Y, Mercado E, Atar D, Weisel Y (2006) Pediatric olecranon fractures: open reduction and internal fixation with removable Kirschner wires and absorbable sutures. J Pediatr Orthop 26:39–42

Hell AK, von Laer L (2014) Growth behaviour after fractures of the proximal radius: differences to the rest of the skeleton. Der Unfallchirurg 117:1085–1091

Marzi I (2016) Kindertraumatologie, 3rd edn. Springer, New York

Metaizeau JP (1988) Ostosynthese chez l'enfant par E.C.M.E.S. Sauramps Médical, Montpellier

Metaizeau J, Lascombes P, Lemelle J, Finlayson D, Prevot J (1993) Reduction and fixation of displaced radial neck fractures by closed intramedullary pinning. J Pediatr Orthop 13:355–360

Narang AM, Pandey AA, Bhat M (2020) Management of severely displaced radial neck fractures in children: a systematic review and meta-analysis of outcomes. Indian J Orthop 54:60–68

Rockwood C, Wilkins KE, King RE (1984) Fractures in children. Lippincott, Philadelphia

Schmittenbecher PP (2008) Osteosynthesen am proximalen Unterarm im Kindesalter. Oper Orthop Traumatol 20:321–333

Schneidmüller D, Gutsfeld P, Woltmann A, Marzi I, Bühren V (2014) Problems and complications of radial neck fractures in children. Obere Extremität 2014:1–4

von Laer L, Kraus R, Linhart WE (2012) Frakturen und Luxationen im Wachstumsalter 6., überarbeitete und erweiterte Auflage 2012 512 S., 1380 Abb. Thieme, Stuttgart

Ulrich D, Voth M, Frank J, Marzi I (2015) Dislocation fractures of the elbow in childhood. Trauma Berufskrankheit 17:253–259

9 Forearm

9.1 Physiological Findings

The radius and ulna begin ossification from the primary ossification centers in the 6th week of gestation. Secondary ossification begins along the distal radius in the first one and half years, and the distal ulna at 4 years. The proximal ossification centers begin ossification between ages 3 and 7 for the radius and between 8 and 10 for the ulna. The proximal epiphyses in the elbow region close somewhat earlier than the distal epiphyses, which ossify between 16 and 19 years of age. The proximal growth plates contribute up to 20%, and the distal up to 80% of forearm length (Fig. 9.1).

Forearm fractures are classified according to localization (Table 9.1) or fracture type (Table 9.2).

9.2 Fracture Types and Localisation of the Forearm

Forearm shaft fractures. The muscles attached to the forearm act as deforming forces when fracture is present.

In proximal fractures (Fig. 9.2a), the supinator and biceps muscles pull the proximal fragment into supination and flexion. The pronator quadratus and teres muscles pronate the distal fragment; thus, immobilization should be carried out in supination to approximate the fracture ends.

For fractures of the mid-shaft (Fig. 9.2b), immobilization should be performed in neutral position or in mild supination. In this case, the

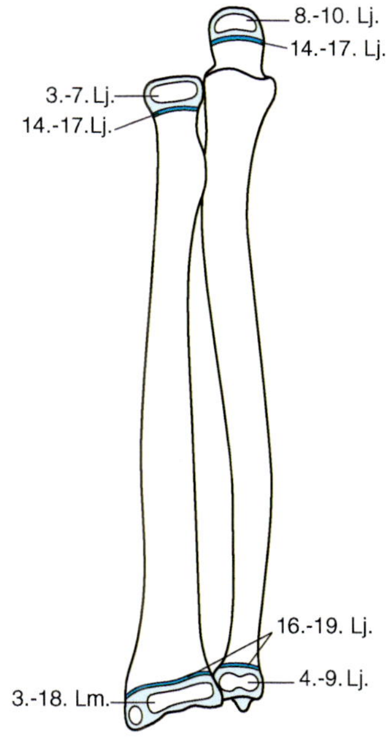

Fig. 9.1 Ossification centers and growth plate fusion. (*Lj*) life year, (*Lm*) life month

I. Marzi et al., *Pediatric Skeletal Trauma*, https://doi.org/10.1007/978-3-030-93685-3_9

Table 9.1 Distribution of forearm fractures according to localization

Proximal third	Isolated radial fractures Fracture of both forearm bones Monteggia injury
Mid-third	Isolated radial fractures Fracture of both forearm bones Greenstick fracture/bowing fracture
Distal third	Isolated radius fractures Fracture of both forearm bones Galeazzi injury

Table 9.2 Distribution of forearm fractures by fracture type

Closed or open fractures
Buckle fracture/compression fracture
Greenstick fractures
Complete forearm fracture
Comminuted fracture

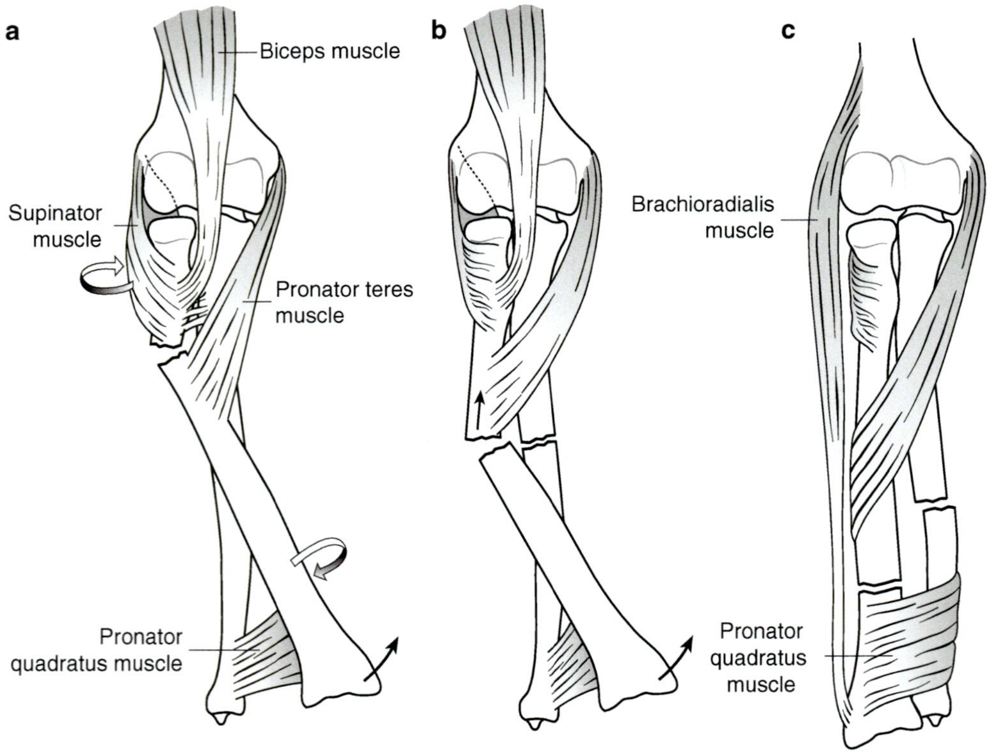

Fig. 9.2 Forearm musculature, displacement of the fracture fragments. (**a**) Proximal forearm fracture, (**b**) Mid-forearm fracture, (**c**) Distal forearm fracture

pronator teres and the supinator neutralize each other, leaving only the biceps acting to flex the proximal fragment.

If the fracture is located in the distal shaft (Fig. 9.2c), the distal fragment supinates due to pull of the brachioradialis muscle. Thus, immobilization in slight pronation is most likely to approximate the fracture ends. However, immobilization for each fracture type should be considered individually and adapted as needed.

Isolated radial fractures have a tendency for valgus deformity, and rarely there is distal ulnar epiphyseal rupture corresponding to a Galeazzi equivalent.

Isolated ulnar fractures tend to a varus deformity and can lead to accompanying radial head dislocation Monteggia fracture).

Angulation of the forearm shaft region corrects only under certain conditions and this usually only to the age of 5 years. Rotational deformities do not correct spontaneously. Both can lead to significant functional deficits in both pronation and supination. Rotational deficits are functionally significant from angulation of 20°; thus, this is the largest tolerance limit for non-operative treatment. The further proximal the angulation, the less it can be tolerated. Similarly, opposing deformations in the shaft region lead to pronounced functional deficits. In contrast, side-to-side shifts will generally compensate spontaneously to a single shaft width.

If correction osteotomies are indicated, mostly due to impaired forearm rotation, it is recommended to perform them as soon as possible, because functional deficits can persist and interfere with operative outcomes (see further Chap. 20).

The cause of this injury is usually a fall onto the outstretched hand. The incidence of mid-shaft fractures peaks between 6 and 8 years and is more common in boys. More distal fractures occur most frequently around the age of 10. Fracture localization depends on the impact but is most common in the distal third. While distal fractures can in part be treated conservatively, fractures of the mid and proximal shaft mostly require surgery.

Greenstick and complete fractures are more common in the shaft region, and torus fractures in the metaphyseal regions. It is important to complete the greenstick fractures in anesthesia in order to achieve a straight healing. Since anesthesia is necessary to correct shaft alignment, definitive treatment should be performed as well. Thus, reduction of greenstick fractures and intramedullary nail fixation for instability should be carried out at the same time. Also, in most other forearm shaft fractures the operative stabilization with intramedullary nailing is the recommended treatment with the highest chance to come out without any functional impairments.

In forearm shaft fractures, the adjacent joints must be visualized on x-ray. In cases of insufficient visualization and clinical symptoms, the elbow joint should be radiographed separately in two planes to avoid overlooking a combination injury. If one of the two forearm bones is fractured and shortened, this suggests dislocation of the proximal or distal radio-ulnar joints. Left untreated, potential consequences include movement deficits, instability, and valgus deformity.

To exclude radial head dislocation, a reference line is drawn through the axis of the proximal radius. This must project to the center of the humeral capitulum in all planes (also oblique views), see Fig. 2.14. If not, a radial head dislocation is present (Fig. 9.3).

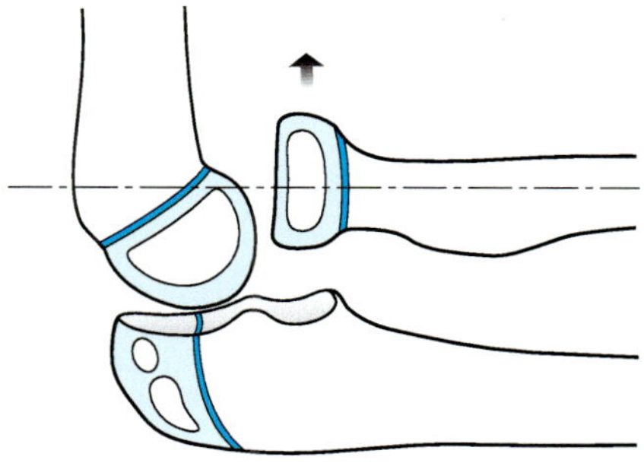

Fig. 9.3 The axial reference line of the proximal radius must project to the center of the humeral capitulum in all planes

The classic Monteggia fracture is an ulnar shaft fracture with radial head dislocation. The ulnar shaft fracture can be located from the middle third all the way proximal, and thus be considered an olecranon fracture. The radial head usually dislocates anteriorly or radially. There are also Monteggia equivalent fractures, for example an ulnar shaft fracture in combination with a radial neck fracture, or complete proximal forearm fractures fitting the definition of a Monteggia fracture (Table 9.3 and Fig. 9.4).

Clinical signs of radial head dislocation are pain, deformity and marked deficits in elbow range of motion with fixed pronated position. The prognosis is good for primarily diagnosed dislocations, when the treatment is correct. This results generally in an anatomical reduction and stabilization of the ulnar fracture and a reduction of the radial head. Sometime, the ulnar fracture is not very good visible, since it is only a bowing fracture with a straight ulna leading to a luxation of the radial head. If a Monteggia injury is missed, the prognosis of this injury is much less favorable and can result in permanent painful movement deficits. Early reconstruction is the only way for rescuing a good function, since late reconstructions are demanding (see Chap. 20).

The Galeazzi fracture and Galeazzi equivalent are rare injuries in children (Table 9.4 and Fig. 9.5). It is typically caused by a fall on the outstretched, pronated hand. The injury occurs

Table 9.3 Monteggia injuries are most commonly classified according to Bado

– Type I Anterior dislocation of the radial head and fracture of the ulnar diaphysis with anterior angulation. 70% of Monteggia injuries in children.
– Type II Posterior or posterolateral dislocation of the radial head and fracture of the ulnar diaphysis with posterior angulation. 6% of Monteggia lesions.
– Type III Lateral or anterolateral dislocation of the radial head with fracture of the ulnar metaphysis. 23% of Monteggia lesions in children.
– Type IV Anterior dislocation of the radial head with fractures of the proximal third of both radius and ulna. Rare injury. About 1% of Monteggia lesions.

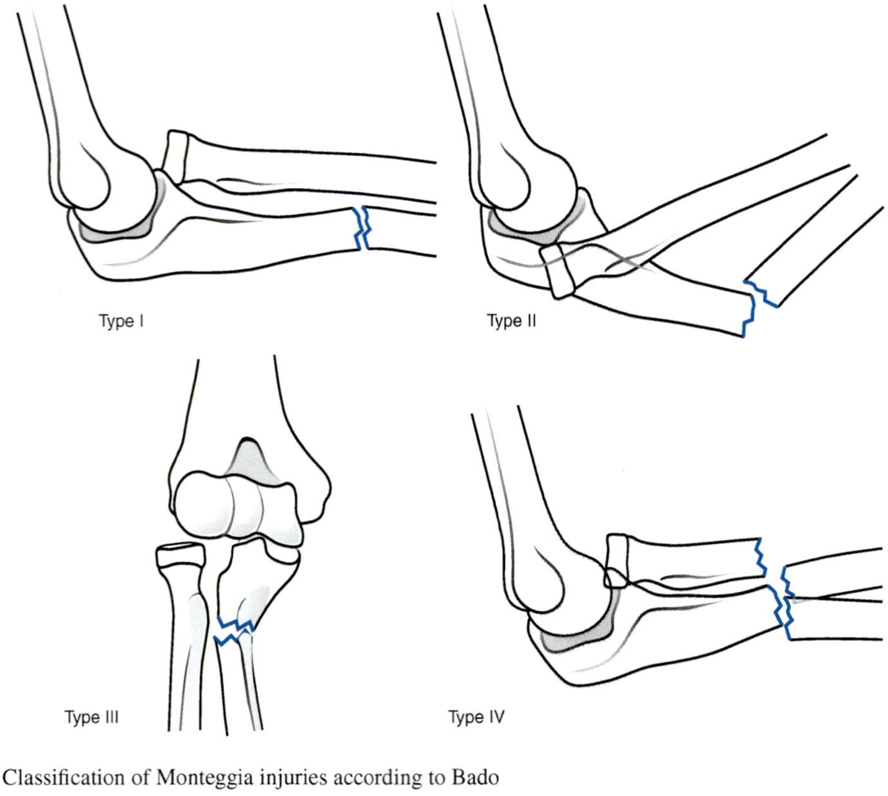

Fig. 9.4 Classification of Monteggia injuries according to Bado

primarily in children between 9 and 12 years of age. Often there is a varus deformity of the forearm with a deformed, swollen, painful wrist. Sometimes there is protrusion of the ulnar head or increased mobility of the distal ulna.

The classic Galeazzi injury is a radial shaft fracture in combination with dislocation of the distal radio-ulnar joint (DRUJ). The radial shaft usually fractures at the intersection of the mid to distal third. In children, the DRUJ dislocates around the ulnar epiphysis because this is weaker than the disco-ligamentous connection; this is called the Galeazzi equivalent. In most cases, this epiphyseal injury is a Salter II/Aitken 1 fracture. The restoration of the precise length of the radius is of outmost importance also for the DRUJ function. Since this injury occurs often in adolescence, a plate osteosynthesis of the radius is a safe solution to restore the correct length of the radius.

Complete dislocation of the distal radio-ulnar joint always includes injury to the triangular fibrocartilaginous complex (TFCC) and is thus an unstable injury. Usually, in children, this might be primarily treated conservatively, but sometimes an MRI and/or arthroscopy in adolescents might be necessary.

The distal forearm shows extraordinary corrective capacity in children under 10–12 years. Beyond that age, spontaneous correction varies considerably and particularly according to the

Table 9.4 Galeazzi fractures and Galeazzi equivalents are classified according to Letts and Rowhani

– Type A Radial fracture at the intersection of the middle and distal thirds and
1. Posterior discoligamentous dislocation of the distal ulna
2. Distal epiphysiolysis of the ulna and posterior metaphyseal displacement
– Type B Fracture of the distal third of the radius and
1. Posterior discoligamentous dislocation of the distal ulna
2. Distal epiphysiolysis of the ulna and posterior metaphyseal displacement
– Type C Greenstick fractures of the radius with posterior angulation and
1. Posterior discoligamentous dislocation of the distal ulna
2. Distal epiphysiolysis of the ulna and posterior metaphyseal displacement
– Type D Distal radius fracture with anterior angulation and
1. Anterior discoligamentous dislocation of the distal ulna
2. Distal epiphysiolysis of the ulna and anterior displacement of the metaphysis.

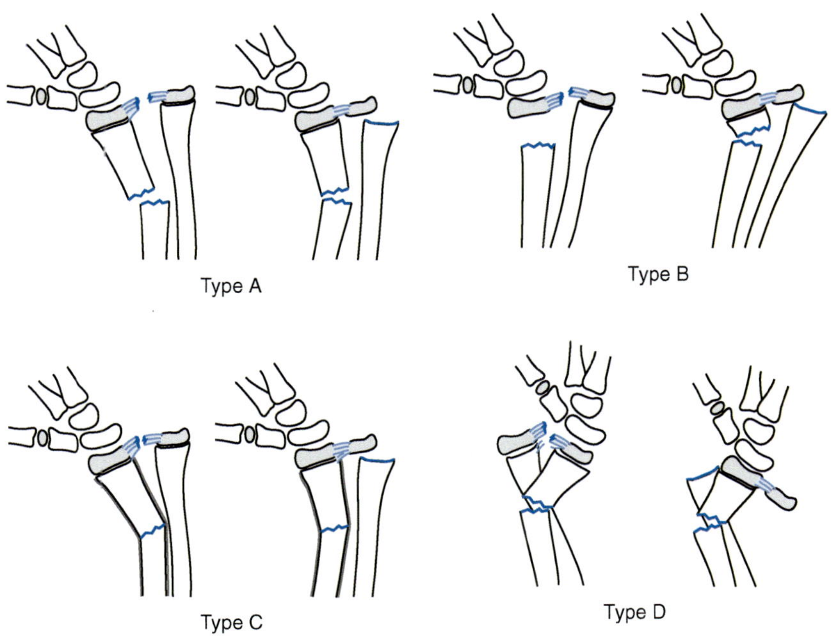

Fig. 9.5 Classification of Galeazzi injuries according to Letts and Rowhani

stage of growth plate development. Thus, up to 30° angulation can be allowed in children under 10 years, however in decreasing degrees with age. In children over 12 years, there is barely any spontaneous correction and angulation should be corrected as much as possible. Because the deformities are sometimes clearly visible, parents should be encouraged not to worry with detailed explanations and close support. However, it should be noted that fractures of the distal or metaphyseal areas of the forearm generally occur in older children (>12 years). In addition, the position of the distal ulna needs to be controlled as well, since remaining growth deformities might result in DRUJ incongruence an rotational deficit.

There are many types of injury of the distal radius, most commonly epiphyseolysis (Salter-Harris-I and II), Buckle Handle fractures and complete metaphyseal fractures. Articular fractures of the joint surface (Salter-Harris III and IV) and metaphyseal greenstick fractures are less common. While the definition of the metaphysis is the square of the width of the distal radius and ulna, the treatment of meta-diaphyseal fractures is difficult to achieve as indicated in the tables.

38% of all pediatric fractures involve the forearm. More than 50% of these are located at the distal forearm. Of all forearm shaft fractures, two thirds are distal and one third are mid-shaft fractures. Fractures of the proximal shaft are rare.

In the following, the typical fracture types of the forearm shaft and the distal forearm are described in the tables and illustrated by the typical x-rays after trauma and during treatment.

9.3 Forearm Fractures

In the following tables, the diagnosis and treatment of forearm fractures are indicated: Tables 9.5, 9.6, 9.7, 9.8, 9.9 and corresponding figures.

Table 9.5 Forearm fractures—greenstick fractures (Fig. 9.6)

Details	Various fracture forms: typical: cortex ruptured on the convex side and intact on the concave side, “Bowing fracture”: no visible fracture line; especially <5 years of age.
Diagnostic assessment	Forearm x-rays A.P. and lateral with adjacent joints and if needed, additional x-rays centered on the adjacent joints to exclude Monteggia or Galeazzi injuries
Goals of treatment/ tolerance limits	Angulation <10° in both planes corrects spontaneously; the younger the child, the greater the potential for correction
Primary treatment	Above-elbow plaster slab, with medical analgesia if needed
Conservative therapy	
Indication	Angulation <10°; only in younger patients with higher corrective potential to <20° if needed
Procedure	3–4 weeks above-elbow cast, with overcorrection of the fracture in anesthesia to complete the fracture (Fig. 9.7) (KT Abb. 15.7). Wedging if necessary on the 5th–8th day to compress the completed fracture line; operative treatment recommended for angulation >10°
Follow-up	Functional, physical therapy is usually not necessary
X-ray controls	Day 5–8 position control; 4th week consolidation control (without cast)
Sports participation	6–8 weeks after consolidation
Operative therapy	
Indication	Angulation >10°; also with less angulation in fractures of both forearm bones
Procedure	Overcorrection of the opposite cortex (completing the fracture in anesthesia) Stabilization with ESIN (elastic stabilizing intramedullary nail) (Figs. 9.8 and 9.9). Should be considered also with bowing fracture (Fig. 9.10)
Follow-up	Functional, if necessary several days of above-elbow plaster slab for analgesia
X-ray controls	Post-operative position control; 4-week consolidation control
Hardware removal	12 weeks post-operatively
Sports participation	8 weeks after consolidation
Complications	Delayed spontaneous correction, increase of the primary deformity, if fracture not completed. Risk of refracture due to consolidation dysfunction in typical greenstick fractures For angulation >20° deficits in pronation and supination
Growth disturbance	Temporary length difference, which usually evens out over time
Follow-up	3–4 weeks until free function
Classification	AO: 22-D/1(2).1-3 LiLa: 2.2.s.2.0-2.

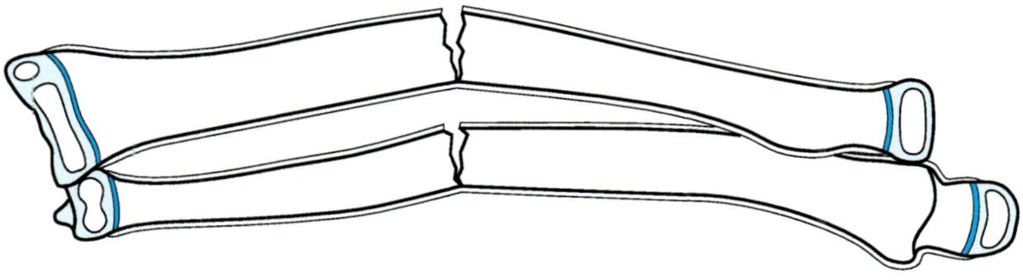

Fig. 9.6 Greenstick fracture of the forearm shaft

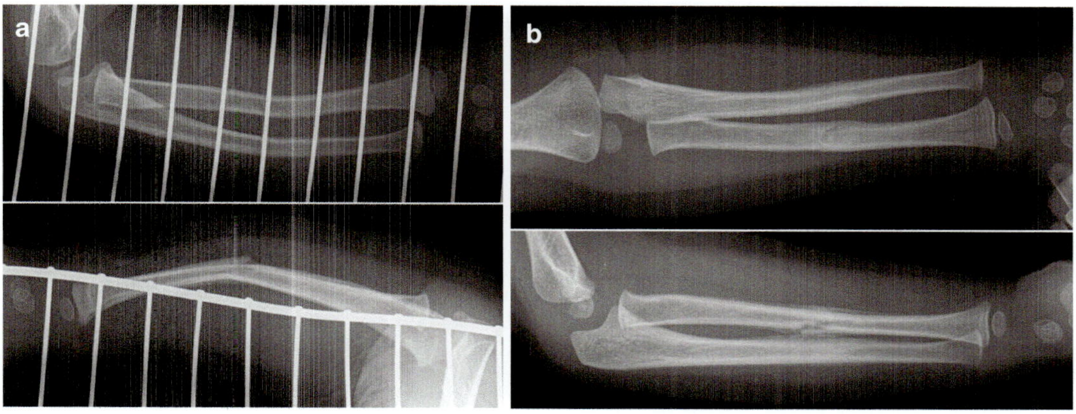

Fig. 9.7 Greenstick fracture of the forearm shaft after fall at home in a 2 year old girl. (**a**) Trauma image, (**b**) 4 Weeks after completion of fracture in general anesthesia and upper arm cast

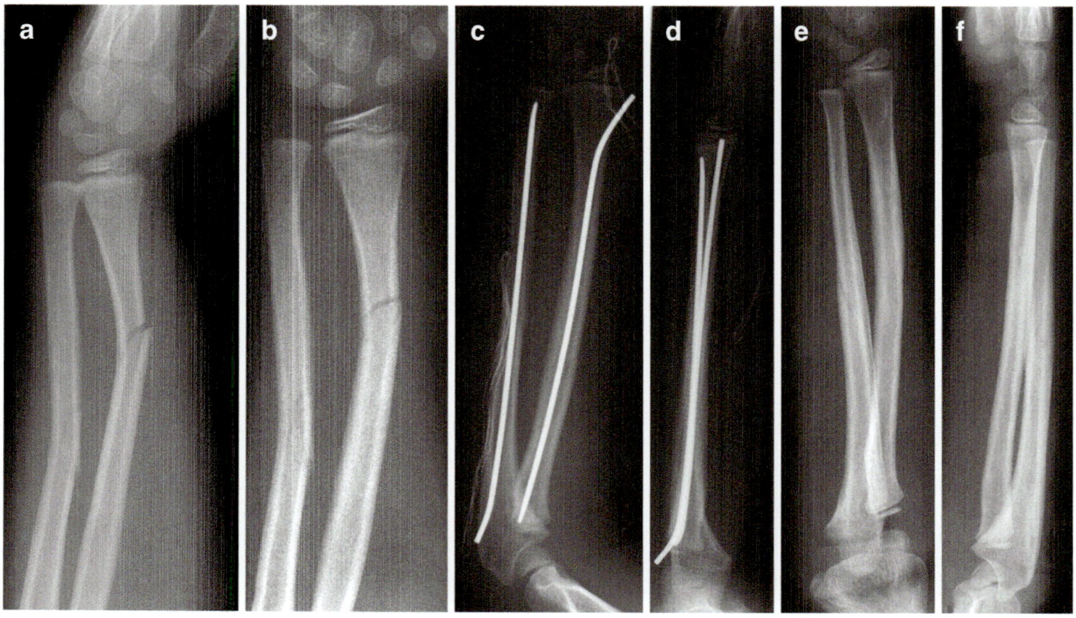

Fig. 9.8 Greenstick fracture of the forearm shaft of a 5 year old girl after fall on the left hand. (**a**, **b**) Trauma image, (**c**, **d**) Osteosynthesis with ESIN after completion of fracture during day of trauma, (**e**, **f**) Complete healing after metal removal

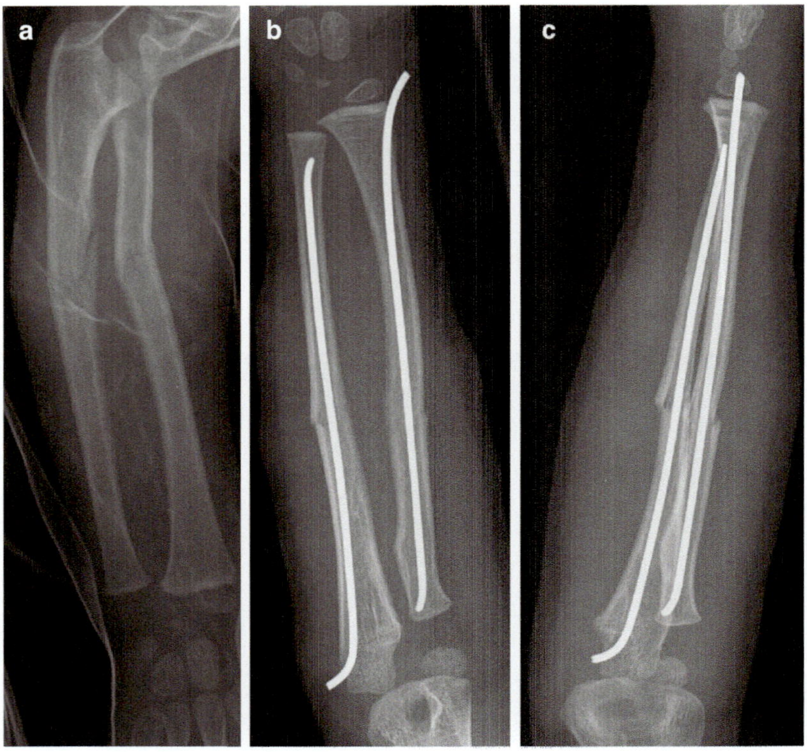

Fig. 9.9 7 Greenstick fracture of the forearm shaft in a 5 year old boy. (**a**) Trauma image, (**b**, **c**) ESIN with 2.0 mm nails on day of accident and functional after treatment

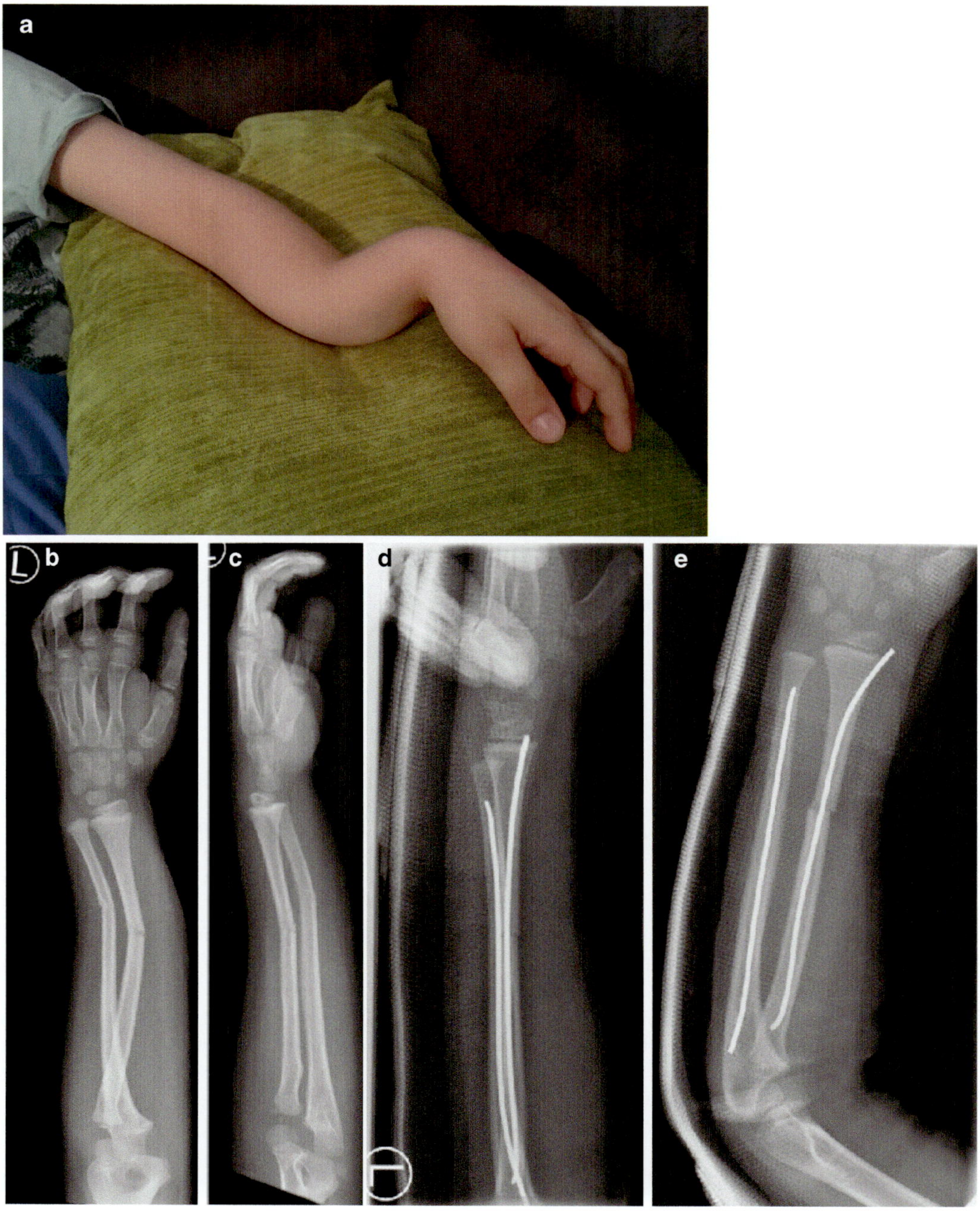

Fig. 9.10 (**a**) Serious dislocation, redressed by the emergency physician; (**b**, **c**) Trauma image Greenstick fracture of the radius, bowing fractures of the ulna; (**d**, **e**) After operative overcorrection and ESIN

Table 9.6 Complete forearm fractures (Fig. 9.11)

Details	Typically above the age of 10–12 years, mostly both forearm bones affected except with direct impact trauma. But also, fractures of the radius or ulna alone can take place.
Diagnostic assessment	Forearm x-rays A.P. and lateral with adjacent joints and if needed, additional x-rays centered on the adjacent joints to exclude Monteggia or Galeazzi injuries (see below) Evaluation of perfusion, motor and sensory function and exclusion of compartment syndrome
Goals of treatment/ tolerance limits	Angulation <10° in both planes, the younger the child, the greater the potential for correction only spontaneous correction of side-to-side shifts is possible
Primary treatment	Above-elbow plaster slab, with medical analgesia if needed
Conservative therapy	
Indication	Angulation <10°; especially in isolated fractures of one forearm bone; in children <5 years
Procedure	3–4 weeks above-elbow cast; if necessary with secondary wedging on the 5th to 8th day, spontaneous axis correction can be expected in small children (Fig. 9.12)
Follow-up	Functional, physical therapy is usually not necessary
X-ray controls	Day 5–8 position control, if needed after wedging; day 14 position control; 4th week consolidation control (without cast)
Sports participation	About 8 weeks after consolidation
Operative therapy	
Indication	Instability in fractures of both forearm bones Angulation ≥10°, rotational deformity, shortening Soft-tissue interposition Second and third grade open fractures, concomitant neurovascular injuries Polytrauma/multiple injuries Malunion, deformity after conservative treatment
Procedure	Closed reduction and fixation with ESIN: Ulna shaft fracture (Fig. 9.13) radius fracture (Fig. 9.14) or complete forearm fracture (Figs. 9.15 and 9.16). Open reduction in cases of impediments (interposed periosteum or muscle) Wound debridement and stabilization possible in open fractures External fixators for multi-fragment and comminuted fractures for which length can't be fixed with ESIN; in open fractures and peri-articular fractures Plate fixation in adolescent older children and in special cases (malunion, corrective osteotomies, peri-articular fractures in adolescents) (Figs. 9.17 and 9.18)
Follow-up	Functional, if necessary several days of above-elbow plaster slab for analgesia Physical therapy is usually not necessary
X-ray controls	Post-operative position control; 4-week consolidation control (without cast)
Hardware removal	12 weeks post-operatively
Sports participation	8 weeks after consolidation
Complications	For angulation >20° deficits in pronation and supination; Malunion, re-fracture risk for early hardware removal (under 3 months) Synostosis formation
Growth disturbance	Temporary length difference and rotational deficits
Follow-up	3–4 weekly controls until free function
Classification	AO: 22-D/4(5).1-3 LiLa: 2.2.s.3(4).0-2.

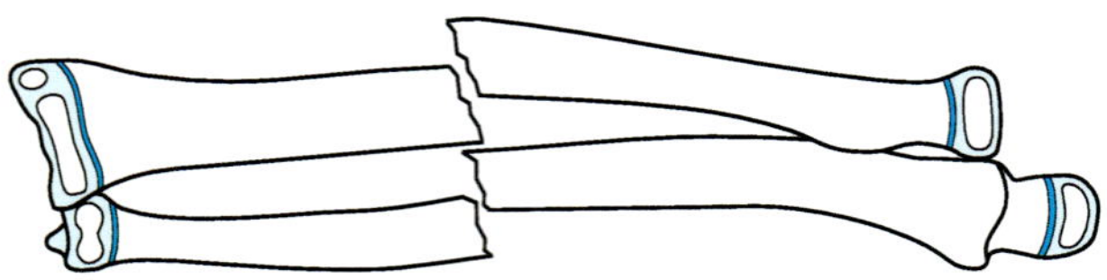

Fig. 9.11 Complete forearm fracture

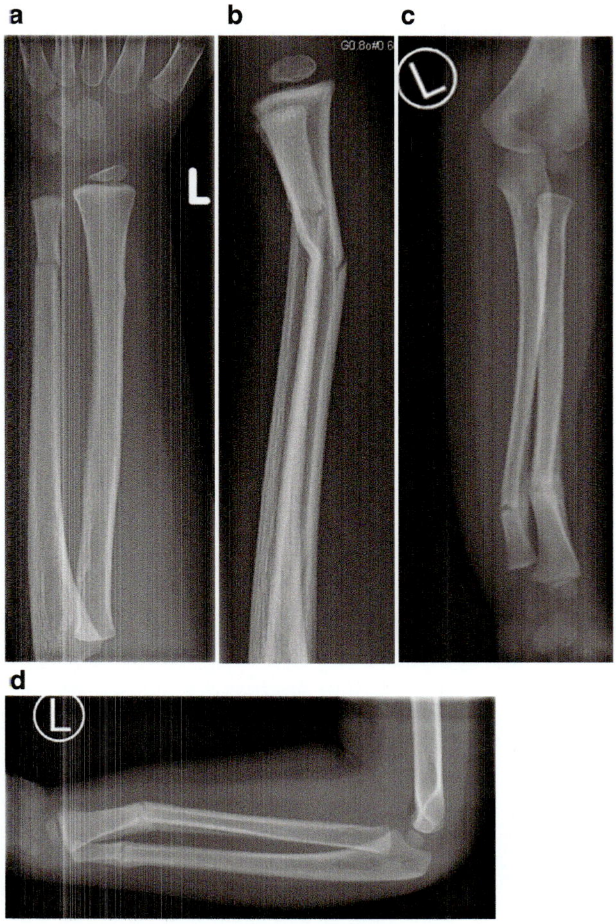

Fig. 9.12 3 year old girl. (**a**, **b**) Trauma Image and upper arm cast; (**c**, **d**) Healing and remodeling after 4 weeks

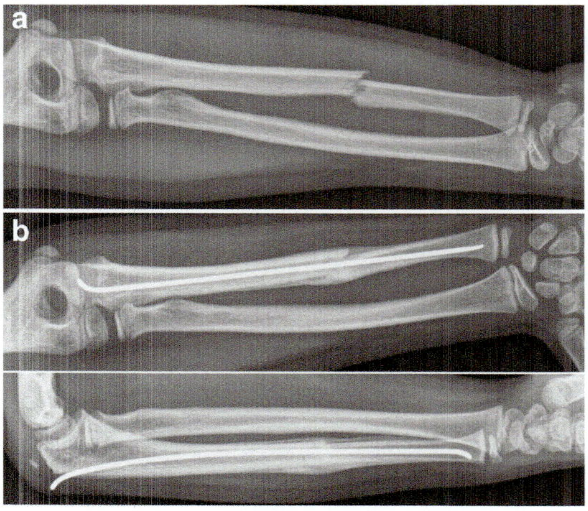

Fig. 9.13 Isolated complete ulna fracture by direct trauma in a 7 year old girl. (**a**) Trauma image, (**b**) 2 Months after ESIN osteosynthesis (2 mm) and functional after treatment

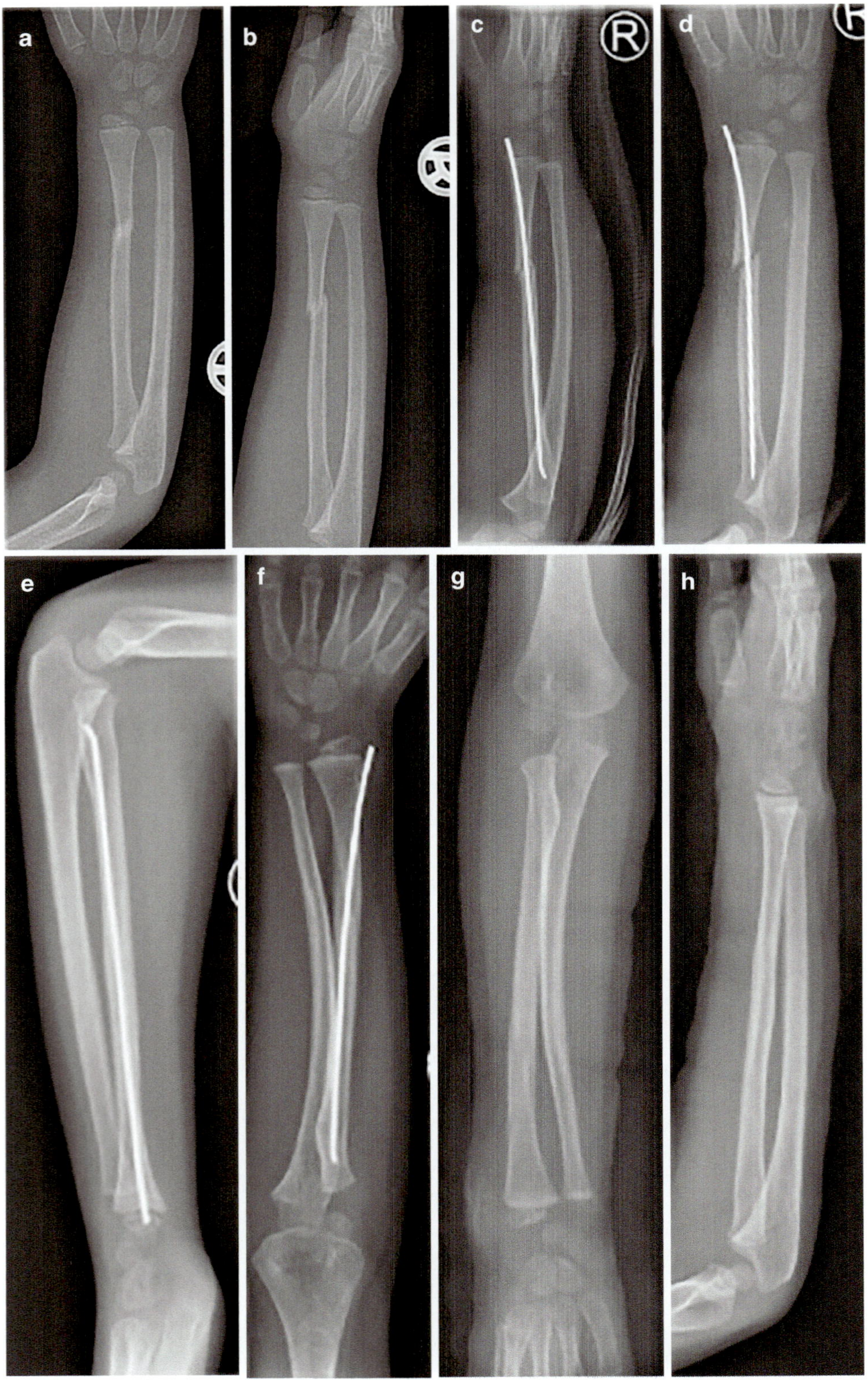

Fig. 9.14 5 year old boy, only radius shaft fracture; (**a**, **b**) Trauma image, (**c**, **d**) Postoperatively with ESIN, (**e**, **f**) Healing of the fracture, (**g**, **h**) After implant removal

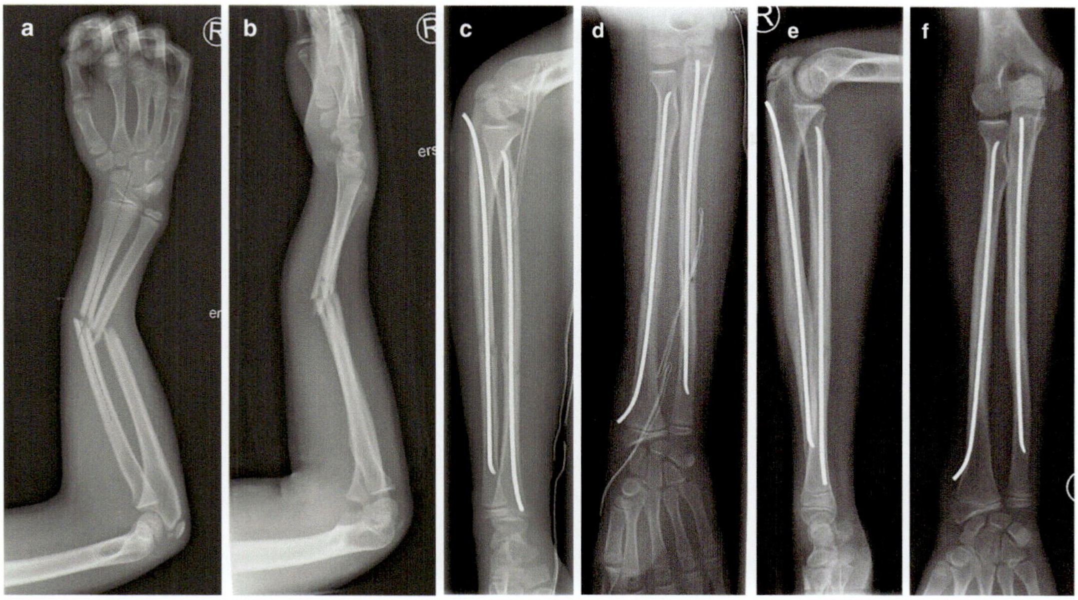

Fig. 9.15 Complete forearm fracture at the same level. (**a**, **b**) Trauma image, (**c**, **d**) After ESIN, (**e**, **f**) healing after implant removal

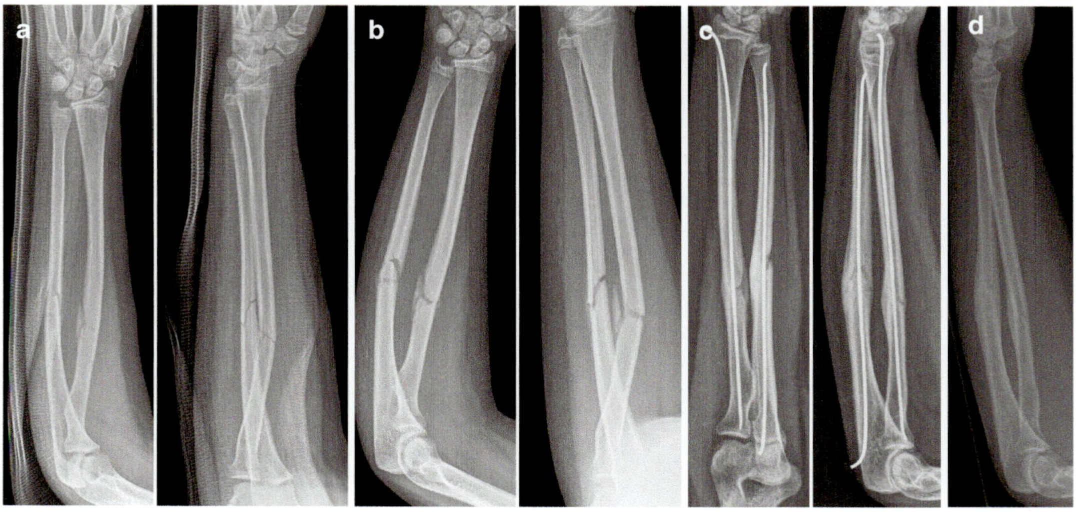

Fig. 9.16 Completely undisplaced fracture of a 13.5 year old girl after fall. (**a**) Trauma image, (**b**) 2.5 Weeks after upper arm cast with progressive dislocation of the radius, (**c**) 4 Months after ESIN osteosynthesis with slow healing, (**d**) 6 Months after osteosynthesis and final healing

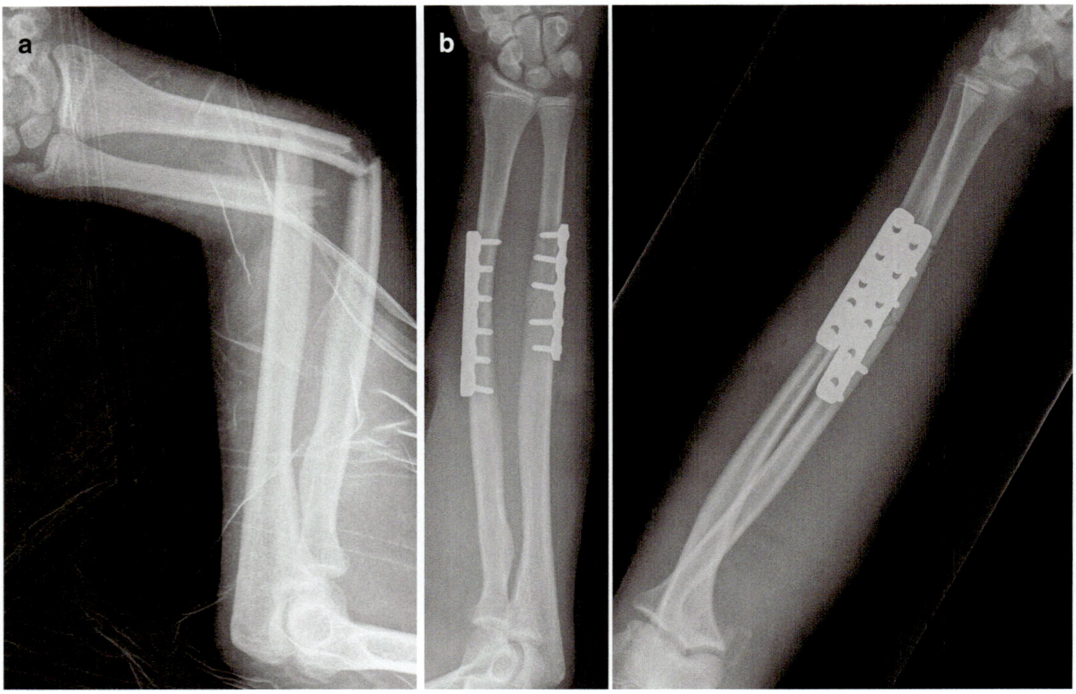

Fig. 9.17 Complete forearm shaft fracture with 90° dislocation in a 15.5 year old boy after Salto jump. (**a**) Trauma image, (**b**) Open reduction and plate osteosynthesis of radius and ulna in adolescence with compression plate

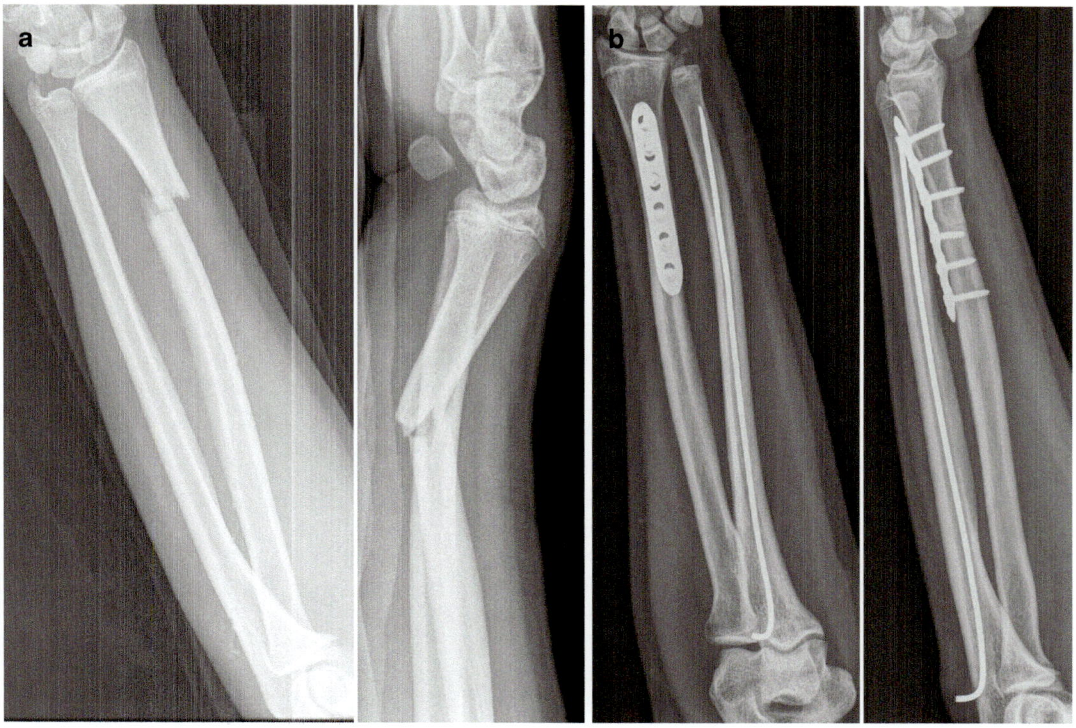

Fig. 9.18 Forearm shaft fracture with complete radius fracture and bowing fracture of the ulna after sports injury in a 16 year old boy. (**a**) Trauma image, (**b**) 2.5 Months after plate osteosynthesis (LC-DCP 3.5 mm) of the radius and ESIN (2.5 mm) of the ulna

Table 9.7 Metaphyseal buckle fracture, compression fracture and greenstick fracture (Fig. 9.19a, b)

Details	Cortex is maintained on both sides in buckle and compression fractures, in metaphyseal greenstick fractures a single cortex is ruptured Occurrence of buckle fractures especially in small children
Diagnostic assessment	X-ray AP and lateral of the wrist
Goals of treatment/ tolerance limits	Compression fractures and buckle fractures are characterized by a preserved periosteal tube that almost always leads to spontaneous correction; this fracture is barely observed in older children (>12 years).
Primary treatment	Above-elbow plaster slab, with medical analgesia if needed
Conservative therapy	
Indication	Mostly conservative for buckle and compression fractures; in young children in part in metaphyseal green stick fractures (Fig. 9.19c, d).
Procedure	2–3 weeks of forearm cast for buckle fractures; 3–4 weeks forearm cast for greenstick fractures (Fig. 9.20)
Follow-up	Functional, physical therapy is usually not necessary
X-ray controls	Usually not necessary for buckle fractures; day 5–8 position control, day 14 position control, 4th week consolidation control for greenstick fractures
Sports participation	2–3 weeks after consolidation
Operative therapy	
Indication	In metaphyseal greenstick fractures, of ulna, radius or both (Figs. 9.21, 9.22 and secondary after conservative treatment in Fig. 9.23).
Complications	Growth disturbance, rarely mobility deficits
Growth disturbance	Premature partial or total growth plate closure; rarely temporary overgrowth, especially of the radius, that is generally compensated for over the course of growth
Follow-up	No additional radiological controls are needed if there is no clinical evidence for poor growth, discharge on pain-free status
Classification	AO: 23-M/2.1-3 LiLa: 2.3.s.2.0-2.

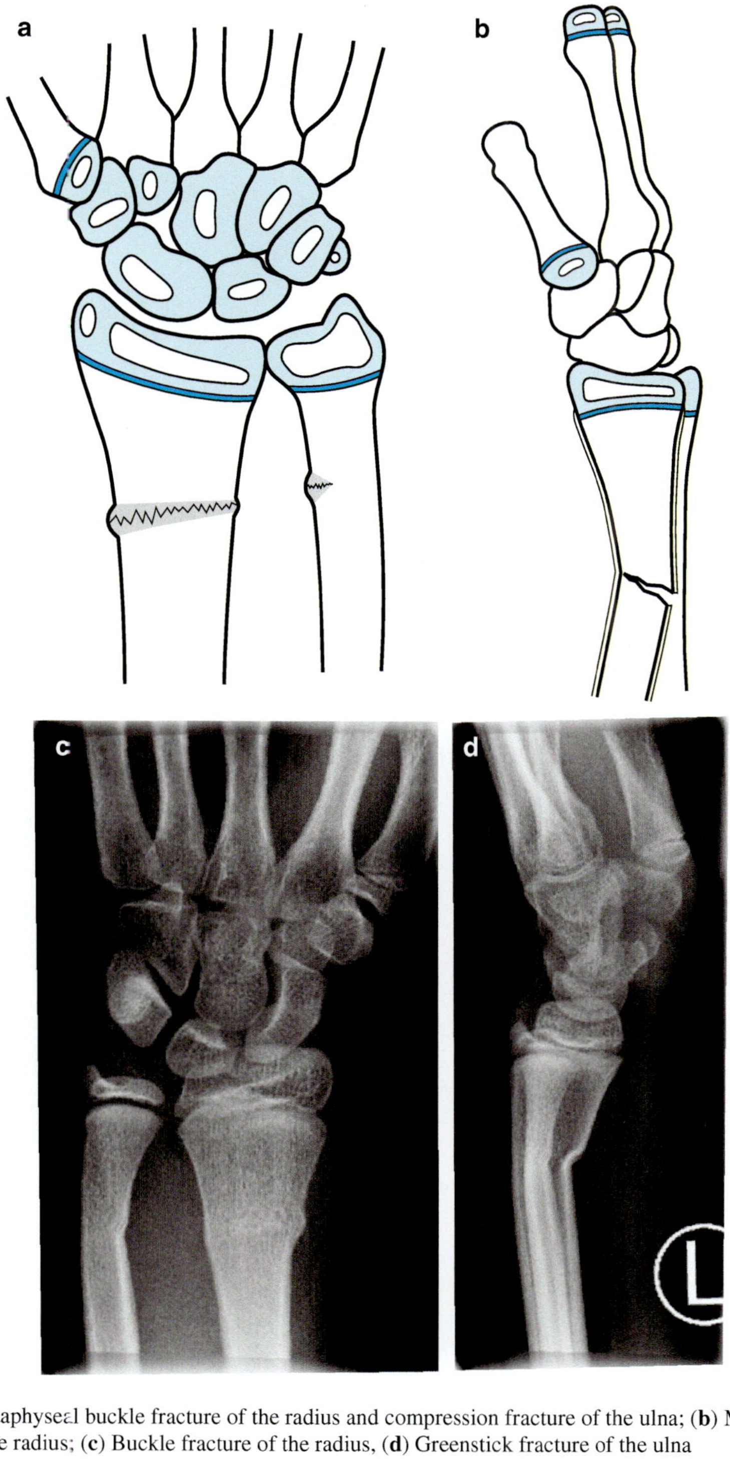

Fig. 9.19 (**a**) Metaphyseal buckle fracture of the radius and compression fracture of the ulna; (**b**) Metaphyseal greenstick fracture of the radius; (**c**) Buckle fracture of the radius, (**d**) Greenstick fracture of the ulna

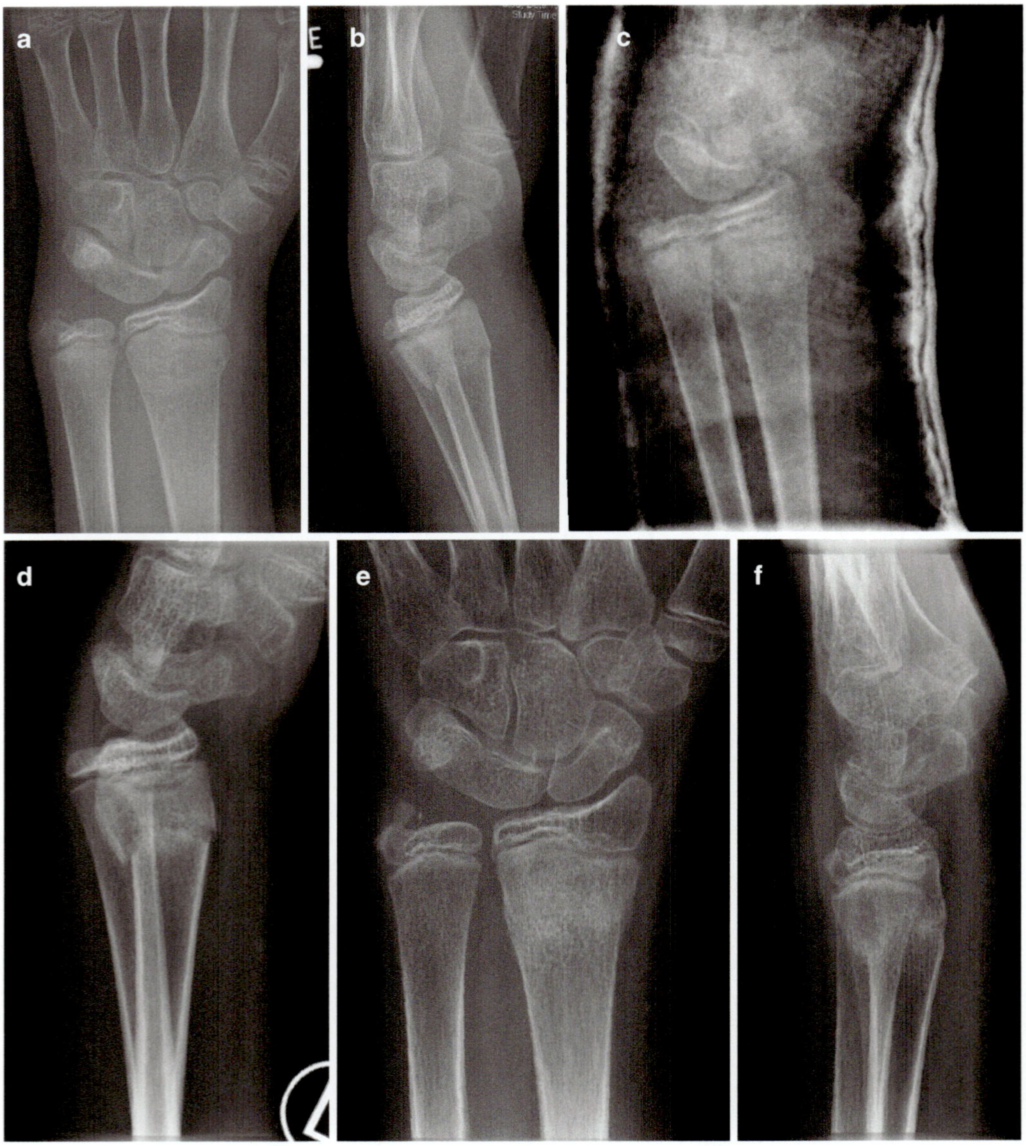

Fig. 9.20 13 year old boy. (**a**, **b**) Trauma image, (**c**, **d**) Conservative treatment in cast, (**e**, **f**) Healing

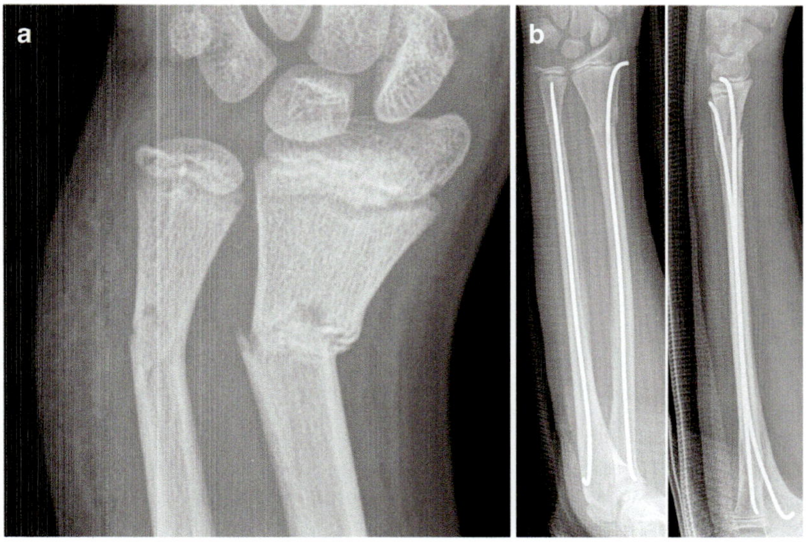

Fig. 9.21 Distal forearm fracture after all of a 3.5 year old boy. (**a**) Trauma image, (**b**) ESIN osteosynthesis

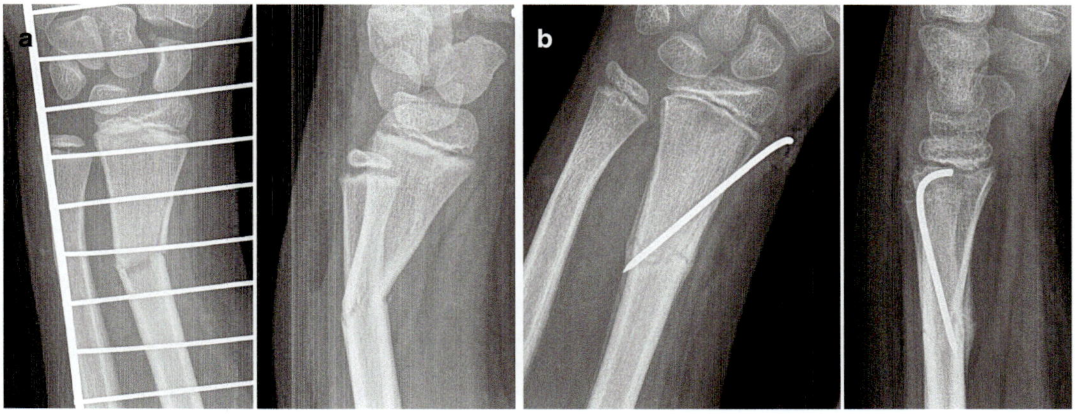

Fig. 9.22 Displaced metaphyseal buckle fracture of the distal radius over 20° in a 11.5 year old boy. (**a**) Trauma image, (**b**) 2 Weeks after closed reduction and K-wire osteosynthesis

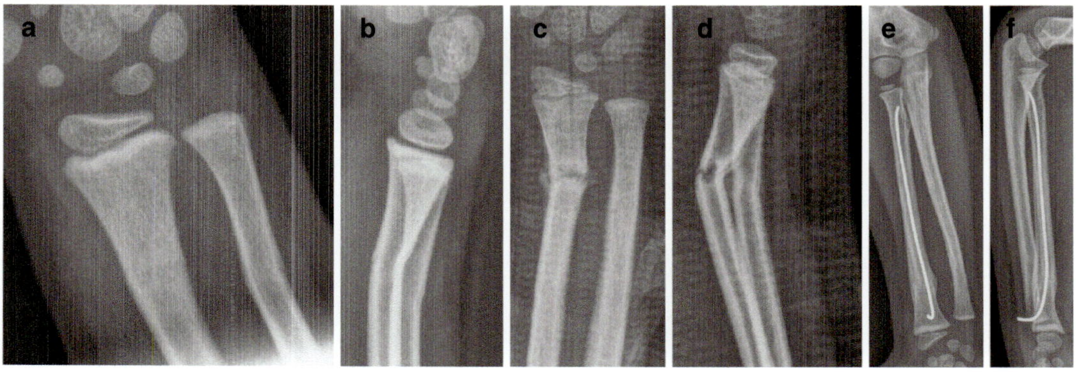

Fig. 9.23 Metaphyseal greenstick fracture of the distal forearm in a 3.5 year old girl. (**a**, **b**) Trauma image and upper arm plaster, (**c**, **d**) Secondary dislocation after 2 weeks above 30°, (**e**, **f**) 10 Weeks after closed reduction and ESIN. Complete fracture of the distal forearm

Table 9.8 Complete fractures of the distal forearm

Details	Marked swelling and pain
Diagnostic assessment	X-ray of the wrist AP and lateral
Goals of treatment/ tolerance limits	<12 years: theoretically possible up to 30°, more in small children >12 years: barely any spontaneous correction (physiological axis should be the goal) side-to-side shifts up to shaft width
Primary treatment	Above-elbow plaster slab, with medical analgesia if needed
Conservative therapy	
Indication	Rare, since reduction is necessary and fixation with K-wire is unproblematic and more stable <12 years: Angulation <30° in the sagittal plane and < 10° in the frontal plane can be left in principle; the closer to 12 years, the more anatomic the position must be. Leaving deformity within the tolerance limits must be carefully discussed with parents and the operative alternative presented (Fig. 9.24). >12 years: Angulation <10° in both planes Side-to-side shifts, tolerance limit to single shaft width
Procedure	4 weeks above-elbow cast; if necessary with secondary wedging on the 5th–8th day if secondary angulation is too much (small children)
Follow-up	Functional, physical therapy is usually not necessary
X-ray controls	Day 8 position control, possibly after cast wedging; 2-week position control, at 4 weeks consolidation control (no cast)
Sports participation	2–3 weeks after consolidation
Operative therapy	
Indication	Side-to-side translation >1/4 shaft width <12 years: Angulation between 30° (small children) and 10° (12-year-olds) in the sagittal plane and >10° in the frontal plane Rotational deformities Unstable fractures Radial shortening >5 mm Concomitant neurovascular injuries Malunion
Procedure	Reduction under anesthesia, secure fixation with K-wires possible Closed reduction K-wire fixation with Kapandji technique (Fig. 9.25) or transepiphyseal over the radial styloid process (Fig. 9.26) With external fixator, mounted as a T-fixator, in distal radius fractures (Fig. 9.27) Small fragment T-plate fixation for adolescents and older children (Figs. 9.28, 9.29, and 9.30)
Follow-up	2 weeks above-elbow cast, 2 weeks forearm cast
X-ray controls	Post-operative position control; 4 weeks consolidation control (without cast)
Hardware removal	4 weeks post-operatively
Sports participation	2–3 weeks after consolidation and hardware removal
Complications	Compartment syndrome Malunion of the radial and ulnar styloid processes Osteosynthesis after conservative treatment with secondary reconstruction (Fig. 9.31).
Growth disturbance	Temporary length difference
Follow-up	2 to 3 weekly controls until free function and acceptable position
Classification	AO: 23-M/3.1-3 LiLa: 2.3.s.3(4).0-2.

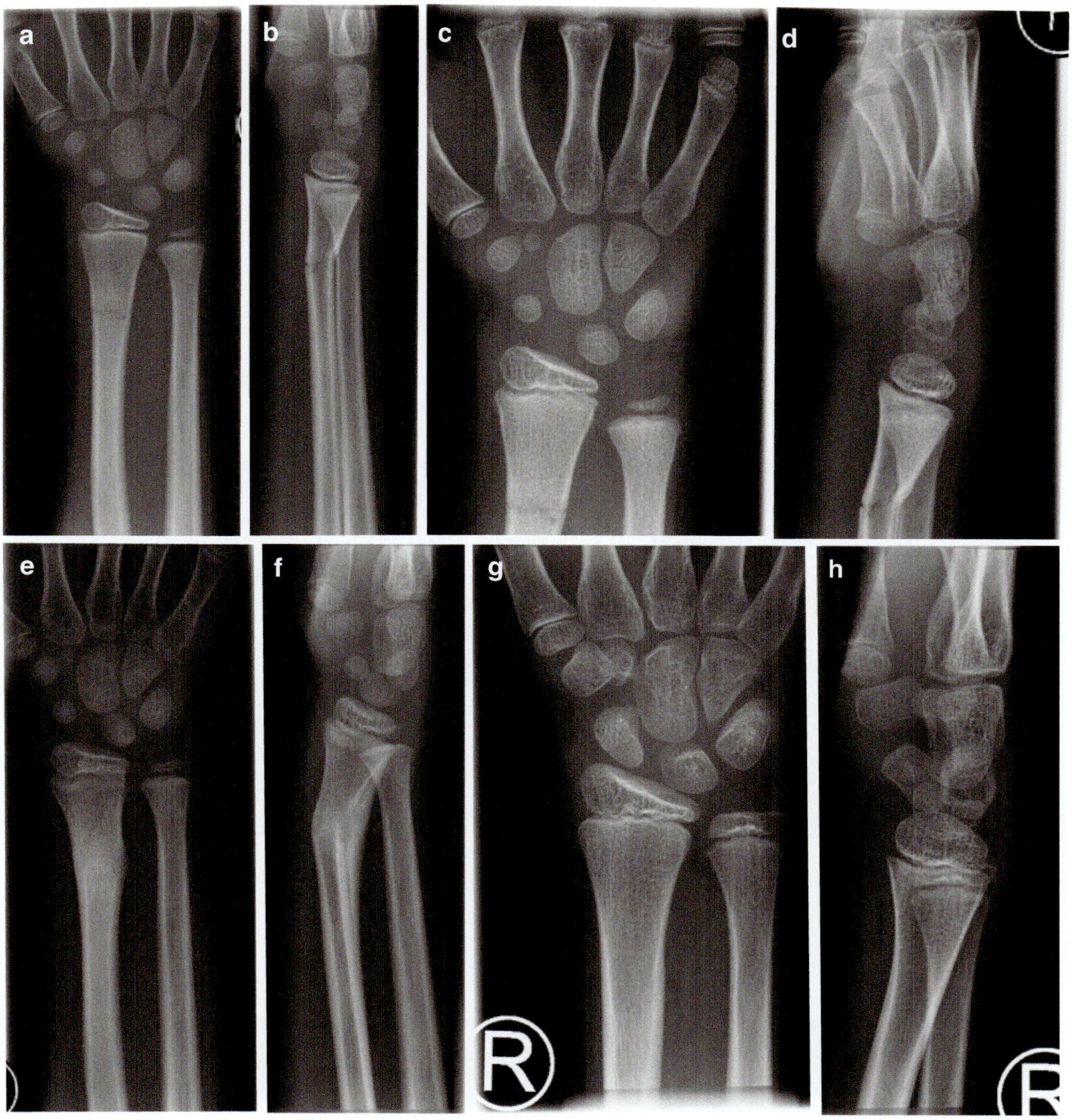

Fig. 9.24 7 year old boy, full radius fracture distally. (**a**, **b**) Trauma image, conservative treatment. (**c**, **d**) During treatment in cast, (**e**, **f**) After consolidation, with remaining angulation, (**g**, **h**) After 3 years and full remodeling

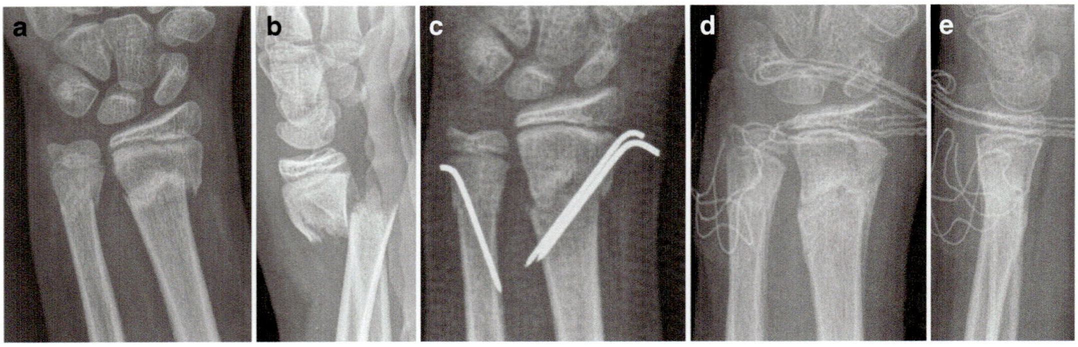

Fig. 9.25 Fracture of the distal metaphyseal radius and ulna after fall in a 11 year old girl. (**a**, **b**) Trauma image, (**c**) 2 Weeks after reduction and K-wire osteosynthesis, (**d**, **e**) Healing 5 weeks after metal removal

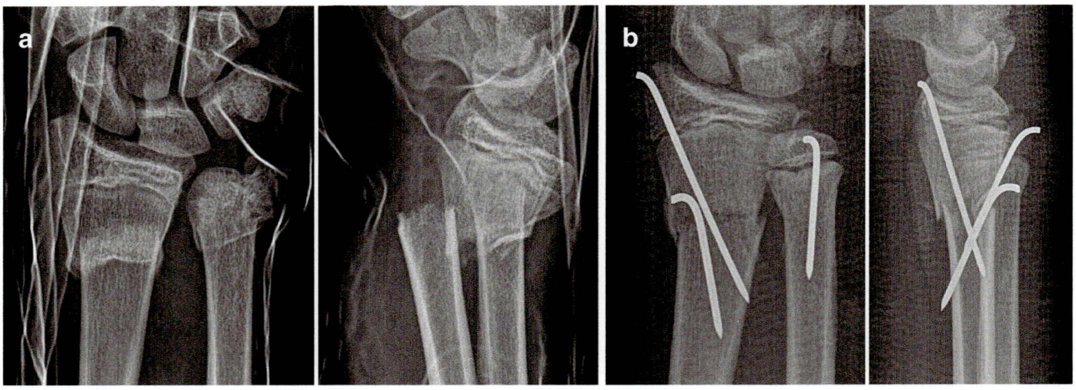

Fig. 9.26 Fracture of the distal forearm (Ulna epiphyseal fracture) after fall in a 16 year old boy. (**a**) Trauma image, (**b**) 2 Weeks after K-wire osteosynthesis (Kapandji technique and cast)

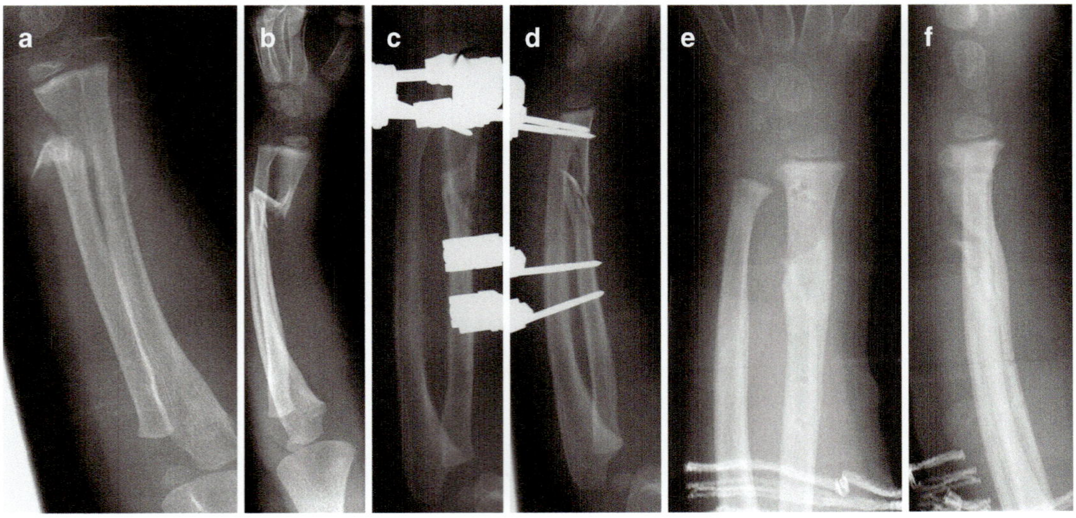

Fig. 9.27 Distal radius fracture, open second grade, and bowing fracture of the ulna after fall from window at 6 m in a 2.5 old boy. (**a**, **b**) Trauma image, (**c**, **d**) After reduction and external fixateur, (**e**, **f**) After 6 weeks complete healing

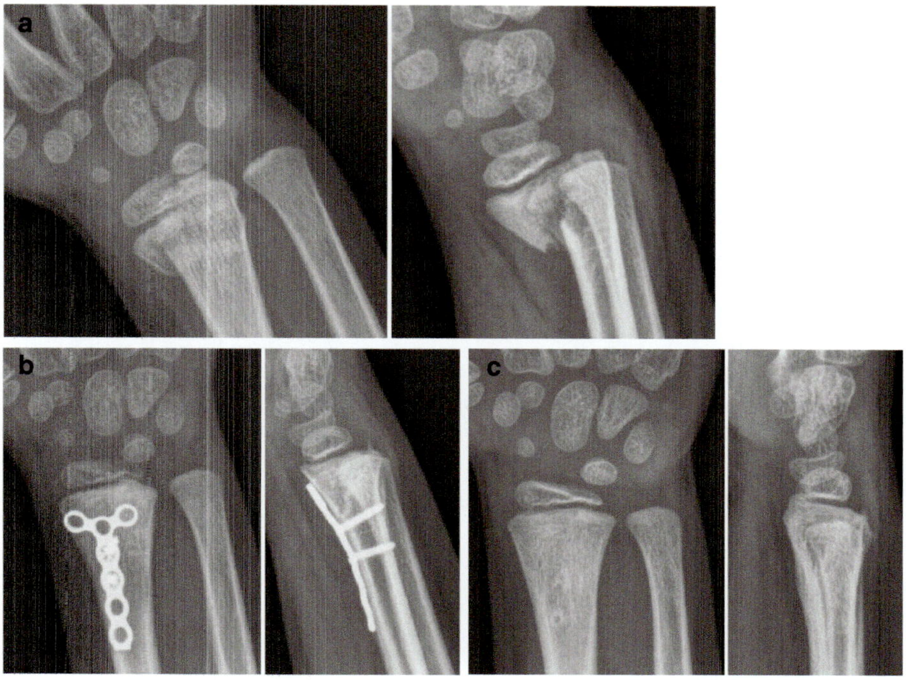

Fig. 9.28 Flection fracture (Salter-Harris II) of the distal radius metaphysis after fall of a 8 years old boy. (**a**) Trauma image, (**b**) Buttress plate palmar of the radius (2 mm) 5 days after trauma, (**c**) Healing 3 months later after metal removal

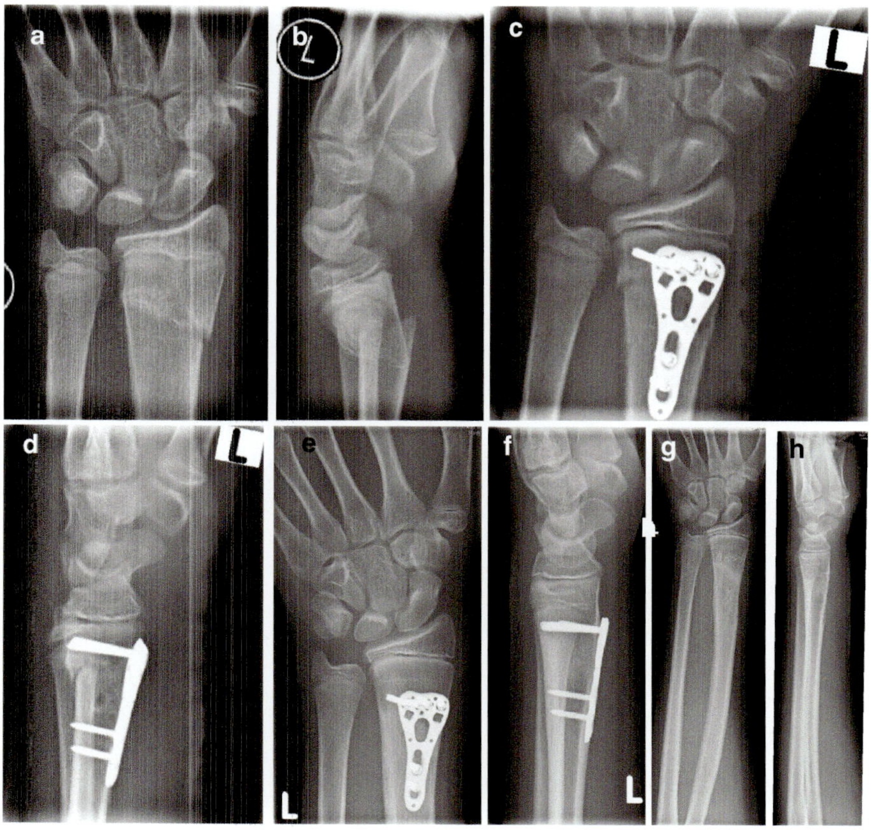

Fig. 9.29 13 Year old boy with displaced dia-metaphyseal fracture. (**a**, **b**) Trauma image, (**c**, **d**) After open reduction and palmar plate—proximal to the growth plate, (**e**, **f**) Healing with plate, (**g**, **h**) After hardware removal

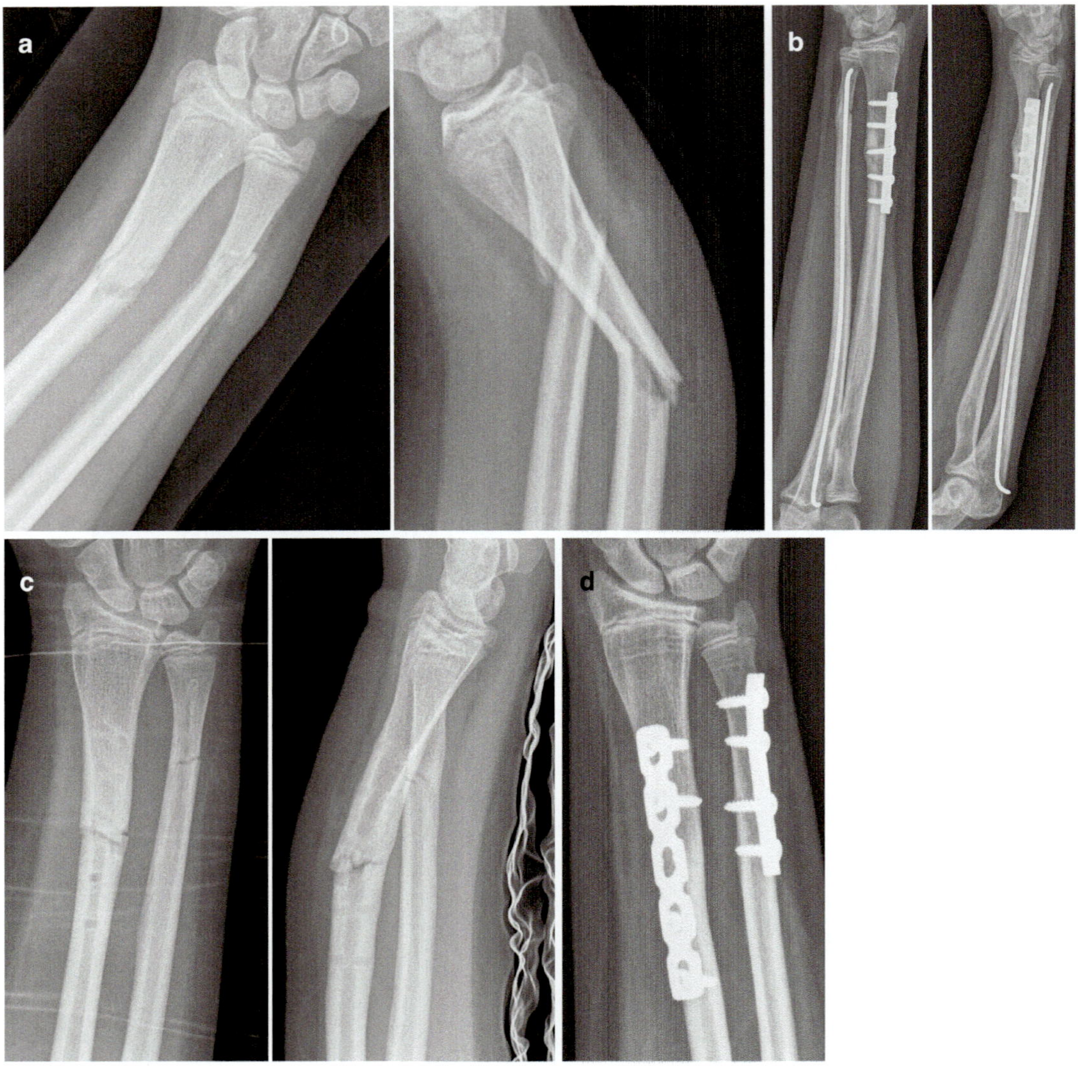

Fig. 9.30 Complete distal forearm fracture after fall (girl 12.5 years). (**a**) Trauma image, (**b**) 8 Weeks after plate osteosynthesis of the radius und ESIN of the ulna, (**c**) Re-fracture 4 months later after metal removal at gymnastics, (**d**) 9 Months after double plate osteosynthesis

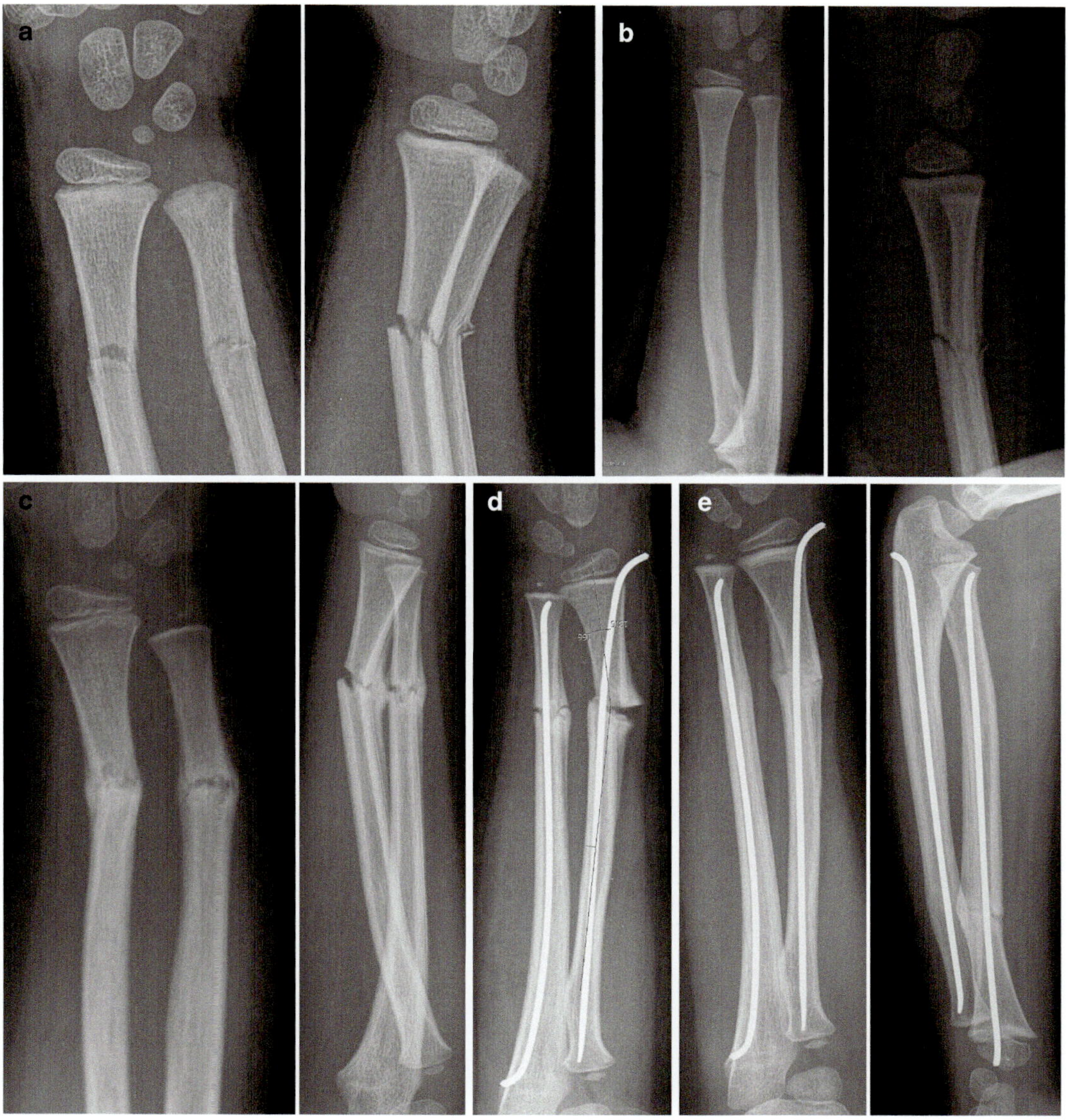

Fig. 9.31 Distal Forearm greenstick fracture in a 5.5 years old boy. (**a**) Trauma image, (**b**) X-ray control after 4 days, (**c**) 4 Weeks later after conservative treatment with increasing dislocation, (**d**) Reduction and ESIN (2 mm), (**e**) Healing 4 months postoperatively

Table 9.9 Epiphyseal injuries of the distal forearm (Fig. 9.32)

Details	Most common location of epiphysiolysis, rarely epiphyseal fractures; often good potential for correction despite significant deformity, but extensive discussion with parents regarding potential for correction, reduction and short-term stabilization can be given as alternative		
Diagnostic assessment	X-ray of the wrist AP and lateral		
Goals of treatment/ tolerance limits	<12 years: to 30° in frontal and to 10° in sagittal plane (decreasing until 12 years) >12 years: barely any spontaneous correction (strive for anatomical reduction) Salter III/IV fractures, transitional fracture: Displacement <2 mm in epiphyseal gap		
Primary treatment	Above-elbow plaster slab, with medical analgesia if needed		
Conservative therapy			
Indication	Within the tolerance limits (Fig. 9.33) Salter III/IV fractures, transitional fractures: Dislocation <2 mm		
Procedure	3 weeks above-elbow cast; if necessary with secondary wedging on the 4th–8th day		
Follow-up	Functional, physical therapy is usually not necessary		
X-ray controls	5th–8th day position control in cast, 4 weeks consolidation control (without cast)		
Sports participation	2–3 weeks after consolidation		
Operative therapy			
Indication	Outside the tolerance limits, Epiphyseal space >2 mm		
Procedure	Closed reduction and definitive treatment with K-wire fixation (Figs. 9.34 and 9.35)		
Follow-up	2 weeks above-elbow cast, 2 weeks forearm cast		
X-ray controls	Post-operative position control; 4-week consolidation control (without cast)		
Hardware removal	4–6 weeks post-operatively		
Sports participation	2–3 weeks after consolidation and hardware removal		
Complications	Compartment syndrome; secondary dislocation after conservative casting order K-wire fixation (Fig. 9.36).		
Growth disturbance	Premature partial or total epiphyseal closure with consequent deformity		
Follow-up	2 to 3 weekly controls until free function and acceptable position		
Classification	AO: 23-E/1.9.1-3	LiLa: 2.3.s.1.0-2	2.3.a.5.0-2.

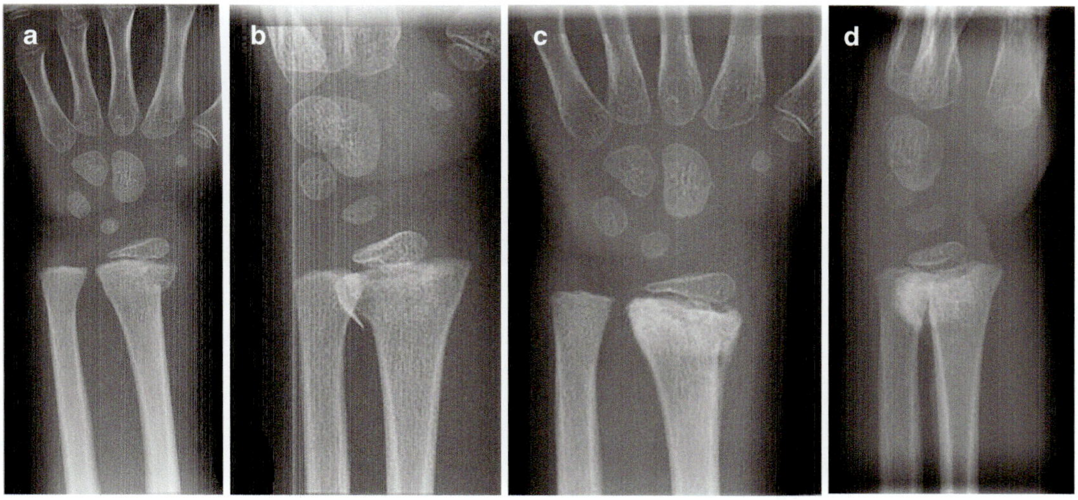

Fig. 9.32 Injury of the epiphysis of the distal radius (here Salter-Harris II). (**a**, **b**) Trauma Image, (**c**, **d**) ongoing consolidation with conservative treatment

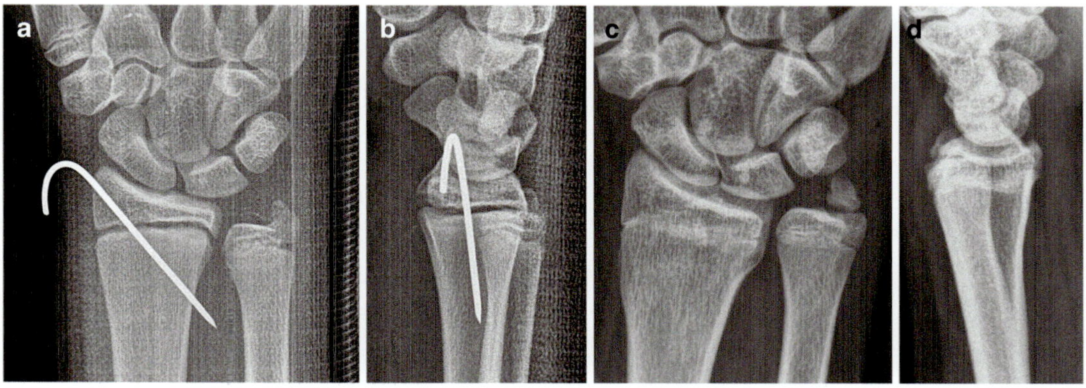

Fig. 9.33 Epiphysiolysis (Salter-Harris II) of the distal radius in a 6 years old boy. (**a**, **b**) Trauma image, (**c**, **d**) Healing after 4 weeks with a forearm plaster

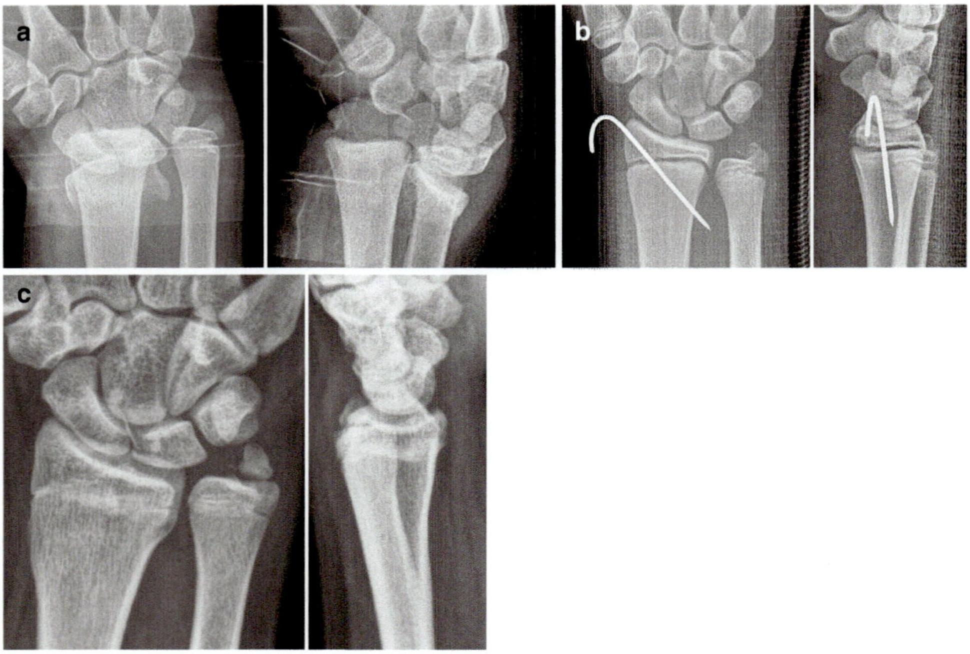

Fig. 9.34 Complete epiphysiolysis (Salter-Harris II) of the distal radius. (**a**) Trauma image, (**b**) After closed reduction and K-wire osteosynthesis from the styloid of the radius. (**c**) Healing after wire removal at 6 weeks

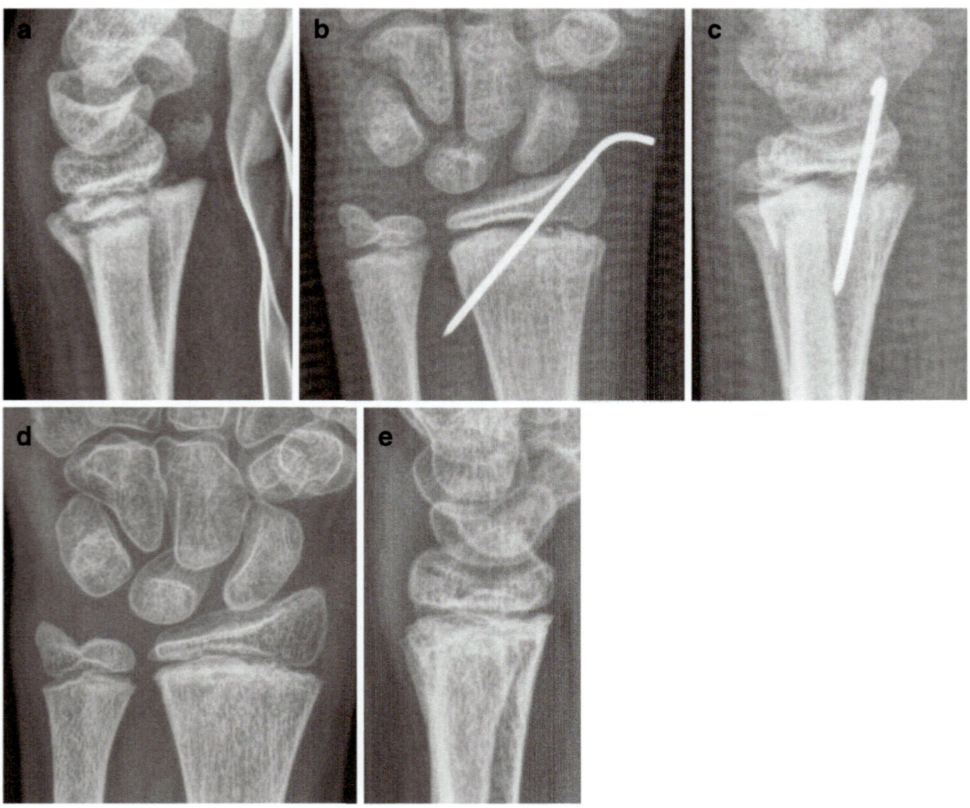

Fig. 9.35 Epiphysiolysis (Salter-Harris II) of the distal radius in a 12 year old boy. (**a**) Trauma image, (**b**, **c**) Closed reduction and percutaneous K-wire fixation through the radial proc. styloideus for 4 weeks and cast (**d**, **e**). Healing after 3 months

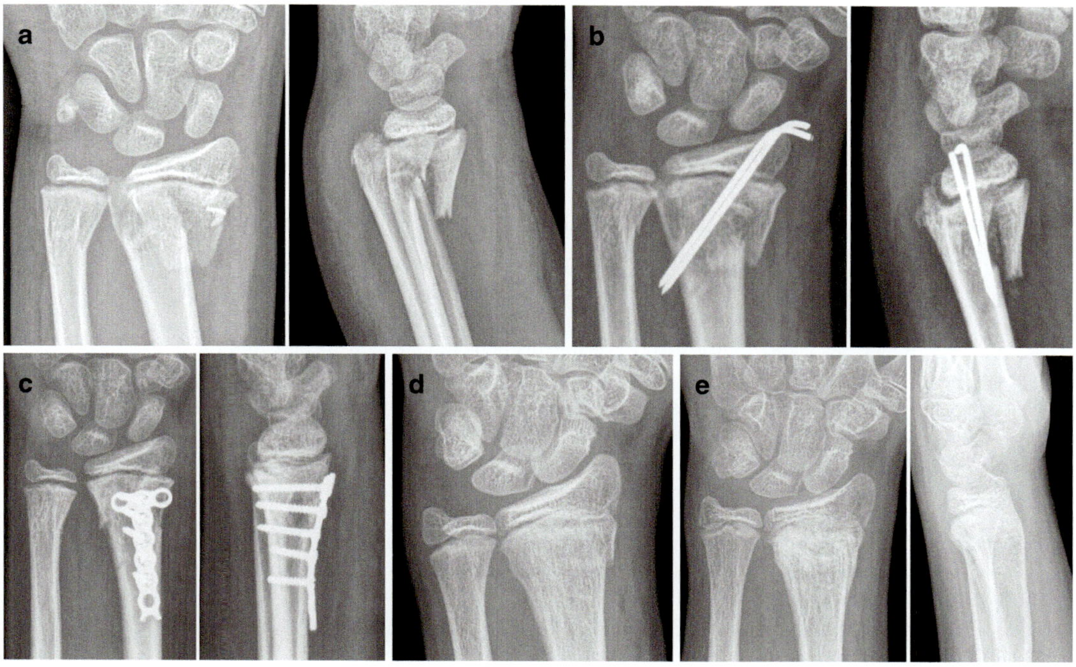

Fig. 9.36 Epiphysiolysis (Salter-Harris II) of the distal radius in palmar direction and dorsal dislocation of the ulna with soft tissue injury after bicycle fall in a 13.5 year old boy (Galeazzi equivalent). (**a**) Trauma image, (**b**) Secondary dislocation after initial reduction and K-wire osteosynthesis, (**c**) Revision surgery with palmar plate osteosynthesis and plate (2.4 mm) removal after 3 months. (**d**) Re-fracture after 24 months. (**e**) Healing after 25 months in slight deformity

9.4 Monteggia Injuries

In this subchapter, the different types of Monteggia Injuries are indicated in tables and corresponding figures (Table 9.10).

Table 9.10 Monteggia injuries (ulnar fracture with radial head dislocation) (Fig. 9.37)

Details	Easily overlooked combination injury of the forearm with severe consequences		
Diagnostic assessment	For every forearm fracture with shortening, there should be additional x-rays of the elbow in two planes (and the wrist if necessary)		
Goals of treatment/ tolerance limits	Radial head reduction, usually through reduction of the ulnar deformity or shortening Congruence of the proximal radioulnar joint is essential for proper rotation; subluxations must also be addressed; later spontaneous corrections are not possible, rather, there is progressive worsening through "pre-growth" of the radial head and further flexion deficits		
Primary treatment	Above-elbow plaster slab, with medical analgesia if needed		
Conservative therapy			
Indication	Occasional indication in small children with moderate dislocation; mostly operative closed reduction of a simple ulnar shaft fracture with reduction of the radial head dislocation (Fig. 9.38)		
Procedure	4 weeks immobilization in above-elbow cast		
Follow-up	Movement as tolerated after cast removal, usually physical therapy not necessary		
X-ray controls	Positional control after reduction; 1 week; 4-week consolidation control (without cast)		
Sports participation	When there is free function, about 5–8 weeks after consolidation		
Operative therapy			
Indication	Unstable ulnar shaft fracture, displaced fractures; mostly necessary to achieve a stable ulnar fixation with appropriate length. Usually closed reduction of the radial head is possible at the same time		
Procedure	Usually closed reduction of the ulna and radial head Open reduction is needed occasionally for interposed soft tissues Goal: anatomic reduction of the ulna and radial head dislocation After reduction of the ulnar fracture, typically there is spontaneous reduction of the dislocated proximal radius Shaft fractures: Closed reduction with overcorrection (fracture completion) of the opposite cortex in greenstick fractures, stabilization with ESIN for functional treatment (Fig. 9.39) In proximal Monteggia fractures, tension bend wiring of the olecranon and reduction (Fig. 9.40) In rare cases, fixation with plate (Fig. 9.41) or external fixator		
Follow-up	Several days of above-elbow cast for analgesia, then functional therapy, if necessary with physical therapy; with K-wire fixation 4 weeks above-elbow cast		
X-ray controls	Post-operative positional control; 2-week control, 4-week consolidation control (without cast)		
Hardware removal	8–12 weeks post-operative (after consolidation control)		
Sports participation	5–8 weeks after consolidation		
Complications	Missed radial head dislocation Damage to the deep radial nerve/ulnar nerve Radial head necrosis Tendency to re-dislocate/subluxated position Synostosis formation Persisting motion deficits of the elbow and forearm (see also Chap. 19)		
Growth disturbance	Growth disturbance of the proximal radial end Potential head reconstruction disturbance with thickening of the proximal radial end with consequent pronation/supination limitations		
Follow-up	3–4 weekly visits until free function, then semi-annually until 2 years post-trauma		
Classification	AO: 22-D/6.1-3	LiLa: 2.2.s.2-4.2.U	2.1.s(a).5.2.U.

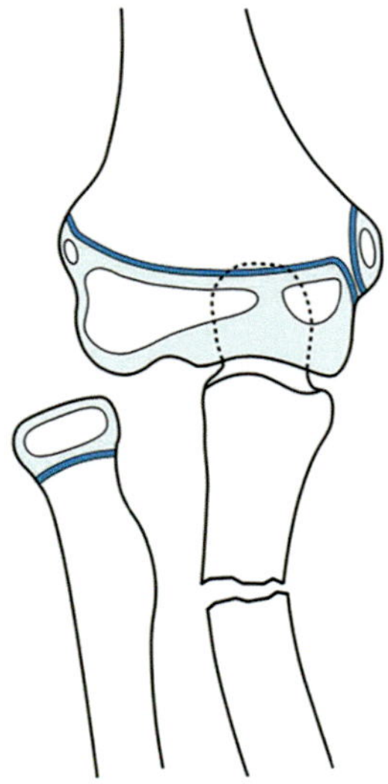

Fig. 9.37 Monteggia—Injury (fracture of the ulna and luxation of radial head)

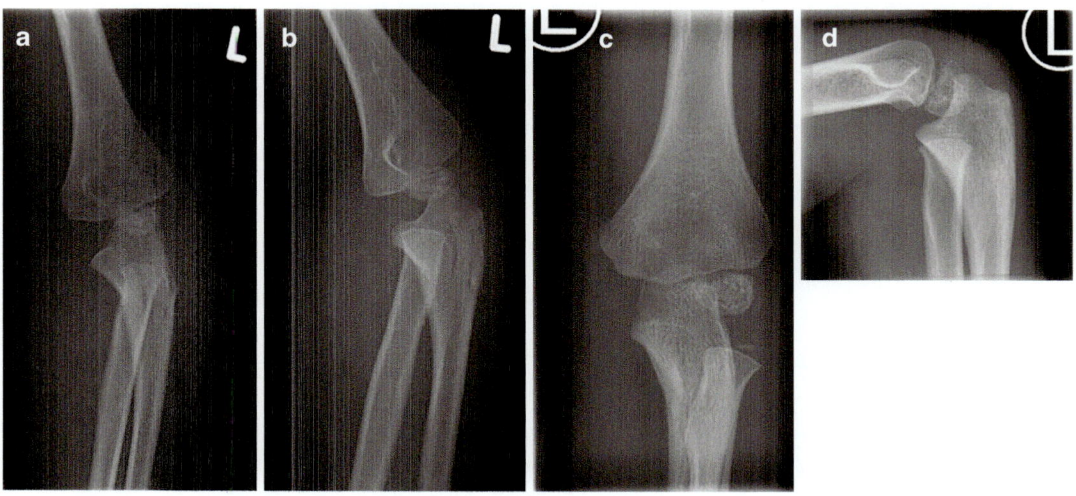

Fig. 9.38 4 Year old girl with proximal ulna fracture and radial head subluxation. (**a**, **b**) Trauma image, (**c**, **d**) Correct consolidation images

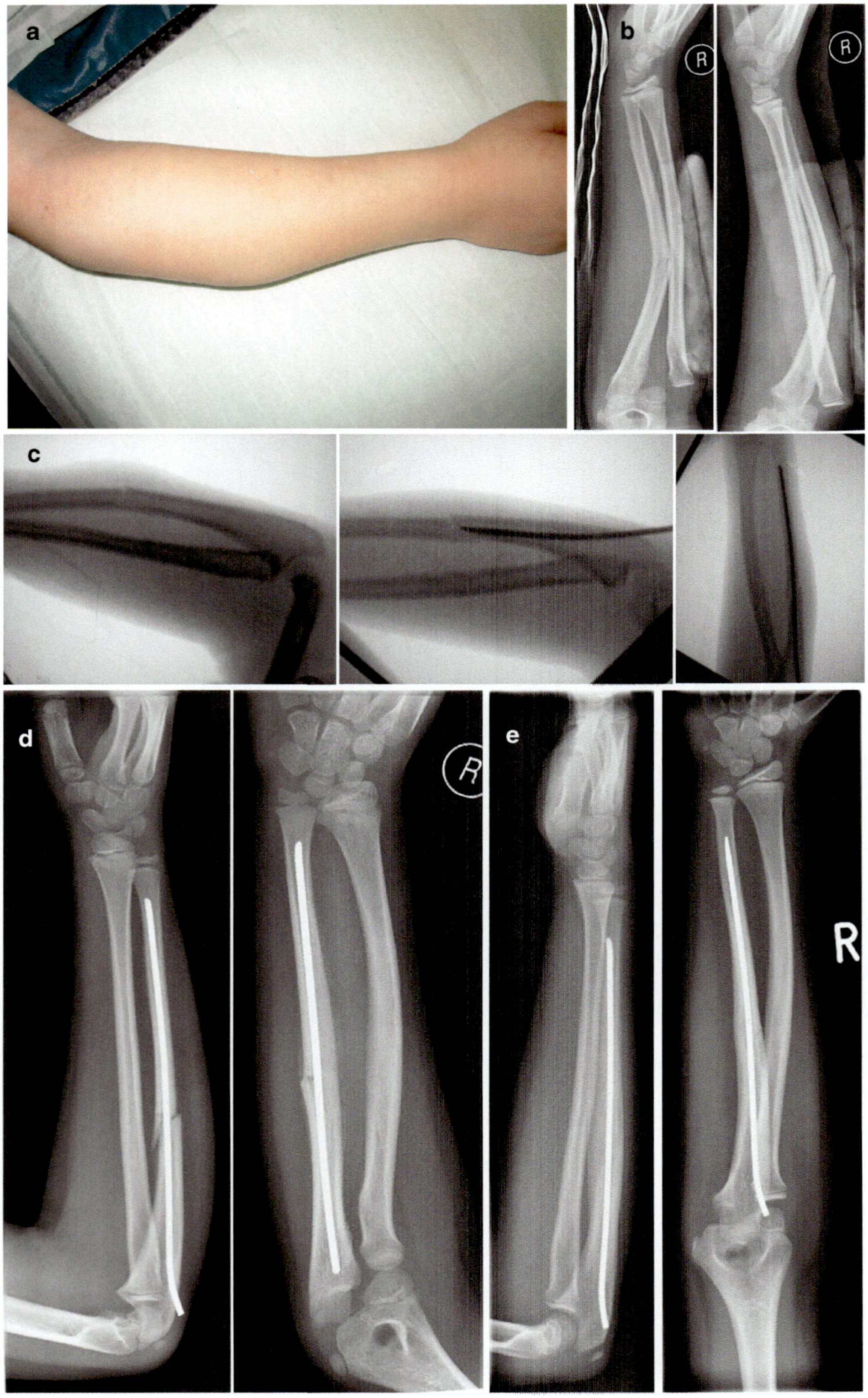

Fig. 9.39 Monteggia lesion of a 7 year old girl. (**a**) Clinical image with swelling and dislocation. (**b**) Trauma image with displaced greenstick fracture of the ulna and radial head luxation, (**c**) Intraoperative reposition and ESiN of the ulna, (**d**) Postoperative image, (**e**) Healing prior metal removal at correct joint position

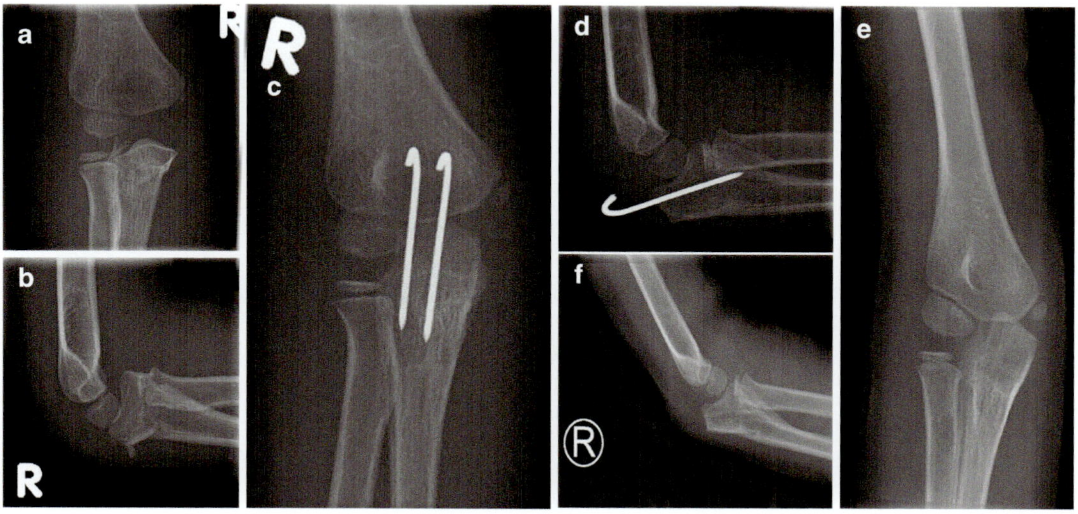

Fig. 9.40 4 Years old girl with prox. Monteggia fracture. (**a**, **b**) Trauma image, (**c**, **d**) Tension band wiring with 2 K-wires and fibersuture, (**e**, **f**) Bony healing in correct position

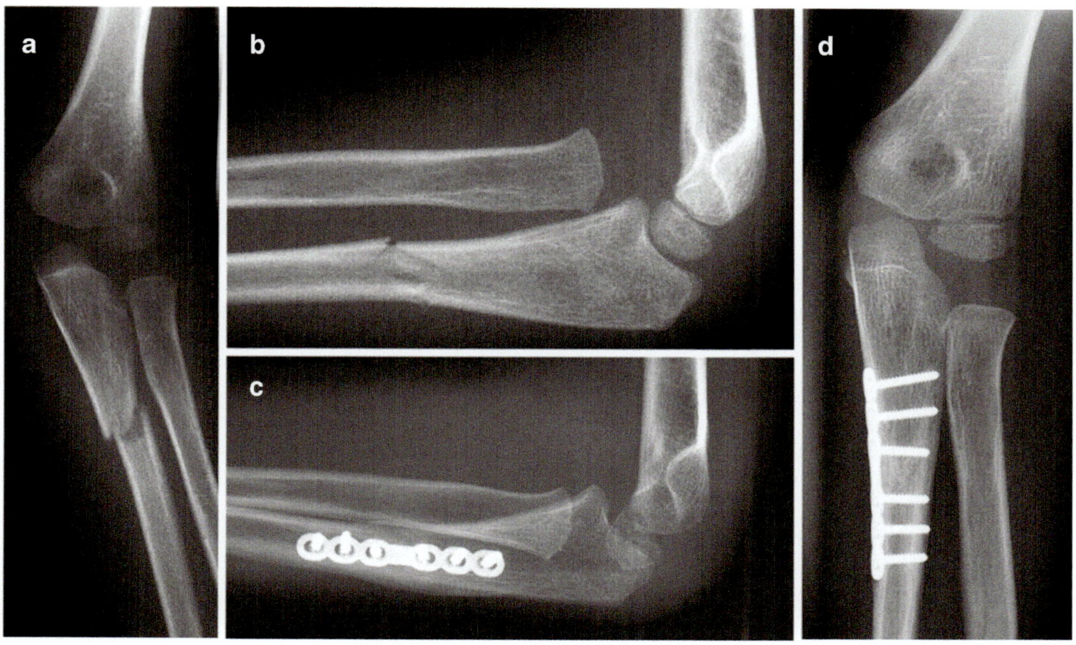

Fig. 9.41 Monteggia injury after fall from roof on the left arm of a 8.5 year old boy. (**a**, **b**) Taurma image with ulna fracture and radial head luxation in ventral position, (**c**, **d**) Open reduction and correct healing with ulna plate

9.5 Galeazzi Injuries

In this subchapter, the different types of Galeazzi Injuries are indicated in tables and corresponding figures (Table 9.11).

Table 9.11 Galeazzi injury (displaced radial fracture and ulnar head dislocation) (Fig. 9.42)

Details	Rare; predominantly >10 years	
Diagnostic assessment	For each displaced forearm fracture, x-ray of the wrist A.P. and lateral (exact lateral)	
Goals of treatment/ tolerance limits	Reduction and stabilization of the radius and thus, indirect correction of distal radioulnar joint incongruence	
Primary treatment	Above-elbow plaster slab, with medical analgesia if needed	
Conservative therapy		
Indication	Stable closed reduction of the radial fracture with reduction of the ulnar head or growth plate injury possible (Fig. 9.43)	
Procedure	4 weeks immobilization in above-elbow cast	
Follow-up	Movement as tolerated after cast removal, usually physical therapy not necessary	
X-ray controls	Day 8 positional control; 2 weeks positional control, 4 weeks consolidation control (without cast)	
Sports participation	When there is free function, about 5–8 weeks after consolidation	
Operative therapy		
Indication	>10° radial angulation Radial shortening Soft-tissue interposition (e.g. communal extensor digitorum tendon between the ulnar epiphysis and metaphysis or pronator quadratus muscle in the radial fracture line)	
Procedure	According to radial fracture type: ESIN, external fixator, rarely plate or K-wires, but the correct length of the radius must be achieved exactly, otherwise the distal ulna position will not be correct. In small children and distal fractures, K-wire fixation after reduction might be sufficient (Fig. 9.44) In older children, plate osteosynthesis outside the growth plate is a safe solution (Fig. 9.45). ESIN in mid-shaft, if the reduction can be securely maintained technically External fixator should be considered especially in distal radius fractures	
Follow-up	3 weeks above-elbow cast in supination (for setting of the distal radioulnar joint), then functional treatment Physical therapy is usually not necessary	
X-ray controls	Post-operative positional control; 2-week positional control, 4-week consolidation control (without cast)	
Hardware removal	4 weeks post-operatively for K-wires and external fixator; ESIN after 3–4 months, plates 8–12 weeks post-operatively (after consolidation controls)	
Sports participation	5–8 weeks after consolidation	
Complications	DRUJ instability with recurrent dislocation or position in subluxation position Deficits in pronation/supination Chronic pain Loss of power	
Growth disturbance	Possible growth disturbances with chronic distal radioulnar joint complaints when there is ulnar growth plate trauma; functional assessments then with MRI or wrist arthroscopy if needed	
Follow-up	3–4 weekly visits until free function, then semi-annually until 2 years post-trauma	
Potential corrections	Radial osteotomy and re-fixation with corrective length according to the distal ulna; wrist arthroscopy and debridement of the TFC complex if needed after growth conclusion; ulnar shortening osteotomy or radial shortening osteotomy after growth conclusion to reset congruence of the distal radioulnar joint. (see Chap. 20)	
Classification	AO: 22-D/7.1-3	LiLa: 2.2.s.2-4.2.

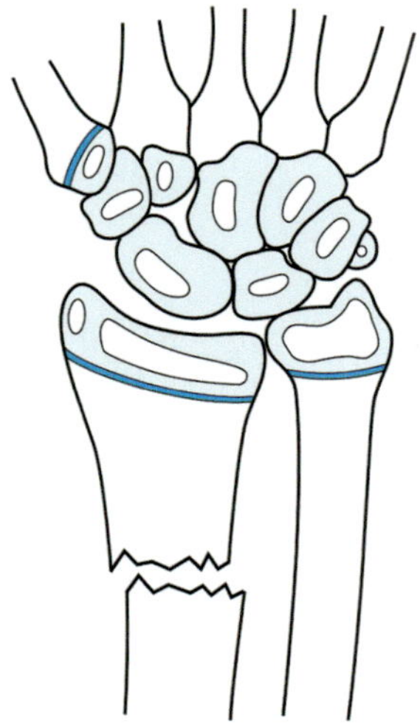

Fig. 9.42 Galeazzi injury—Displaced radial fracture and ulnar head dislocation

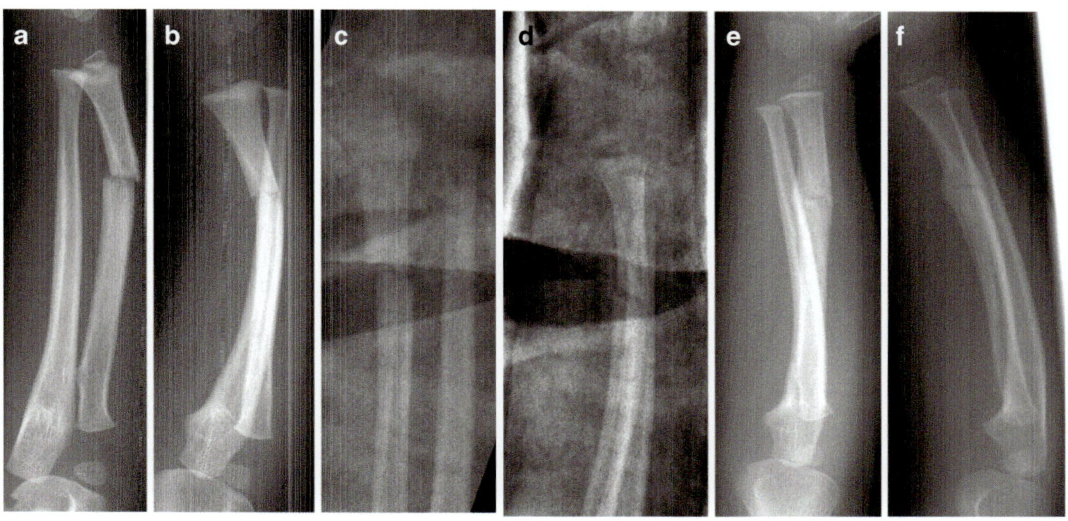

Fig. 9.43 Galeazzi fracture in complete radial shaft fracture, girl, 2 year, fall from a window 5 m high. (**a**, **b**) Trauma images. (**c**, **d**) Cast wedging after swelling decrease with initial angulation >20°. (**e**, **f**) Healed images

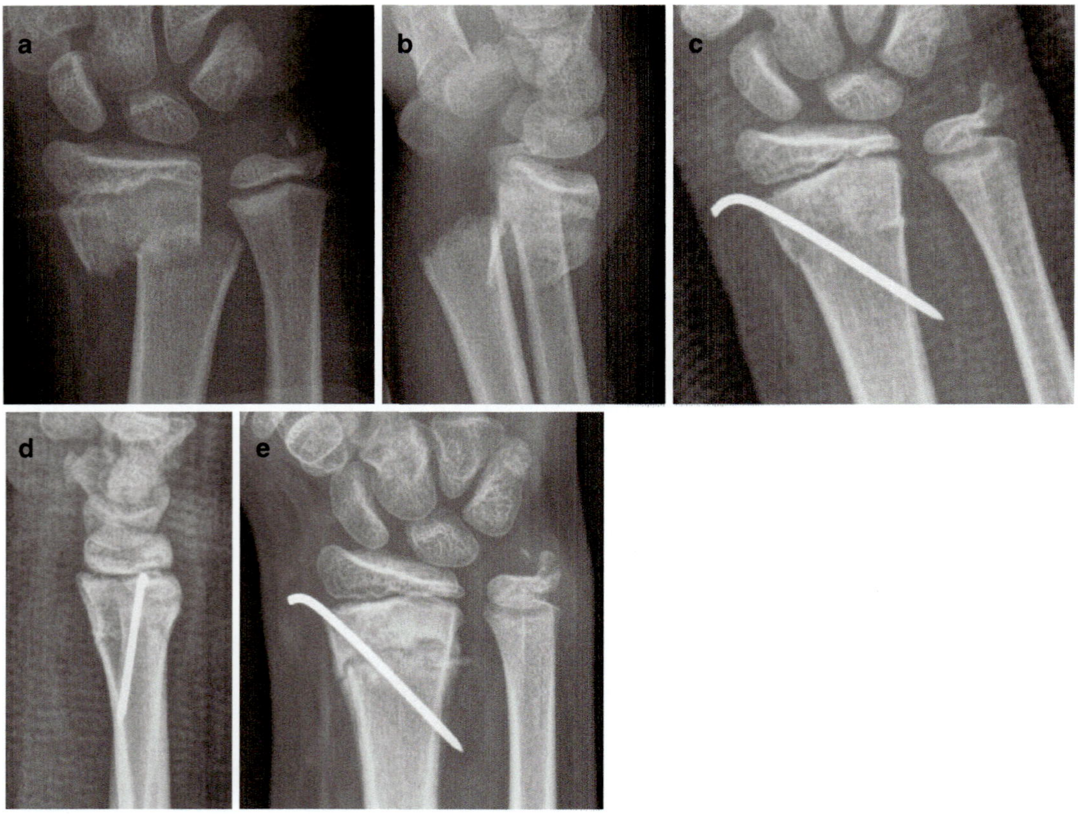

Fig. 9.44 Distal metaphyseal displaced radius fracture with rupture of styloid proc. Of the ulna and distended distal radio-ulnar joint after skater fall. Galeazzi equivalent in a 10.5 year old boy. (**a**, **b**) Trauma image, (**c**, **d**) 1 Week after closed reduction and K-wire osteosynthesis. (**e**) 4 Weeks postoperative with good healing, prior to metal removal

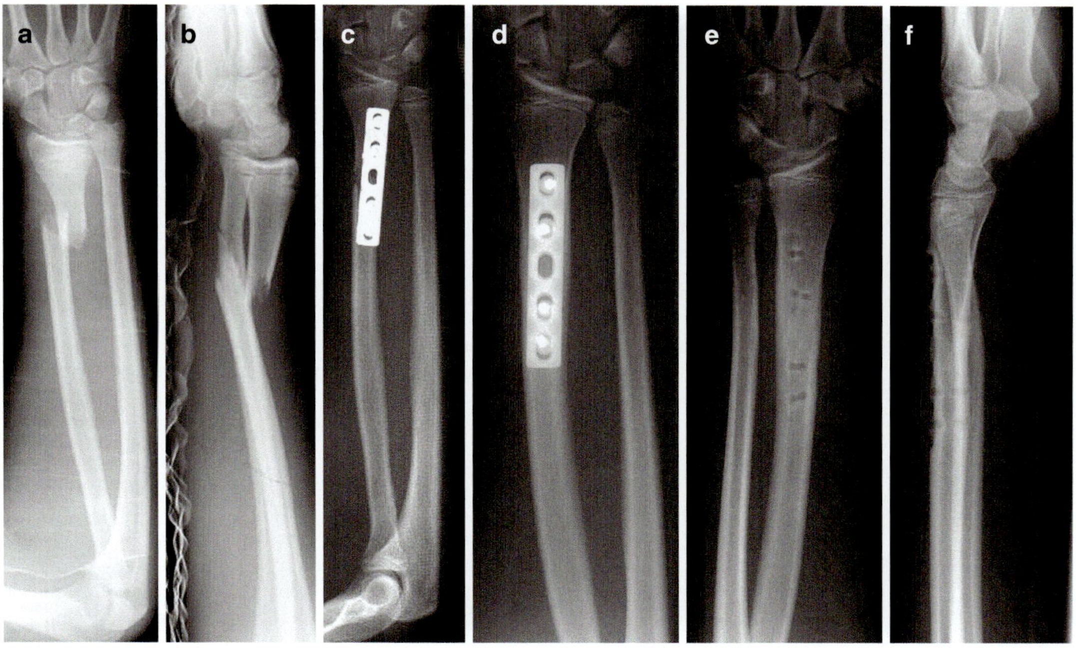

Fig. 9.45 Galeazzi injury, boy, 14 year, backwards fall from a height onto both arms. (**a**, **b**) Trauma images. (**c**, **d**) Corrective lengthening of the radius with a plate. (**e**, **f**) Good healing and function

9.6 Technical Considerations

In this subchapter, technical steps for the treatment of forearm fractures are given in Table 9.12, 9.13, 9.14 with the corresponding figures.

Table 9.12 Technical considerations forearm

A forearm fractures—ESIN	
Material	Elastic tension nail size 2.0/2.5/3.0 mm, implant size should correspond to one third of the medullary canal If possible two nails with the same diameter for simultaneous lengthening and support
Positioning	Supine, trans-illuminating arm board on the operating table, movable draping above the elbow joint
Approach	Radius: Recommended approach → radial incision of 2–3 cm, beginning about 2 cm proximal to the distal epiphyseal plate (Fig. 9.46) → Visualization and protection of the superficial branch of the radial nerve Alternative, but more dangerous entry approach: → Dorsoradially between the third and fourth extensor compartments after visualization of the tendons, leaving the nail protruding over the tendons; caution: extensor pollicis longus tendon Ulna: → Entry point is approximately 2 cm distal to the olecranon apophysis, more dorsally, corresponding skin incision with protection of the apophysis (Fig. 9.47)
Special explanation	Injury to the superficial radial nerve during fixation of the radius, extensor tendons as well with the posterior approach during hardware removal
Operative principle	Symmetrical tension of two metaphyseal-introduced elastic nails, each with three support points in the bone and thus, offering bending stability, axial stability, translational stability, and rotational stability (Fig. 9.48) Intramedullary stabilization creates tension forces within compression forces, and thus helps support callus formation. Operative case: Fig. 9.49a, b trauma image of forearm fracture in a 7 year old boy; Fig. 9.50 sequential insertion of ESIN in radius; Fig. 9.51 sequential insertion of ESIN in ulna.
Hardware removal	After 3–4 months → Nail ends cleanly visualized → Caution: superficial radial nerve can grow into the scar!
Other particulars	None

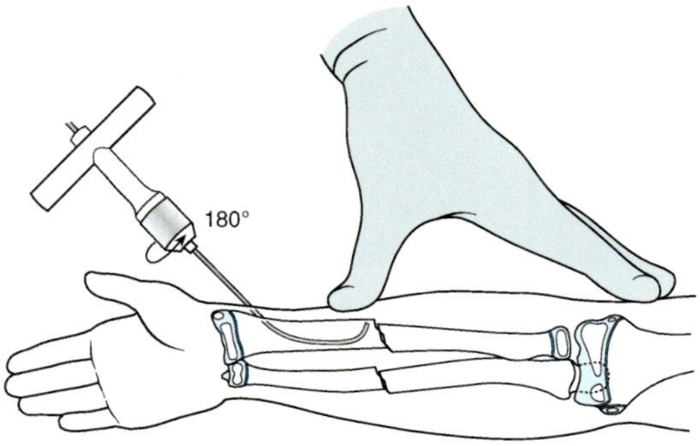

Fig. 9.46 ESIN of the forearm; radial approach

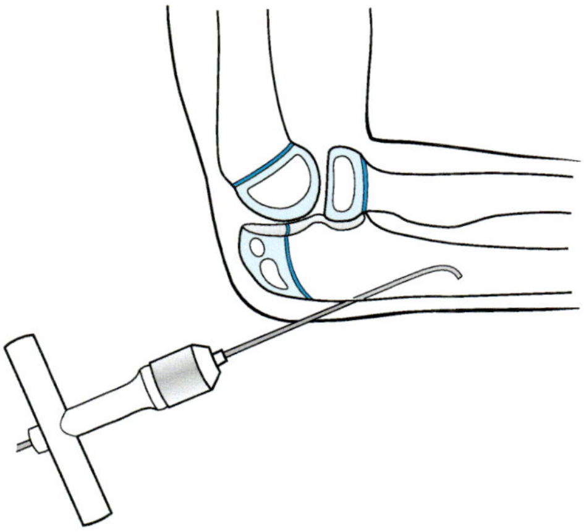

Fig. 9.47 ESIN of the forearm; ulnar approach

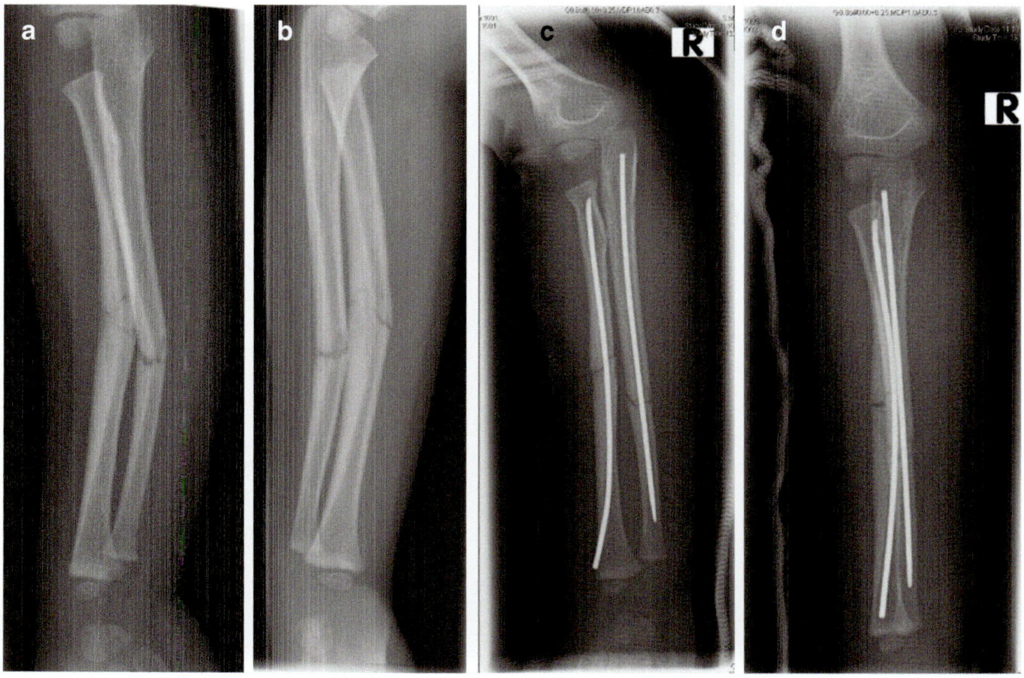

Fig. 9.48 5 year old boy with complete forearm fracture. (**a**, **b**) Trauma image, (**c**, **d**) Postoperative after ESIN of radius and ulna. The first days a cast might be useful for pain relief

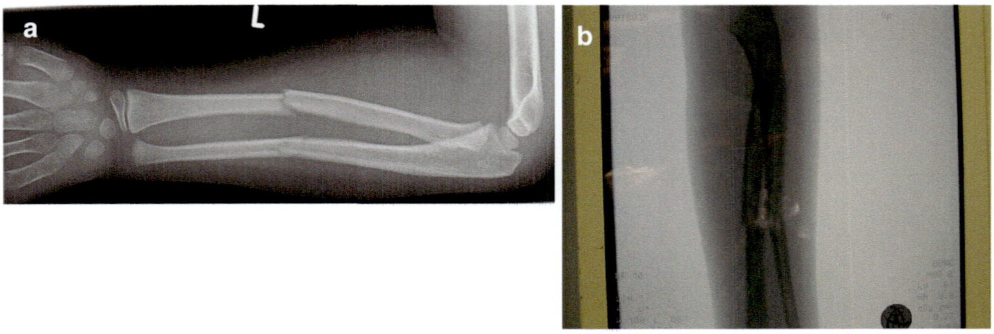

Fig 9.49 (**a**, **b**) Trauma image of forearm fracture in a 7 year old boy

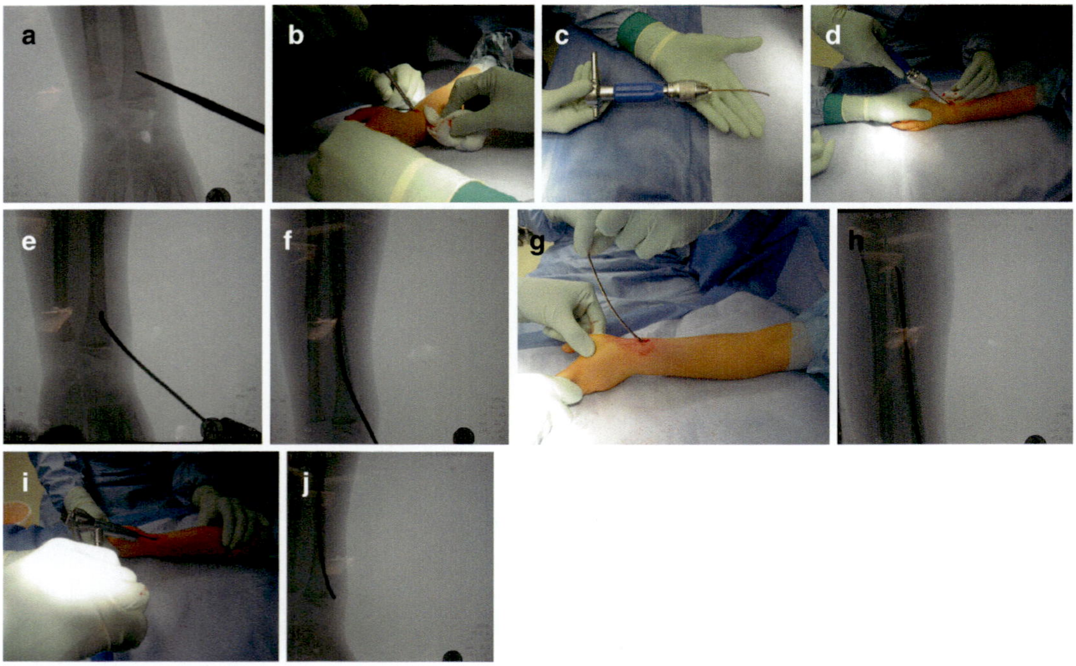

Fig. 9.50 Sequential insertion of ESiN in radius

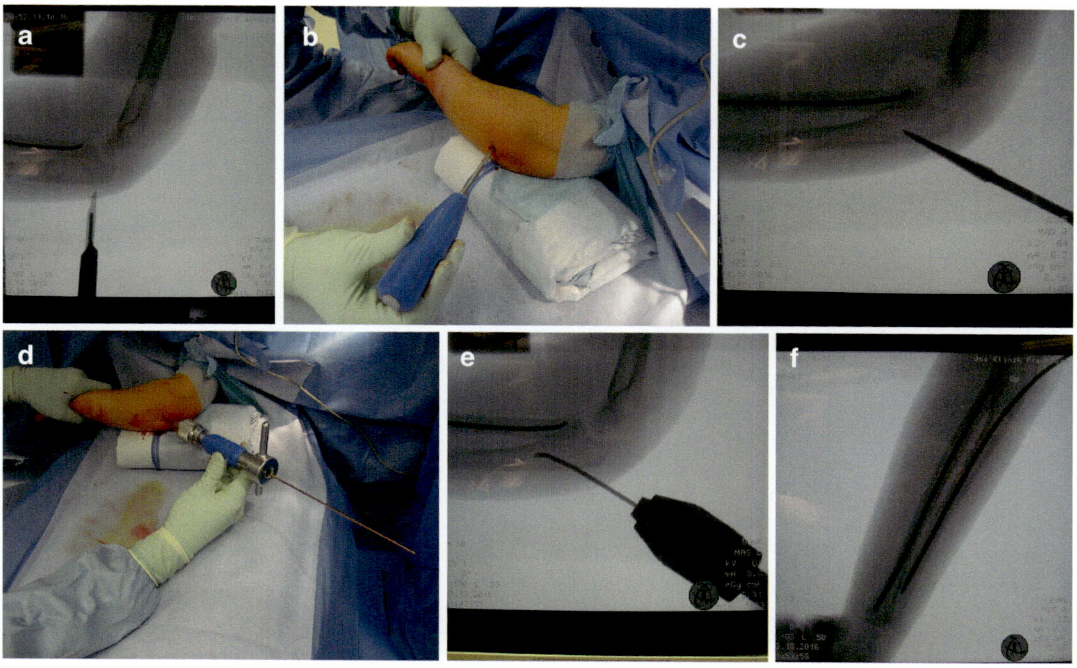

Fig. 9.51 Sequential insertion of ESiN in ulna. (**a**) Localiation with x-ray, (**b**, **c**) opening of the ulna and corresponding x-ray, (**d**, **e**) inseration of elastic nail and corresponding x-ray, (**f**) finale x.ray with both ESIN in place

Table 9.13 Fracture of the distal forearm—Kapandji technique (Fig. 9.52)

Principle	Indirect realignment of the fracture without affecting the epiphysis
Material	2 size-adapted K-wires (usually 1.4 mm)
Positioning	Supine, trans-illuminating operative table with arm board, moveable draping above the elbow joint.
Operative principle	Dorsal skin incision Introduction of a K-wire from proximal into the fracture line Reduction of the fracture in the sagittal plane by advancing the wire distally Introduction of a second K-wire from lateral into the fracture line Reduction in the second plane Stabilization through drilling into the opposing cortex, without wide perforation (Fig. 9.52) Wires left percutaneously, so that hardware can be removed without repeat anesthesia (Fig. 9.53). Alternative procedure—K-wire fixation through the radial styloid processus (Fig. 9.54) Percutaneous K-wire fixation over the radial styloid process; (Fig. 9.55) the wires can remain epicutaneous for easier take out. However, the growth plates must never be drilled through here (!) because of the risk of premature closure and only one trial.
Special explanation	Injury to the superficial radial nerve during fixation of the radius
Hardware removal	At 4 weeks, ambulatory, repeat anesthesia unnecessary
Other particulars	None

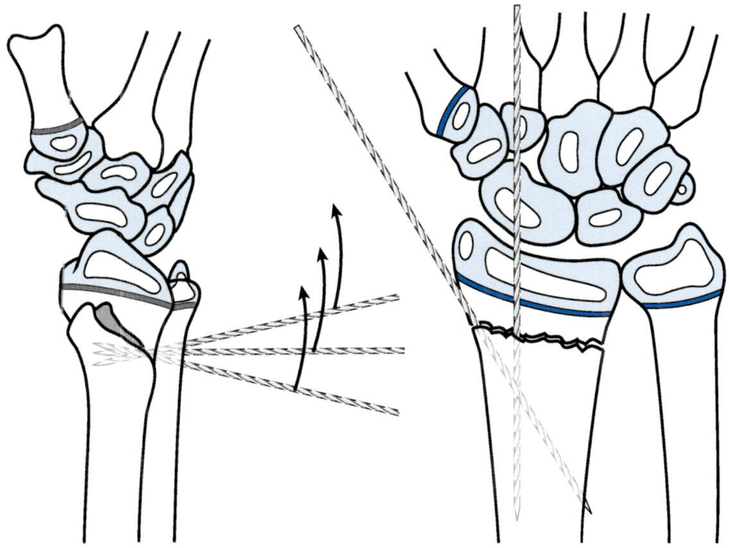

Fig. 9.52 Kapandji technique. Dorsal skin incision. Introduction of a K-wire from proximal into the fracture line. Reduction of the fracture in the sagittal plane by advancing the wire distally. Introduction of a second K-wire from lateral into the fracture line. Reduction in the second plane. Stabilization through drilling into the opposing cortex, without wide perforation. Wires left percutaneously

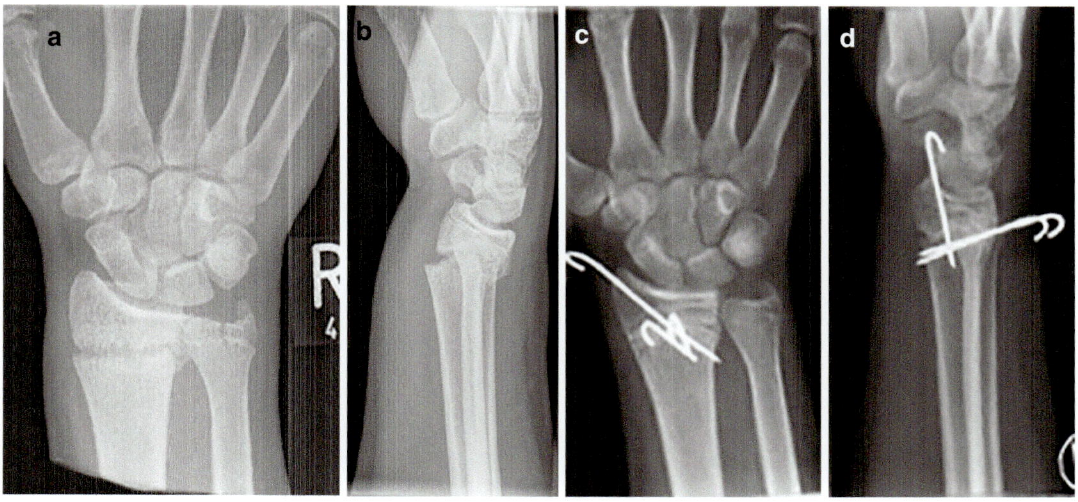

Fig. 9.53 15 year old boy with dorsally dislocated radius fracture. (**a**, **b**) Trauma image, (**c**, **d**) Indirect reduction acc. to Kapandji with 1 dorsal K-wire and 1 radial K-wire, without touching the growth plate; the ulna fracture was treated together with the cast for 4 weeks

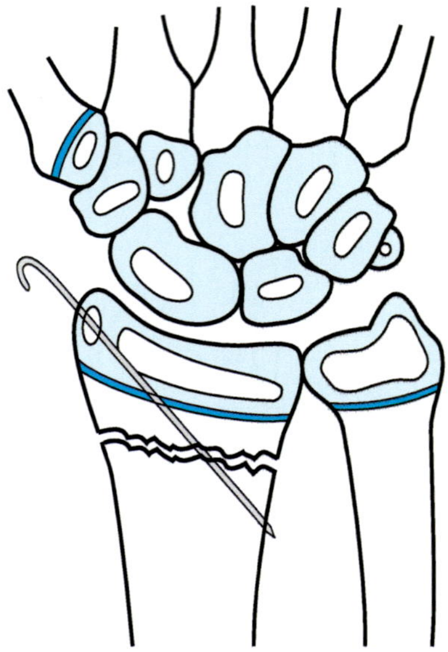

Fig. 9.54 Percutaneous K-wire osteosynthesis via the radial styloid processus with perforation of the growth plate with one or occasionally 2 wires. The growth plate should not perfused several times in order not to harm

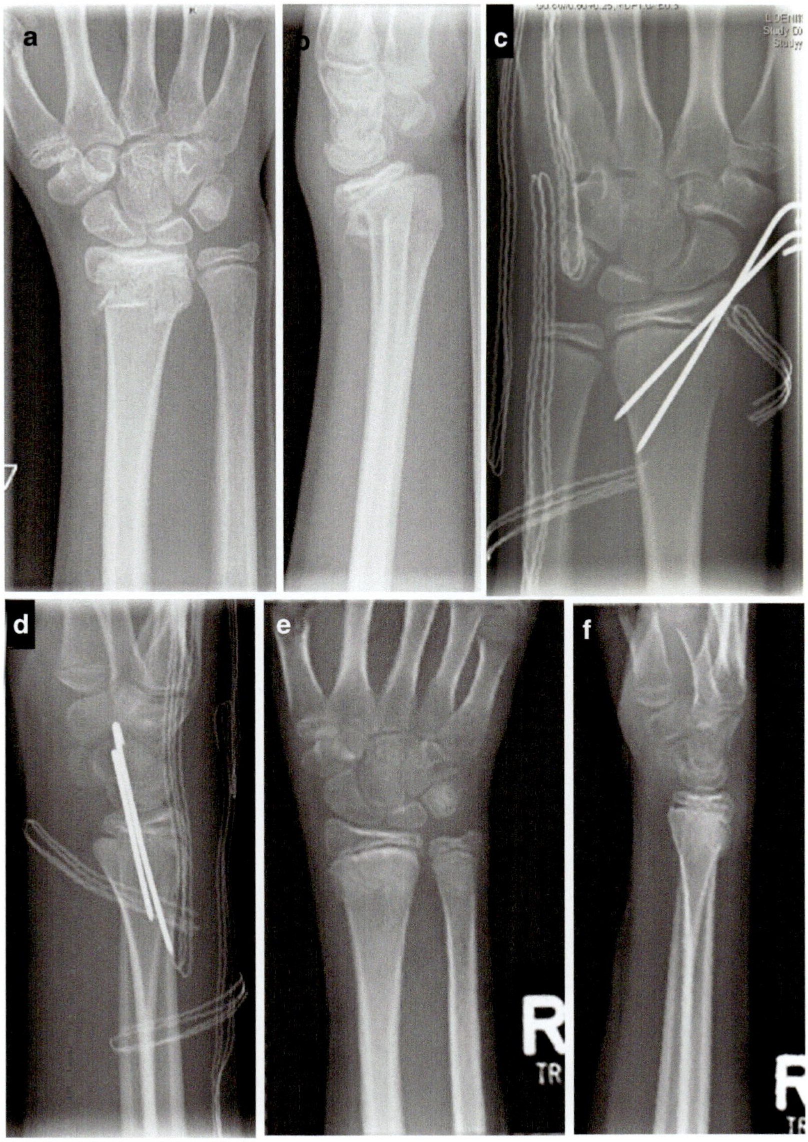

Fig. 9.55 12 year old girl after inline skating. (**a**, **b**) Trauma image, (**c**, **d**) Percutaneous fixation via the growth plate after reduction, (**e**, **f**) Consolidation after metal removal after 4 weeks. The wires can remain over the skin for easier take out

Table 9.14 Technical aspects of the treatment of Monteggia injuries

Material	Size adapted plate fixation (e.g., 2.4 mm) Hand or foot implant (Fig. 9.56)
Positioning	Supine, trans-illuminating operative table with arm board, moveable draping above the elbow joint.
Approach	Posterior approach to the ulnar shaft: 1. Incision over the dorsal ulnar edge 2. Splitting of the forearm fascia and the periosteum between the flexor carpi ulnaris and the extensor carpi ulnaris muscles 3. Sub-periosteal release of the flexor carpi ulnaris and lateral positioning 4. Release of the extensor carpi ulnaris and anconeus muscles Anterolateral approach to the radial head when open reduction of the radial head is necessary 1. Incision from the lateral epicondyle towards the ulnar edge 2. Incision of the fascia between the extensor digitorum muscle and the extensor carpi radialis 3. Vertical incision of the capsule
Special explanation	Injury of the radial nerve in supinator incision
Operative principle	Reduction of the radial head through stabilization of the ulnar fracture in anatomic position
Hardware removal	After definitive consolidation, usually after 3–4 months
Potential corrections	Ulnar osteotomy and re-fixation with correct proportion to the radius with repaired radial head, to compensate for the spontaneous ulnar correction; promising procedure, best performed with an external fixator, in two stages (see Chap. 19)
Follow-up	Functional
Hardware removal	After definitive consolidation, usually after 3–4 months

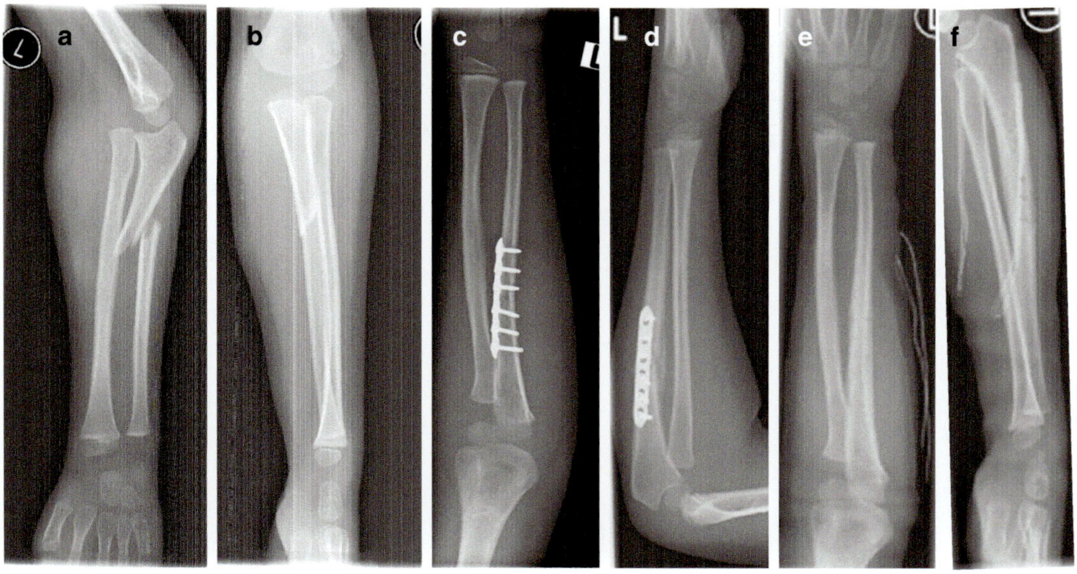

Fig. 9.56 5 year old boy with Monteggia lesion. (**a**, **b**) Trauma image, (**c**, **d**) Open reduction of ulna with plate osteosynthesis and thereby indirect closed reduction of the radial head, (**e**, **f**) Healing in correct position after metal removal

Recommended Literature

Chirurg PSD (2017) Frakturen der oberen Extremität im Kindes-/Wachstumsalter. Orthopäde. Thieme, Stuttgart. https://doi.org/10.1007/s00104-017-0420-5

Dietz HG, Schmittenbecher PP, Illing P (1997) Intramedulläre Osteosynthese im Wachstumsalter. Urban & Schwarzenberg, Munich

Dietz HG, Schmittenbecher PP, Slongo T, Wilkins KE (2006) Elastic stable intramedullary nailing (ESIN) in children. Thieme, Stuttgart

Frank J, Sommer K, Sander AL, Marzi I (2018) Soft tissue reconstruction of hands and feet in childhood. Trauma Berufskrankheit 48:2119–2110

Hubbard J, Chauhan A, Fitzgerald R, Abrams R, Mubarak S, Sangimino M (2018) Missed pediatric Monteggia fractures. JBJS Rev 6:e2

Kraus R (2014) Distal radial fractures in growing children. Trauma Berufskrankheit 16:53–60

Kruppa C, Bunge P, Schildhauer TA, Dudda M (2017) Low complication rate of elastic stable intramedullary nailing (ESIN) of pediatric forearm fractures. Medicine 96:e6669

Lieber J (2014) Growth behavior after fractures of the distal forearm: reasons for the high rate of overtreatment. Unfallchirurg 117:1092–1098

Lieber J, Sommerfeldt DW (2011) Diametaphyseal forearm fracture in childhood. Pitfalls and recommendations for treatment. Unfallchirurg 114:292–299

Marzi I (2016) Kindertraumatologie, 3rd edn. Springer, Berlin

Metaizeau JP (1988) Ostosynthese chez l'enfant par E.C.M.E.S. Sauramps, Montpellier

Peterlein C-D, Modzel T, Hagen L, Ruchholtz S, Krüger A (2019) Long-term results of elastic-stable intramedullary nailing (ESIN) of diaphyseal forearm fractures in children. Medicine 98:e14743

Schmittenbecher PP (2008) Osteosynthesen am proximalen Unterarm im Kindesalter. Oper Orthop Traumatol 20:321–333

Sinikumpu JJ, Nietosvaara Y (2021) Treatment of distal forearm fractures in children. Scand J Surg 110(2):276–280. https://doi.org/10.1177/1457496920983104

Stragier B, Smet LD, Degreef I (2018) Long-term follow-up of corrective ulnar osteotomy for missed Monteggia fractures in children. J Shoulder Elbow Surg 27:e337–e343

Weinberg A-M, Castellani C, Amerstorfer F (2008) Elastisch-stabile intramedulläre Marknagelung (ESIN) von Unterarmfrakturen. Oper Orthop Traumatol 20:285–296

van Delft EAK, Vermeulen J, Schep NWL, van Stralen KJ, van der Bij GJ (2020) Prevention of secondary displacement and reoperation of distal metaphyseal forearm fractures in children. J Clin Orthop Trauma 11:S817–S822

Hand

10

10.1 Carpal Fractures and Dislocations

After birth, the entire carpus is composed of cartilage, and the gradual ossification occurs according to a particular pattern with mild variations between girls and boys. First, the ossification center of the capitate is visible, followed by the hamate. Then, areas of the triquetrum become visible at 1½–2½ years, the lunate at 4 years, and the trapezium, trapezoid, and scaphoid at 4–5 years. The ossification center of the pisiform is visible at approximately 10 years, and ossification of the carpus is completed at approximately 15 years (Fig. 10.1).

Because the scaphoid ossifies from distal to proximal, the joint line between the lunate and scaphoid appears wide in children (Pseudo Terry Thomas Sign). At age 7, it measures approximately 9 mm, and at 15, it reaches approximately 3 mm. This can complicate the evaluation for ligament injuries. Pediatric scaphoid fractures also show the particular nature of the ossification sequence. About half of all fractures occur in the distal third, with dorsoradial avulsion fractures the most common. One third of fractures occur in the scaphoid body due to larger forces. Thus, one must be observant for accompanying injuries such as capitate fractures.

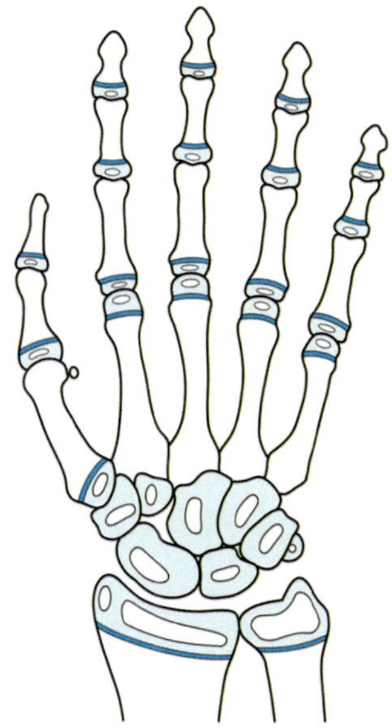

Fig. 10.1 Ossification centers of the hand

I. Marzi et al., *Pediatric Skeletal Trauma*, https://doi.org/10.1007/978-3-030-93685-3_10

Incidence, Mechanism of Injury and Clinical Picture

Carpal injuries are rare in children; carpal fractures make up approximately 0.4% of all pediatric fractures. Scaphoid fractures usually occur between the ages of 15 and 30, and in children mainly between 10 and 15 years. In recent years, carpal and ligament injuries have received increased attention. Improved and more widely applied imaging (MRI) and experience with wrist arthroscopy have contributed to this.

Fractures and ligament ruptures rarely occur in children because the carpal complex consists almost entirely of cartilage. Increasing age means increased ossification, and then similar injury patterns to those in adults occur in adolescents and young adults. Thus, in this age group, there is also avascular necrosis, for example of the lunate bone.

The mechanism of injury in the carpus is generally a fall, for example from a bike or while skating. Carpal fractures often occur in combination with distal radius fractures, and the fractures themselves are generally of the scaphoid, capitate, and lunate bones. Fracture dislocations of the carpus do not often occur.

Classification

The types of fractures around the carpus correspond to those of adults, with fractures occurring within the corresponding centers of ossification. Thus, fractures in children are more likely to be found in distal areas, e.g. the scaphoid, because ossification begins there. Classification is strictly adapted to the individual carpal bones, and then characterized by fracture anatomy. Complex injuries with ligament instability are found in adolescents, as well as peri-lunar fracture dislocations. They are classified as in adults. The Mayo Clinic Classification is used according to the pattern of injury, especially in cases of complex carpal injuries with tearing of the interosseous ligaments and subsequent carpal tilting (Tables 10.1 and 10.2). A classification for more common (scaphoid, capitate, triquetrum) and more complication-prone (lunate, hamate) fractures is listed in Table 10.3.

Table 10.1 Classification of carpal injuries

Category I Chronicity	Category II Constancy	Category III Etiology	Category IV Location	Category V Direction	Category VI Pattern
Acute (<1 week)	Predynamic dynamic	Congenital Traumatic Inflammatory Arthritic	Radiocarpal Proximal Intercarpal Midcarpal	VISI rotation DISI rotation Ulnar translation Radial translation Volar translation Dorsal translation Proximal translation Distal translation	Carpal instability dissociative (CID)
Subacute	Static, reducible	Neoplastic Iatrogenic Miscellaneous	Distal intercarpal Carpometacarpal Specific bones		Carpal instability non-dissociative (CIND) Carpal instability complex (CIC) Carpal instability adaptive (CIA)
Chronic (>6 weeks)	Static, not reducible				

CIA carpal instability, adaptive, *CIC* carpal instability, complex, *CID* carpal instability, dissociative, *CIND* carpal instability, non-dissociative, *DISI* dorsal intercalated segment instability, *VISI* volar intercalated segment instability

Table 10.2 Mayo classification of carpal injuries according to injury pattern

Pattern	Injury
I. CID	CID of the proximal carpal row (scaphoid fracture, SL dissociation, LT dissociation) CID of the distal carpal row (axial radial tearing, axial ulnar tearing) Combined proximal and distal CID
II. CIND	Radiocarpal CIND (volar ligament rupture, dorsal ligament rupture) Midcarpal CIND (ulnar MCI, radial MCI ligament as well as combined MCI and volar or dorsal ligament lesions) Combined radiocarpal and midcarpal CIND
III. CIC	Perilunar and radiocarpal instability Perilunar and axial instability Radiocarpal and axial instability SL dissociation and lunotriquetral dissociation
IV. CIA	Deformity with malunion/nonunion of the radius, scaphoid, or lunate fractures Madelung deformity

CIA carpal instability, adaptive, *CIC* carpal instability, complex, *CID* carpal instability, dissociative, *CIND* carpal instability, non-dissociative, *MCI* mid-carpal instability, *S* scaphoid, *L* lunate, *Tq* triquetrum

Table 10.3 Classification of common (scaphoid, capitate, triquetrum) and frequently complicated (lunate, hamate) carpal fractures

Scaphoid	Type A	Stable fracture A1 tubercle fracture A2 incomplete body fracture
	Type B	Unstable fracture B1 distal oblique fracture B2 complete body fracture B3 proximal pole fracture B4 perilunar fracture dislocation
	Type C	Delayed healing
	Type D	Pseudarthrosis
Lunate	Type I	Fracture of the volar pole
	Type II	Chip fracture
	Type III	Fracture of the dorsal pole
	Type IV	Sagittal fracture
	Type V	Transverse fracture
Triquetrum		Dorsal avulsion fracture Body fracture
Hamate		Body fracture Articular surface fracture Hamulus fracture
Capitate		Proximal pole fracture Body fracture Trans-scaphoid, trans-capitate fracture

Diagnostic Assessment

In cases of an appropriate trauma history with corresponding swelling and protective positioning of the wrist, carpal injuries must be ruled out along with radius fractures. Typical tenderness over the corresponding carpal bone is often difficult to discern because of smaller proportions, and the structures can be obscured by fat distribution. Typical stress tests (e.g. Watson test, scapholunate ballottement, lunotriquetral ballottement) are rarely possible and must be carefully interpreted in children and adolescents whose ligaments remain lax. However, this should not be an excuse to avoid performing a complete examination. The specific structures such as the snuffbox and also the distal scaphoid pole can be palpated, and fingertip percussion can serve as a helpful provocation test. The examination should be completed with tests of motion. Here, comparison to the other side can be particularly helpful to assess the motion of the carpus on the radial joint surface and the ulnar joint compartment. Carpal injury assessment is problematic in that the distance between the individual to-be-ossified bones varies with age, and thus, correct distance and axis are difficult to measure.

Because of the lack of ossification, injuries or fractures of the carpal bones can be easily overlooked on standard radiographs. Scaphoid, capitate, and lunate injuries are more common. In the scaphoid, the distal third in particular must be observed. With corresponding trauma and clinical suspicion then, repeat radiographs should be performed after 1–2 weeks, combined with an additional dorsovolar x-ray in pronation/ulnar deviation or an MRI.

As in adults, the basic goal of therapy for carpal injuries in children is to restore carpal stability. An interruption in the chain of loading leads to severe functional deficits. The choice between conservative and operative therapy depends on the localization of the fracture and the degree of displacement. As with adults, 1 mm displacement can be used as the limit for surgical indication. It must be borne in mind that these injuries are correlated with increasing ossification and thus, are usually found in adolescents. Limits for correction can't be specified in detail. According to case reports, remodeling is possible up to about age 10 years. Primary treatment depends on the symptoms, and until definitive diagnosis there should be immobilization and pain control with a plaster splint.

Conservative Therapy

The more frequently occurring fractures of the distal scaphoid and avulsion fractures of the distal pole can be treated conservatively (Figs. 10.2 and 10.3) as well as undisplaced stable fractures of the scaphoid waist (Fig. 10.4). The same applies for undisplaced capitate fractures, the second most common carpal fracture in children. Isolated capitate fractures are less common. They tend to occur in combination with scaphoid frac-

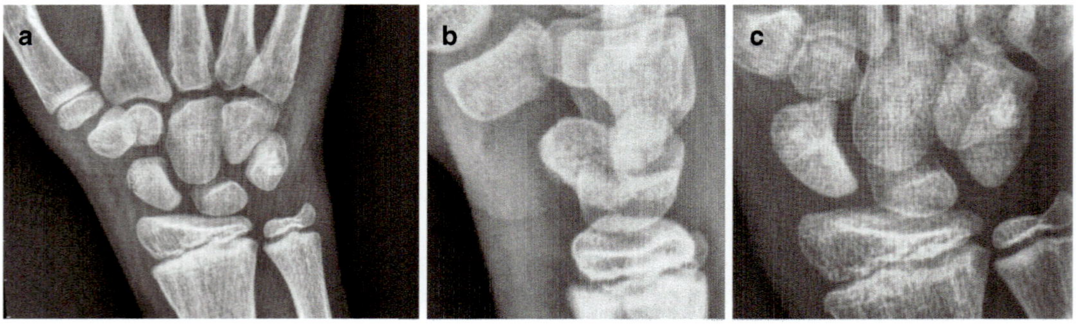

Fig. 10.2 8 Year old boy with undisplaced distal scaphoid fracture after fall. (**a**, **b**) Trauma image, (**c**) Healing after 4 weeks immobilisation with Rehbein plaster

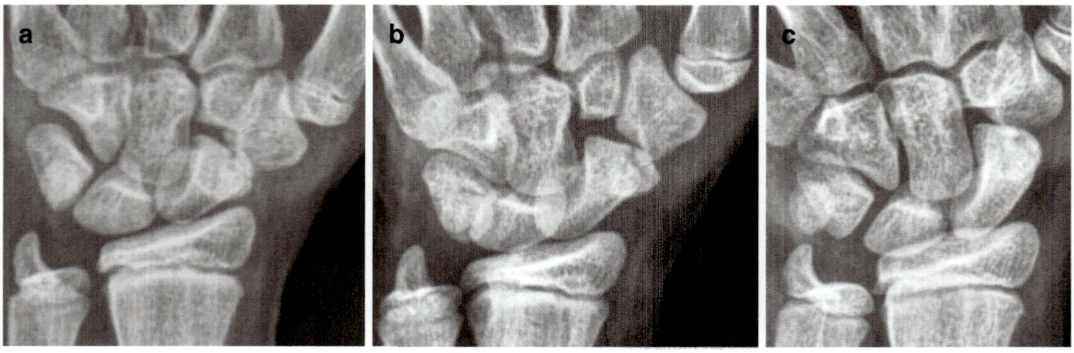

Fig. 10.3 11 Year old girl with distal scaphoid fracture after skate board accident. (**a**, **b**) Trauma image, (**c**) Painless free function after after 2 weeks of Rehbein plaster

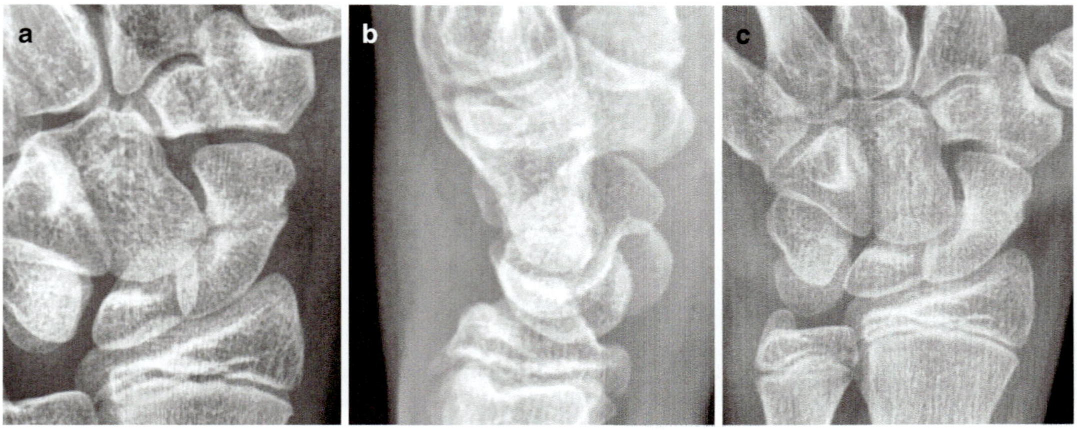

Fig. 10.4 13 Year old boy with undisplaced scaphoid waist fracture after fall. (**a**, **b**) Trauma images, (**c**) Healing after 8 weeks of Rehbein plaster

tures, called the scaphocapitate syndrome. In extreme cases, this pattern of injury leads to a hamate fracture. Triquetrum fractures, which also occur in adults, are worth mentioning as well. Generally, these are dorsal avulsion fractures of the triquetrum when there is a fall on the outstretched hand in ulnar deviation. This causes carpal impingement on the distal ulna.

Immobilization is carried out for 4–6 weeks with a forearm cast including the thumb. In small children, generally an overarm cast is indicated, since forearm casts fall off. If the fracture is detected late—after more than 10 days—the immobilization should be extended to 10 weeks. After casting, the injury is treated functionally. Physical therapy is initiated when the patient can't make a complete fist or when there are marked mobility deficits persisting longer than two weeks. The wrist should not be loaded over 5 kg for three months. Afterwards, normal sport activities can be resumed, but contact sports or martial arts and sports with excessive hand loading (tennis) should be suspended for six months.

Operative Therapy

Operative treatment is carried out for unstable and displaced carpal fractures. These are usually scaphoid (Fig. 10.5a) or capitate fractures. The

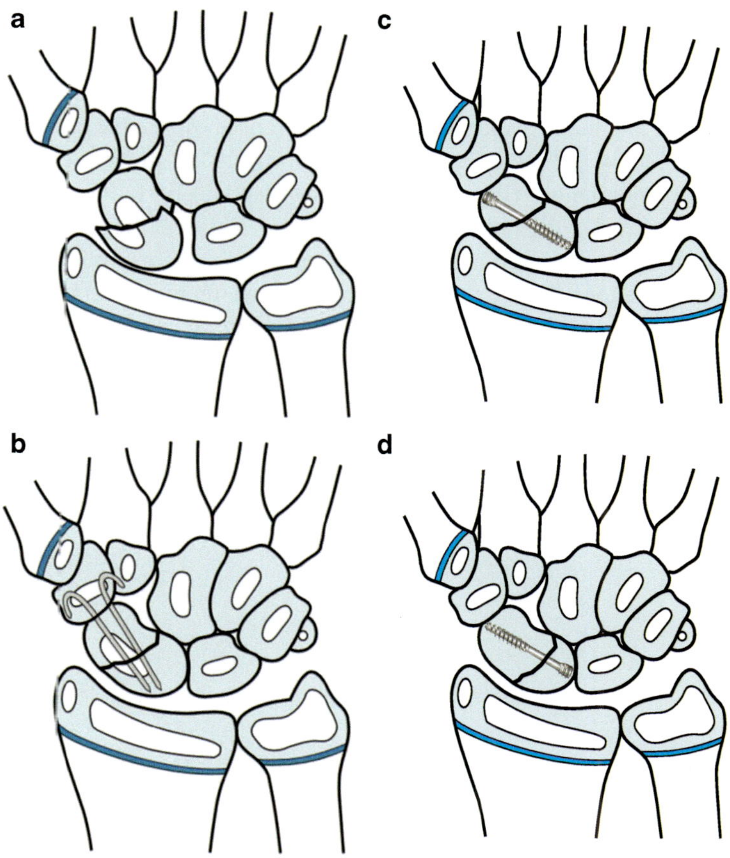

Fig. 10.5 Displaced scaphoid fracture. (**a**) Displaced transverse fracture, (**b**) K-wire stabilization in a child, (**c**) Sunk Herbert screw fixation from distal, (**d**) Sunk Herbert screw fixation from proximal. Indication in older children and adolescents

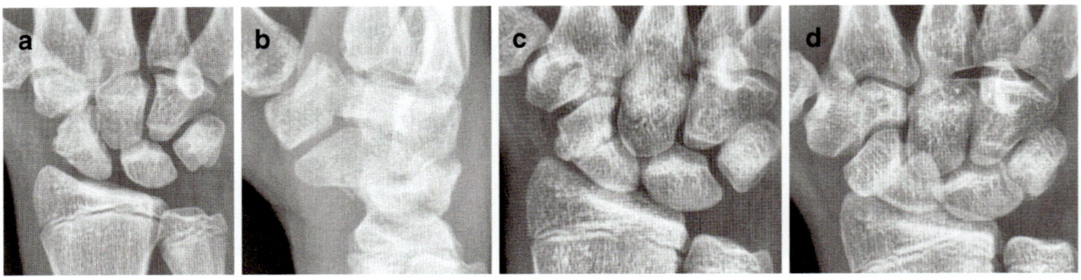

Fig. 10.6 17 Year old boy with fall playing football and undisplaced scaphoid waist fracture. (**a**, **b**) Trauma images, conservative treatment in Rehbein plaster for 10 weeks, (**c**, **d**) Slow healing with slight displacement after 12 weeks painless free wrist function after 16 weeks

procedure of choice for pediatric carpal fractures is K-wire fixation (Fig. 10.5b), or Herbert screw fixation in older children from distal (Fig. 10.5c) or proximal (Fig. 10.5d). Care should be taken in adolescents with seemingly stable undisplaced fractures of the scaphoid in order to avoid secondary dislocations in this active groupe of patients which might lead to non-union (Fig. 10.6). Ligament injuries such as SL dissociation are treated surgically with ligament suture and temporary K-wire transfixation for 6 weeks. Transfixation should secure two joints. Thus, in cases of SL dissociation, transfixation of the scapholunar and scaphocapitate joints is necessary.

Internal fixation is combined with six weeks of cast immobilization including the thumb. Forearm or above-elbow cast is suitable depending on age. Cast immobilization and hardware removal should be followed up with functional treatment. Physical therapy is initiated when the patient can't make a complete fist or when there are marked mobility deficits persisting longer than two weeks.

Complications/Growth Disturbances

Classical complications such as malunion or aseptic bone necrosis must also be considered in pediatric injuries. These have been observed in case studies of the lunate (Kienboeck's disease) or the proximal scaphoid (Preiser's disease). In cases of persistent carpal instability, operative fixation of the carpal malformation may be necessary. Here, volar flexion and lunar subluxation are recognized after distal radius fracture.

In cases of **conservative therapy**, the unstable scaphoid fracture can result in malunion in flexion, leading to dorsal tilting of the lunate. The major difference compared to adults is that such a flexion deformity can correct itself until about 10 years of age. In children, complications of malunion and osteonecrosis can both respond well to and resolve after immobilization.

After **surgical intervention**, there should be careful observation regarding tendon and nerve irritation. With a volar approach to the scaphoid, for example, the tendons of the flexor carpi radialis or the flexor pollicis longus are vulnerable. In adults, ruptures have been reported after bony extraction in the carpal area. The dorsal approach to the wrist, commonly used for ligament injuries, proximal scaphoid fractures, or problems in the lunate area, can lead to problems with the extensor pollicis longus in particular. Carpal stabilization with K-wires, as is often done, runs the risk of injuring the cutaneous branches of the radial and ulnar nerves. The long-term prognosis is markedly better in children, and healing can be expected.

Conservative and operatively treated carpal injuries should be checked clinically and radiologically at six months and one year. Special attention should be paid to signs of refracture or malunion, such as deformities and cyst formation along the scaphoid, for example. Other complications such as aseptic osteonecrosis can then also be detected at an early stage and treated as needed in a timely manner.

An overview for scaphoid fractures is given in Table 10.4.

Besides carpal fractures, complex luxation and luxation fractures (Table 10.5) occur rarely in children (Fig. 10.13). In particular, perilunar luxations or trans-scaphoideal luxation fractures might be observed, mostly in adolescents.

Table 10.4 Scaphoid fractures (Fig. 10.7)

Special features	Usually after the age of 15 with ossification of the scaphoid, thus more distal fractures
Diagnostic assessment	Clinical examination, radiographs of the wrist in two planes, when needed dorso-volar views in pronation and ulnar deviation, MRI
Goals of therapy/limits for correction	Anatomical reduction, loading of the carpus, prevention of osteonecrosis
Primary treatment	Pain therapy, elevation, measures to decrease swelling, splint immobilization
Conservative therapy	
Indication	Generally, with the more common distal scaphoid fractures (Fig. 10.8), but also in oblique fractures without larger displacement (Fig. 10.9)
Procedure	Forearm cast with thumb, in small children above-elbow cast with thumb, immobilization for 4–6 weeks, up to 10 weeks with delayed diagnosis (Fig. 10.10)
Follow up	Functional follow up with gradual and full loading till the 10–12th week, after delayed treatment until the 16th week
X-ray control	After 2 weeks and after cast removal
Resuming sports	After 12 weeks
Operative therapy	
Indication	Displacement of the fracture >1–2 mm and instability Bone defect of cystic alterations at the fracture side
Procedure	K-wire fixation in small In adolescents mostly from palmar retrograde distal screw fixation (Fig. 10.11) in proximal fractures, also an antegrade fixation from dorsal is possible
Follow up	According to age, forearm or above-elbow casting for six weeks, then functional therapy and gradual loading until the 12th postoperative week
X-ray control	After approximately two weeks at cast change and prior to hardware removal at six weeks
Hardware removal	K-wires at six weeks, screws are generally left in place
Resuming sports	After 12 weeks, with excessive hand loading after six months
Complications	Malunion, osteonecrosis; in these cases (Fig. 10.12) occasionally a bone graft might be required.
Growth disturbances	Not to be expected
Follow up	At 6 and 12 months

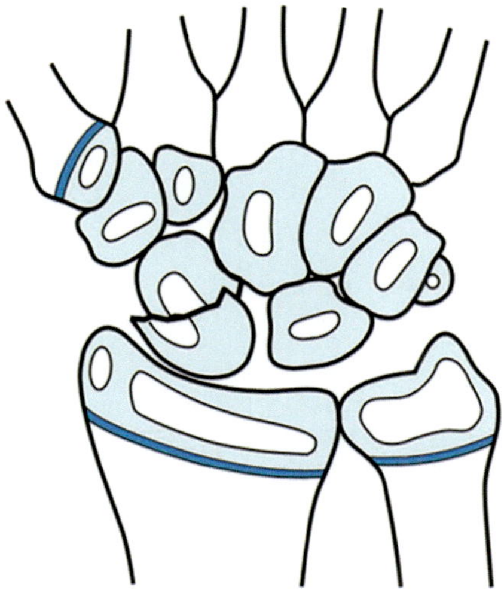

Fig. 10.7 Scaphoid fracture

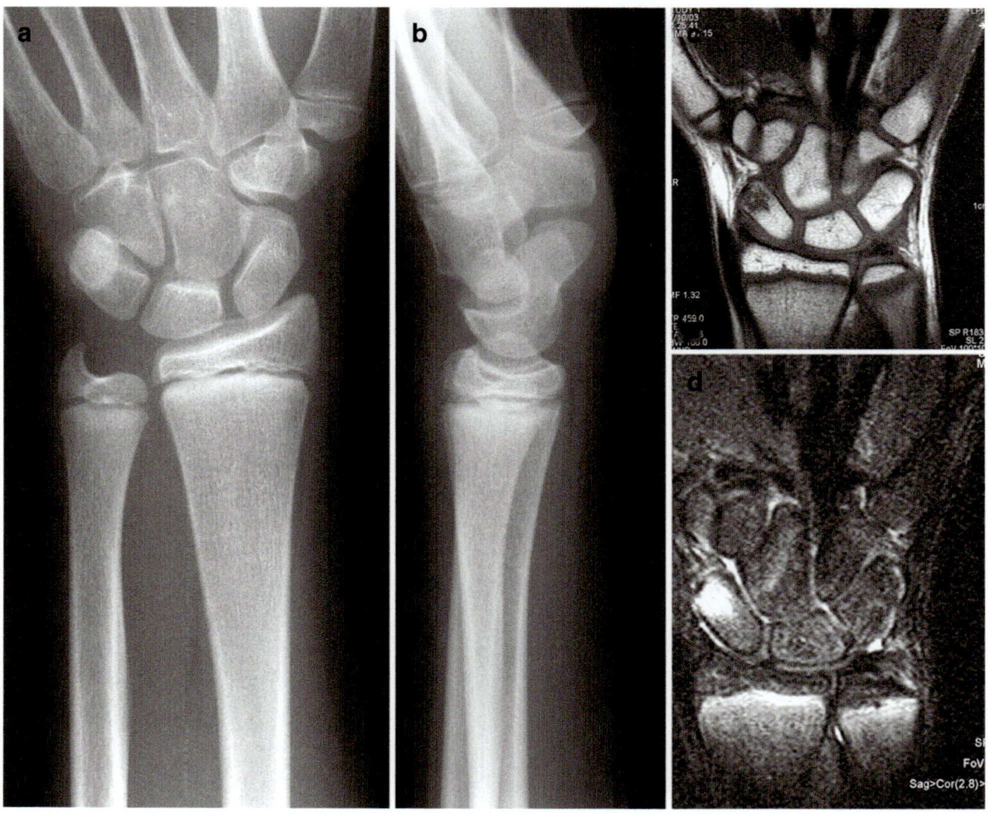

Fig. 10.8 Distal scaphoid fracture (**a**, **b**) X-ray, (**c**, **d**) MRI

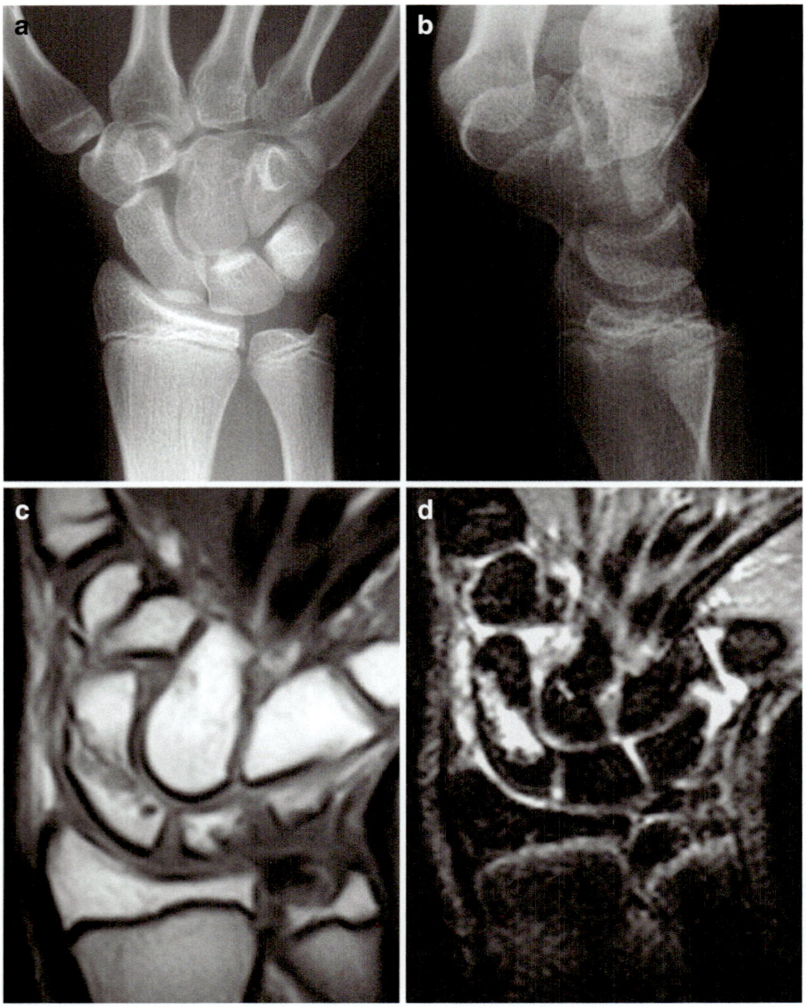

Fig. 10.9 Oblique scaphoid fracture with slight displacement and conservative treatment. (**a**, **b**) X-ray (**c**, **d**) MRI

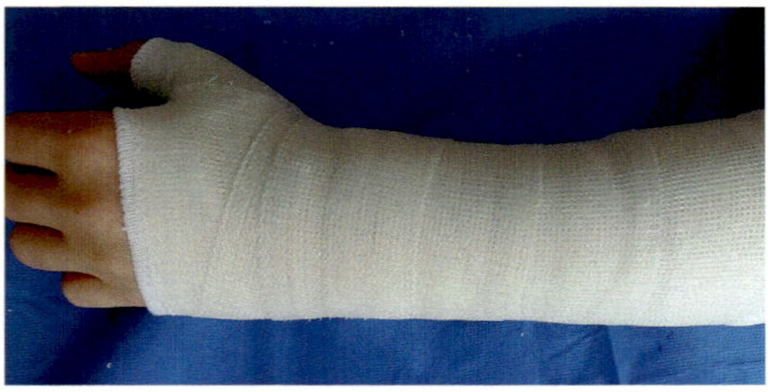

Fig. 10.10 Scaphoid cast of a children with basis bone of the thumb

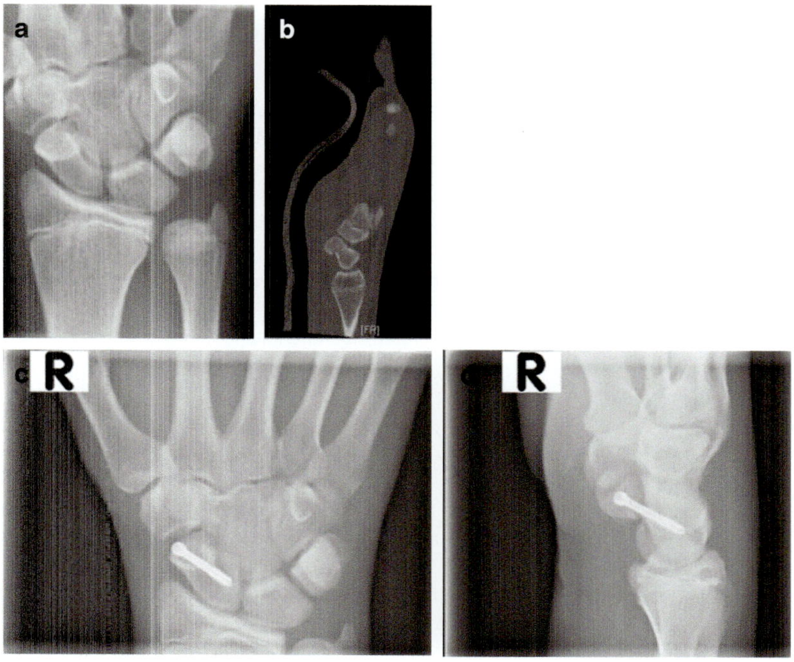

Fig. 10.11 Scaphoid malunion at the border to the distal third (**a**, **b**) Scaphoid cyst with fracture on CT, (**c**, **d**) Retrograde screw fixation (Herbert screw) with cancellous bone

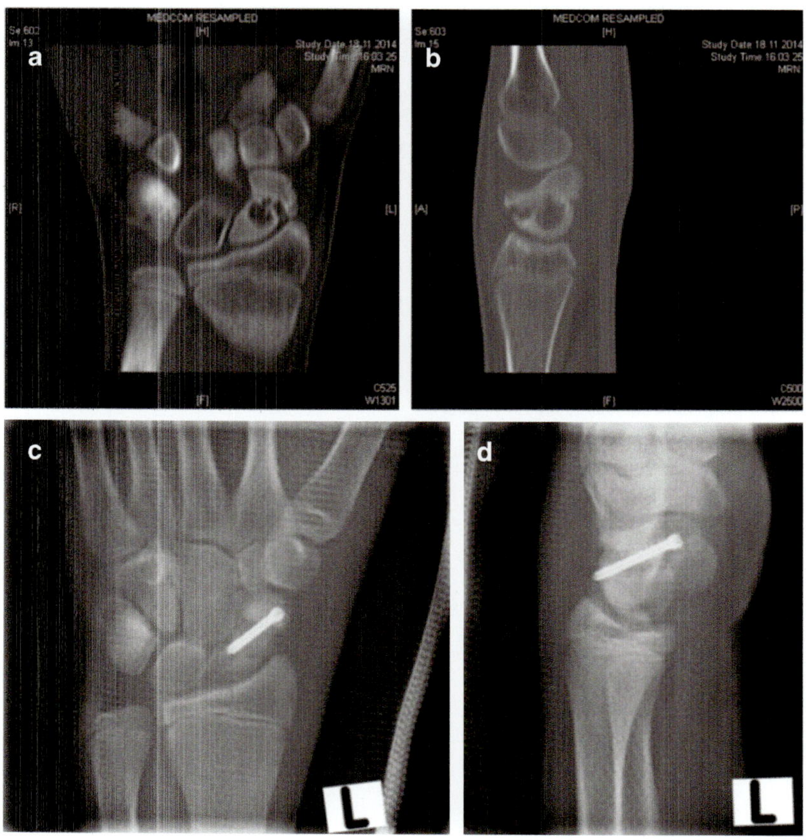

Fig. 10.12 Scaphoid fracture (**a**, **b**) Old fracture with cysts, (**c**, **d**) After open reduction with retrograde screw fixation (Herbert screw)

Table 10.5 Carpal dislocation and luxation fractures

Special features	Generally occurs with 15 years or older
Diagnostic assessment	Marked swelling of the hand, radiographs of the wrist in two planes, CT or MRI when unclear
Goals of therapy/limits for correction	Anatomic reconstruction, carpal stability, full reconstruction
Primary treatment	Elevation, cooling, immediate assessment, urgent surgery in cases of dislocation
Conservative therapy	
Indication	Only with anatomic reduction in both planes and dynamic exclusion of ligament instability (carpal transillumination)
Procedure	Forearm cast until swelling is reduced, then up to six weeks forearm cast with thumb base included.
Follow up	Splint for 2–4 weeks after cast removal and gradual loading till the 12th week
X-ray control	At 14 days and 6 weeks
Resuming sports	After 12 weeks
Operative treatment	
Indication	Dislocation of a carpal bone (Fig. 10.14), or peri-lunar trans-scaphoid fracture-dislocations (Fig. 10.15).
Procedure	Open dorsal reduction of the carpus, transfixation with 1.4 to 1.6 mm K-wires Cast immobilization for 6–8 weeks or external fixator from the radius to the second metacarpal bone
Follow up	Wound checks, forearm cast for 14 days, then 4–6 weeks of closed cast with thumb
X-ray control	Post-operatively and at 6 weeks
Hardware removal	At 6–8 weeks
Resuming sports	After 12–16 weeks
Complications	Unstable reduction and transfixation, delayed ligament healing with need for secondary reconstruction, secondary deformity
Growth disturbances	Unlikely
Follow up	At 6 and 12 months

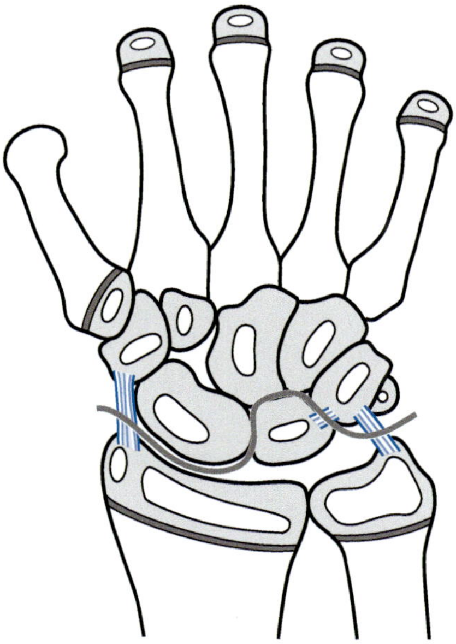

Fig. 10.13 Carpal dislocation

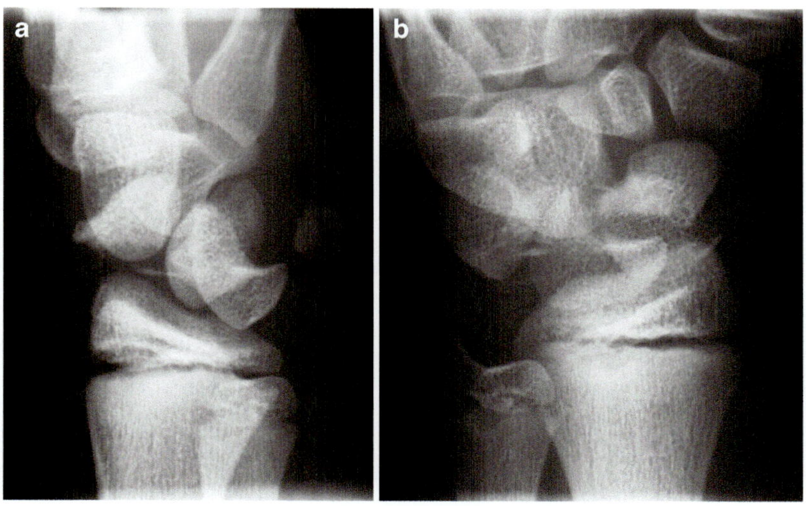

Fig. 10.14 Perilunar luxation of the carpal bones (**a**) lateral view, (**b**) A.P. view

10.2 Metacarpal Fractures

Incidence, Mechanism of Injury and Clinical Picture

Fractures of the metacarpals and fingers in children have historically remained in the domain of conservative therapy. However, some fractures require a more aggressive approach to achieve better results. It must be stressed here that the hand is the most often injured body part in children. Various investigations of risk have yielded an incidence over 0.25% for pediatric hand fractures.

Cartilaginous bone is initially relatively stable, and fractures are thus somewhat rare. Beginning at approximately 8 years of age, the incidence of fractures rises significantly, reaching a maximum at 13 years. However, this appears to be due not only to increasing ossification but also to increased activity and participation in more risky sport activities. Significantly more boys are affected. American football is the most common, but also basketball, wrestling, hockey and skiing must be mentioned.

With certain injury patterns, the possibility of physical abuse must also be considered.

Classification

Injuries around the epiphyseal plate are classified using the systems of Aitken or Salter-Harris. For this, the fractures are classified according to fracture anatomy and distinguished as intraarticular or extraarticular. In addition, fractures are classified according to stability/instability. Another classification considers localization.

Metacarpal head fractures:

- Epiphyseal fractures (Salter-Harris III)
- Ligament avulsion
- Osteochondral shear
- Boxer fracture
- 2-fragment fracture (sagittal, coronal, transverse)
- Comminuted fracture
- Defect fracture
- Compression fracture with avascular necrosis

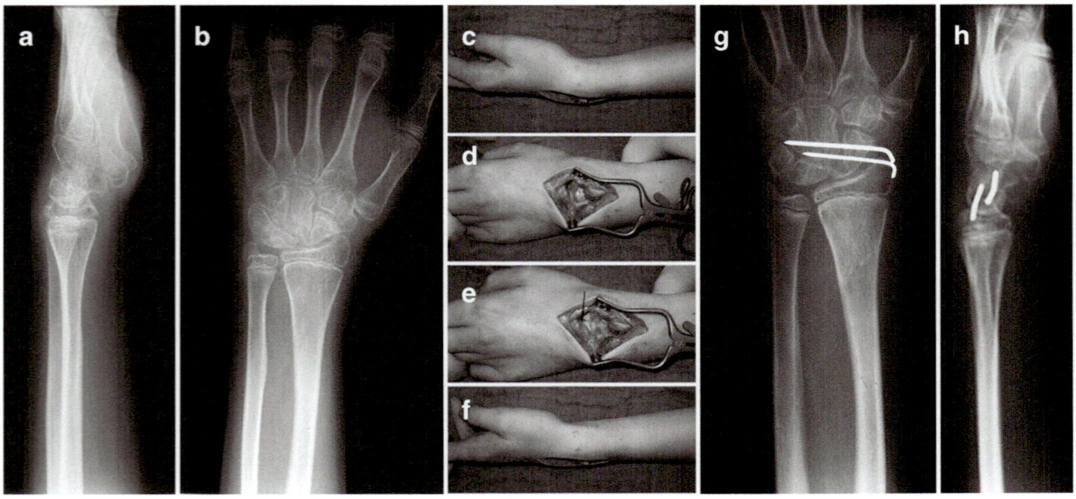

Fig. 10.15 Palmar flexion and lunar subluxation after distal radius fracture (**a**, **b**) Trauma images, (**c**) Clinically evident palmar axis deformity, (**d–f**) Lifting of the lunate under tension, (**g**, **h**) Transfixation with K-wires

Shaft fractures:

- simple fracture, comminuted fracture, compression fracture, defect fracture
- Transverse fracture, angled fracture, spiral fracture, avulsion fracture

The epiphyses are present at both ends of the metacarpals; however, there is no secondary ossification center in the proximal metacarpal. The collateral ligaments and volar plate of the metacarpophalangeal joint (MCP joint) are almost exclusively located on the opposing epiphysis. Thus, the growth plate is less protected by the soft tissues, which explains the high proportion of Salter-Harris II and III fractures. This is different than injuries in the finger joints (interphalangeal or IP joints).

Diagnostic Assessment

Assessment first requires accurate collection of the trauma history, previous injuries, known deformities, and other health issues. Especially deformities can complicate assessment, for example, brachydactyly can simulate a fracture-related shortening of the metacarpal.

The clinical examination of the injured hand is especially difficult in children. The patient is often uncooperative, cries, and suffers from the pain. In addition, there is the fear of the child and often insecurity of parents or responsible companions. Specific tests evaluating hand function and joint/bone stability are difficult to perform. The particular laxity of the ligament structures, loose connective tissue and fat padding of small hands also complicate assessment. Finally, there is generally an enormous size disparity between the hand of the patient and that of the examiner. Thus, exact localization of tenderness is very difficult.

Examination begins when entering the treatment room. The behavior, use of the extremity, and interaction between the child and his/her companion must be closely monitored. The potential need for sedation and anesthesia should be considered early in the examination. Thus, it's essential to assess for neurological deficits early. The particularly valuable assessment with 2-point discrimination is often impossible. In cases of open injuries of a region where nerve injuries are common, operative revision is necessary. In closed injuries in the hand and finger area, children can generally be expected to recover. Assessment of swelling and exclusion of compartment syndrome are of primary importance. The "wrinkle test" can be useful here for certain cases. For this, the fingers are soaked in warm water for 5 minutes. Afterwards, the presence (innervated) or absence (denervated) of wrinkling offer important information.

Then, adequate sedation or anesthesia can be carried out and the examination and further assessments are often easier. The hand can be better positioned and redundant radiographs, which are generally adequate to evaluate bony hand injuries, can be avoided.

Goals of Therapy/Limits for Correction

In cases of hand fractures, the effects and the potential for correction of traumatic deformities in the metacarpals and fingers must be considered when choosing treatment. Sagittal deviation after sub-capital and shaft fractures can be well corrected; some authors accept deformities up to 70° after sub-capital fractures in small children. Shortening and rotational deformities cannot be compensated for. Considering function, similar measures to those used in adults can be applied. A rotation deformity of 1° leads to 5° rotation of the fingertip, rotation deformity of 5° can yield up to 1.5 cm crossing of the fingers, and shortening of 2 mm can result in 7° loss of extension. The goal of treatment should thus be to avoid sagittal volar tilt of more than 30°, rotation of the fingertip more than 10°, and shortening of the finger more than 5 mm.

Conservative Therapy

Metacarpal injuries without significant rotation deformity (< 10°), volar tilt (< 30°) or loss of length (< 5 mm) can be treated conservatively. Reduction, such as in a shaft fracture, can be performed conservatively when there is no longer a tendency toward displacement. Experience teaches that unstable subcapital metacarpal fractures that are reduced primarily and immobilized in a cast will return to their primary deformity. Functional treatment can avoid this; however, this can only be implemented in adolescents and not for children under 10–12 years. Spiral fractures that carry a high risk for rotation deformities must be monitored closely since they heal quickly when there is sufficient immobilization because of the large amount of bone contact. A transverse fracture in the shaft area can be difficult to treat in a cast. For this, mandatory early follow up must provide and answer whether conservative therapy is adequate.

The procedure of choice is immobilization in a plaster splint in intrinsic-plus position of the finger (flexion of the MCP joint to 70° and complete extension of the long finger with wrist extension of about 20–30). This is not possible in toddlers because of the small hand size; here, a fist cast can be used. The cast should be left for three weeks, and four weeks in transverse shaft fractures.

Uncomplicated fractures like buckle fractures, non-displaced subcapital metacarpal fractures as well as stable base fractures don't require further radiographs with clinical follow up. Spiral fractures, transverse shaft fractures, and fractures that underwent primary reduction should be x-rayed at one week and after cast removal.

Operative Therapy

Injuries of the carpometacarpal joint (CMC joint) or the long finger MCP joints are rare and should be stabilized additionally with K-wires when there are two or more dislocated joints. There are more frequent injuries in the area of the thumb CMC joint, most commonly metaphyseal fractures (Salter-Harris II) of the proximal phalanx and less commonly Bennett fractures through the epiphysis (Salter-Harris III). The metaphyseal base fracture with the common lateral deviation can be reduced and treated in a plaster cast. If reduction is prevented by the fragment or the periosteum, or if there is medial deviation, open reduction becomes necessary. For this, K-wire fixation is carried out. Bennett fractures in children also require anatomic reduction.

Shaft fractures and subcapital metacarpal fractures leading to relevant rotational deformity or to marked shortening for which reduction can't be held in a cast will undergo open reduction as needed and stabilized with K-wires.

In cases of displacement greater than 1 mm, joint fractures require an open approach with stabilization.

With appropriate indications, injuries to the CMC joints of the long fingers or thumb are stabilized with K-wires after open or closed reduction. In cases of open approach, K-wires can stabilize through the neighboring ray. In cases of Bennett fractures, thin K-wires can be used to fix the epiphyseal fragment parallel to the ray. Close to skeletal maturity, transarticular K-wire fixation can be performed.

Shaft fractures can be stabilized with crossed K-wires over the collateral recess of the metacarpal head, sub-capital fractures with intramedullary splinting over the metacarpal base. Intermetacarpal fixation is always a possibility as well.

In cases of joint fractures, stabilization can be carried out with K-wires or with special mini-screws. In cases of multiple metacarpal fractures, metacarpal stability can also be achieved using plate fixation. Recent thin plate systems take little space and thus, barely disturb the soft tissues. This is not possible in toddlers, however.

Complications/Growth Disturbances

Delayed fracture healing or malunion is extremely rare and then often only in combination with high-speed trauma or metacarpal crush injury. Axis deviation and rotational deformities are possible and can interfere with hand function. Deviation, for example volar deviation of the metacarpal head, can cause pain with gripping. Rotational deviation, leading to finger crossing, is also a risk. For this, corrective osteotomy within the metaphysis of the metacarpal base is recommended. Fractures, particularly ephiphyseal fractures of the II, III, and IV rays associated with axial forces have higher risk of resulting growth disturbances. It must be explained early to the parents that despite anatomic reduction, good functional results cannot be guaranteed. This is particularly true in cases of open reduction and stabilization in the joint area, where adhesions and irritation of tendons and tendon sheaths can easily lead to deficits in motion.

K-wire infections are common at the skin level. This rarely leads to osteitis but can result in severe bone destruction when it occurs.

Most uncomplicated fractures do not require follow up. Intraarticular fractures should be monitored at six months and one year to evaluate for avascular necrosis. Mild post-traumatic deformities that don't yet require operative correction should be monitored at six months and then annually to rule out increasing deformity with growth.

An overview of metacarpal base fractures is given in Table 10.6.

Table 10.7 gives an overview about the Metacarpal shaft fractures.

Subcapital metacarpal fractures and the treatment options are indicated in Table 10.8.

Table 10.6 Metacarpal base fractures (Fig. 10.16)

Special features	Most occur from the age of 8 years with increasing physical activity
Diagnostic assessment	Clinical and radiographic examination of the hand in dorso-volar, oblique, and lateral views if necessary
Goals of therapy/limits for correction	No tilting >30°, no rotation deformity at the fingertip >10°, no shortening >5 mm, no dislocation of the adjacent carpometacarpal joint
Primary treatment	Pain therapy, elevation, measures to decrease swelling, splint immobilization
Conservative therapy	
Indication	Fractures within the tolerance limits (Fig. 10.17)
Procedure	Plaster splint in intrinsic-plus position of the finger, fist cast in toddlers, immobilization for 3 weeks (Fig. 10.18)
Follow up	Functional treatment with gradual to full loading until the sixth week
X-ray control	Not required for uncomplicated fractures, at one week with displacement risk, and after cast removal
Resuming sports	After 8 weeks
Operative therapy	
Indication	Dislocation, tilt, rotation deformity and shortening over the tolerance limits
Procedure	K-wire fixation (Figs. 10.19 and 10.20). In bennet fracture, a plate osteosynthesis might be necessary (Fig. 10.21)
Follow up	Plaster splint in intrinsic-plus position of the finger, fist cast in toddlers, immobilization for 4 weeks then functional treatment and gradual loading until the eighth postoperative week
X-ray control	At one week during cast change and prior to hardware removal at four weeks
Hardware removal	At 4 weeks
Resuming sports	After 8 weeks
Complications	Tendon injuries and adhesions, finger motion deficits, persisting deformity, K-wire infections
Growth disturbances	Not to be expected
Follow up	Most fractures don't need follow up, if increased deformity is feared, at 6 months and one year

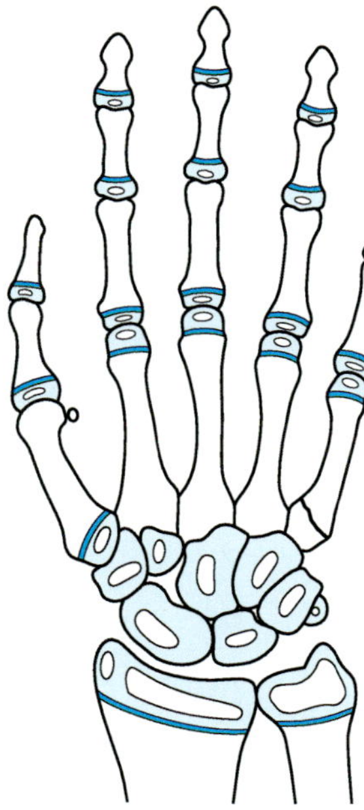

Fig. 10.16 Metacarpal base fractures

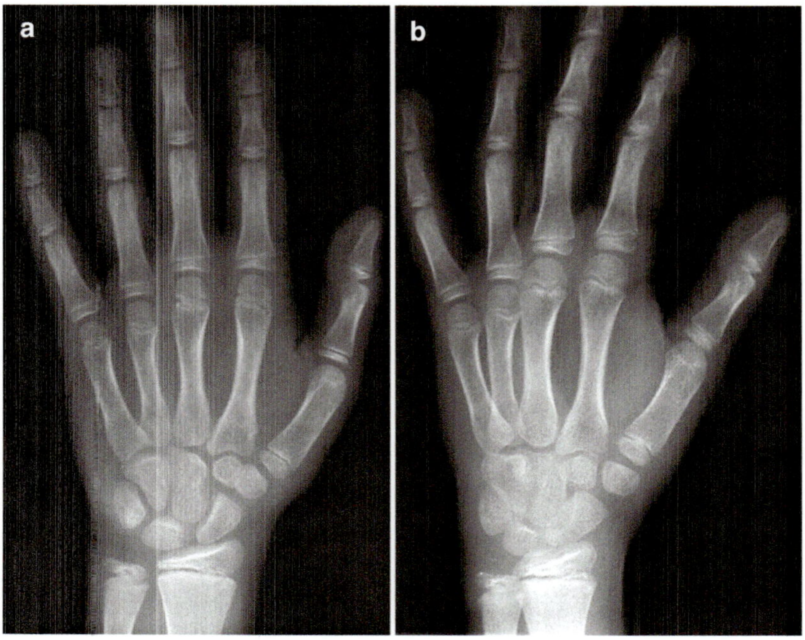

Fig. 10.17 (**a**, **b**) Non-displaced and uncomplicated fracture of the second metacarpal base

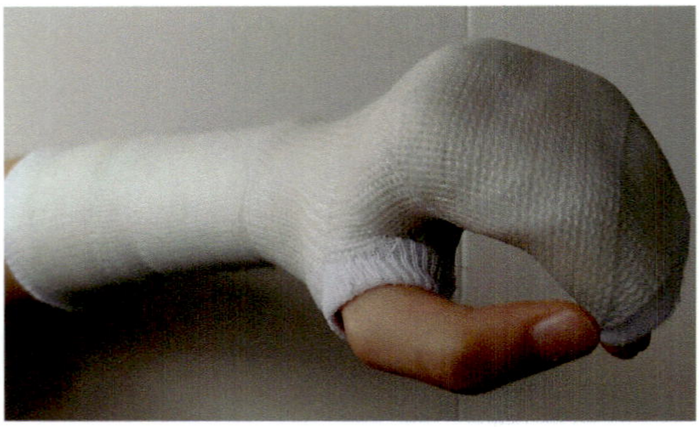

Fig. 10.18 Plaster splint in intrinsic-plus position of the finger

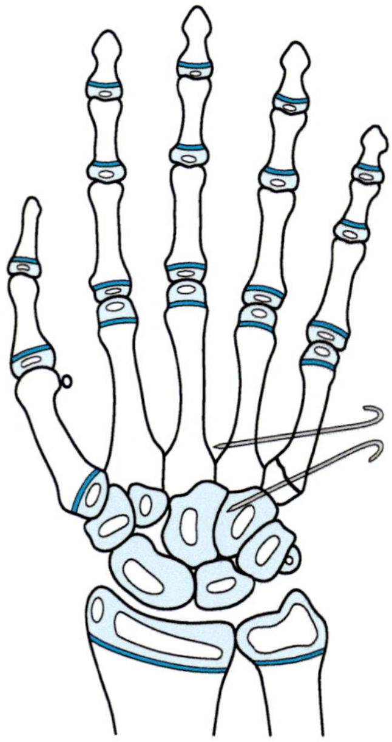

Fig. 10.19 Principle of transfixation to the fourth metacarpal bone in proximal fractures of the 5th metacarpal

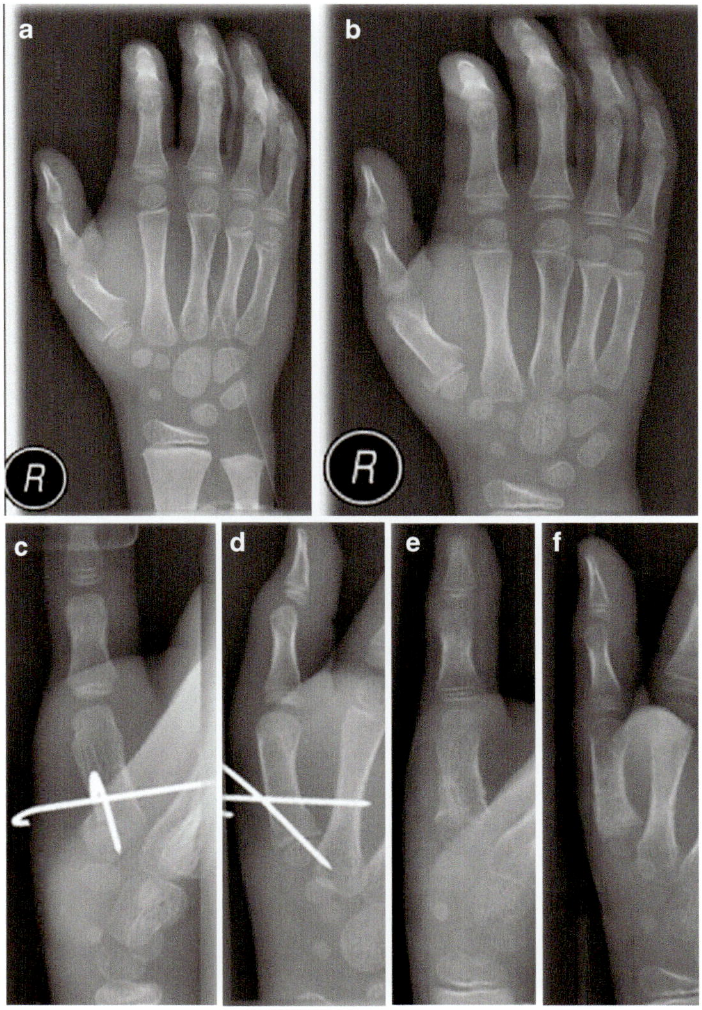

Fig. 10.20 (**a–f**) Fracture of the first metacarpal base. (**a**, **b**) Preoperatively, (**c**, **d**) After reduction and percutaneous transfixation, (**e**, **f**) Healing

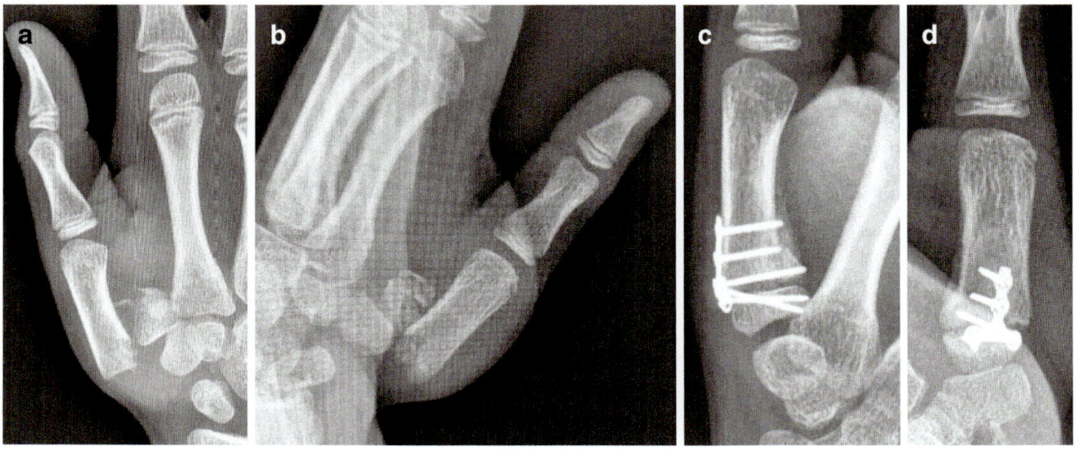

Fig. 10.21 Fracture of the first metacarpal bone. Largely displaced Bennet fracture, (**a**, **b**) Trauma image, (**c**, **d**) Reduction and plate fixation

Table 10.7 Metacarpal shaft fractures (Fig. 10.22)

Special features	Most occur from the age of 8 years with increasing physical activity
Diagnostic assessment	Clinical and radiographic examination of the hand in dorso-volar, oblique, and lateral views if necessary
Goals of therapy/limits for correction	No tilting >30°, no rotation deformity at the fingertip >10°, no shortening >5 mm
Primary treatment	Pain therapy, elevation, measures to decrease swelling, splint immobilization
Conservative therapy	
Indication	Normally for fractures within the tolerance limits, in cases of displacement or difficult to treat in cast
Procedure	Plaster splint in intrinsic-plus position of the finger, fist cast in toddlers, immobilization for 4 weeks
Follow up	Functional treatment with gradual to full loading until the sixth week
X-ray control	Not required for uncomplicated fractures, at one week with displacement risk, and after cast removal (Fig. 10.23)
Resuming sports	After 8 weeks
Operative therapy	
Indication	Displacement, tilting, rotation deformities and shortening over the tolerated limits
Procedure	K-wire fixation, in older children screw or plate fixation (Fig. 10.24)
Follow up	Plaster splint in intrinsic-plus position of the finger, fist cast in toddlers, immobilization for 4 weeks then functional treatment and gradual loading until the eighth postoperative week
X-ray control	At 1 week with cast change and prior to hardware removal at 4 weeks
Hardware removal	At 4 weeks, with screws or plates optional after 6 months (Fig. 10.25).
Resuming sports	After 8 weeks
Complications	Tendon injuries and adhesions, finger motion deficits, persisting deformity, K-wire infections
Growth disturbances	Not to be expected
Follow up	Most fractures do not require follow up. If there is risk for increasing deformity, then at 6 months and one year

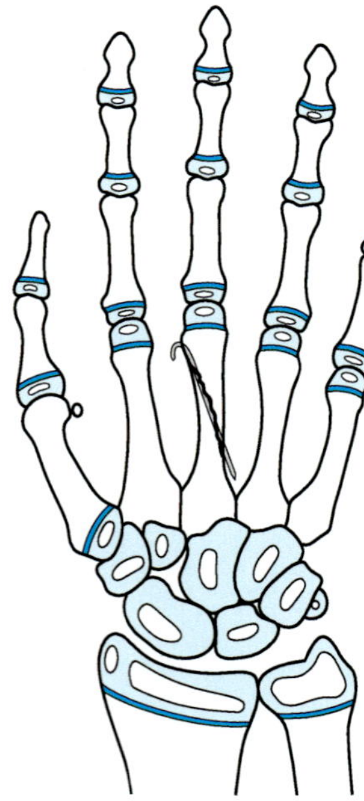

Fig. 10.22 Shaft fractures of metacarpal bones

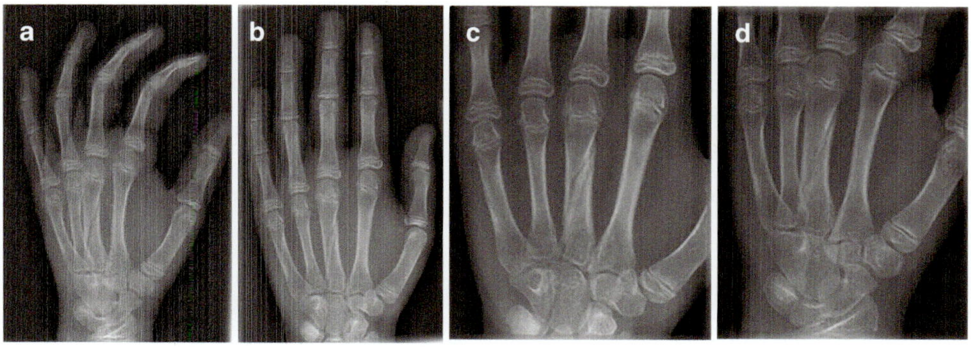

Fig. 10.23 Metacarpal shaft fracture of the third metacarpal bone with conservative treatment in intrinsic plus cast. (**a**, **b**) Trauma image, (**c**, **d**) Complete anatomical healing

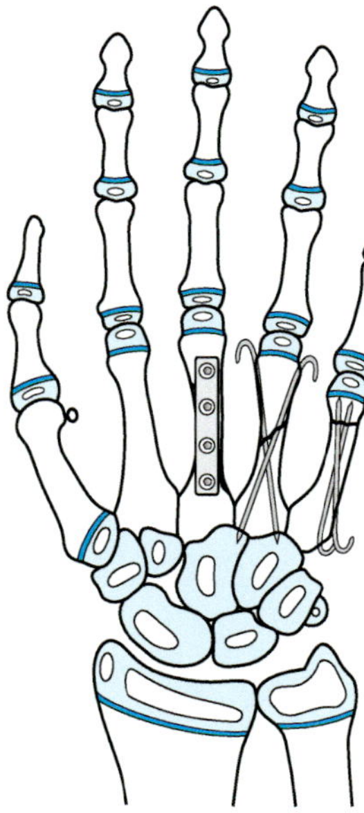

Fig. 10.24 K-wire fixation or plate osteoynthesis in metacarpal fractures, depending on the fracture type and age

Fig. 10.25 Shaft fracture of the fourth metacarpal (**a**) Trauma image, (**b**, **c**) Postoperative with plate osteosynthesis, not touching the growth plate

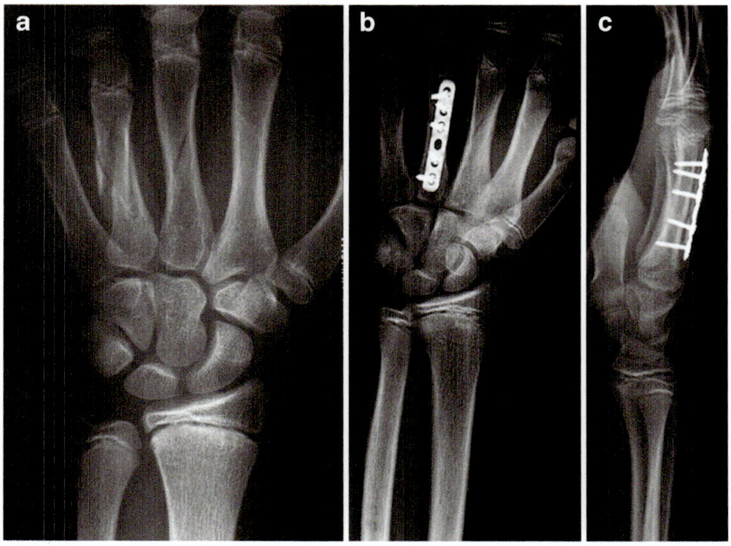

Table 10.8 Subcapital metacarpal fractures (Fig. 10.26)

Special features	Most occur from the age of 8 years with increasing physical activity
Diagnostic assessment	Clinical and radiographic examination of the hand in dorso-volar, oblique, and lateral views if necessary
Goals of therapy/ limits for correction	Tilting <30–50°, rotation deformity of the fingertip <10°, shortening <5 mm
Primary treatment	Pain therapy, elevation, measures to decrease swelling, splint immobilization
Conservative therapy	
Indication	Fractures within the tolerance limits (Fig. 10.27)
Procedure	Plaster splint in intrinsic-plus position of the finger, fist cast in toddlers, immobilization for 3 weeks
Follow up	Functional treatment with gradual to full loading until the sixth week
X-ray control	Not required for uncomplicated fractures, at one week with displacement risk, and after cast removal
Resuming sports	After 8 weeks
Operative therapy	
Indication	Displacement, tilting, rotation deformities and shortening over the tolerated limits
Procedure	K-wire fixation (Figs. 10.28 and 10.29).
Follow up	Plaster splint in intrinsic-plus position of the finger, fist cast in toddlers, immobilization for 4 weeks then functional treatment and gradual loading until the sixth postoperative week
X-ray control	At 1 week with cast change and prior to hardware removal at 4 weeks
Hardware removal	After 4 weeks
Resuming sports	After 8 weeks
Complications	Tendon injuries and adhesions, limitations in finger motion, persisting deformity, K-wire infections, osteonecrosis with joint surface involvement
Growth disturbances	Not to be expected
Follow up	Most fractures do not require follow up. If there is risk for increasing deformity or osteonecrosis, then at 6 months and one year

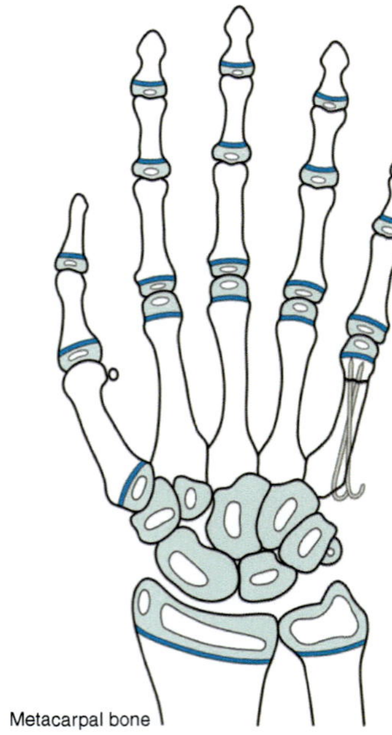

Fig. 10.26 Subcapital fracture of the fifth metacarpal

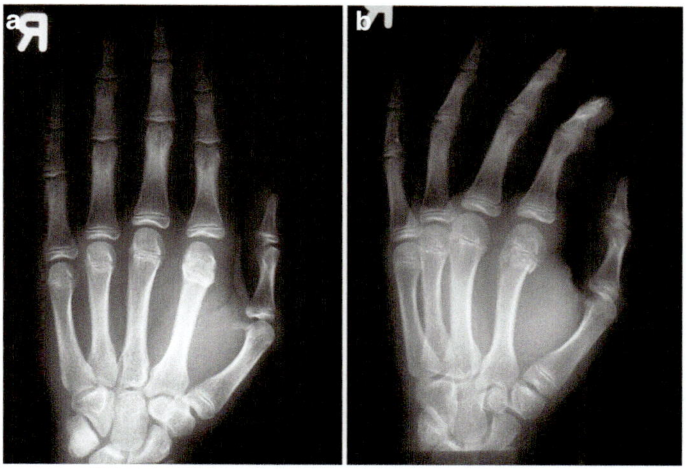

Fig. 10.27 (**a**, **b**) Sucapital metacarpal fracture without relevant displacement

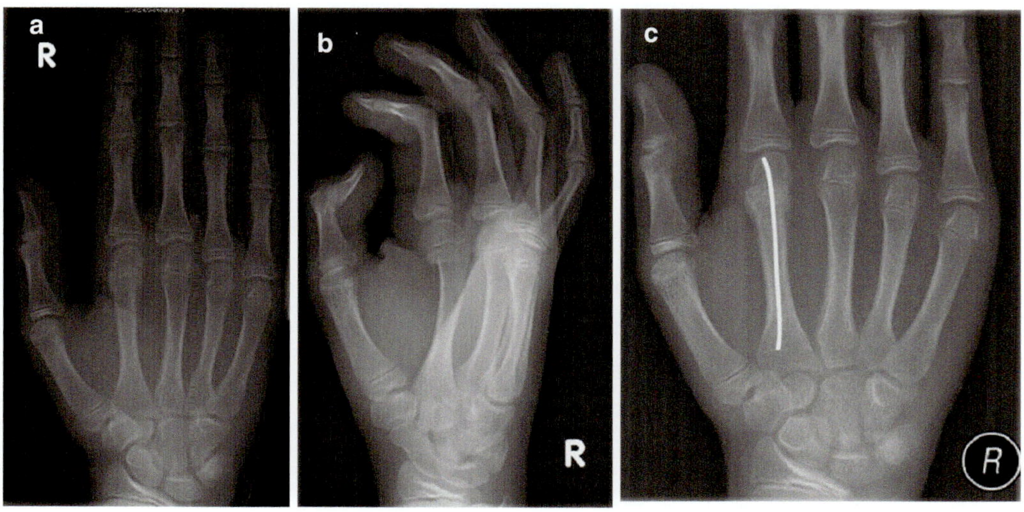

Fig. 10.28 (**a–c**) Subcapital second metacarpal fracture. (**a**, **b**) Preoperative, (**c**) After K-wire fixation

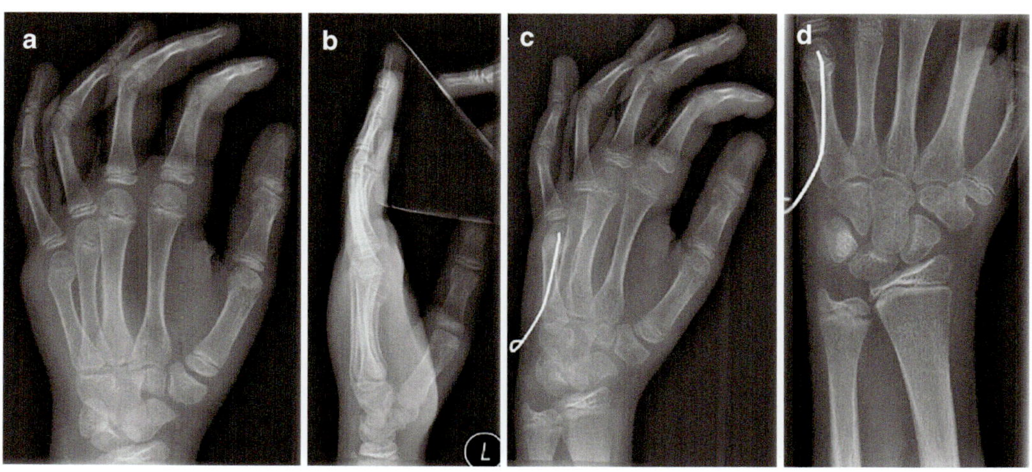

Fig. 10.29 (**a–d**) Subcapital fracture of the fifth metacarpal (**a**, **b**) Preoperative, (**c**, **d**) Fixation

10.3 Finger Fractures and Dislocations

Incidence, Mechanism of Injury and Clinical Picture

Injuries of the phalanges are the most common injuries of the child's hand. The causes of injury correspond essentially to those of metacarpal fractures. For finger fractures, the marginal rays (index and little finger) are more commonly affected. Phalangeal fractures are slightly more common than metacarpal fractures, with a marked frequency around the MCP joint. MCP joint dislocations are the most common hand joint dislocations in children. The thumb is most commonly affected, and it is often impossible to reduce the dislocated MCP of the index finger. Dislocation results from forced hyperextension with rupture of the volar plate (palmar fibrocartilage). Dislocations or lesions of the volar plate of the proximal interphalangeal joint (PIP joint) occur increasingly as skeletal maturity nears.

Up to more than 30% of finger fractures are epiphyseal injuries. Injury to the proximal phalanx (Salter-Harris II) is thus the most common, apart from bruises of the distal phalanx and the large variety of fingertip injuries (Figs. 10.30, 10.31, and 10.32).

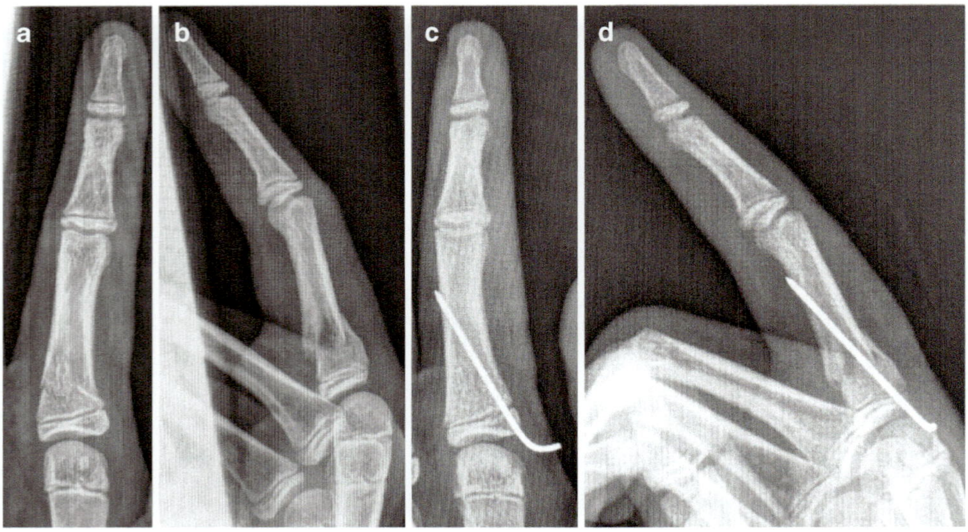

Fig. 10.30 13 Year old boy with severe distortion of index Salter-Harris II. Rotation and axial deviation. (**a**, **b**) Preoperatively, (**c**, **d**) 4 Weeks K-wire fixation with external protection

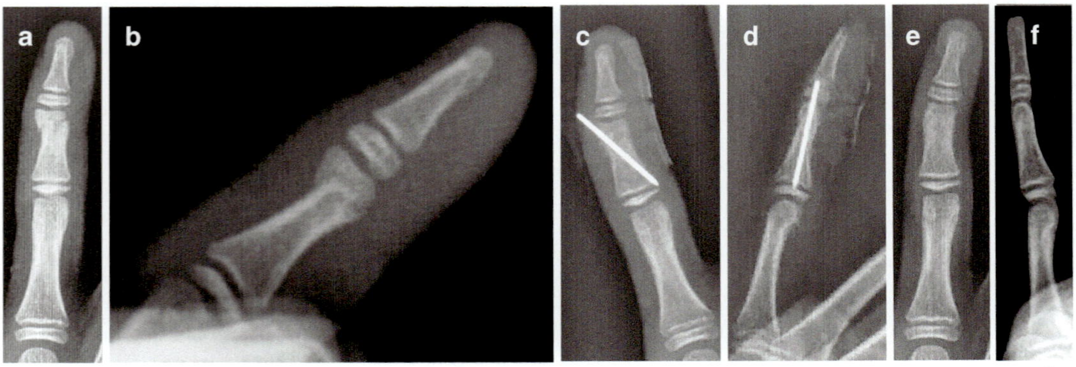

Fig. 10.31 Subcapital finger fracture, (**a**, **b**) Trauma image, (**c**, **d**) After reduction and K-wire fixation, (**e**, **f**) Healing images

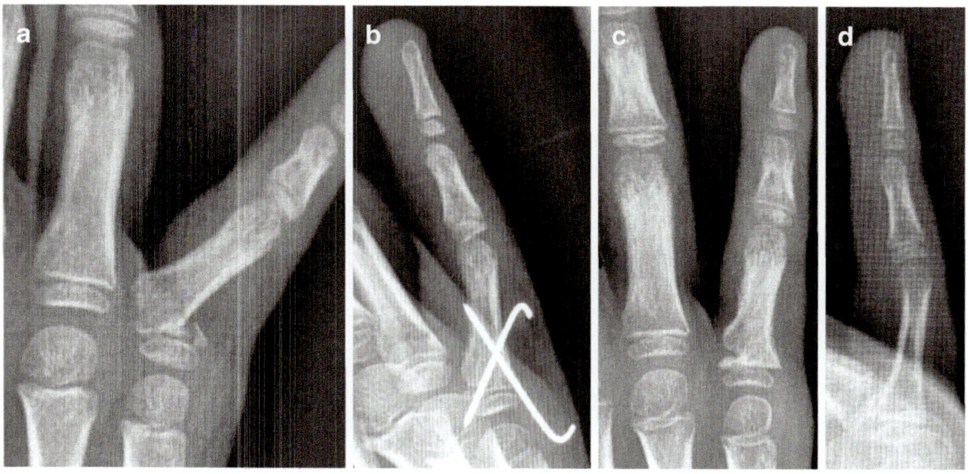

Fig. 10.32 8 Year old boy, fall during running with severely displaced transepiphyseal fracture of little finger. (**a**) Trauma image, (**b**) After reduction and K-wire fixation, (**c, d**) X-ray of healing

Classification

Injuries around the epiphyseal plate are classified using the systems of Aitken or Salter-Harris. For this, fractures are classified according to fracture anatomy and distinguished as intraarticular or extraarticular. In addition, stable and unstable fractures are differentiated. Further classification of finger fractures and dislocations is given in Table 10.9.

As with the metacarpals, epiphyses are found on both bone ends. Secondary ossification centers are missing on the distal ends of the first metacarpal and the distal phalanges. In contrast to the MCP joints, there is broad surface coverage of the IP joints by ligamentous structures, with fibers extending to the metaphyses. In addition, there are stable connections to the volar plate. The joints are surrounded by the flexor and extensor tendons. The extensor tendons insert at the epiphyses, and the flexor tendons extend to the metaphyses of the corresponding distal or middle phalanx. In the area of the middle phalanx, the superficial flexor tendon covers over 50% of the entire length. This anatomical structure protects the joint from fracture. The thick periosteum contributes to stability but can also—particularly in long spiral fractures—present a barrier to reduction.

The anatomical structure described leaves a certain vulnerability to force directed in the movement axis of the joint. This is particularly true for the distal phalanx. Here, the stabilizing effect fails when there is forced flexion or extension. In younger patients, Salter-Harris I and II type injuries occur and in patients closer to skeletal maturation, Salter-Harris III type injuries are more common.

In finger fractures, shaft fractures of the middle phalanx require more time for stable and loadable healing because of the high cortical composition. In children, however, healing occurs very quickly overall, which must be considered during follow up, since the time to make adjustments is short. The ability to remodel after healing depends on age, fracture localization regarding the growth plates, as well as the magnitude and level of deformity.

Table 10.9 Finger fractures and dislocation (Fig. 10.33)

Fractures	
Distal phalanx	Tuft fracture (simple, comminuted)
	Shaft fracture (transverse, longitudinal)
	Articular fracture: – Volar (flexor tendon avulsion) – Epiphyseal fracture – Dorsal (mallet fracture)
Proximal and middle phalanx	Epiphyseal fracture
	Simple fracture, comminuted fracture, compression fracture, defect fracture
	Transverse fracture, angled fracture, spiral fracture, avulsion fracture
PIP dislocations	
Type I	Non-displaced disruption of the volar plate
Type II	Dissociation of the main and accessory collateral ligaments; bony displacement <1 mm
Type III	Complete dissociation, bony fragment turned 90°, joint instable
Type IV	Additional rupture of the collateral ligament, instability in two planes
Type V	Dislocation towards the flexor side with lesions of the central slip and collateral ligament
Type VI	Collateral ligament and volar plate torn in opposition

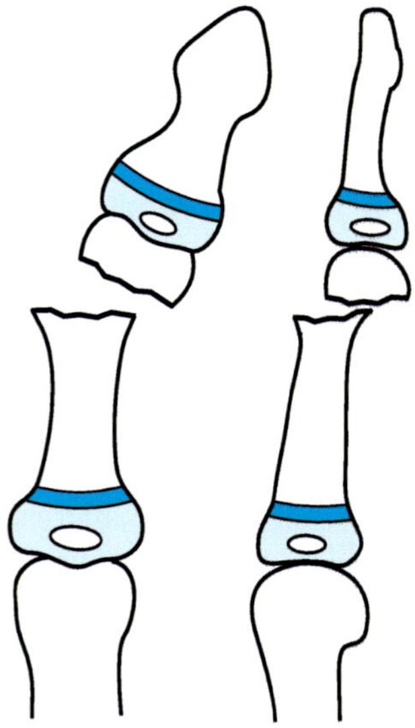

Fig. 10.33 Subcapital finger fractures

Diagnostic Assessment

Assessment first requires accurate collection of the trauma history, previous injuries, known deformities and other health issues. Malformations such as Kirner syndrome can simulate a fracture-induced radial deformity of the distal phalanx, and injury-induced flexion contractures of the PIP joint can be confused with camptodactyly, if the parents haven't noticed it prior to finger trauma.

A mechanism of injury suggesting extreme hyperextension can result in volar plate rupture, particularly in the area of the metacarpophalangeal joint, but also of the proximal interphalangeal joint. The joints are more often affected in children, resulting in the metacarpal head being trapped between the flexor tendons and the tendons of the lumbricals. The finger is then supinated in ulnar deviation, and the PIP joint is inflected because of the increased tension of the flexor tendon. The metacarpal head is also markedly palpable in the palm and the dorsal skin is rippled because of its absence. Like MCP dislocations, this injury also occurs to the thumb. In this case, ulnar instability of the thumb CMC joint must be particularly assessed during the examination for stability. Gamekeeper's thumb (also called skier's thumb), the injury of the ulnar collateral ligament, and the less common lesion of the radial collateral ligament, are usually found as avulsion fractures of the epiphysis and not as intra-ligamentous ruptures in the immature skeleton.

Dislocations of the PIP joints are markedly less common in children than in adults and often reduce spontaneously on presentation. However, the collateral ligaments and the volar plate are injured. In addition to conspicuous swelling and tenderness to palpation, particularly at the palmar aspect of the PIP joint, lateral x-ray of the affected finger often shows fine separation or fracture of the epiphysis. Dislocation of the distal joint through hyperextension or loading of the bent distal phalanx is extremely rare.

The most common finger fracture at the base of the proximal phalanx (Salter-Harris II) is often recognizable from the swelling and pain symptoms, as well as the "sticking out" position of the finger. Similar to dislocation, x-rays should be performed with dorso-volar and oblique views. A strict lateral view of the affected finger is necessary to visualize the area distant to the mid-proximal phalanx and to assess palmar deviation at the level of the metacarpal head.

Injuries to the fingertip can be very complex due to involvement of the nail and the nailbed. Fractures of the distal phalanx can be divided into lesions with involvement of the growth plates, and lesions without. Involvement of the nailbed with subungual hematoma is clinically evident, as well as swelling and deformity of the fingertip. On radiographs, one must assess for accompanying tuft fractures.

Goals of Therapy/Limits for Correction

The goal of therapy is to prevent sagittal tilt more than 30°, rotation of the fingertip more than 10°, and shortening of the finger more than 5 mm. In cases of dislocation and fractures in the finger joint areas, the goal is anatomic reduction of the articular relations and surfaces.

Deformities at the level of the joint axes correct themselves. In cases of linear deviation (abduction or adduction), predictions are unreliable. This problem increases with increasing distance from the joint. Sub-capital fractures of the phalanges undergo only mild remodeling.

During primary care, the most difficult aspects are adequate pain therapy and the associated assessment. Splint immobilization in a functional position must be carried out until definitive therapy can be performed, whether that is conservative closed or operative open reduction. If the child is too small, a fist bandage with cotton padding can be applied as protection. Particularly in cases of finger dislocation, adequate local anesthesia should be given early.

Conservative Therapy

In cases of MCP dislocation, operative reduction is often necessary, especially when reduction is prevented by additional entrapment of the volar plate. However, reduction maneuvers are indicated. Reduction of proximal (PIP) and distal (DIP) interphalangeal joints is easy once adequate sedation and local anesthesia have been applied. Most phalangeal fractures can be treated conservatively. For children under 10 years of age, deformity up to 30° in the plane of motion can be accepted.

For reduction of the MCP joint, first intraarticular anesthesia is applied followed by hyperextension (in dorsal dislocations in relation to the distal finger portion). Thus, the volar plate can be pushed slowly volar on the metatarsal head and sometimes reduction is attained. Longitudinal traction must be avoided, as it increases tension of the tendons and thus, reinforces the entrapment. Dislocation of the PIP and DIP joints can usually be reduced easily with longitudinal traction on the corresponding finger (Fig. 10.34). In small children, local anesthesia is sometimes impossible and thus, sedation or anesthesia becomes necessary.

The procedure of choice for finger fractures is immobilization with plaster splint in intrinsic-plus position of the finger (70° flexion of the MCP joint and complete extension of the long finger with approximately 20–30° wrist extension. This is not possible in toddlers because of the small hand size; here a fist cast can be used. As with the common proximal phalanx fracture, reduction is generally attained by flexion of the MCP joint and finger traction. In cases of shaft fractures, conservative therapy can often be carried out because of the good soft tissue splinting (flexor tendon sheath).

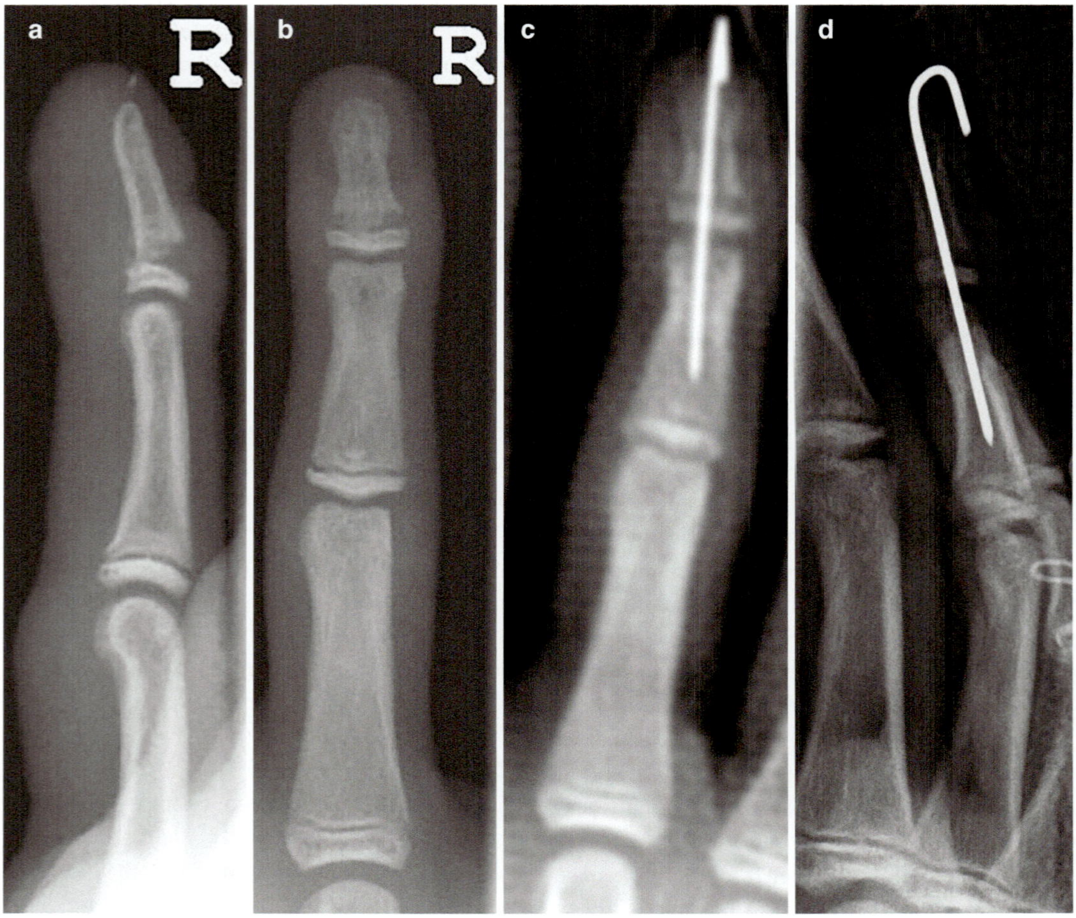

Fig. 10.34 Dislocation of the growth plate of the end phalanx, (**a**, **b**), Trauma Images, (**c**, **d**). Fixation with K-wire after reduction

Cast check is performed the following day to check for finger position and possible pressure points. The cast should remain for 3 weeks, for 4 weeks in shaft fractures (especially transverse fractures), and 6 weeks for fractures in the middle phalanx area.

In MCP and PIP joint dislocations, there should be early mobilization after a short phase of immobilization not more than 7 days. For better protection and to avoid hyperextension, "buddy splints" can then be applied (Fig. 10.35). Thumb MCP joint dislocation is immobilized for 3 weeks with a thumb splint. The MCP joint is mildly flexed. For this, the correct position must be used to ensure there is no overstretching of the collateral ligaments.

Operative Therapy

MCP joint dislocations that can't be reduced closed must be openly reduced. Instability after PIP joint dislocations is possible in adolescents, and these cases must be treated operatively. If the volar plate, the collateral ligament, or osteochondral fragments prevent reduction, surgery is also indicated. Palmar PIP dislocations do not occur in children.

For finger fractures, surgery is indicated when there is more than 25% joint involvement and more than 1.5 mm displacement. Overall, however, phalangeal fractures only rarely require operative treatment, apart from severe and open crush injuries. However, interposition of periosteum, tendons, or tendon sheaths can hinder reduction and lead to a need for operative intervention (Fig. 10.36). Shaft fractures that can't be held after conservative man-

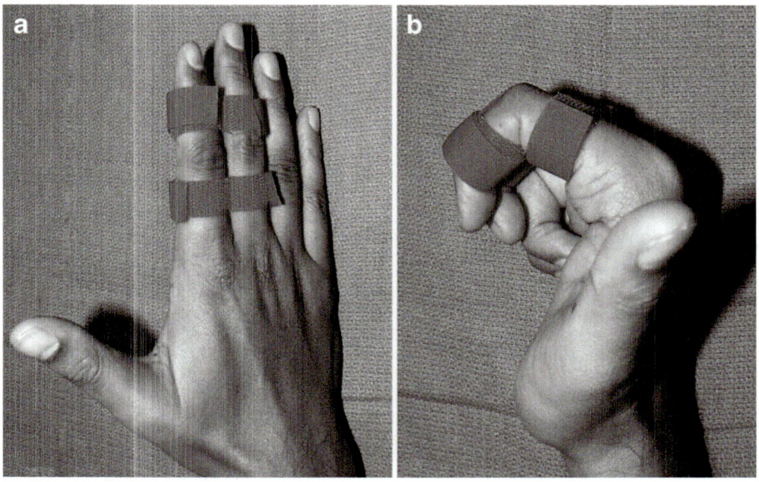

Fig. 10.35 (**a**, **b**) Buddy splints to stabilize neighboring finger, synchronous motion of the two fingers is possible

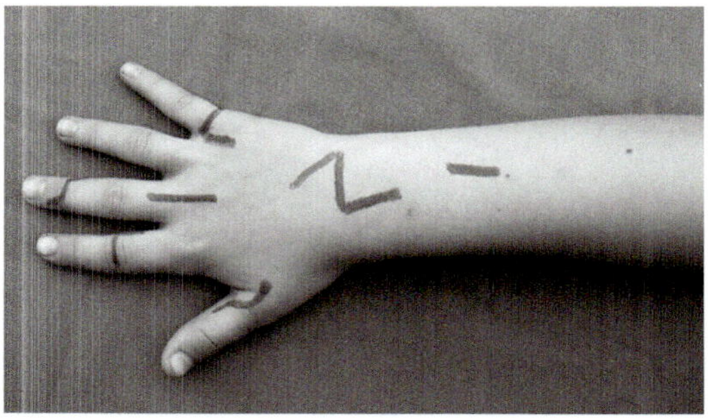

Fig. 10.36 Dorsal approach to the hand and fingers

agement or those in which rotation deformity develops after treatment should be stabilized operatively.

Fingertip injuries must be treated operatively when the hematoma overtakes the entire nail and raises it or when a tuft fracture is recognizable on x-ray. Smaller hematomas can be treated with drilled cannulas.

MCP joint dislocations can be well visualized using a volar approach. This often requires the release and if needed, separation of the A1 ring ligament and longitudinal incision of the volar plate. Occasionally, incision of the superficial transverse metacarpal ligament is necessary. The digital nerves within the subcutaneous tissues are particularly vulnerable during this approach. When there are additional bony injuries, the dorsal approach is recommended. The entire joint can be visualized in flexion through the longitudinal incision of the extensor apparatus. Using a dissector, it is often possible to reduce the volar plate and occasionally also the dorsally displaced flexor tendons and to eliminate the dislocation. In cases of chronic dislocation, often both approaches must be used for reduction.

Phalangeal fractures are primarily stabilized with K-wires after reduction (Fig. 10.37). The proximal phalanx can generally be accessed through a dorsal approach. The extensor apparatus can be split, or the peri-tendinous periosteum stripped. The main concern is that the extensor apparatus is recentered at the end of the procedure.

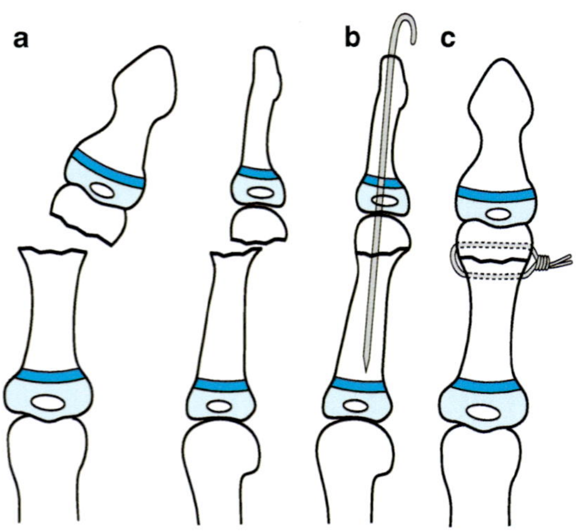

Fig. 10.37 (**a**) Schematic representation of one potential operative treatment for subcapital fracture of the middle phalanx. The reduction can be held with K-wire (**b**) or with an intraosseous suture (**c**)

Sub-capital and condylar fractures are particularly challenging. These fractures must be anatomically reduced and fixed because of their high instability. If closed reduction is not successful, open reduction through a dorsal or lateral approach must be performed, offering easier access to this fracture on the middle phalanx (Fig. 10.38).

Significant injuries of the nail bed must be treated like an open fracture The nail must be lifted, the nailbed washed and closed with resorbable 5.0 suture. The suture itself and the subsequent splinting with the cleaned fingernail is often the best treatment of the accompanying tuft fracture. Transverse, oblique, or comminuted fractures must be reduced and stabilized with fine K-wires if necessary. When the epiphyseal plate is involved, this is considered mallet finger. When there is extensor tendon involvement and displacement of the epiphysis or a dorsal epiphyseal fragment, reduction and stabilization is necessary.

Follow up of MCP joint dislocation involves early mobilization after a short phase of immobilization no longer than 7 days (Fig. 10.39).

For better protection and to avoid hyperextension, "buddy splints" can then be applied. In cases

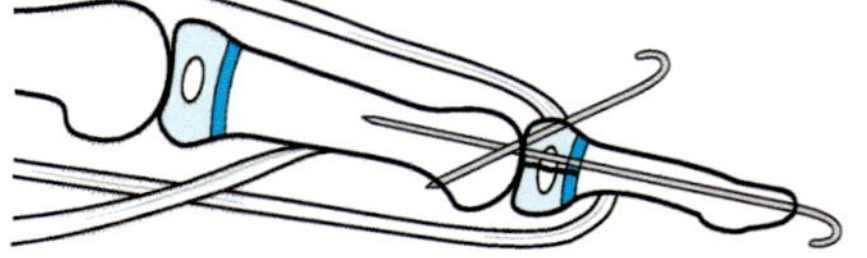

Fig. 10.38 (**a**, **b**) Schematic representation of the operative treatment of a displaced mallet finger of the distal phalanx (**a**) with K-wires (**b**)

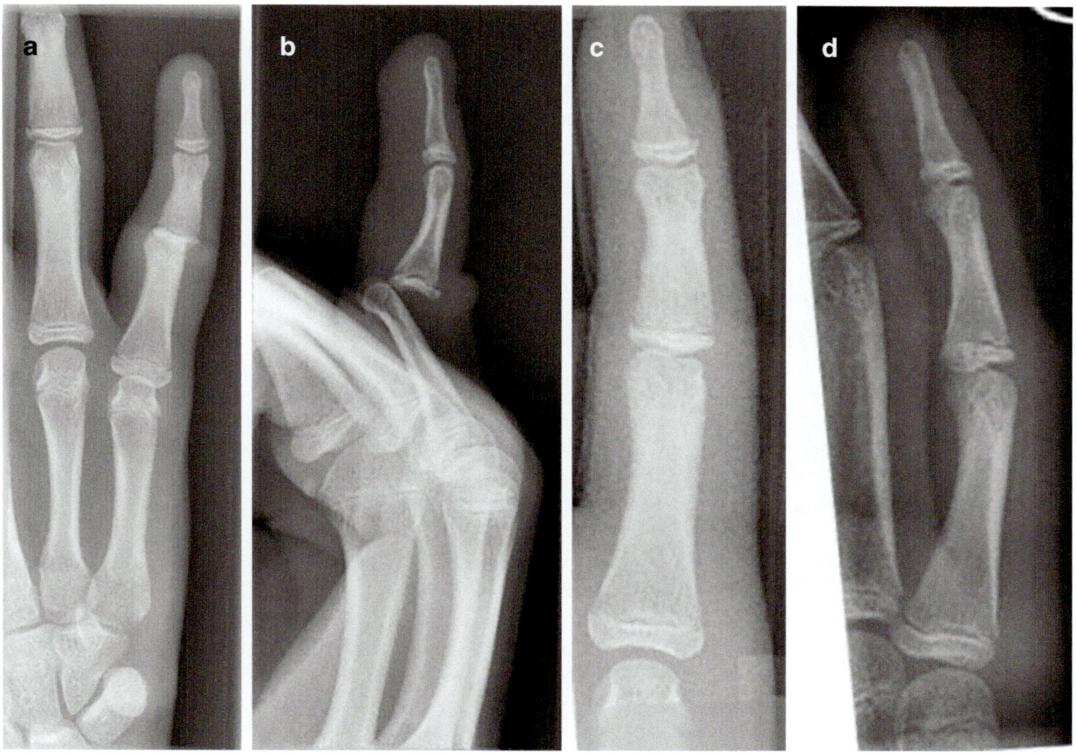

Fig. 10.39 Luxation of the PIP joint (**a**, **b**) Trauma image, (**c**, **d**) After closed reduction

of K-wire fixation, accompanying immobilization is carried out corresponding to conservative fracture treatment: a plaster splint in intrinsic-plus position of the finger or a fist cast bandage in toddlers. Fractures in the distal phalanx area are treated post-accident and in the first week after surgery with a 3-finger or age-appropriate splinting. For the remaining 3 weeks, often a finger splint reaching over the distal phalanx, sparing the other digits, is sufficient. The size of the finger must be noted here; in toddlers a fist cast might be necessary for immobilization.

Complications/Growth Disturbances

Delayed fracture healing and non-unions are extremely rare and often occur only in combination with high-speed trauma or finger crush injuries. Axial deviation and rotation deformities are possible and can interfere with hand function. Rotational deviations are generally caused by inadequate reduction, and axial deviations often result from growth disturbances.

K-wire infections at the skin level are common after operative treatment. They seldom lead to osteitis, but in individual cases can result in severe bone destruction.

Particularly in the treatment of joint dislocations and intraarticular fractures recognized after a delay, the children and parents must be advised of the risks of motion deficits, premature epiphyseal closure, and avascular bone necrosis. Clinodactyly is the most common deformity after articular fractures and can occur in up to 20% of these cases. If there is less than 10° deviation, generally no limitations result. A high grade deformity can lead to overlapping of the fingers.

Motion deficits, deformity, and ossification of the sub-condylar recess can easily occur in sub-capital and condylar fractures, which are particularly difficult to treat. A flexion deficit must be treated operatively for functional improvement, usually from volar. The accessory collateral ligament is released and the excess bone resected.

Most uncomplicated fractures do not require follow up. Intraarticular fractures should be seen at six months and one year to catch avascular necrosis. Mild post-traumatic deformities that don't require operative correction should be seen at six months and then annually to exclude increasing deformity with growth (Table 10.10).

Table 10.10 Finger fractures

Special features	30% of epiphyseal injuries, when not crush injuries generally the proximal phalanx, often the small or index fingers
Diagnostic assessment	Clinical examination and dorso-volar and lateral x-rays of the affected finger
Goals of therapy/limits for correction	No tilt >30°, no rotation deformity of the fingertip >10°, no shortening >5 mm, anatomic joint relations, good correction in the plane of the joint axis, unclear correction potential for axial deviation, low correction potential for sub-capital fractures
Primary treatment	Pain therapy, elevation, measures to decrease swelling, splint immobilization
Conservative therapy	
Indication	Usual treatment for fractures within the limits of tolerance, in cases where there is no step formation and joint incongruence (Fig. 10.40)
Procedure	Plaster splint in intrinsic-plus position of the finger, fist cast in toddlers, immobilization for 3 weeks, 4 weeks for shaft fractures, 6 weeks for shaft fractures of the middle phalanx. If there is a deviation of the axis, exact reduction if possible in locale anesthesia is necessary!
Follow up	Functional follow up with gradual to full loading until the eighth week
X-ray control	Not necessary in uncomplicated fractures, at 1 week and at cast removal after reduction and with risk of displacement (oblique, transverse shaft fractures)
Resuming sports	After 8 weeks, after 12 weeks for middle phalanx fractures
Operative therapy	
Indication	Displacement, tilt, rotation deformities and shortening over the tolerance limits; joint dislocation and joint involvement >25° with displacement >1.5 mm.
Procedure	K-wire fixation, rarely mini-screws for articular fractures approach, small incisions or dorsally
Follow up	Plaster splint in intrinsic-plus position of the finger, fist cast in toddlers, immobilization for 3 weeks, 4 weeks for shaft fractures, 6 weeks for shaft fractures of the middle phalanx
X-ray control	At one week and prior to hardware removal of K-wires at 3–4 weeks
Hardware removal	After 3–4 weeks, 6 weeks for middle phalanx shaft fractures (>5 years)
Resuming sports	After 8 weeks
Complications	Tendon injuries and adhesions, limitations in finger motion, persisting deformity, K-wire infections, osteonecrosis with joint surface involvement
Growth disturbances	Not to be expected
Follow up	Most fractures do not require follow up, follow up at 6 months and one year for intraarticular fractures if there are risks for increased deformity or osteonecrosis

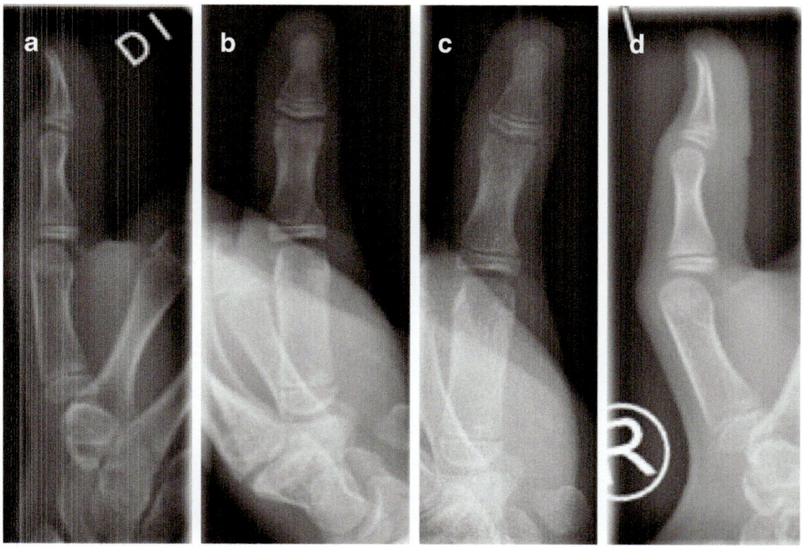

Fig. 10.40 Salter-Harris II fracture of the basis of the thumb, (**a**, **b**). Trauma image, (**c**, **d**) Healing after conservative treatment in cast

Recommended Literature

Campbell RM (1990) Operative treatment of fractures and dislocations of the hand and wrist region in children. Orthop Clin North Am 21(2):217–243

Fitoussi F (2013) Finger bone and joint trauma of the hand in children. Chir Main 32(Suppl 1):S7–S15

Frank J, Sommer K, Sander AL, Marzi I (2018) Soft tissue reconstruction of hands and feet in childhood. Trauma und Berufskrankheit Springer Medizin 48:2119–2110

Franz T, Jandali AR, Jung FJ, Leclère FM, Wartburg von U, Hug U (2013) Functional-conservative treatment of extra-articular physeal fractures of the proximal phalanges in children and adolescents. Eur J Pediatric Surg 23(4):317–321

Hohendorff B, Weidermann C, Burkhart KJ, Rommens PM, Prommersberger KJ, Konerding MA (2010) Lengths, girths, and diameters of children's fingers from 3 to 10 years of age. Ann Anat 192(3):156–161

Lieber J, Härter B, Schmid E, Kirschner HJ, Schmittenbecher PP (2012) Elastic stable intramedullary nailing (ESIN) of pediatric metacarpal fractures: experiences with 66 cases. Eur Pediatric Surg 22(4):305–310

Light TR (2000) Carpal injuries in children. Hand Clin 16(4):513–522

Matzon JL, Cornwall R (2014) A stepwise algorithm for surgical treatment of type II displaced pediatric phalangeal neck fractures. J Hand Surg 39(3):467–473

Nellans KW, Chung KC (2013) Pediatric hand fractures. Hand Clin 29(4):569–578

Seymour N (1940) Juxta-epiphyseal fractures of the terminal phalanx of the finger. J Bone Joint Surg 22:436–441

Sivit AP, Dupont EP, Sivit CJ (2014) Pediatric hand injuries: essentials you need to know. Emerg Radiol 21(2):197–206

Voth M, Lustenberger T, Frank J, Marzi I (2017) Pediatric finger and hand injuries: an epidemiological study. Chirurg 88:871–878

Weber DM (2011) Scaphoid fractures in childhood. Unfallchirurg 114(4):285–291

11 Hip

11.1 Physiological Findings

The blood supply to the proximal femur changes as a child grows. Until the age of 8, the vessels of the ligamentum teres contribute little to the circulation of the head. At birth, the branches of the medial and lateral circumflex arteries are responsible for this. These vessels are less important after infancy, when the growth plate forms a perfusion barrier. At this time, the lateral epiphyseal vessels become more prominent, and they alone supply the femoral head. After age 3 or 4 years, the lateral, posterior and superior vessels also supply the anterior and lateral sections of the femoral head and the epiphysis. The posterior-inferior and posterior-superior arteries supply the femoral head and are present throughout our lifespan. The medial femoral circumflex artery is also responsible for supplying the head (Fig. 11.1).

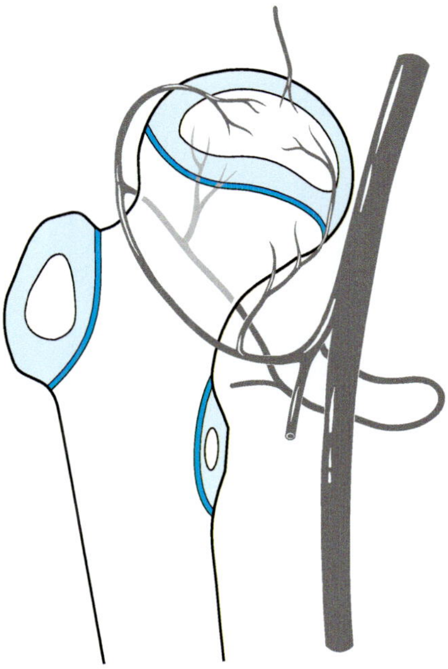

Fig. 11.1 Vascular supply of the femoral head

The secondary ossification centers generally begin developing between 5 and 8 months after birth (Fig. 11.2). The hemispherical contours of the proximal femoral epiphyses have emerged between 6 and 8 years, and the epiphysis of the greater trochanter separates from that of the femoral neck. Thus, it is no longer involved in longitudinal growth and becomes an apophysis. Injury to the apophysis before the age of 8 leads to a shortened greater trochanter and Coxa valga. Sometimes, between the ages of 7 and 10, an accessory bone appears close to the trochanteric apophysis. This should not be confused with a traumatic apophyseal disruption. Plate closure occurs between the ages of 14 and 17 years (Fig. 11.3).

I. Marzi et al., *Pediatric Skeletal Trauma*, https://doi.org/10.1007/978-3-030-93685-3_11

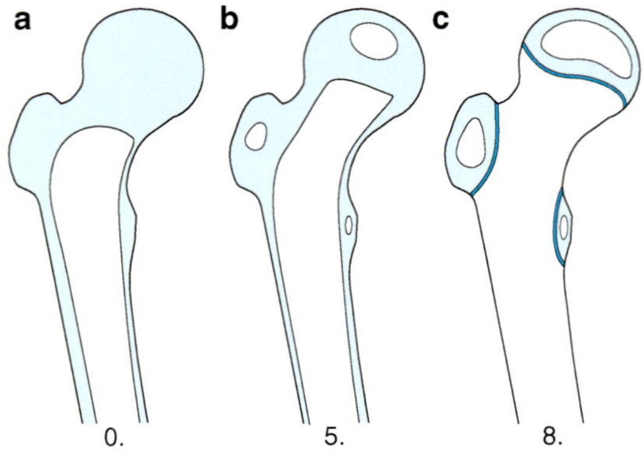

Fig. 11.2 Development of ossification centers of the proximal femur. (**a**) Proximal femoral epiphysis, 5th–8th month, (**b**) Greater trochanter: 3–5 years, (**c**) Lesser trochanter: 10–11 years

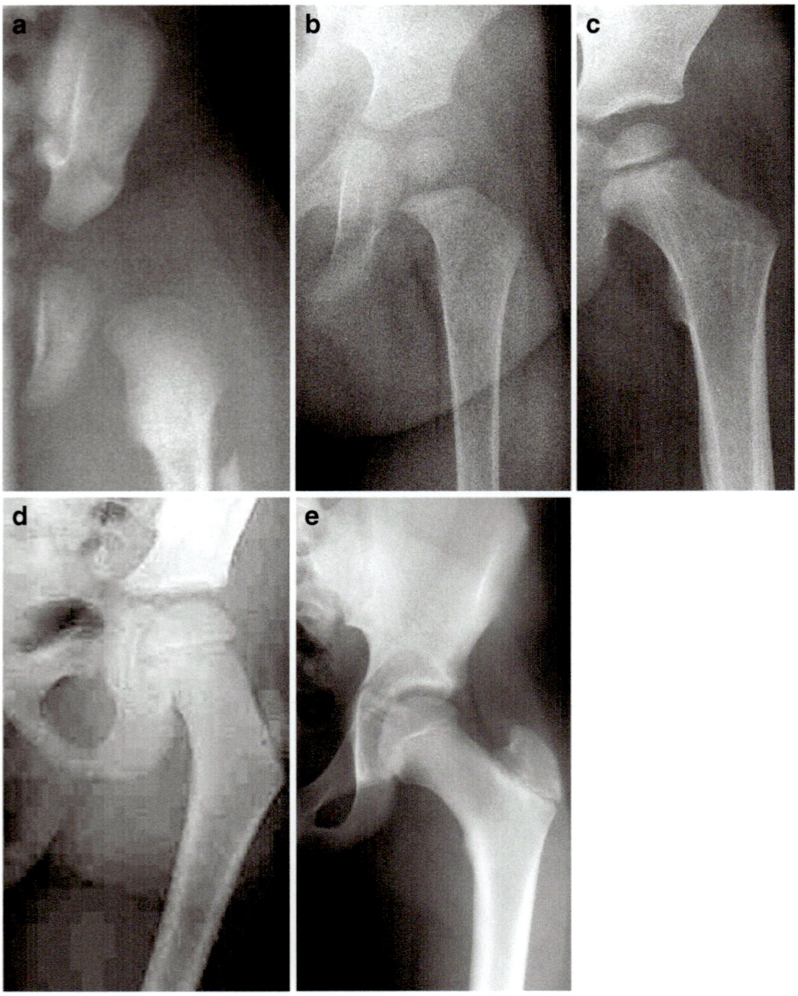

Fig. 11.3 Development of the proximal femur on x-ray. (**a**) Newborn, (**b**) 1½ Years, (**c**) 5 Years, (**d**) 8 Years, (**e**) 9 Years

11.2 Proximal Femur Fractures

Incidence, Mechanism of Injury, and Clinical Presentation

Proximal femur fractures are extremely rare during childhood. Incidence is <1%.

In children, the bone is more robust than in adults, so only massive trauma will result in a proximal femur fracture. Concomitant injuries must always be suspected and excluded. Because of the vascular supply to the femoral head and neck, these injuries can have serious consequences.

Classification

The Delbet and Colonna Classification (Fig. 11.4) divides proximal femur fractures into four types: Type I (transepiphyseal fractures), Type II (transcervical fractures), Type III (cervicobasal fractures), and Type IV (intertrochanteric fractures). The newly developed AO Classification for pediatric fractures is based on this system and distinguishes epiphyseal from transcervical, cervicobasal, and pertrochanteric fractures (Fig. 11.5).

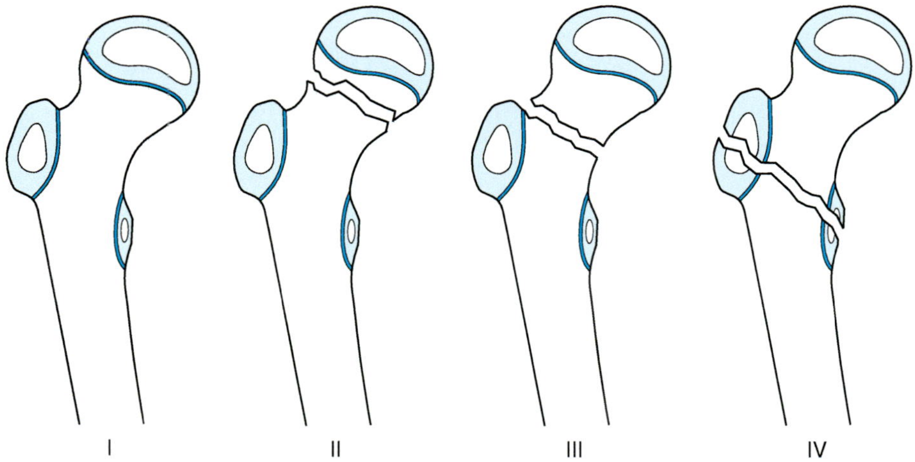

Fig. 11.4 Delbet and Colonna classification: Type I transepiphyseal, Type II transcervical, Type III cervicobasal, Type IV intertrochanteric

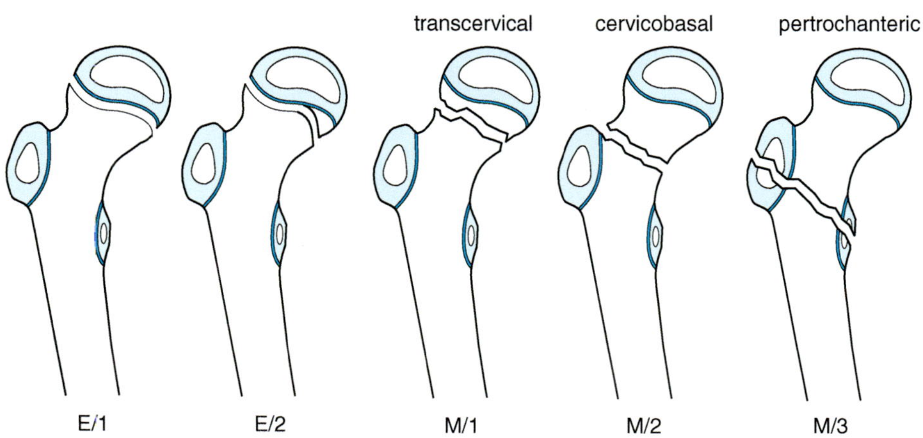

Fig. 11.5 AO classification in childhood. E/1 epiphysiolysis, E/2 epiphysiolysis with metaphyseal wedge, M/1 transcervical, M/2 cervicobasal, M/3 intertrochanteric

Type I Fractures

Type I fractures are extremely rare (8%) and are mainly seen in birth trauma and abuse. As a rule, they only occur in infants and toddlers (Fig. 11.6). Type I fractures must often be reduced and fixed with K-wires. The reduction with K-wires must also be immobilized in a hip spica cast for 3–4 weeks.

Type II Fractures

Type II fractures make up about half of all proximal femur fractures and occur in small and school-aged children after massive trauma. Displaced type II fractures can still be stabilized with K-wires after open reduction in very young children. However, screw fixation should be attempted to achieve adequate stability or com-

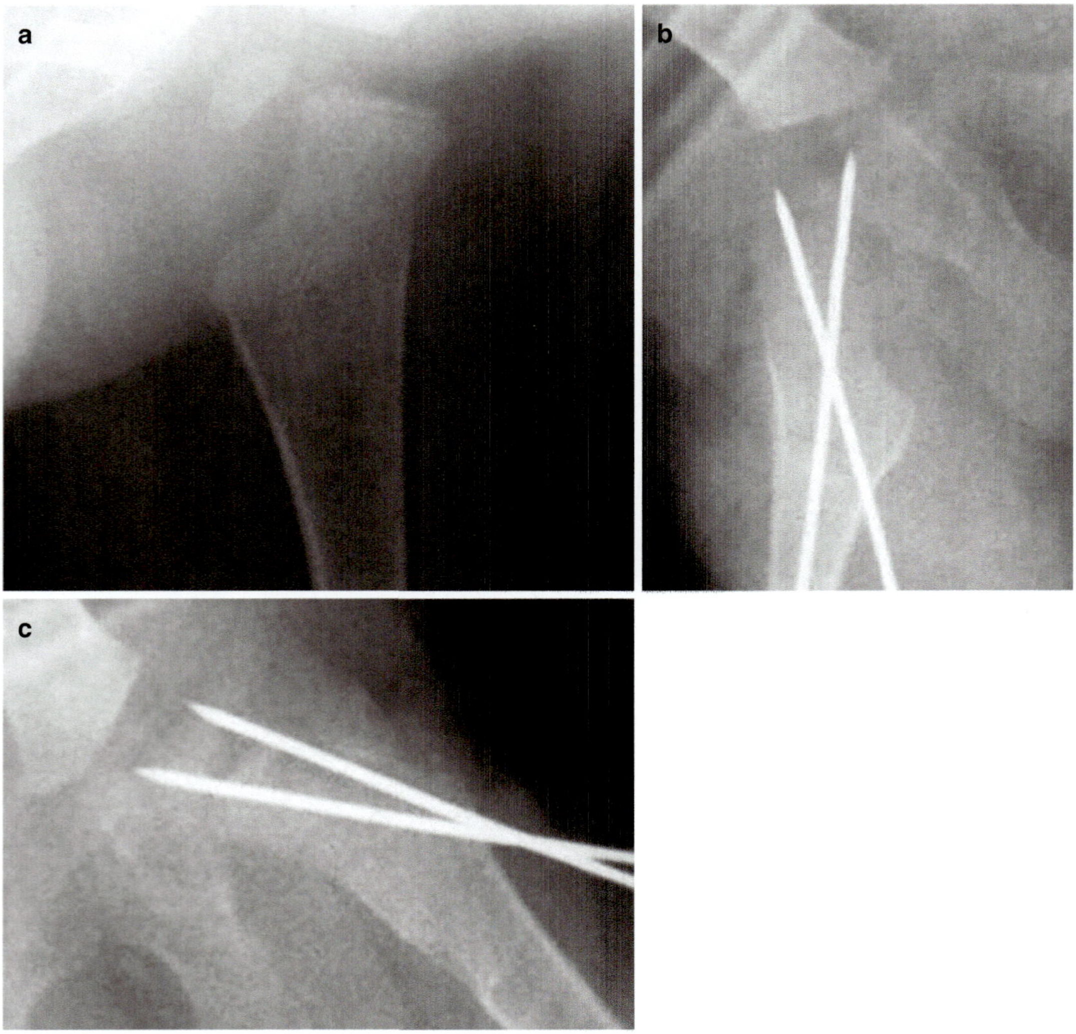

Fig. 11.6 Proximal femur fracture type I, boy, 1½ years, injury during physical therapy. (**a**) Trauma image, (**b**, **c**) After reduction and K-wire fixation

pression when the fracture allows. Good results have been reported recently with cannulated and self-tapping hollow screws, and crossing the growth plate can be avoided, depending on fracture course. At least two screws have been firmly inserted for fixation, thus allowing functional after-treatment. However, if necessary, the growth plate has to be crossed, but metal removal should be performed as early as possible (Fig. 11.7).

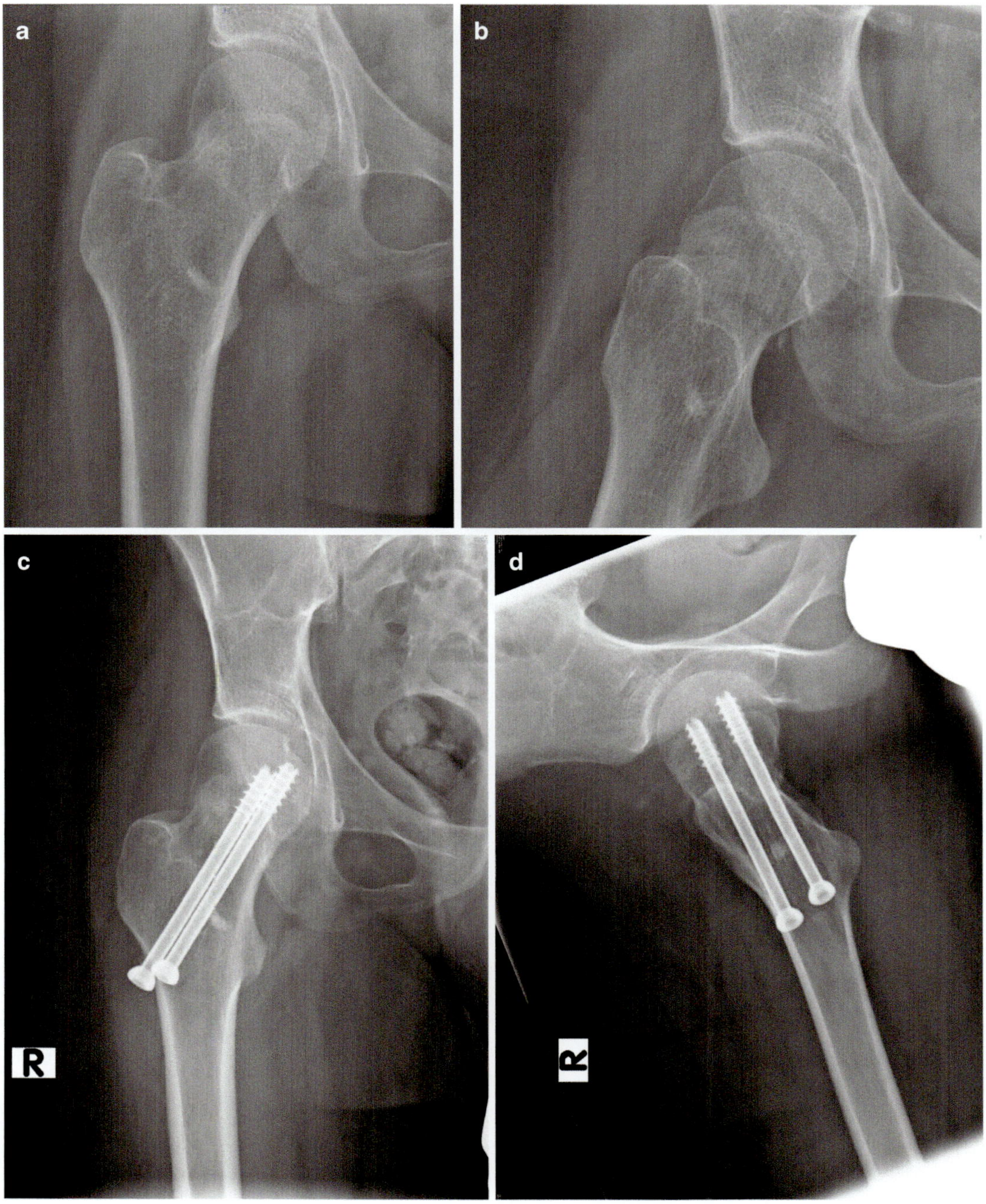

Fig. 11.7 Medial transcervical femoral neck fracture after fall of a girl. (**a**, **b**) Trauma image, (**c**, **d**) Stabilization with 2 cannulated screws, crossing the almost closed growth plate

Type III Fractures

Type III fractures (Fig. 11.8) make up approximately 30% of all proximal femur fractures. Type III fractures are also only treated conservatively in exceptional cases, in incomplete, stable fractures. Cannulated screws work well for operative fixation, and immobilization is then only necessary in exceptional cases (for K-wire fixation in small children). It is sometimes possible, to end the screws just before the growth plate (Fig. 11.9).

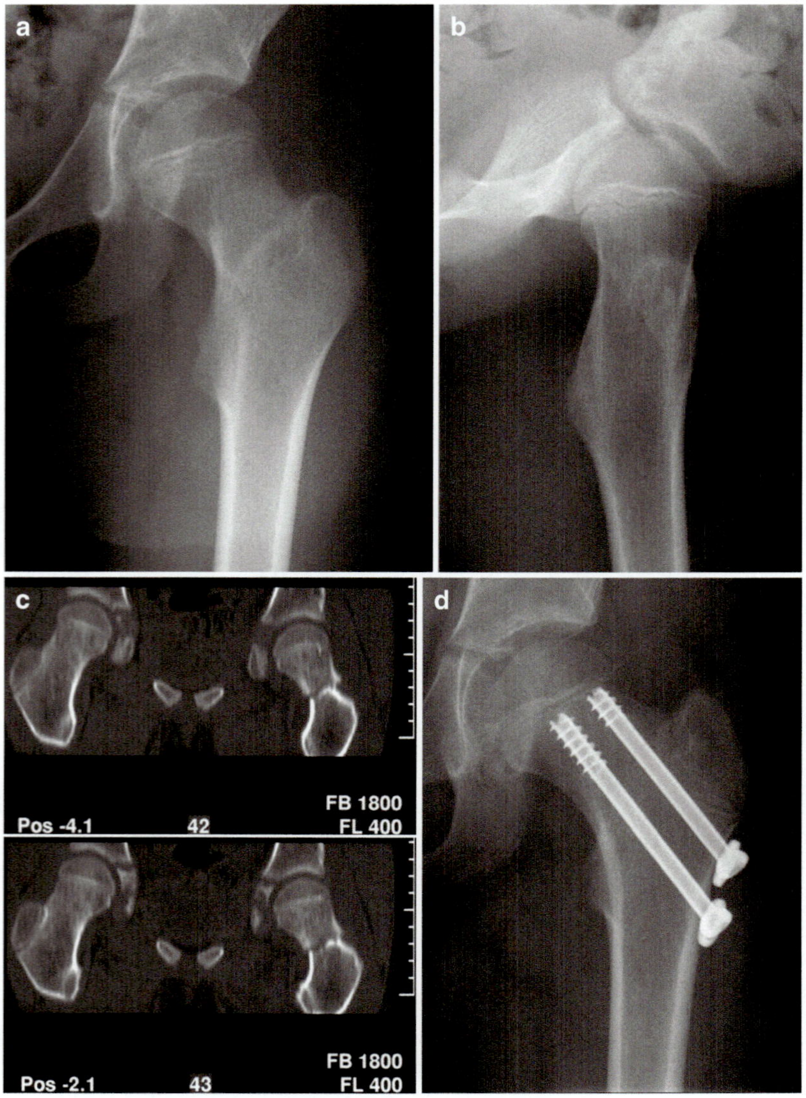

Fig. 11.8 Proximal femur fracture type III, boy, 16 years, fall from horse. (**a**, **b**) Trauma images, x-ray. (**c**) Trauma image, CT. (**d**) Screw fixation

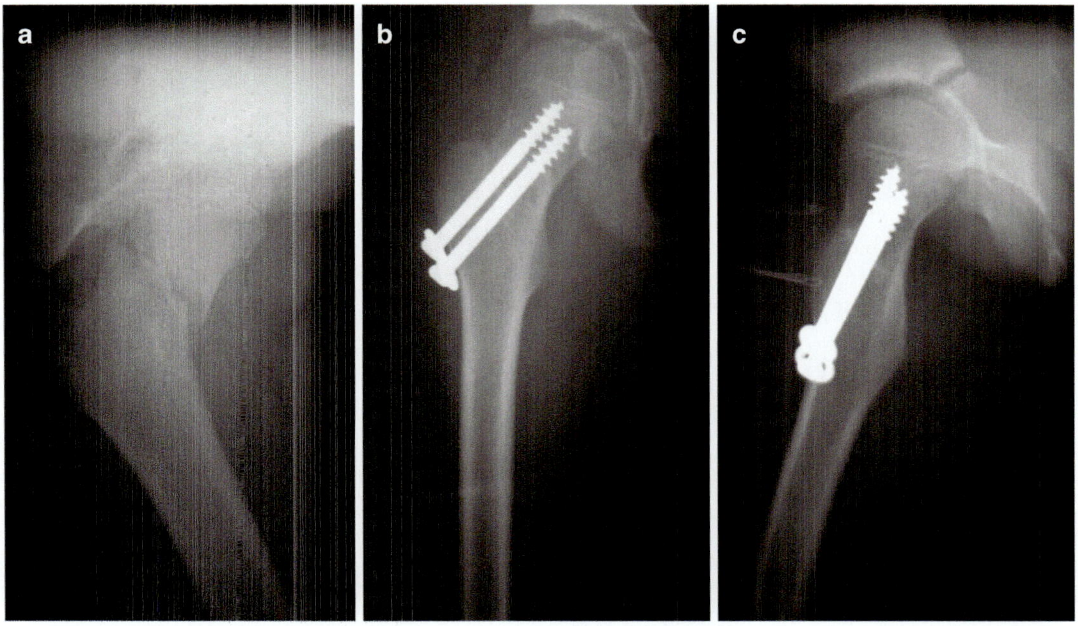

Fig. 11.9 Proximal femur fracture type II, girl, 12 years, fall while ice skating. (**a**) Trauma image, (**b**, **c**) Screw fixation

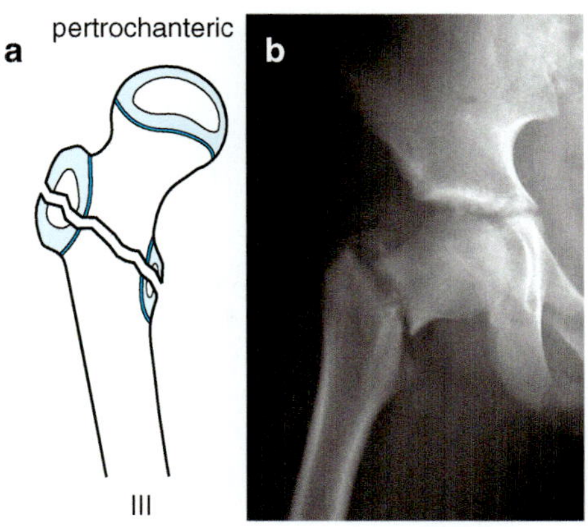

Fig. 11.10 Proximal femur fracture, type IV, M/3. (**a**) classification scheme, (**b**) radiological view

Type IV Fractures

Type IV fractures (Fig. 11.10), the intertrochanteric and pertrochanteric fractures, make up approximately 8% of proximal femur fractures. The prognosis is more easily assessed than in Type I–III fractures. In small children with good fracture position, type IV fractures can be treated conservatively in a hip spica cast. In certain cases, particular if the fractures is per- to subtroachanteric, retrograde intramedullary nailing is an option (Fig. 11.11). A pediatric angular stable plate is an alternative, and K-wires or screw fixation can be used in exceptional cases (Fig. 11.12).

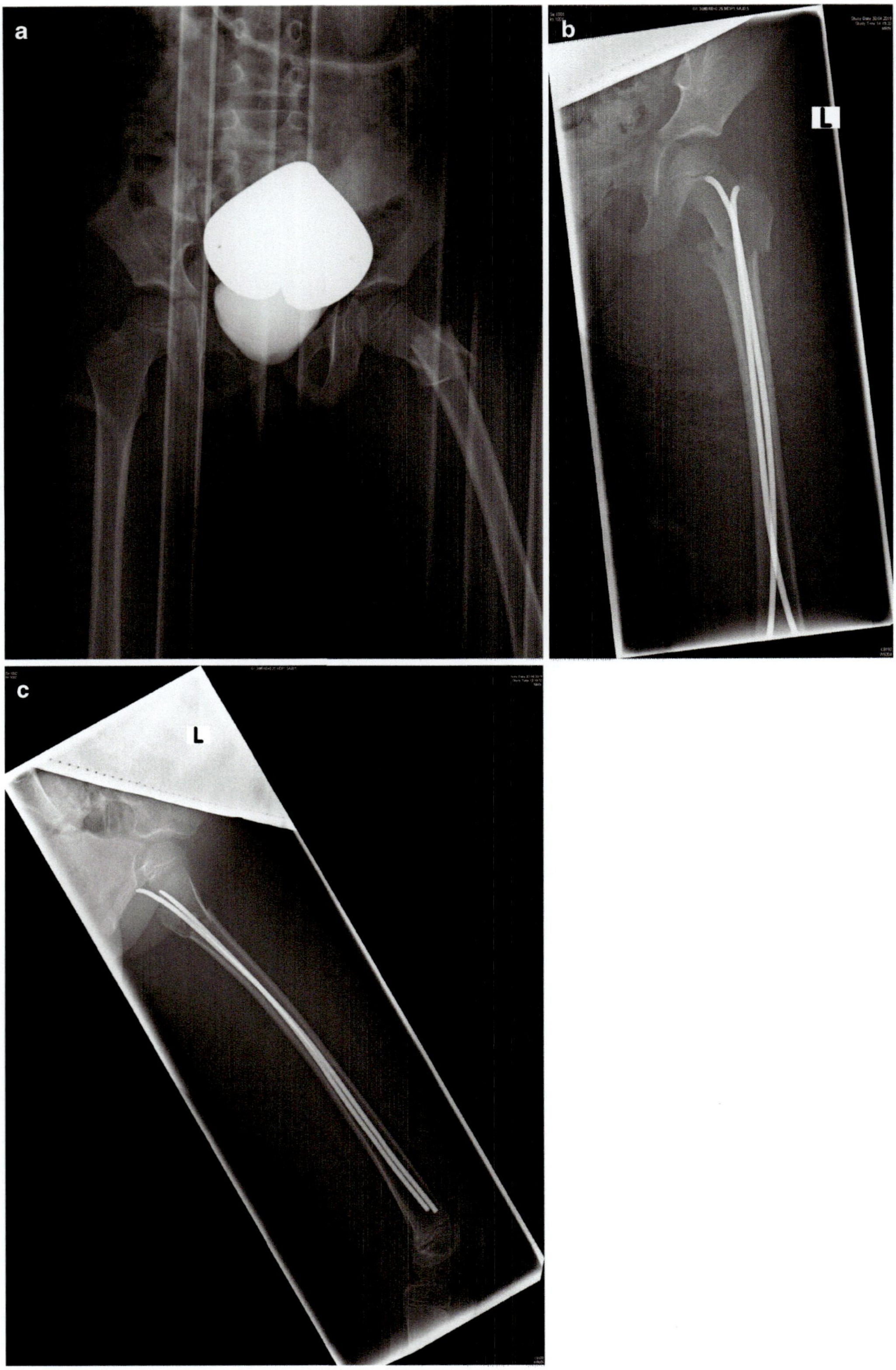

Fig. 11.11 5 Year old boy with per- to subtrochanteric fracture. (**a**) Trauma image, (**b**, **c**) Postoperative with retrograde ESIN

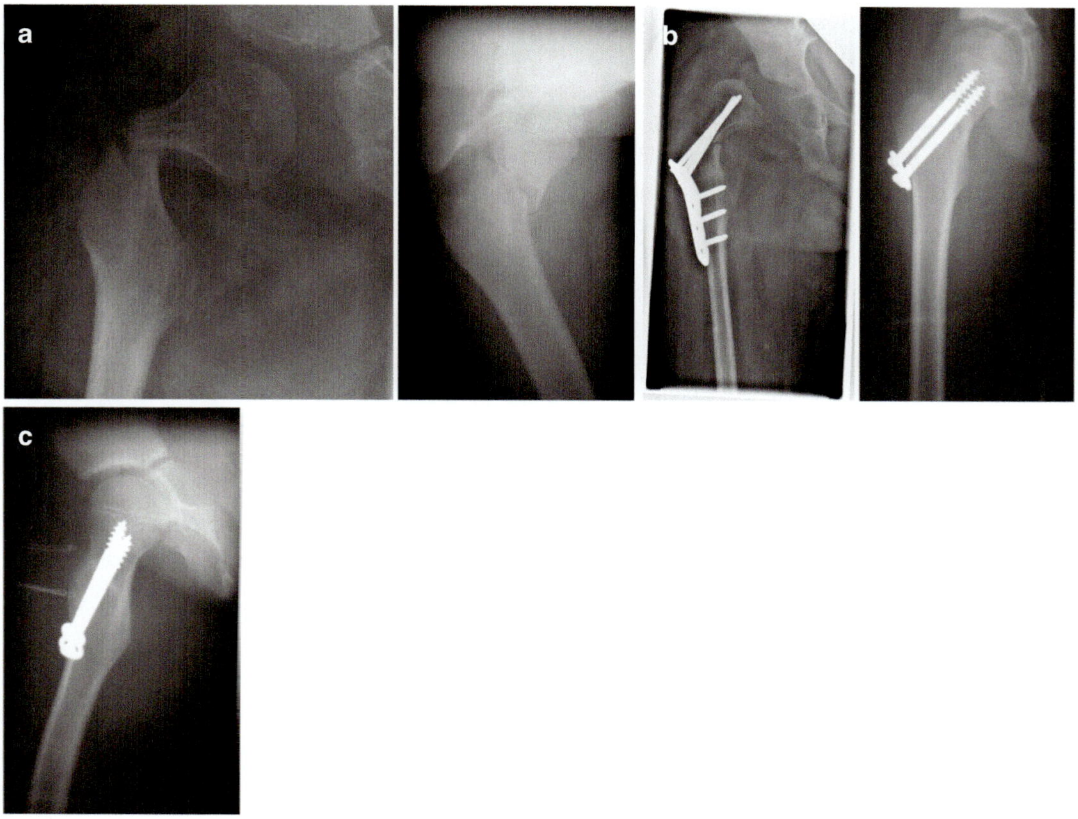

Fig. 11.12 8 Year old girl with Hamartom-tumor-syndrome, osteosynthesis with an angular stable plate. (**a**) Trauma image, (**b**, **c**) Postoperative with angular stable plate

Treatment Objective

The goal of treatment is to restore femoral neck anatomy and retain the reduction while protecting head circulation as much as possible. Because the fracture is rare and affects a small number of patients, there are no current evidence-based treatment recommendations.

The essential factor determining the outcome of proximal femur fractures is the integrity of the vascular system in the femoral neck. The most common complications are head and neck necrosis as well as, rarely, non-union and Coxa vara. Because patient numbers are so small, the extent to which prognosis is influenced by emergency surgical therapy cannot be definitively answered. Recent studies have reported positive results for surgery performed within 12 h of trauma, especially in fracture types II and III. Cases with Ratliff grade I head and neck necrosis exhibit the most severe, negative clinical course (Table 11.1).

Prognosis is challenging because small collectives have been treated with varying approaches over long periods. While type I fractures have almost 100% poor results, the rate of head necrosis in type IV fractures approaches zero. A different evaluation approach was suggested more recently by Gill, where the presence or lack of bleeding after drilling of the femoral head is observed to identify good or poor prognosis. Vitality checks of the femoral neck with MRI should be carried out within 12 months or when symptoms are present (Table 11.2).

Table 11.1 Risk of avascular femoral head necrosis

Rate der avasuläre Nekrose nach Frakturtyp	Ratliff Classification	Prognosis	
Typ I 100%	I	bad	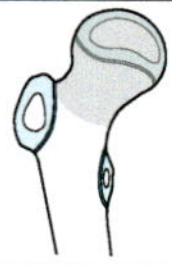
Typ II 52%	II	batter than type I	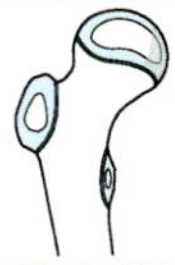
Typ III 27%	III	best	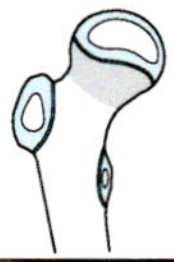

Table 11.2 Proximal femur fractures

Special features	Rare (<1%); most commonly from high-speed trauma (often with polytrauma)
Diagnostic approach	A.P. x-ray, axial (Lauenstein) view if possible
Treatment objective/ limits of correction	Anatomical repositioning while protecting head circulation
Primary treatment	Analgesia
Conservative treatment	
Indication	Non-displaced fractures
Approach	Hip spica cast for 4–6 weeks Hemarthrosis aspiration (decompression of the vessels → necrosis prophylaxis)
Follow up	After cast removal, weight-bearing as tolerated, physical therapy if needed
Radiological controls	Position check after 1 week, consolidation check at 4–6 weeks (cast-free), MRI at 12 months or for symptoms
Return to sports	When symptom-free, with unlimited function
Operative treatment	
Indication	Displaced and instable fractures, urgent indication
Approach	Open reduction and internal fixation age-dependent with K-wires and usually screws depending from the age; if possible stable fixation with screws. Anterolateral approach (Watson-Jones) Ventral capsule incision and fracture exposure Care for the growth plates (exception: epiphysiolysis) Intraoperative imaging to exclude head perforation with K-wire, exclusion documented; sometimes, a perforation of the growth plate is necessary to achieve enough stability. For medial and lateral femoral neck fractures – Cannulated screw osteosynthesis (Fig. 11.13) – Cannulated screw osteosynthesis and ESIN femur (Fig. 11.14) – Dynamic hip screw (Fig. 11.15) – Screw osteosynthesis in lateral femoral neck fracture (Fig. 11.16) – Fixed angular plate (Fig. 11.12) Type IV fractures: also retrograde ESIN, fixed-angle plates
Follow up	Partial weight-bearing (rolling) for 4–6 weeks
Radiological controls	Postoperative, consolidation check (cast-free), MRI at 12 months or for symptoms
Hardware removal	½–1 year post-surgery
Return to sports	When symptom-free, with unlimited function
Complications	Femoral head or neck necrosis, non-union, varus deformity
Growth disturbance	Femoral neck shortening
Follow up	x-ray check at 3 weeks and before full weight-bearing (4–6 weeks), repeat x-ray check at 6–12 months or before hardware removal MRI at 12 months or for symptoms, ½-year clinical checks for 2 years post-trauma
Classification	AO: 31-E/1-9.1-3 31-M/3.1-3.I–III LiLa: 3.1.a.5.0-2. 3.1.s.1-5.0-2.

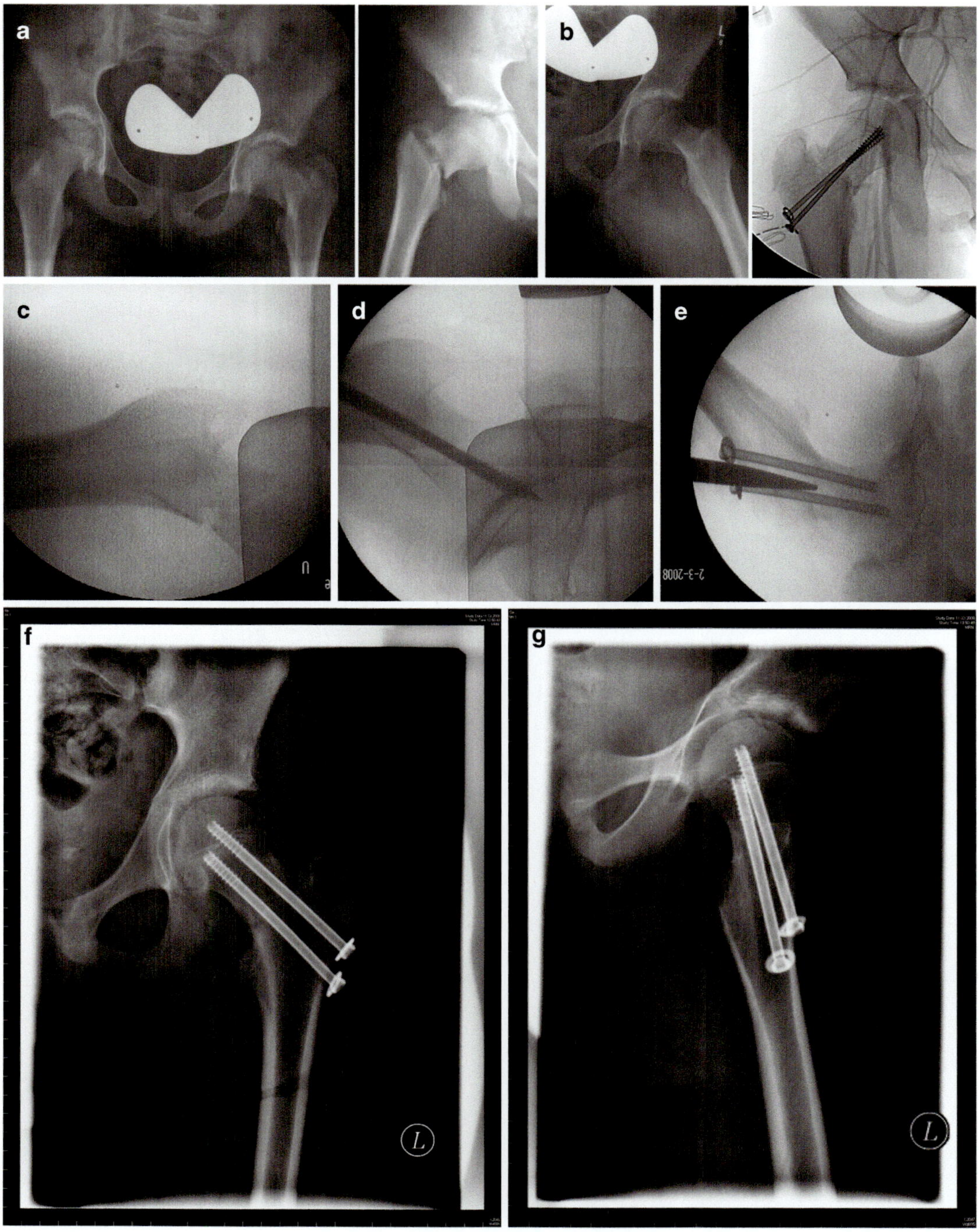

Fig. 11.13 Girl with oblique fracture of the femoral neck (type 2/3). (**a**, **b**) Trauma image, (**c**) Indirect reduction, (**d**) Screw osteosynthesis via K-wire, (**e**) Opening of the capsula of hematoma, (**f**, **g**) Healing with 2 lag screws, one crossing the growth plate

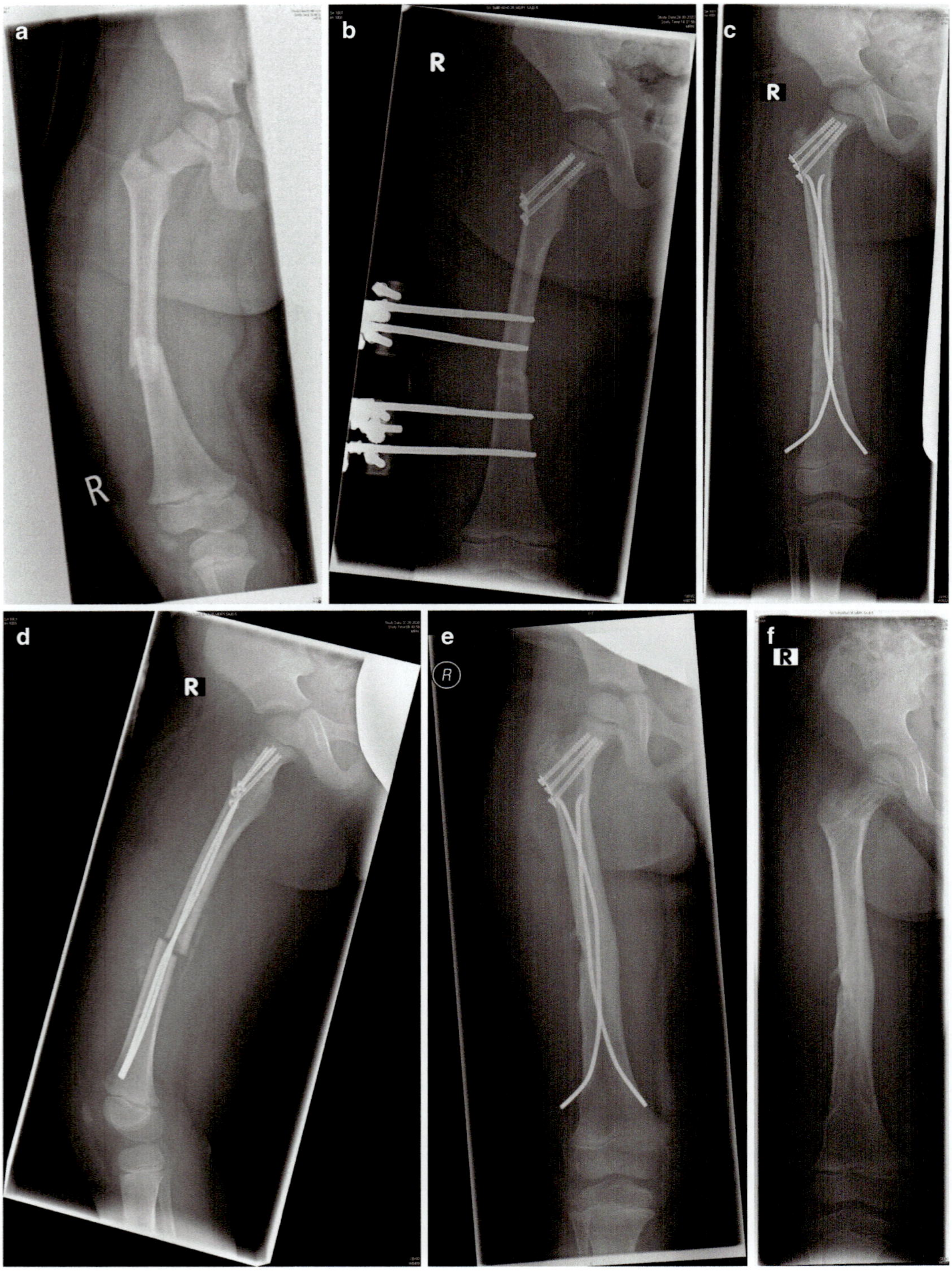

Fig. 11.14 3 Year old boy with combined lateral femoral neck fracture and femur shaft fracture. (**a**) Trauma image, (**b**) Reduction and primary screw osteosynthesis of the femoral neck and ext. fix. For the femur shaft, (**c**, **d**) Change of external fixateur to retrograde ESIN, (**e**, **f**) Complete healing and metal removal

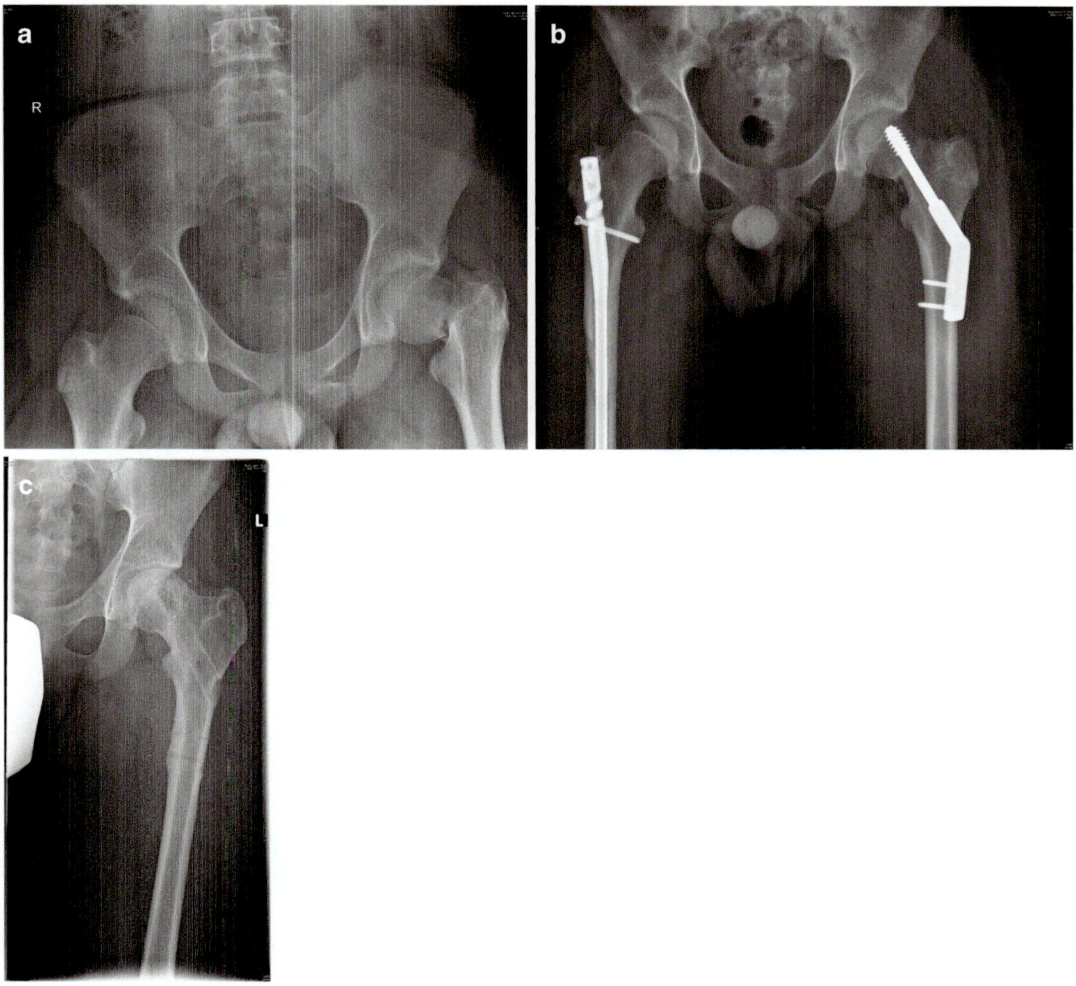

Fig. 11.15 15 Year old boy with displaced lateral femur fracture. (**a**) Trauma image, (**b**) After reduction and dynamic hip screw, (**c**) After metal removal and complete healing

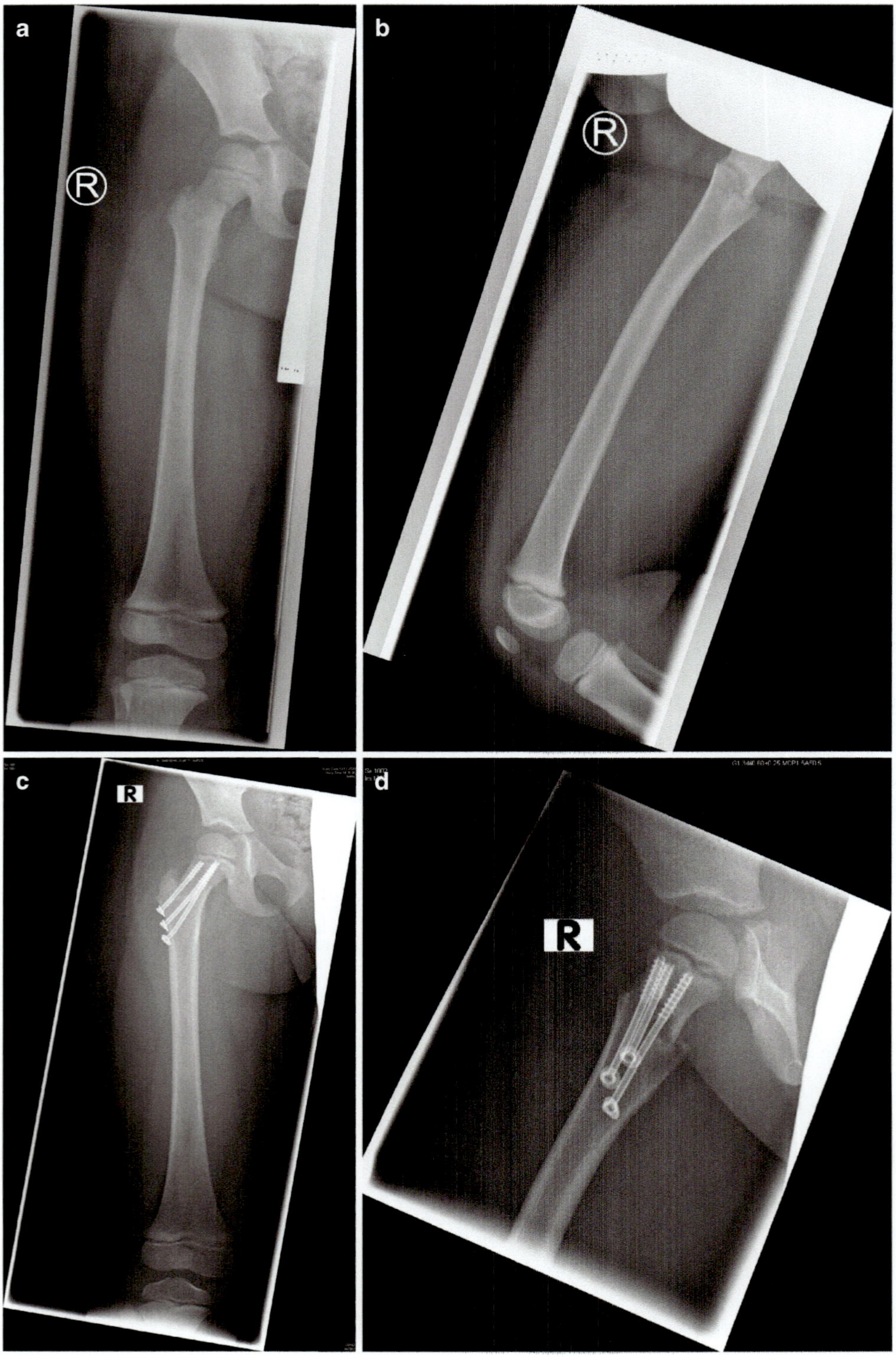

Fig. 11.16 Lateral femoral neck fracture in a 4 year old boy. (**a**, **b**) Trauma image, (**c**, **d**) Osteosynthesis with 3 screws, ending just next to the growth plate

11.3 Apophyseal Avulsions

Apophyseal avulsions of the greater or lesser trochanters are uncommon and usually occur prepuberty, after sudden stress to the gluteus medius or iliopsoas muscles. Avulsion of the lesser trochanter can be treated conservatively, but the grossly-displaced avulsions of the greater trochanter must be re-fixed. Severe growth disturbances do not generally occur because neither of these apophyses is involved in longitudinal growth by this time. Femoral head necrosis is still possible with damage to the vascular supply (Table 11.3).

Table 11.3 Apophyseal avulsions of the proximal femur (Fig. 11.17)

Special features	Uncommon; direct trauma; sudden muscle strain (iliopsoas → lesser trochanter; gluteus medius → greater trochanter)
Diagnostic approach	Hip x-rays in two planes
Primary treatment	Analgesia
Conservative treatment	
Indication	All lesser trochanter fractures; minimally-displaced greater trochanter fractures (Fig. 11.18).
Approach	Lesser trochanter: unloading with forearm crutches for 5–6 weeks; greater trochanter: hip spica cast when non-displaced and in small children
Follow up	Mobilization as tolerated
Radiological controls	Consolidation check with x-ray at 5–6 weeks
Return to sports	When symptom-free with unlimited function
Operative treatment	
Indication	Displaced greater trochanter avulsions
Approach	Open reduction and tension-band fixation
Follow up	Tension-band: functional
Radiological controls	Postoperative, consolidation check at 5–6 weeks
Hardware removal	At 12 weeks
Return to sports	When symptom-free with unlimited function
Complications	Femoral head necrosis
Growth disturbance	Rare
Follow up	Until unlimited function and symptom-free
Classification	AO: 31-M/7.1-3 LiLa: 3.1.s.5.0-2.

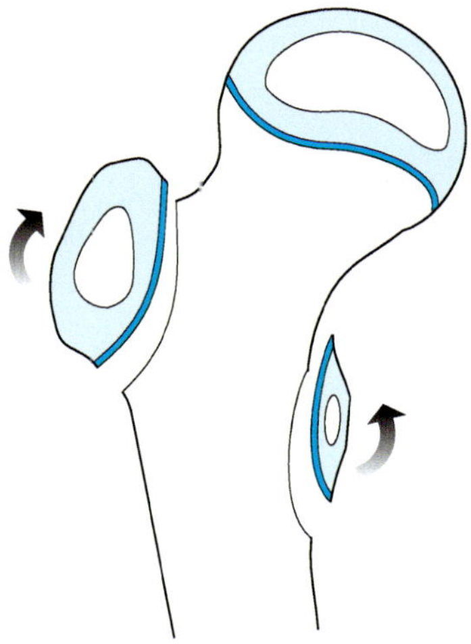

Fig. 11.17 Apophyseal avulsions of the proximal femur

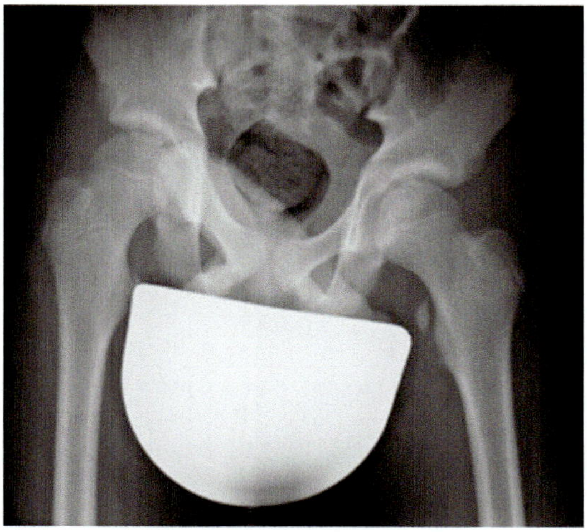

Fig. 11.18 Avulsion of the apophysis of the minor trochanter left side; conservative treatment

11.4 Traumatic Hip Dislocations

Traumatic hip dislocation is one of the rarest pediatric injuries (Table 11.4). Unlike in adults, it can occur not only as a result of high-speed trauma but also during relatively ordinary injuries (during play or sports activities). To prevent perfusion issues and reduce the risk of femoral head necrosis, the most rapid and careful reduction possible must be performed within 6 h under anesthesia. Delayed reductions (>24 h) usually need to be performed open and have a worse prognosis than primary closed reductions. Open reduction may also be necessary if there are interposed soft tissues (capsule, labrum), which can be detected as joint widening on x-ray (after successful joint aspiration). MRI can be carried out post-reduction to exclude capsular ligament or labral injury. It can also be performed to evaluate blood supply, if necessary, before or after reduction. Growth disturbances are possible, especially with vascular injuries, usually leading to shortening of the femoral neck and a resulting elevated trochanter. Vascular injury very often results in femoral head necrosis.

Table 11.4 Traumatic hip dislocation (Fig. 11.19)

Special features	<0.5% of all lower extremity injuries; usually posterior-superior, more rarely an anterior or central dislocation
Diagnostic approach	Deformity and limited range of motion lead to clinical diagnosis; posterior dislocation (90%): leg in adduction, flexion and internal rotation; anterior dislocation: Leg in abduction, extension and external rotation; x-rays of pelvis and femur
Treatment objective/limits of correction	Rapid reduction, prevent femoral head necrosis Hip dislocation Reduction of posterior dislocation: pull anteriorly with hip and knee in flexion External rotation (Fig. 11.20) Reduction of an anterior dislocation: Longitudinal traction with hip extension and knee flexion Internal rotation
Primary treatment	Reduction under general anesthesia with "maximal" relaxation of the patient, emergency indication
Conservative treatment	
Indication	Usually conservative
Approach	Effusion aspiration
Follow up	Unloading with 4 weeks of bed rest or crutches for school-aged children
Radiological controls	Reduction control with MRI, and CT if needed, to rule out associated or acetabular injuries
Return to sports	At approx. 6 weeks, when symptom-free with unlimited function
Operative treatment	
Indication	In cases of interpolation or central dislocation, delayed reduction (>24 h), associated acetabular injury
Approach	Open reduction, with internal fixation if necessary Open reduction over a posterolateral approach (Kocher-Langenbeck) Caution: exposure of the sciatic nerve Common obstacle to reduction: impinged piriformis tendon, capsule, or impinged labrum
Follow up	Unloading with 4 weeks of bed rest or crutches for school-aged children
Radiological controls	Position check with MRI and CT if needed to exclude associated injuries
Hardware removal	–
Return to sports	At approx. 6 weeks, when symptom-free with unlimited function
Complications	Femoral head necrosis; posterior dislocation: sciatic nerve lesion, central dislocation: triradiate cartilage disruption; associated injuries: femoral shaft fracture, acetabular injuries (partially non-ossified), pelvic fractures, recurrent dislocations, osteoarthritis
Growth disturbance	With premature growth plate fusion, possible femoral neck shortening
Follow up	MRI at 4–6 weeks and as needed to exclude head necrosis, ½-year clinical checks for 2 years post-trauma

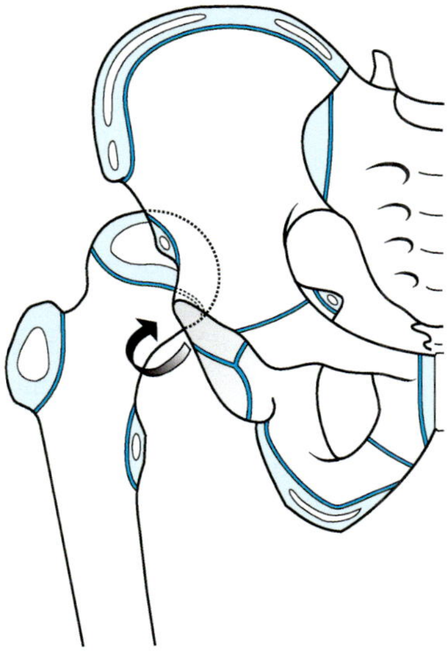

Fig. 11.19 Traumatic hip dislocation

Fig. 11.20 Traumatic hip luxation. (**a**) Trauma image, (**b**) After reduction

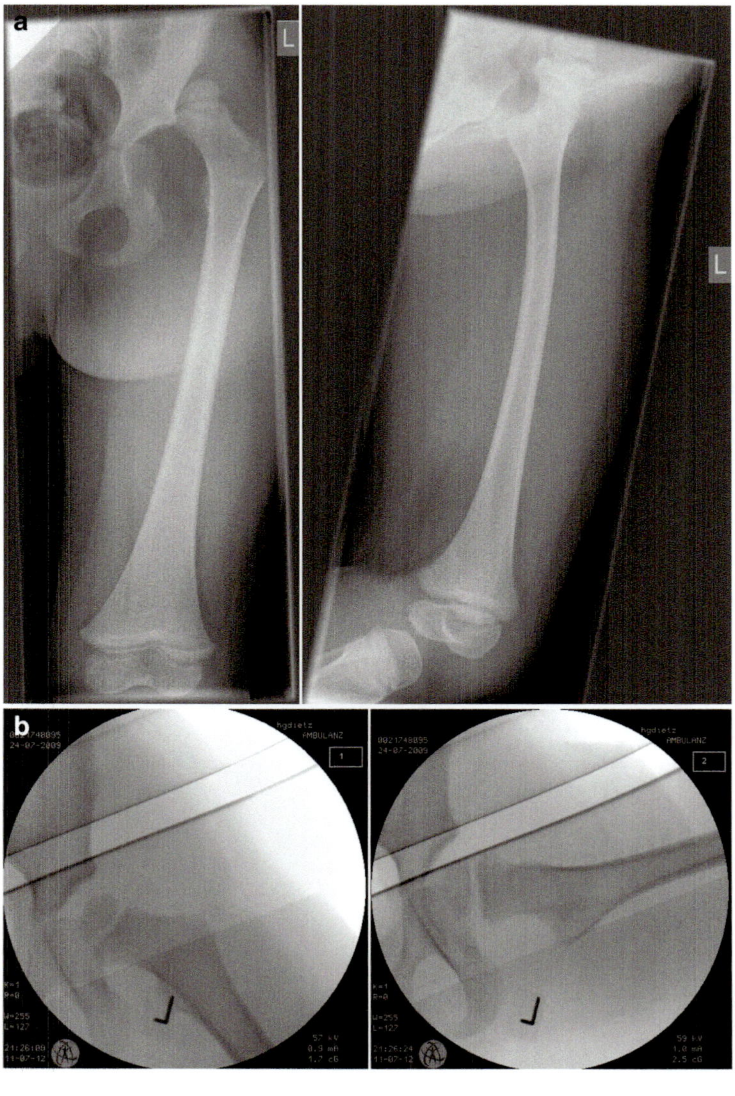

11.5 Transient Synovitis, Legg–Calvé–Perthes Disease (LCPD), and Slipped Capital Femoral Epiphysis (SCFE)

In the differential diagnosis of hip injuries, pathologies such as transient synovitis, Legg–Calvé–Perthes disease, or atraumatic epiphysiolysis of the proximal femur must also be considered, especially because the medical history does not always reveal a specific traumatic event. The main symptom of hip diseases is functional limitation and restricted range of motion (positive FABER test). In contrast to adults, children often experience pain in the thigh or leg rather than in the hip area itself.

Specific radiological methods can help with diagnosis. An early "slipping" epiphysis is challenging to recognize on x-ray; indirect signs such as relative epiphyseal height decrease and widening of the growth plate as well as the Little tangente line can indicate epiphysiolysis (Fig. 11.21). There are broad indications today to perform MRI for diagnosis.

These clinical presentations show typical age distributions and special features, shown in Table 11.5. The following summary provides a simple overview. For more detailed information, we recommend referring to the corresponding specialist literature.

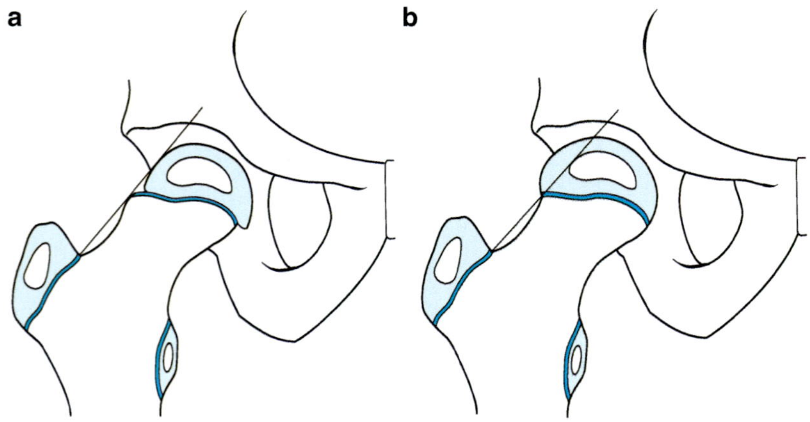

Fig. 11.21 Small tangent line. This line is placed on the external cortex of the femoral neck on the A.P. view image and normally intersects the epiphysis (**a**); In epiphysiolysis, the tangent no longer intersects the epiphysis (**b**)

Table 11.5 Differential diagnosis of orthopedic hip diseases

	Transient synovitis (toxic synovitis, coxitis fugax) Table 11.6	Legg–Calvé–Perthes disease Table 11.8	SCFE Table 11.9
Peak ages (years)	5–6	5–7	12–14
Gender distribution	♂: ♀ 2–3:1	♂: ♀ 4:1	♂: ♀ 3:1
Special features	More cases in spring History of infection in the nasopharynx	15% bilateral	40% bilateral Often associated with obesity, genital underdevelopment
Clinical	Limp Pain in hip and thigh Limited range of motion (positive FABER sign) Sometimes tenderness over the capsule	Limited ROM (positive FABER sign, decreased internal rotation) Limp Sometimes hip, knee, thigh pain	Often mild symptoms External rotation, leg shortening Positive Drehmann sign SCFE unstable SCFE stable SCFE acute
Diagnostic approach	Serology: Sometimes elevated ESR Ultrasound: effusion, capsular swelling If signs of infection are present a bacterial infection is suspicious (Table 11.7)	X-ray in two planes: effusion-condensation-fragmentation-repair	X-ray in two planes: dorsocaudal slipping of the epiphysis
Treatment	Symptomatic, NSAIDs if necessary	Staged treatment: observation, conservative, surgical	Stage-dependent: screws or K-wire fixation

Table 11.6 Transient synovitis (toxic synovitis, coxitis fugax) (Fig. 11.22)

Special features	Common (1:1000), peak age 5–6 years of age (1–12 years), hip involvement during or following a typical virus infection (history: illness in the past 4 weeks, usually upper respiratory or gastrointestinal tract infections) Pain (hip, thigh), restricted range of motion (positive FABER test)
Diagnostic approach	Clinical diagnosis of exclusion Hip ultrasound: effusion or capsular swelling (Fig. 11.23) Serology: inconspicuous or mild inflammatory parameter increases (previous viral infection), exclusion of bacterial septic arthritis with MRI or joint aspiration if necessary to exclude empyema
Conservative treatment	
Indication	Always
Approach	Symptomatic, non-steroidal anti-inflammatory drugs for 2 days (e.g., ibuprofen); illness duration: approx. 1 week
Follow up	None
Radiological controls	None
Return to sports	–
Complications	Other hip diseases; further diagnosis with complaints persisting after 2 days; possible association with Legg–Calvé–Perthes disease
Growth disturbance	None
Follow up	In cases of persistent or "recurrent transient synovitis" radiology to exclude Legg–Calvé–Perthes Other (less common) differential diagnoses: SCFE, leukemia, rheumatoid arthritis, inflammatory bowel disease (Crohn's/ulcerative colitis), epiphyseal dysplasia

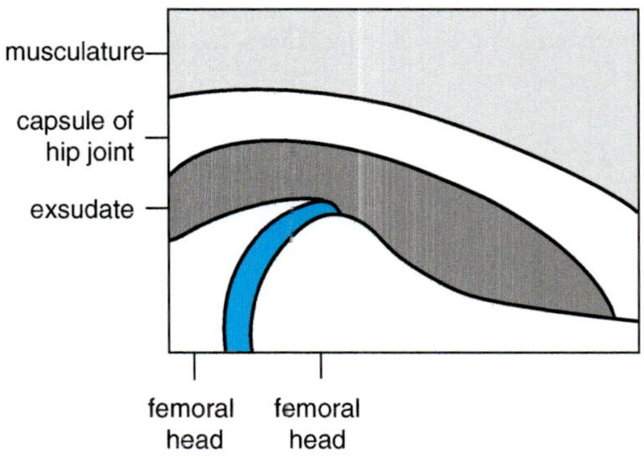

Fig. 11.22 Fluid in hip joint—coxitis fugax

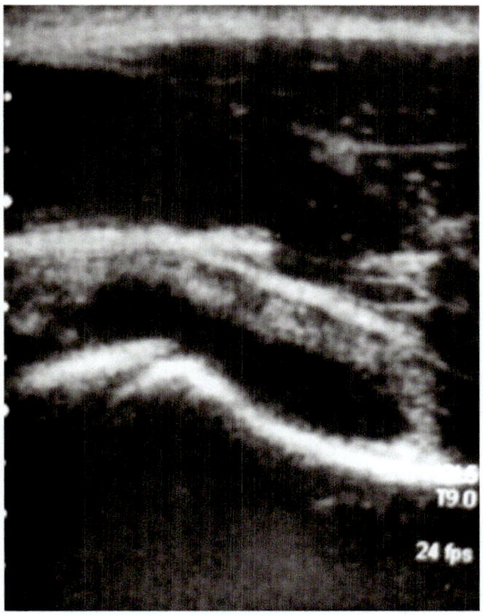

Fig. 11.23 Ultrasound with fluid in hip joint in coxitis fugax

Table 11.7 Bacterial septic arthritis

Special features	Occurs rarely, most often in newborns and infants; usually occurs with hematogenous spread
Diagnostic approach	History: generalized infection; lack of movement, pseudoparalysis, swelling and protective posture, generalized symptoms with fever, ill-appearance and insufficient drinking laboratory: increased CRP and ESR, leukocytes, left shift in the differential blood cell count ultrasound shows arthritis with capsular swelling and effusion (see transient synovitis), x-ray (distension of the joint, late osteolysis) (Fig. 11.24a) and MRI! (Fig. 11.24b); bone scan if necessary (multiple foci possible—10%)
Treatment objective/limits of correction	Treatment of infection, preventing joint damage
Primary treatment	Emergency indication, antibiosis (e.g., cephalosporin, clindamycin)
Operative treatment	
Indication	Always
Approach	Emergency arthrotomy or arthroscopy with joint irrigation, cultures, and immediate antibiotic therapy (e.g., clindamycin 40 mg/kg body weight/24 h) for at least 3 weeks, termination of therapy when laboratory parameters indicate normalization
Follow up	Change of antibiotic therapy according to sensitivity panel
Radiological controls	–
Hardware removal	–
Return to sports	When symptom-free with unlimited function
Complications	Deformity of the femoral head and acetabulum up to complete joint destruction is possible, including growth plates and growth disturbances
Growth disturbance	Possible
Follow up	Clinical controls to exclude growth disturbances up to 2 years

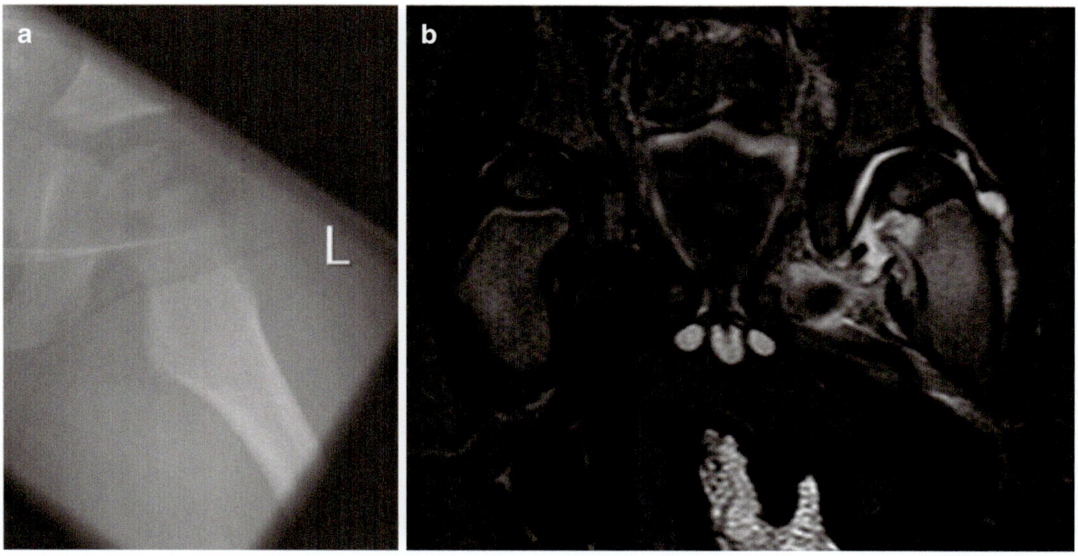

Fig. 11.24 (**a**) X-ray of septic bacterial coxitis with distension of the joint. (**b**) MRI of septic bacterial coxitis of the left side

Table 11.8 Legg–Calvé–Perthes disease (pediatric aseptic femoral head necrosis) (Fig. 11.25)

Special features	Rare (0.8%); also called Perthes or Legg-Perthes disease Peak age: 5–7 years; 15% are bilateral; ♂: ♀ = 4:1 Etiology unclear, possibly a vascular disorder Classification I–V: femoral head shape from spherical to aspherical and incongruent
Diagnostic approach	Clinical: especially thigh and knee pain, limp Examination: limited abduction and internal rotation, leg-length difference, Trendelenburg's sign Hip x-rays in two planes: Initial stage: suspended epiphyseal growth → apparent widened joint space Condensation stage: consolidation of the epiphysis Fragmentation stage: shrinkage and loosening of the epiphysis, flattening, lysis, and fragmentation Regeneration stage: appearance of new ossification centers, atypical growth plate End-stage (Fig. 11.26) – physiological congruence – pathological congruence – incongruence Poor prognosis: Age > 6 years Sex: ♀ Lateral calcification Subluxation Poor ROM
Treatment objective/limits of correction	Prevention of femoral head deformity and restoration of joint congruence with preservation or restoration of unlimited ROM
Conservative treatment	
Indication	Usually conservative
Approach	Symptom-free: observation and care Non-steroidal anti-inflammatory medications, physical therapy, extension, unloading for pain (crutches), night splints
Follow up	Clinical follow up every 6 months (every 3 months if ROM is limited)
Radiological controls	Every 6 months (every 3 months if ROM is limited)
Return to sports	When symptom-free with unlimited function, complete restoration of the femoral head
Operative treatment	
Indication	Persistent limitations in ROM, "hinge abduction phenomenon," risk factors (lateralization of the head, lateral calcification, metaphyseal involvement)
Approach	Joint restoration (centering of the femoral head, unloading): tenotomy, varus intertrochanteric osteotomy, pelvic osteotomy, combination
Follow up	Depends on procedure, intensive physical therapy to maintain mobility
Radiological controls	Postoperative, in regular intervals (every 6 months) until healed
Hardware removal	1 year post-surgery
Return to sports	When symptom-free with unlimited function, complete restoration of the femoral head
Complications	Femoral head deformity, limited range of motion, hinge-abduction phenomenon
Growth disturbance	Possible: femoral neck shortening with elevated trochanteric position
Follow up	Clinical and radiological every 6 months, every 3 months if limited ROM, until healed

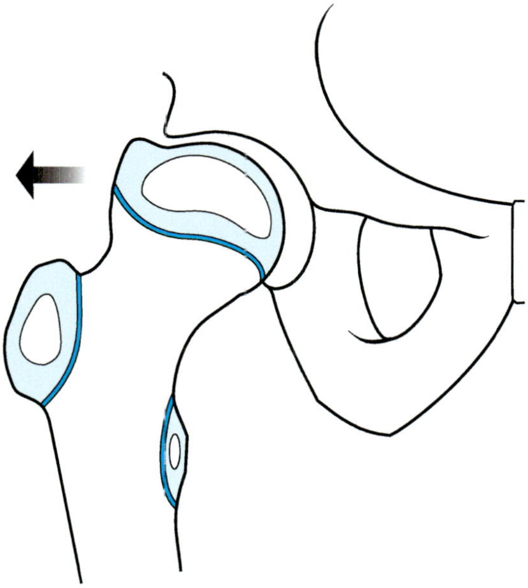

Fig. 11.25 Morbus Perthes (pediatric aseptic necrosis of the head of the hip)

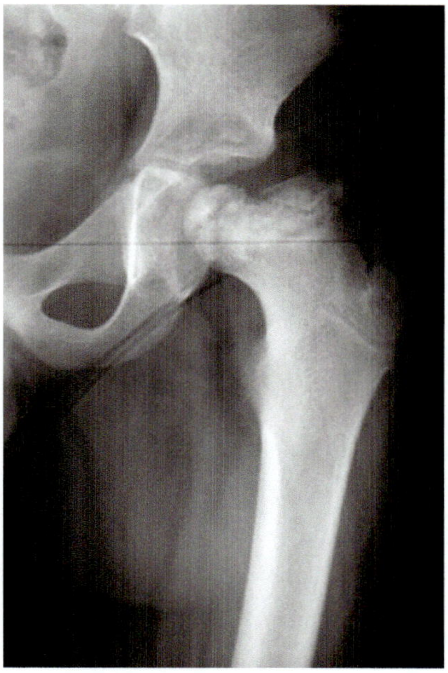

Fig. 11.26 Late stage of Morbus Perthes

Table 11.9 Slipped Capital Femoral Epiphysis (SCFE) (Fig. 11.27)

Special features	Very rare (1:10000) usually occurs in boys with certain features (obesity, underdeveloped genitals) (♂: ♀ = 1.5:1) Occurrence during puberty (approx. 10–15 years), bilateral occurrence: ♂: ♀ = 4:1 Acute: history <2 weeks Chronic: history >2 weeks Acute to chronic: history >2 weeks with sudden deterioration and inability to ambulate Stable: preserved ambulation Unstable: unable to ambulate
Diagnostic approach	Clinical: external rotation and shortening, rapid fatigue Positive Drehmann sign: deviation in external rotation when the hip is flexed Chronic SCFE: often mild symptoms, e.g., limp, with or without hip or thigh pain A.P. and Lauenstein x-ray views: dorsocaudal epiphysiolysis, indirect signs: relative epiphyseal loss of height, plate widening, and little tangent (see Fig. 11.22). MRI if needed to evaluate blood flow
Treatment objective/limits of correction	Reduction of the epiphysis or prevention of further slipping
Primary treatment	SCFE acute: indication for urgent surgery
Conservative treatment	
Indication	Once diagnosis is made, no conservative treatment
Operative treatment	
Indication	Acute SCFE: emergency; chronic SCFE
Approach	Unstable: <40°: careful closed reduction and fixation with K-wire/screws (Fig. 11.28) >40°: open reduction trochanter flip osteotomy) or subcapital wedge osteotomy, in situ fixation in case of disturbed circulation if needed (Fig. 11.29) Stable: <40°: screws or K-wire fixation >40°: open reduction (trochanter flip osteotomy) or subcapital wedge osteotomy, screw fixation in case of disturbed circulation if needed After growth plate fusion: Subcapital wedge osteotomy or valgus flexion derotation osteotomy (Imhäuser) if needed Treatment of the contralateral side: Prophylactic screws/K-wire
Follow up	6 weeks unloading with forearm crutches, physical therapy
Radiological controls	Postoperative, every 6 months, during growth spurt every 3 months
Hardware removal	Once the growth plate is closed, K-wire change if necessary
Return to sports	When symptom-free, unlimited function
Complications	Femoral head necrosis, chondrolysis (Waldenstrom syndrome), arthritis
Growth disturbance	Possible
Follow up	Clinical and radiological controls every 6 months (every 3 months during growth spurt) until plate closure

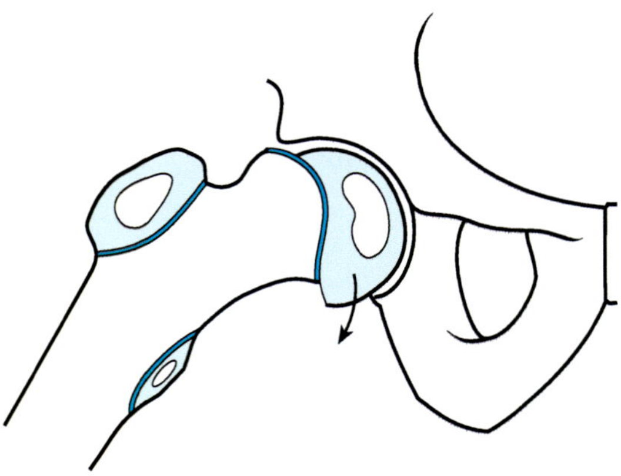

Fig. 11.27 Slipped Capital Femoral Epiphysis (SCFE)

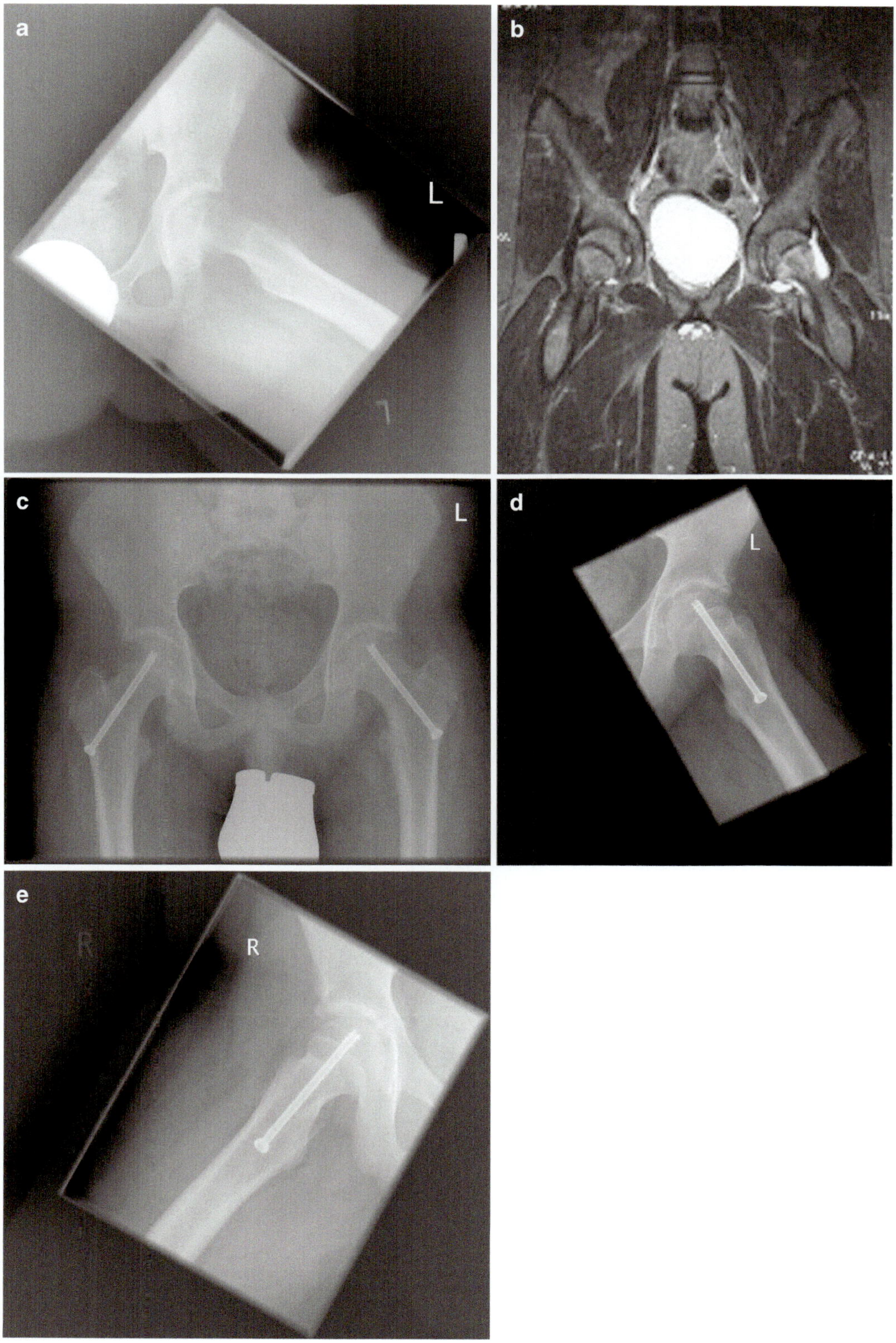

Fig. 11.28 Acute Slipped Capital Femoral Epiphysis (SCFE). (**a**) MRI left jip with dislocation, (**b**) MRI, (**c**–**e**) Closed reduction and fixation with central screw left side and prophylactic fixation of the right side

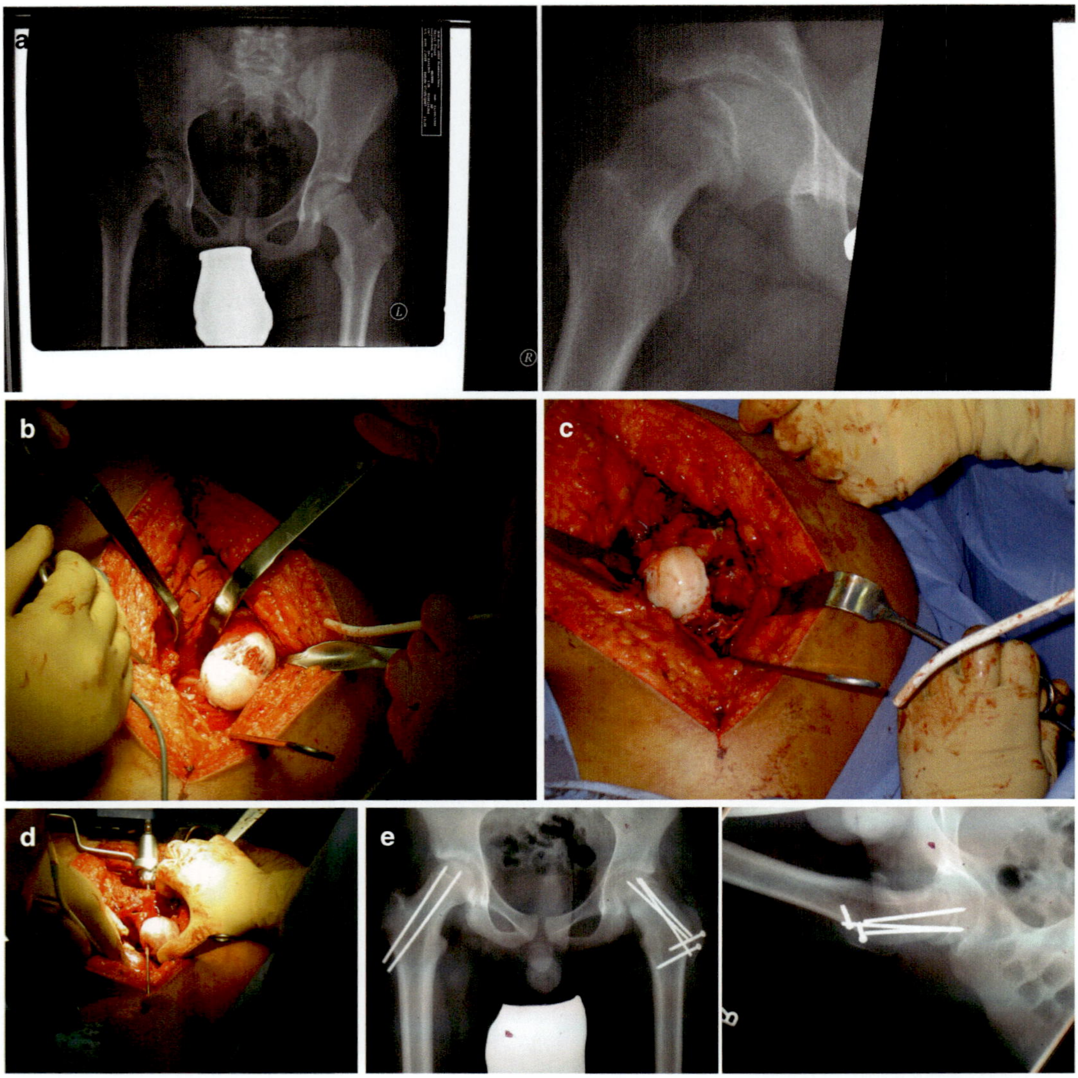

Fig. 11.29 Slipped Capital Femoral Epiphysis (SCFE) treated with surgical hip dislocation and trochanteric flip osteotomy. (**a**) X-ray, (**b**) Intraoperative femur head during surgical luxation, (**c**) Shaping of the femoral neck bumb, (**d**) Intraoperative osteosynthesis, (**e**) Postoperative x-ray with fixation of the femoral head left side and 2 screws to fix the trochanter; prophylactic fixation of the other side

Recommended Literature

Atsumi T, Yamano K, Muraki M, Yoshihara S, Kajihara T (2000) The blood supply of lateral epiphyseal arteries in Perthe's disease. J Bone Joint Surg Br 82:392

Kurz W, Grumbt H (1988) The femoral neck fracture in childhood. Zentralbl Chir 113(14):881–892

Mayr J, Hirner V, Styhler W, Posch E, Jelen M, Linhart WE, Kohlmaier W, Neubauer T, Schwarz N (1998) Femoral neck fractures in childhood. Unfallchirurg 101(6):426–432

Parsch K, Savvidis E (1997)Die Koxitis beim Neugeborenen und Säugling. Diagose und Therapie. Orthopäde. Springer, New York 26(10):838–847

Ratliff AHC (1974) Fractures of the neck of the femur in children. Orthop Clin N Am 5:903

Shah AK, Eissler J, Radomisli T (2002) Algorithms for the treatment of femoral neck fractures. Clin Orthop Related Res 399:28–34

Wiedmann H, Parsch K (1990) Schenkelhalsfraktur bei Kindern. Z Orthop 128:418–421

12 Femur

12.1 Physiological Findings

The femur is the longest and strongest long bone of the body. The shaft shows physiological anteversion and slight lateral bending. The epiphysis of the distal femur is the only one radiologically visible at birth and is a sign of neonatal maturity (Figs. 12.1 and 12.2). The epiphyseal plate and the apophyses of the proximal femur form a functional growth unit. Integrity of these plates is required to achieve appropriate length and femoral neck development.

During infancy, the femur consists primarily of woven bone. This later remodels to harder lamellar bone. Femoral shaft diameter increases with increasing cortical diameter during growth, while canal diameter proportionally decreases. Thus, fracture risk decreases in older children with a corresponding increase in bony stability.

Individual variation must be considered when assessing post-traumatic leg-length discrepancy and rotation deformities. Physiologically, leg length can vary 0.5 to 1 cm, and antetorsion up to 20° in every fifth child.

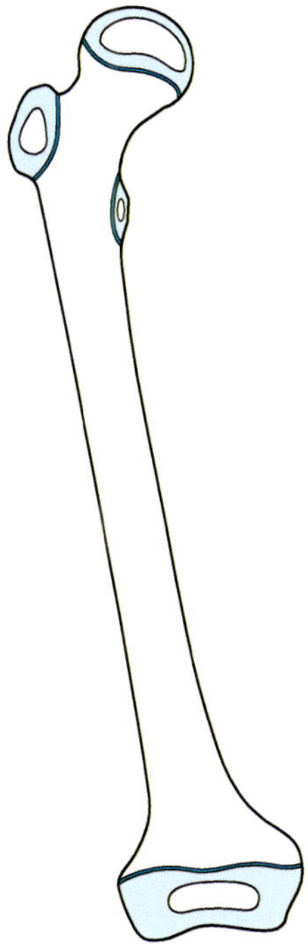

Fig. 12.1 Femoral ossification centers: femoral shaft in the eighth gestational week, distally in the 39th fetal week, femoral head at 4 months, greater trochanter at age 4–6 years, lesser trochanter at 11–12 years

I. Marzi et al., *Pediatric Skeletal Trauma*, https://doi.org/10.1007/978-3-030-93685-3_12

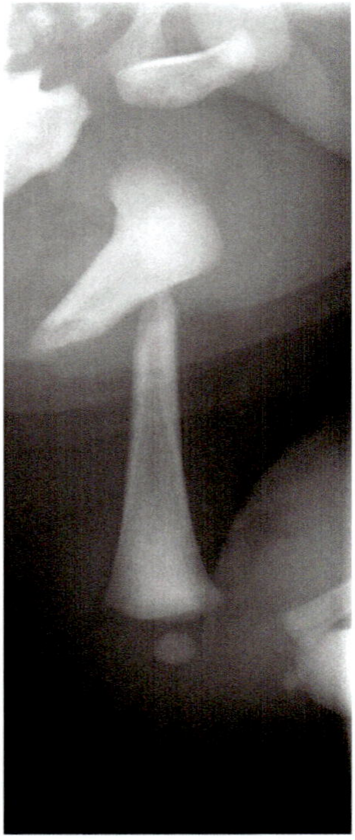

Fig. 12.2 Birth trauma femoral fractures with visible epiphyseal cores along the distal femur. Apophyses and further epiphyseal cores are not yet recognizable

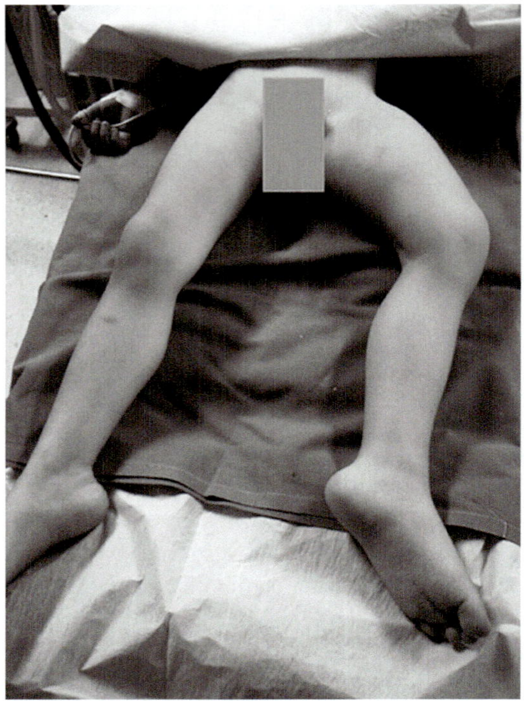

Fig. 12.3 Displaced femur fracture with external rotation after motor vehicle accident

12.2 Femoral Shaft Fractures

Incidence, Mechanism of Injury and Clinical Picture

The incidence of femoral shaft fractures is approximately 1.3%. These fractures usually occur as a result of direct trauma, for example, to cyclists or pedestrians in traffic accidents, or after falls from a height. Femur fractures occur often in seriously injured children. Thus, it is important to consider additional injuries, shock with blood loss, and soft-tissue, nerve and vascular injuries. An x-ray overview of the adjacent hip and knee joints is useful.

Child abuse must be considered in infants and small children, in addition to falls from the changing table. Further injuries and signs of abuse should be considered along with hematomas.

Femoral shaft fractures are clinically evident from local swelling, shortening and rotational deformity of the affected leg (Fig. 12.3). In obviously displaced fractures, it's not necessary to x-ray in the second plane if there is risk of further displacement and pain. Most fractures are in the middle third of the shaft. Oblique and spiral fractures are the most common with 50%, followed by transverse fractures in approximately 30%.

Fractures consolidate rapidly in children, usually with pronounced callus formation. Axial deviation can correct itself with growth, but the corrective potential for rotational deformity is less clear and up to 20° is still considered tolerable. Because of muscle distribution, varus deformities correct better than valgus deformities. The more proximal the deformity, the worse the corrective potential. Deformities of the proximal femur should not be accepted, for the sake of hip joint function alone. Length can be expected to increase an average one cm up to a year post-trauma, and this must be observed during follow-up. Growth stimulation increases with greater need for remodeling, if the fracture is not well reduced. Spontaneous correction is difficult to predict and thus, cannot be accounted for during surgical planning. Best possible reduction and stability should always be the goals of surgery. Depending on magnitude, leg-length discrepancy can lead to pelvic obliquity, with consequent limp and scoliosis.

Treatment of femoral shaft fractures depends primarily on patient age. In infants and toddlers, conservative therapy is the treatment of choice. In newborns and small infants, immobilization in a hip spica cast is primarily used, when the fracture is roughly in the axis. As alternative approache the use of Pavlik bandage was recommended. Primary cast immobilization is not recommended for open and soft-tissue injuries and mostly not in displaced fractures with shortening greater than 2 cm or a strong axis deviation (Fig. 12.2). Overhead non-invasive skin traction can be used up to two years of age with good compliance in cases of large axial deviation or shortening. It can be replaced after 7–10 days with a hip spica cast, when the bones have at least stable contact. In these cases of newborns and infants a rapid re-orientation of the shaft can be observed within a few weeks (Fig. 12.4).

For children between two and three years, operative therapy with the elastic stable intra-

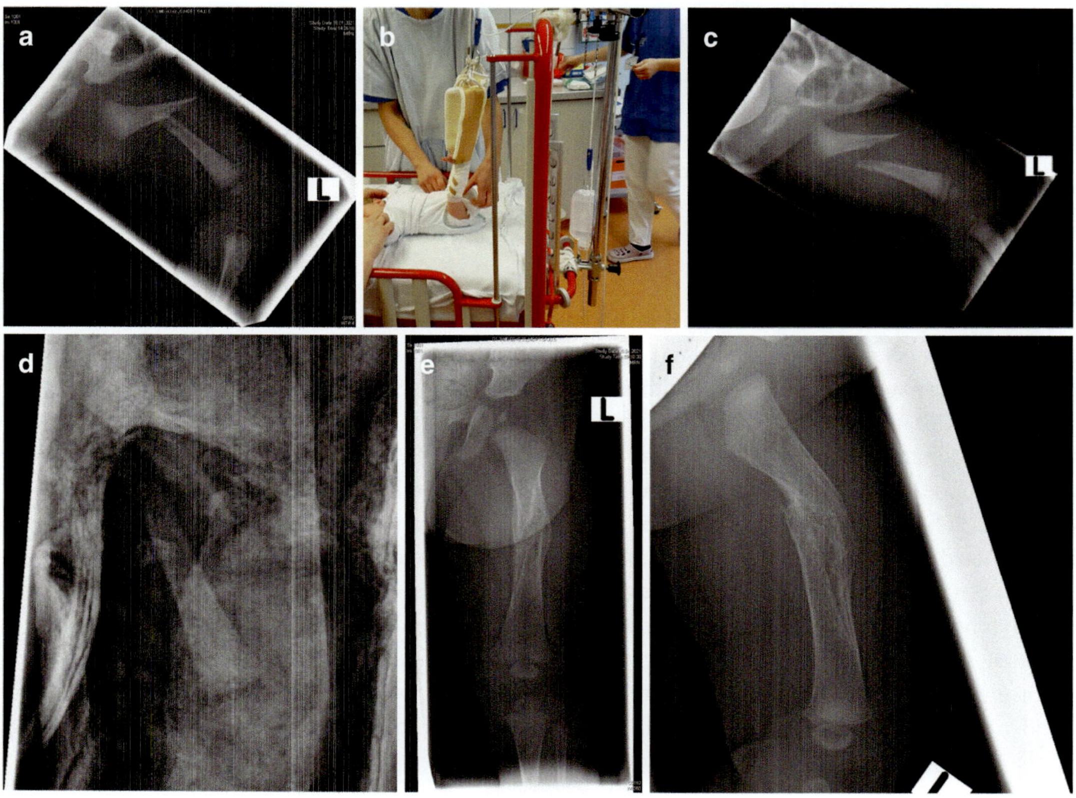

Fig. 12.4 Displaced, oblique femur shaft fracture in a newborn girl (**a**) Trauma image, (**b**) Overhead extension for axis correction. (**c**) X-ray after 2 weeks, (**d**) X-ray in pelvic-hip spica cast, (**e**, **f**) Healing with good axis in x-ray after 3 months

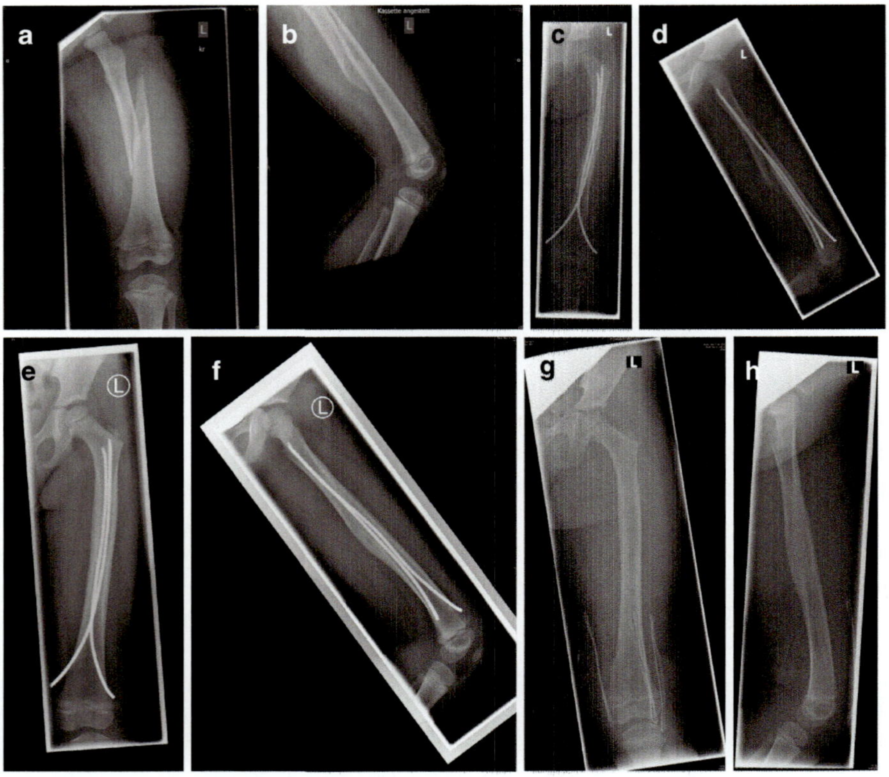

Fig. 12.5 Displaced long spiral fracture of a 4 year old girl, (**a**, **b**) Trauma image, (**c**, **d**) Stable, but not ideal reduction and fixation, (**e**, **f**) Regular healing after 4 months, (**g**, **h**) After metal removal

medullary nail (ESIN) is clearly favored. This procedure can be applied for fractures of almost any type (transverse, oblique) at almost any position (proximal or distal). However, the technical demands such as size of the nails, entry point selection and positioning and fixation have to be done properly (Fig. 12.5). It can also be used for open fractures when safe soft-tissue management might be achieved. ESIN can also be used in selected patients under two years of age when there is marked or painful deformity, heavy weight or high activity of the child.

External fixators are an alternative to ESIN used increasingly for pediatric polytrauma, with extensive soft-tissue damage or unstable oblique or multi-fragment fractures. The external fixator is particularly advantageous compared to ESIN when there is a lack of strut capability, because it is better at maintaining leg length, rotation, and prevents telescoping of the fracture (Fig. 12.6). It is also very well tolerated in children and results in good healing.

Plate fixation is reserved for individual cases, especially when x-ray can't be performed (polytrauma with multiple parallel procedures), or in

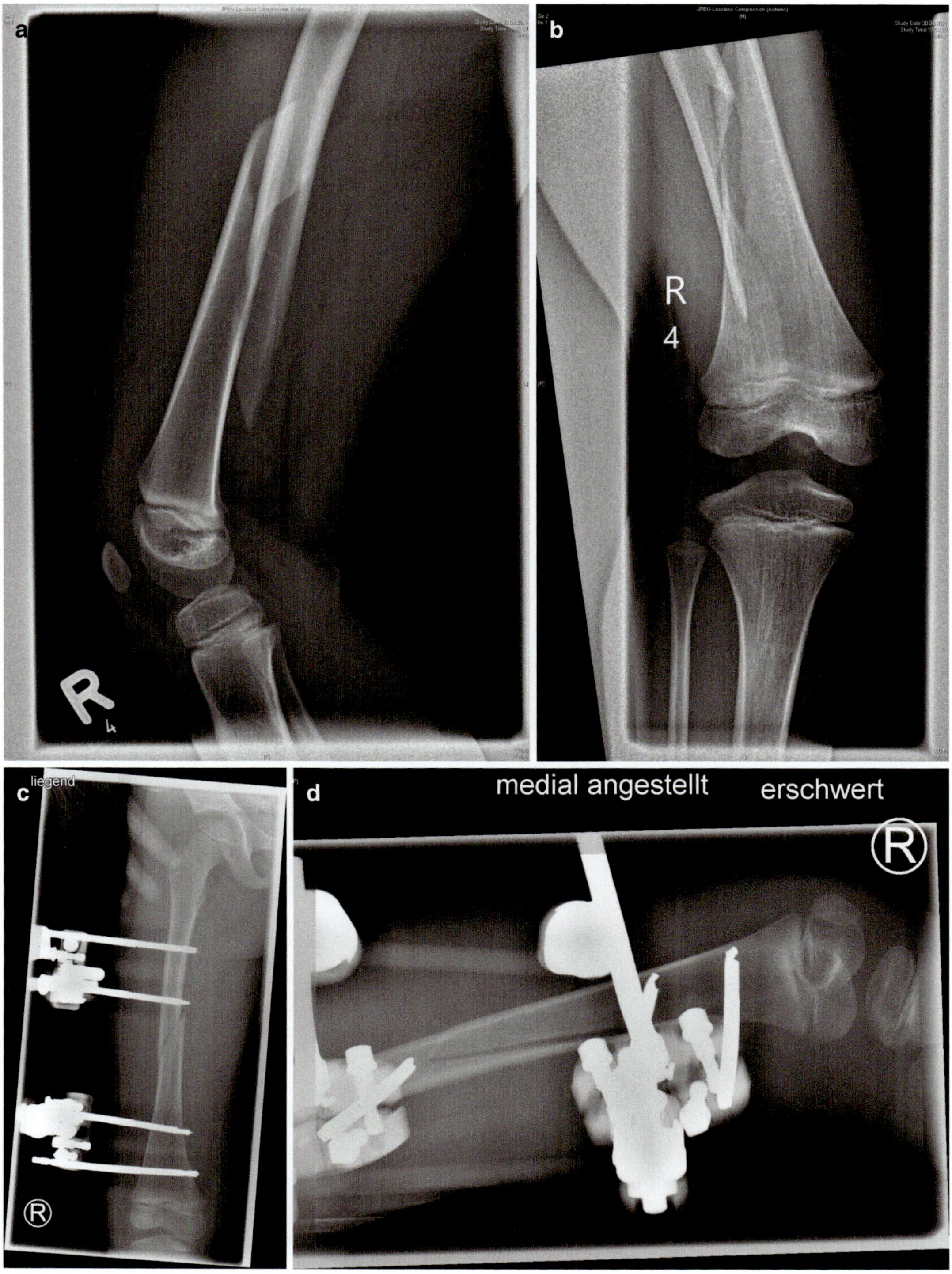

Fig. 12.6 Femur spiral fracture of a boy, fallen due to a dog attack. (**a**, **b**) Trauma image, (**c**, **d**) Initial and definitive stabilization with monoliteral external fixateur

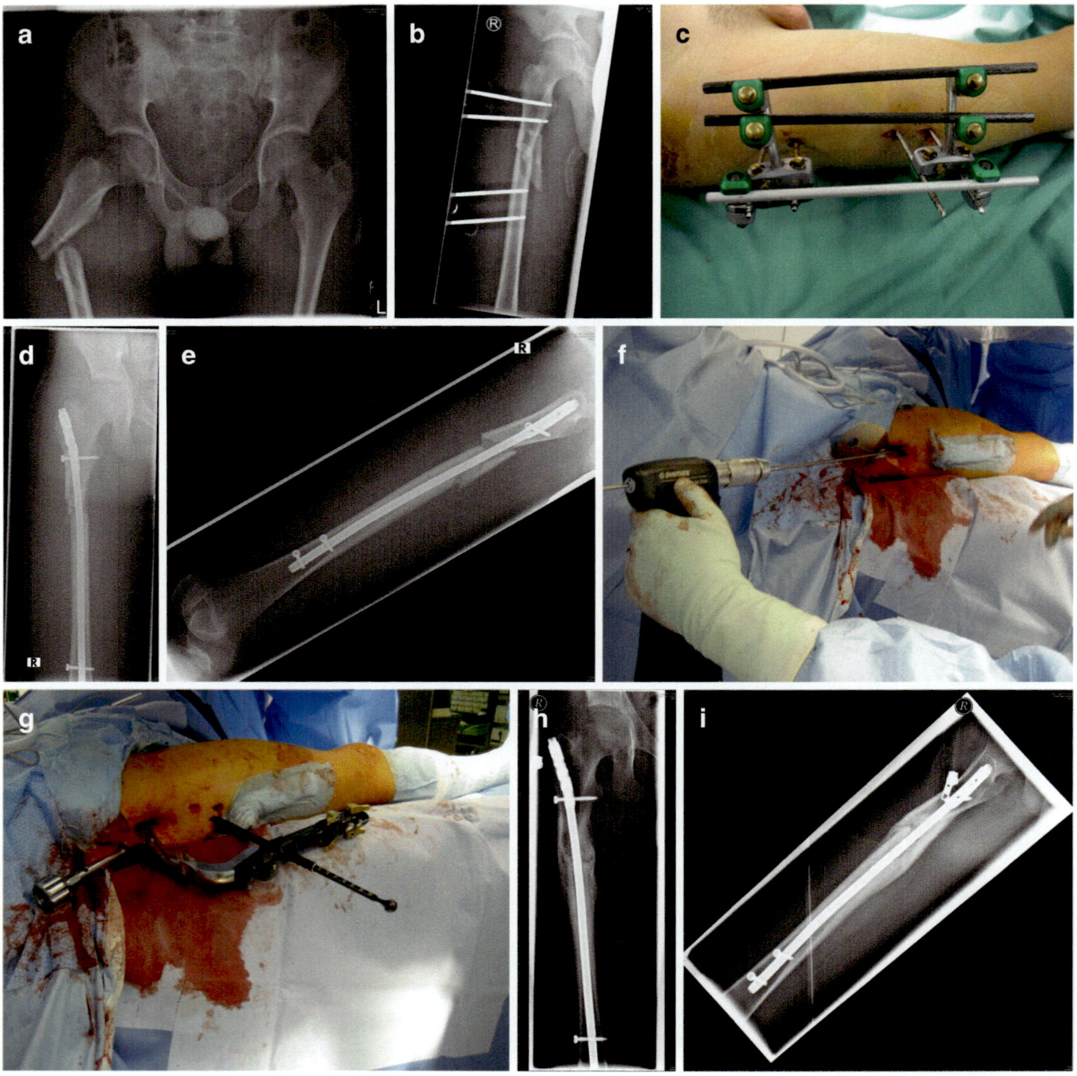

Fig. 12.7 15 Year old boy with multiple injuries and proximal femur fracture. (**a**) Trauma image, (**b**, **c**) Immediate stabilization with external fixateur, (**d–g**) Second operation with removal of external fixateur, reaming and inseration of anterolateral femur nail for adolescdents, (**h**, **i**) Bony healing with nail in situ

fractures close to the hip requiring exact reduction. In adolescents with open growth plates, a special smaller anterolateral intramedullary nail for adolescents (ALFN) can be used, protecting the important growth plates (Fig. 12.7). During growth, there is a risk of femoral head necrosis from vascular disruption when introducing the nail via the piriform fossa. Thus, in adolescents, a lateral approach over the greater trochanter is recommended. In adolescents with completely closed growth plates, a regular locking intramedullary nail can be used.

Subtrochanteric Fracture

Pediatric femoral fractures are mainly classified according to the fracture type and morphology according to the AO and Pediatric Classification. Open and closed injuries must be differentiated regarding soft-tissue damage. For this, the Gustilo and Anderson Classification can be used. The treatement differs in particular related to the age, with infants up to 2 years, when conservative management is still possible, even not always practicle. Above the age of 2 years, basically all treatment options are operative and depend largely on the location and the fracture type. We differentiate proximal, subtrochanteric, fractures (Table 12.1), shaft fractures (Tables 12.2, 12.3 and 12.4) and distal fractures (Table 12.5) of the femur in the following tables and figures. Also the technical aspects are shown in Table 12.6.

Table 12.1 Subtrochanteric femur fractures (Fig. 12.8)

Special features	No spontaneous correction	
Diagnostic assessment	X-ray: AP (+ lateral) Clinical: Usually evident displacement with shortening and rotational deformity	
Goals of treatment/ limits of correction	No axial deviation can be allowed, because no spontaneous correction occurs!	
Primary treatment	Inpatient admission, analgesia	
Conservative therapy		
Indications	Rarely non-displaced fractures <2–3 years	
Procedure	Hip spica cast 4 weeks (Figs. 12.9 and 12.10)	
Follow-up	Wheel chair in small children; sitting once 90° hip flexion is attained, physical therapy for mobilization	
X-ray follow-up	Consolidation check after cast removal	
Return to sports	Symptom-free and full function (up to about 4 weeks after consolidation)	
Operative therapy		
Indications	≥3 years of age or displaced fracture	
Procedure	Closed reduction and retrograde ESIN (Figs. 12.11, 12.12, 12.13, and 12.14). If needed, open reduction and fixed angled plate or a pediatric hip plate might be necessary (Fig. 12.15).	
Follow-up	Stable range of motion, partial weight-bearing with crutches If necessary, gait training with crutches	
X-ray follow-up	Post-operative position check; consolidation check at 4 weeks	
Hardware removal	4–6 months post-operatively (after consolidation check)	
Return to sports	Approximately 6 weeks after consolidation; with free function	
Complications	Rare: Compartment syndrome, cortical perforation by ESIN, excessive callus formation, pseudobursa/infection at the ESIN entry site, secondary displacement with incorrect implant positioning/size, impaired movement of the hip joint initially.	
Growth disturbance	Rare, <10 years lengthening, >10 years shortening	
Follow-up	Twice per year until two years post-trauma with leg-length discrepancy, 1–2 year controls until growth is completed	
Classification	AO: 32-D/1–9.1–3	LiLa: 3.2.s.3(4).0–2.

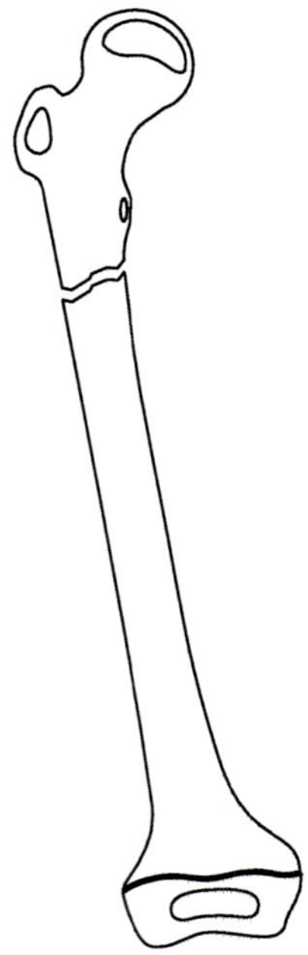

Fig. 12.8 Proximal and subtrochanteric femur fracture

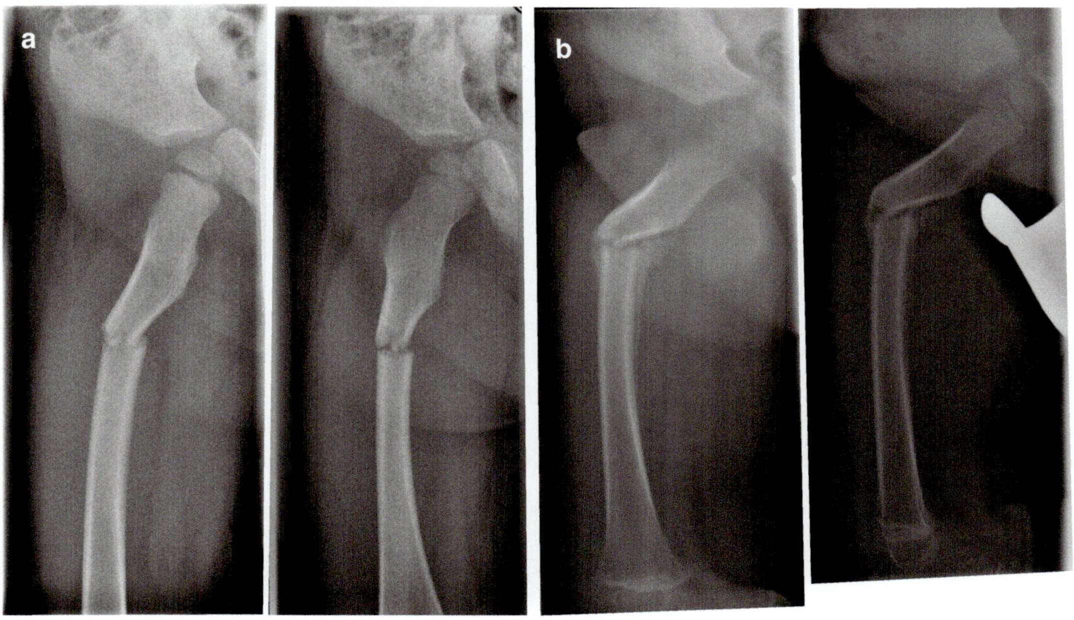

Fig. 12.9 Dislocated proximal femur fracture in a 2 year old boy. Conservative treatment with spica hip cast. To note a high correction potential in this age. (**a**) Trauma image, (**b**) Ongoing callus formation to correct the axis

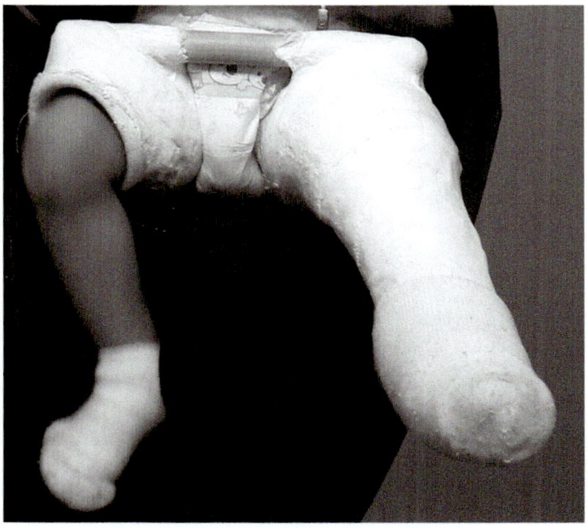

Fig. 12.10 Hip spica cast. For stability it is recommended to fix the proximal other femur as well; optional a woden handle can be included

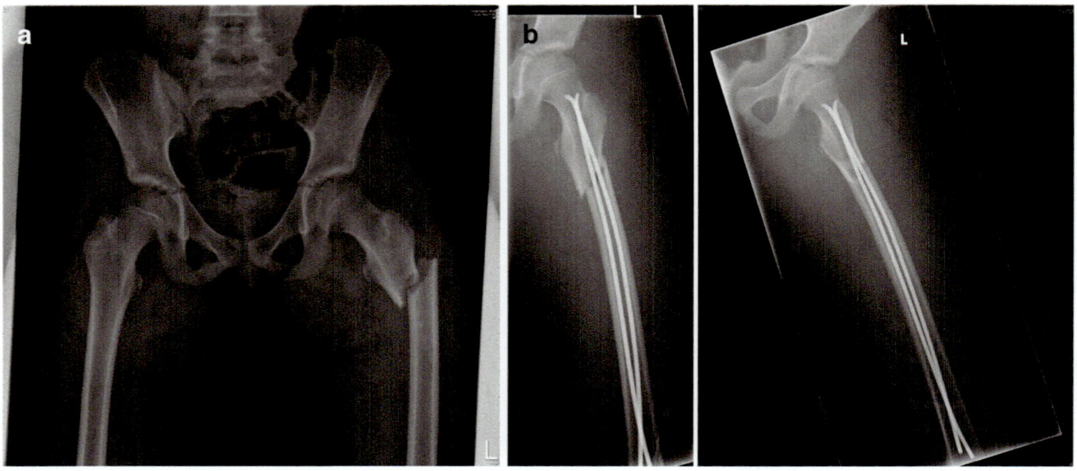

Fig. 12.11 Subtrochanteric femur fracture with short oblique fracture line. (**a**) Trauma image, (**b**) Postoperative x-ray after retrograde ESIN

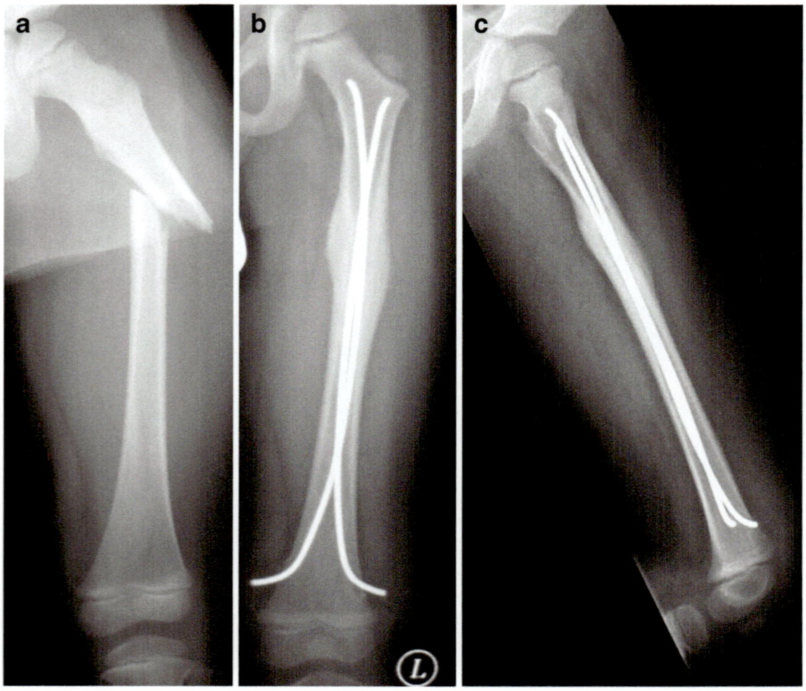

Fig. 12.12 Proximal femur shaft fracture after traffic accident of a 3 year old boy. (**a**) Trauma image, (**b**, **c**) Retrograde ESIN, here already with good callus formation and stability

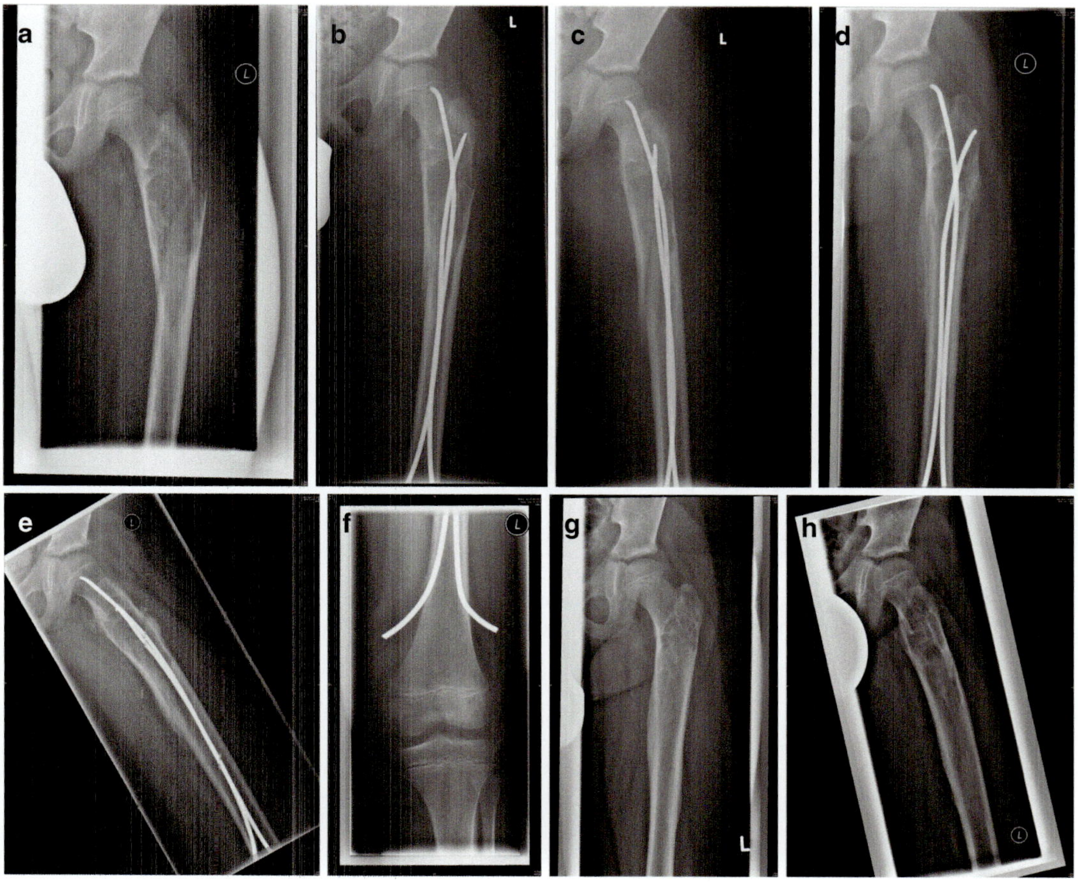

Fig. 12.13 11 Year old boy with fall, without adequate trauma (**a**) Trauma image with juvenile bone cyst, (**b**, **c**) Postoperative after retrograde ESIN, (**d**, **e**, **f**) Subsequent healing with ESIN, (**g**, **h**) Complete healing after metal removal

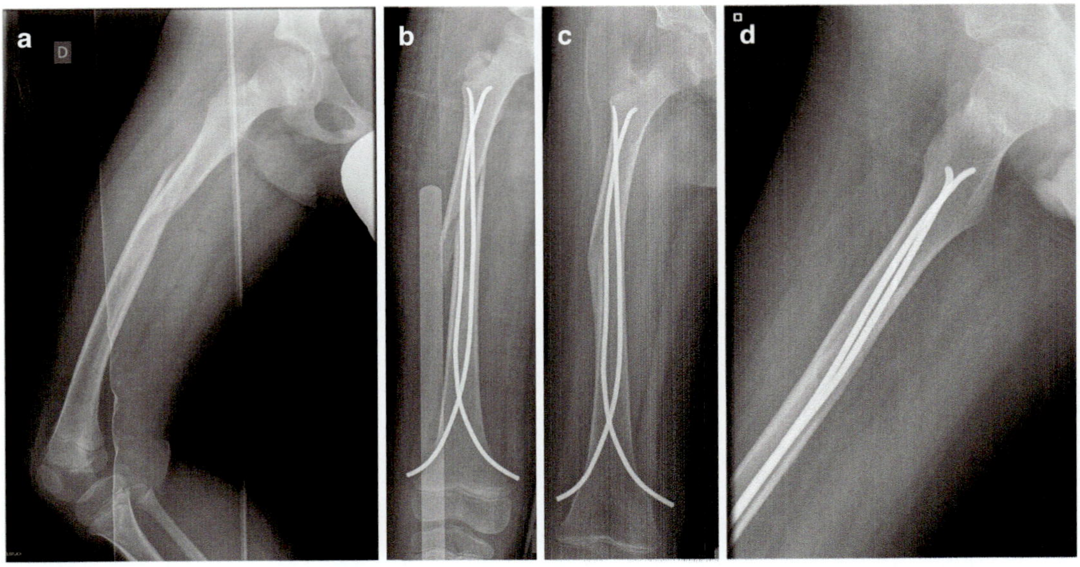

Fig. 12.14 Proximal long oblique fracture of the femur after fall from swing, 8 year old boy. (**a**) Trauma image, (**b**) 5 Days postoperatively, (**c**, **d**) Consolidation x-ray after 8 months prior metal removal

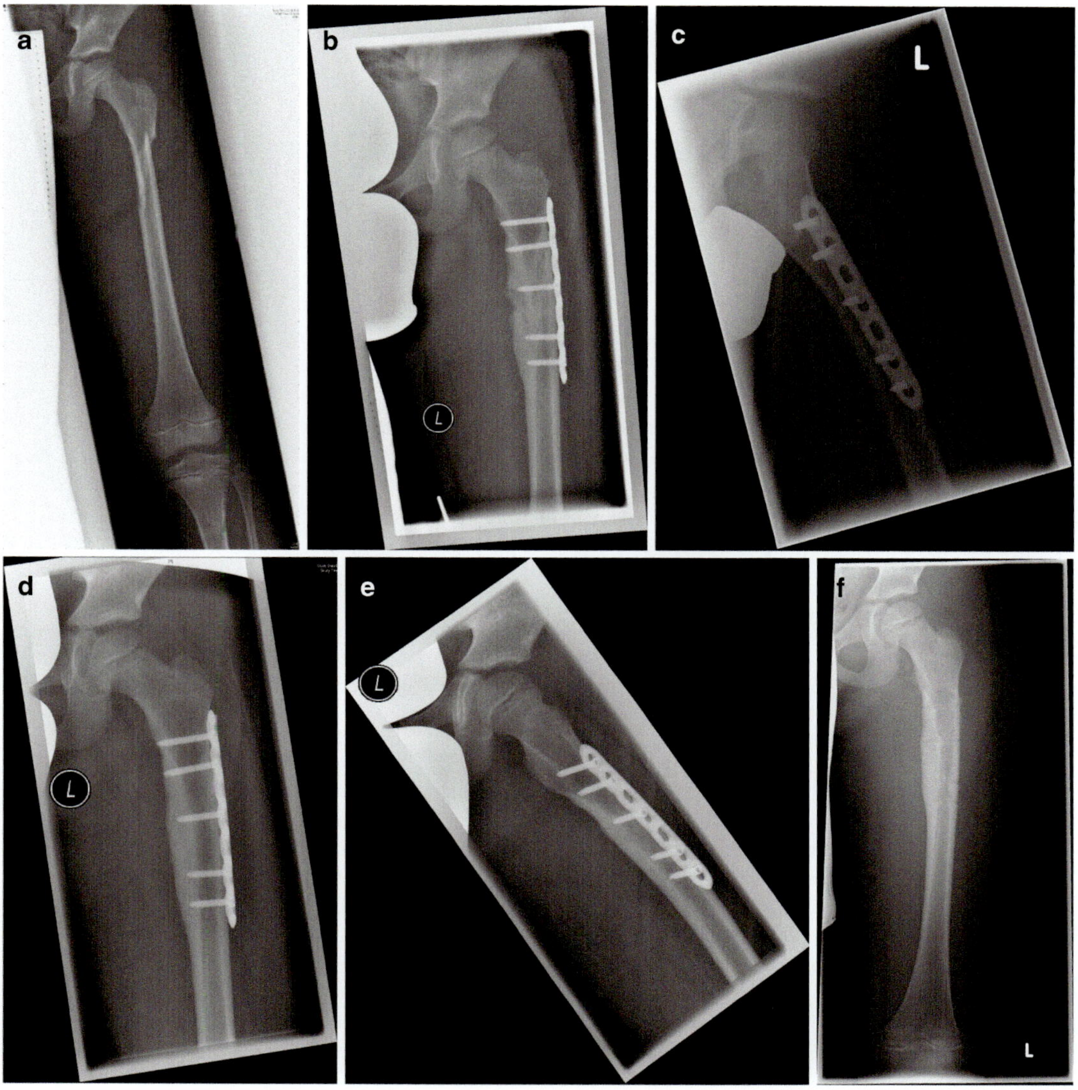

Fig. 12.15 Polytrauma as pedestrian catched by a car; boy, 7 year (**a**) Trauma image, (**b**, **c**) Postoperative proximal plate, (**d**) X-ray of healing, (**e**, **f**) Complete healing after metal removal

Transverse Fractures

Table 12.2 Transverse femoral shaft fractures Fig. 12.16

Special features	30% of femoral shaft fractures, especially direct trauma, usually in the middle third	
Diagnostic assessment	X-ray AP (+ lateral), generally one plane is sufficient Clinical: Usually evident displacement with shortening and rotational deformity	
Goals of treatment/ limits of correction	Rotation deformity 20° for <3 years, 10° for >3 years Varus 20° for <3 years, 10° for >3 years Valgus to 10° Anteversion 10°/retroversion none Ad latus displacement shaft width for <3 years, to ½ shaft width for >3 years	
Primary treatment	Inpatient admission, analgesia, femoral splint as needed	
Conservative therapy		
Indications	<2 years usually conservative, attention to limits of correction	
Procedure	4 weeks of hip spica cast with tolerable deformity2 weeks overhead traction +2 weeks hip spica cast	
Follow-up	Loading as tolerated after cast removal, physical therapy usually not necessary	
X-ray follow-up	Consolidation check at 4 weeks	
Return to sports	Symptom-free and full function (up to about 4 weeks after consolidation)	
Operative therapy		
Indications	>2 years or exceeding limits of correction; but also in smaller children, when the tolerance to a spika cast is not given or the situation not appropriate	
Procedure	Usually closed reduction, open reduction may be required when something (muscle) blocks reduction or excessive fluoroscopy time Retrograde ESIN for fractures of the proximal and middle thirds (Figs. 12.17, 12.18, and 12.19) External fixator: For open fractures or polytrauma if needed (Fig. 12.20)	
Follow-up	With correct implant position, full weight-bearing as tolerated post-operatively Physical therapy usually not necessary (if needed, initial gait training)	
X-ray follow-up	Position check post-operatively; consolidation check at 4–6 weeks and 3–4 months	
Hardware removal	4–6 months post-operatively (after consolidation check)	
Return to sports	Approximately 6 weeks after consolidation	
Complications	Rare: Compartment syndrome, cortical perforation with ESIN, excessive callus formation, pseudobursa/infection at ESIN entry point, painful irritation of the iliotibial band with protruding ESIN, secondary displacement in cases of incorrect implant position/size	
Growth disturbance	Rare, <10 years lengthening, >10 years shortening	
Follow-up	Twice per year until two years post-trauma With leg-length discrepancy, checks every one to two years until growth is completed	
Classification	AO: 32-D/4.1–3	LiLa: 3.2.s.3.0–2.

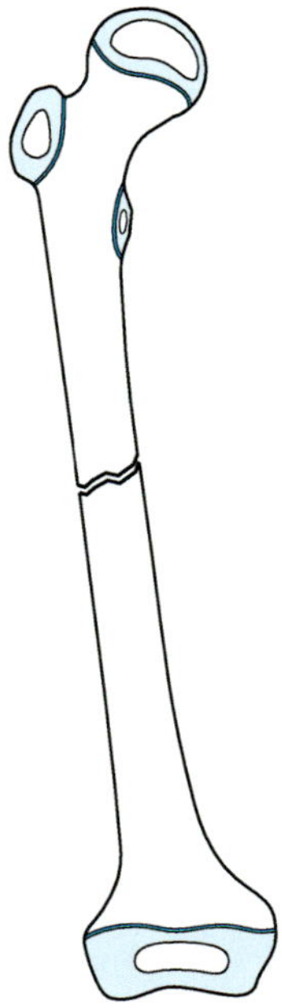

Fig. 12.16 Transverse femur fracture

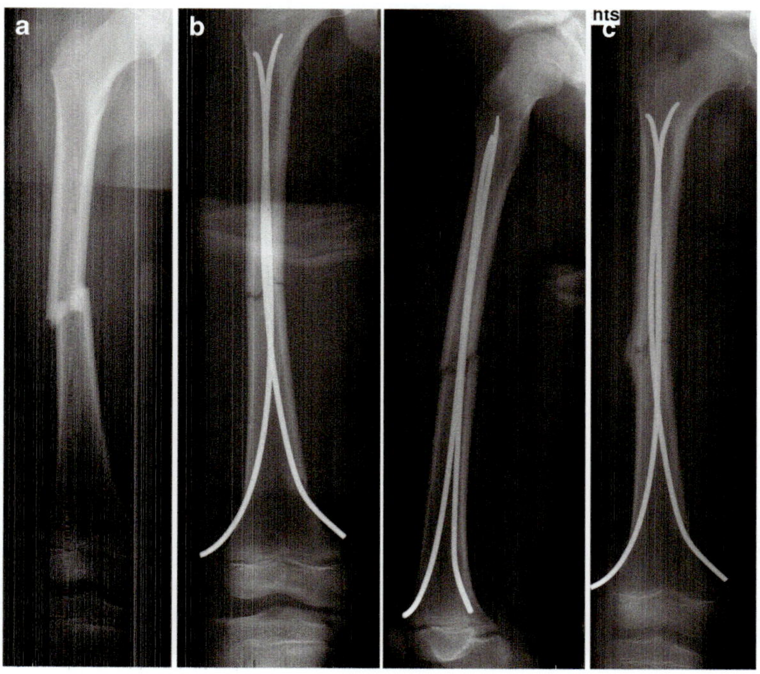

Fig. 12.17 Femur fracture of a 8 year old boy, (**a**) Trauma image, (**b**) After retrograde ESIN, (**c**) Consolidation of fracture with ESIN

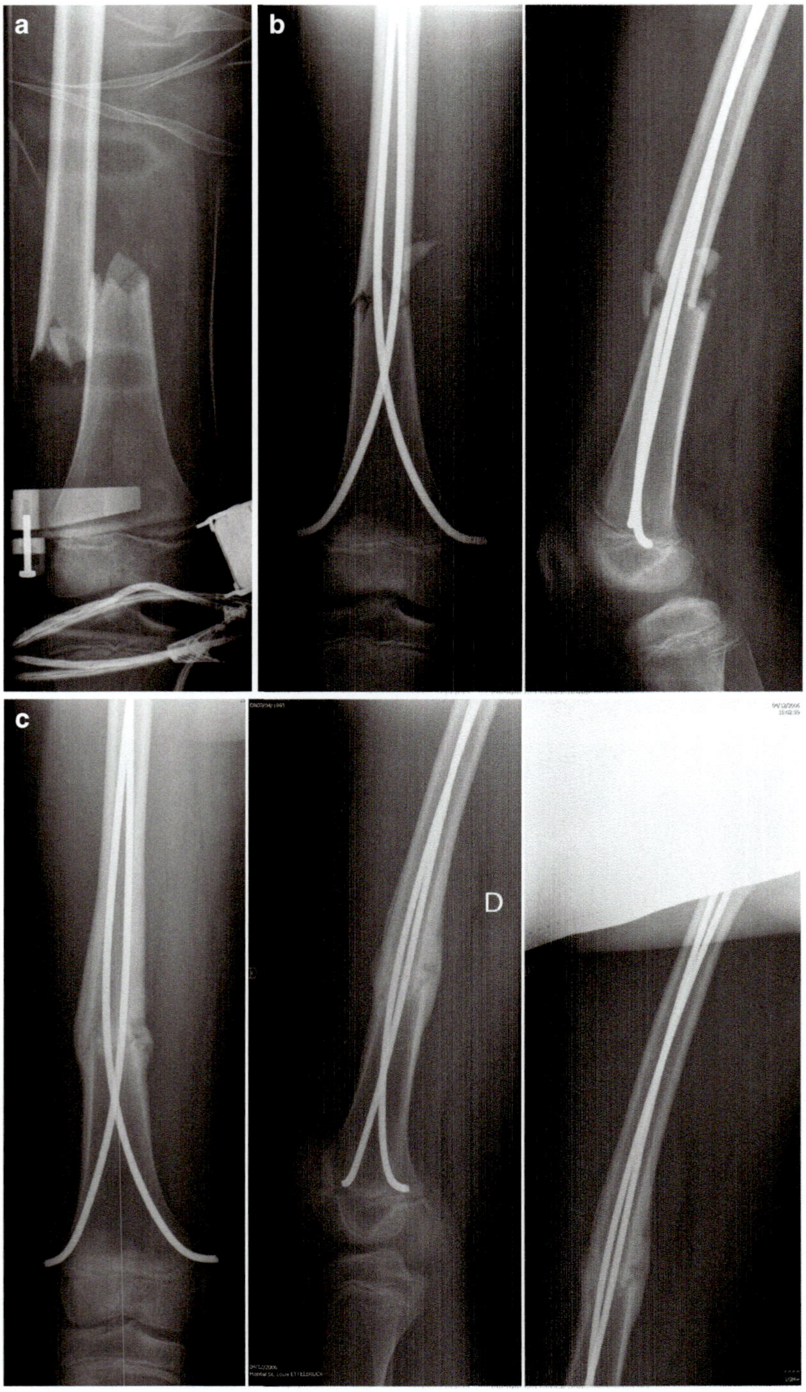

Fig. 12.18 Distal transverse fracture of the femur in a 13 year old girl after bike accident with shortening. (**a**) Trauma image, (**b**) After retrograde ESIN, (**c**) 6 Months with good consolidation

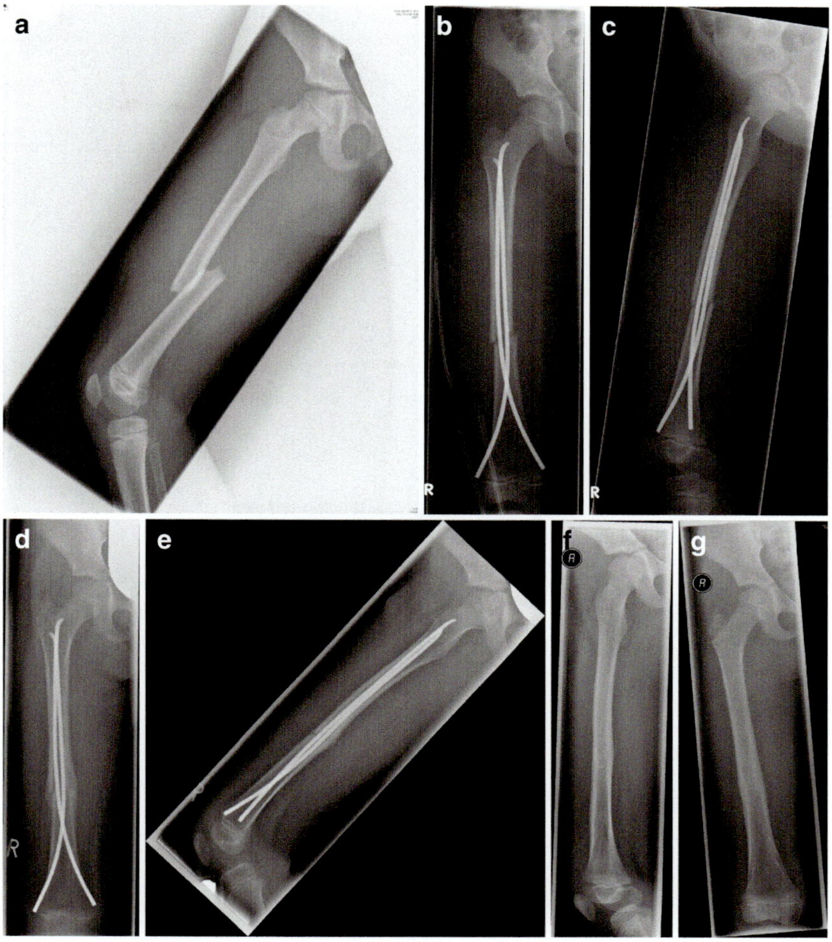

Fig. 12.19 6 Year old girl after fall from tree with transverse femur fracture (**a**) Trauma image, (**b**, **c**) After retrograde ESIN, (**d**, **e**) Consolidation after few weeks, (**f**, **g**) Complete healing after metal removal

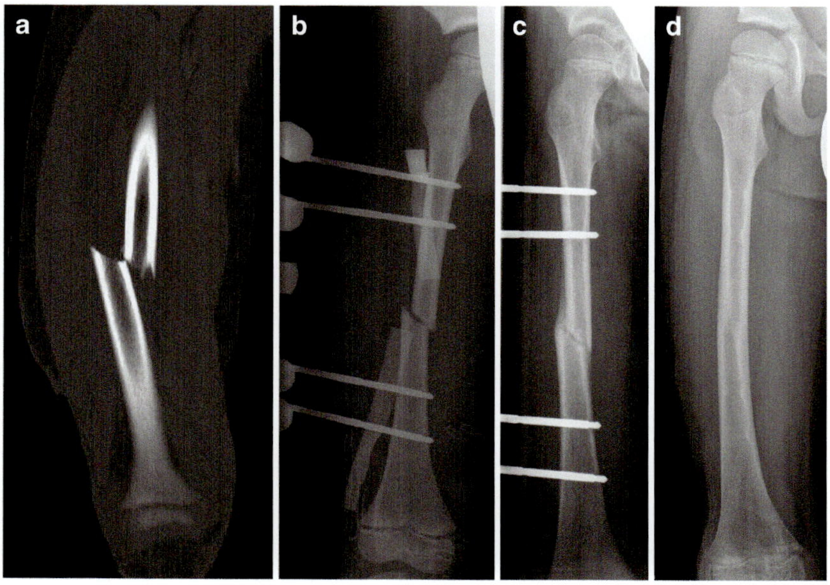

Fig. 12.20 Transverse fracture after overall injury by a truck. (**a**) Trauma image in trauma CT scan, (**b**) Stabilization with fix. ext. (**c**) Healing after 4 months, (**d**) X-ray after 15 months

Oblique and Spiral Fractures

Table 12.3 Oblique femoral shaft fractures (Fig. 12.21)

Special features	Together with spiral fractures account for 49% of all femoral shaft fractures, especially from direct trauma, usually in the mid-third.	
Diagnostic assessment	X-ray AP (+ lateral), second plane is useful to differentiate oblique/spiral fractures and length of the fracture zone, sometimes only feasible under general anesthesia	
Goals of treatment/limits of correction	Rotation deformity 20° for <3 years, 10° for >3 years Varus 20° for <2–3 years, 10° for >2–3 years Valgus to 10° Anteversion 10°/retroversion none Ad latus displacement shaft width for <3 years, to ½ shaft width for >3 years	
Primary treatment	Inpatient admission, analgesia, femoral splint as needed	
Conservative therapy		
Indications	<3 years usually conservative, attention to limits of correction	
Procedure	Over-head extension for a few days until fracture is fixed by cartilage; this is followed by a hip spica cast 3–4 weeks for tolerable deformity 2 weeks overhead traction +2 weeks hip spica cast (Figs. 12.22 and 12.23).	
Follow-up	Loading as tolerated after cast removal, physical therapy usually not necessary	
X-ray follow-up	Consolidation check at 4 weeks	
Return to sports	Approximately 6 weeks after consolidation	
Operative therapy		
Indications	>2 years surgical treatment is indicated	
Procedure	Usually closed reduction Open reduction only in exceptional cases with obstructed reduction or excessive fluoroscopy time Retrograde ESIN for fractures of the proximal and middle thirds (Figs. 12.24 and 12.25) An external fixator (see Fig. 12.6) Or ESIN fixation of the shaft with threaded caps to avoid telescoping are good alternatives for difficult-to-retain, extensive oblique/spiral, and open fractures (see Fig. 12.26)	
Follow-up	Partial weight-bearing 4–6 weeks post-operatively depending on fracture treatment Physical therapy is usually not necessary, initial gait training as needed	
X-ray follow-up	Position check post-operative and at 4–6 weeks; consolidation check at 3–4 months	
Hardware removal	ESIN removed after consolidation check 4–6 months post-surgery, external fixator after consolidation check at approximately 8–12 weeks.	
Return to sports	Approximately 8 weeks after consolidation	
Complications	Leg shortening due to lack of support for oblique/spiral fractures treated with ESIN Rare: Compartment syndrome, cortical perforation with ESIN, excessive callus formation, pseudobursa/infection at ESIN entry point, painful irritation of the iliotibial band with protruding ESIN, secondary displacement in cases of incorrect implant position/size	
Growth disturbance	Rare, <10 years lengthening, >10 years shortening	
Follow-up	Twice per year until two years post-trauma with leg-length discrepancy, controls every one to two years until growth is completed	
Classification	AO: 32-D/5.1–3	LiLa: 3.2.s.3.0–2.

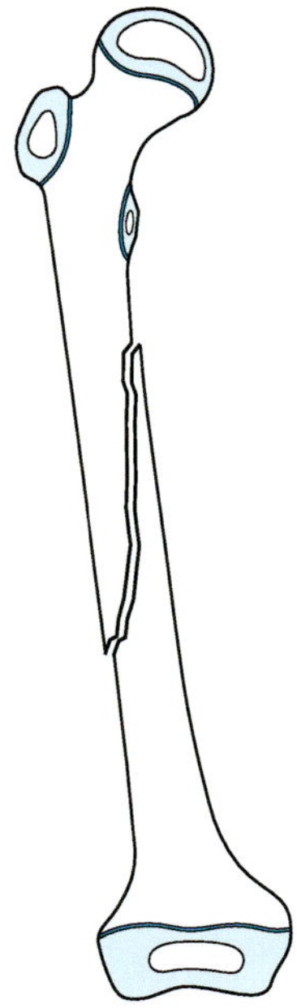

Fig. 12.21 Oblique fracture of the femur

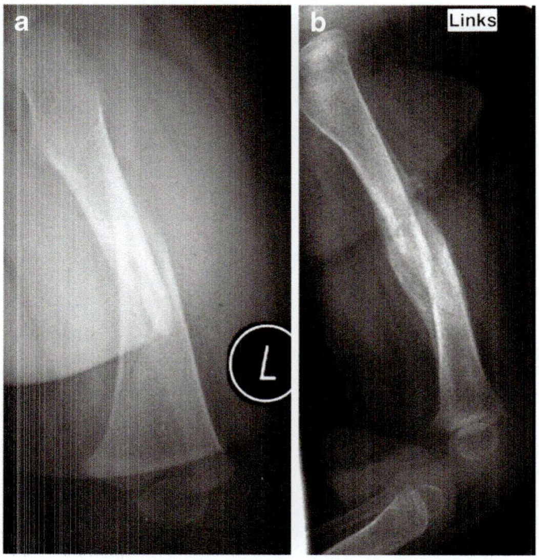

Fig. 12.22 Battered child, 7 months old. (**a**) Trauma image, (**b**) Good callus formation in overhead-extension and conservative therapy

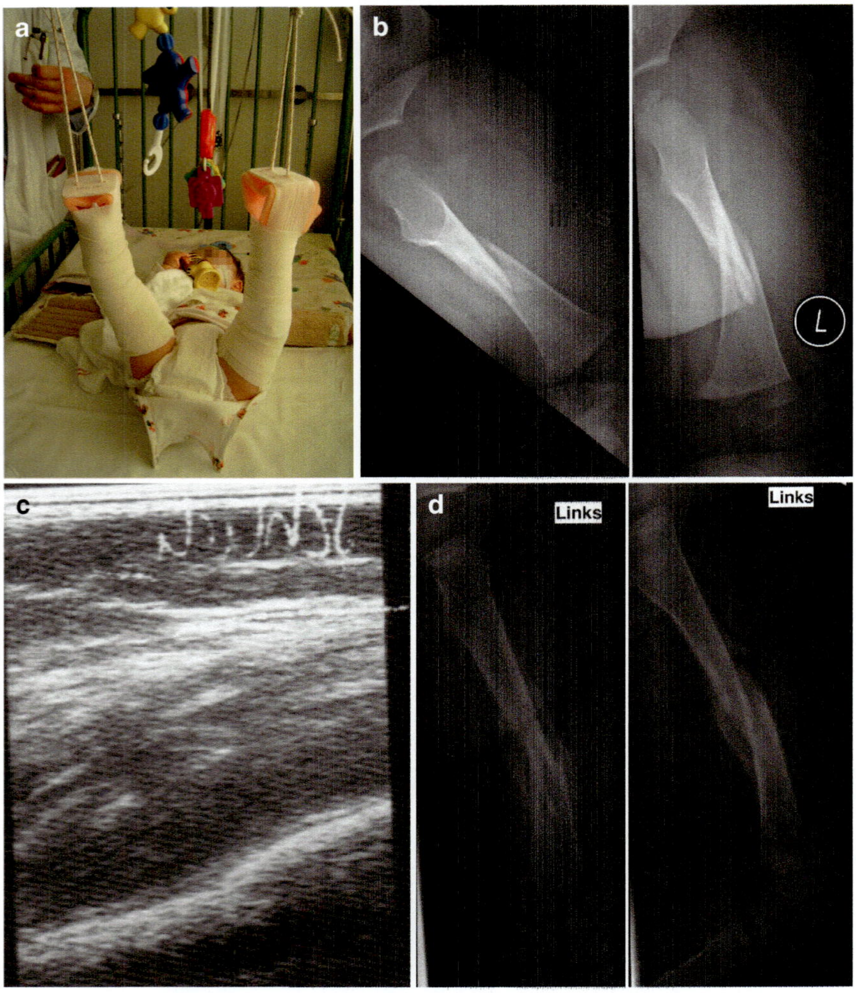

Fig. 12.23 Long spiral fracture of the femur in at 18 months. (**a**) Overhead extension, (**b**) Trauma image, (**c**) Callus formation with ultrasound, (**d**) Ongoing callus formation in good axis for the age

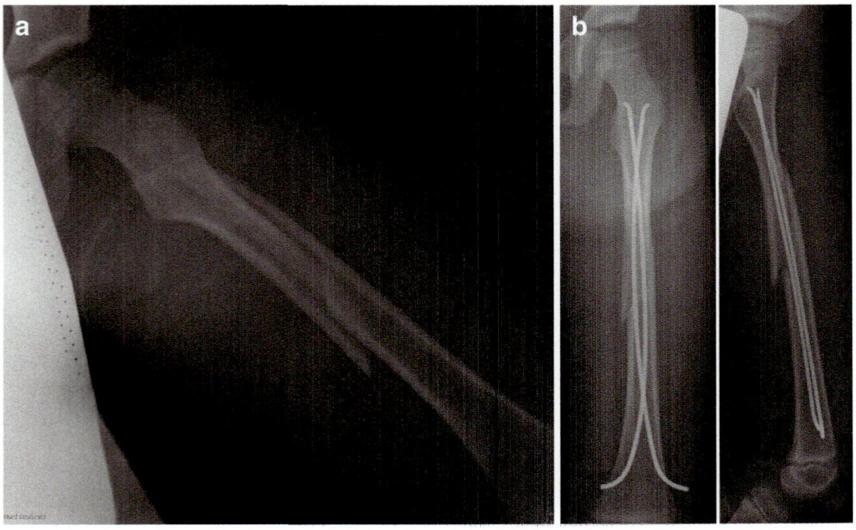

Fig. 12.24 Femur shaft fracture, oblique in a 6 year old boy (**a**) Trauma image, (**b**) Stabilization with retrograde ESIN

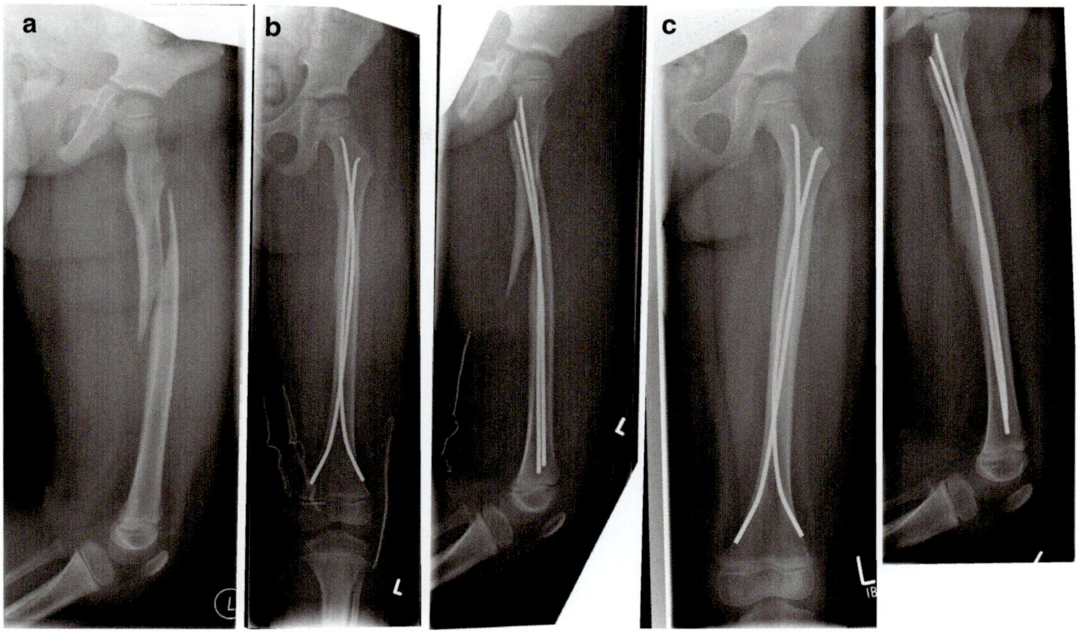

Fig. 12.25 Long spiral fracture in a 4 year old girl. (**a**) Trauma image, (**b**) Retrograde ESIN after closed reduction with control of axis, length and rotation, (**c**) Good bony healing

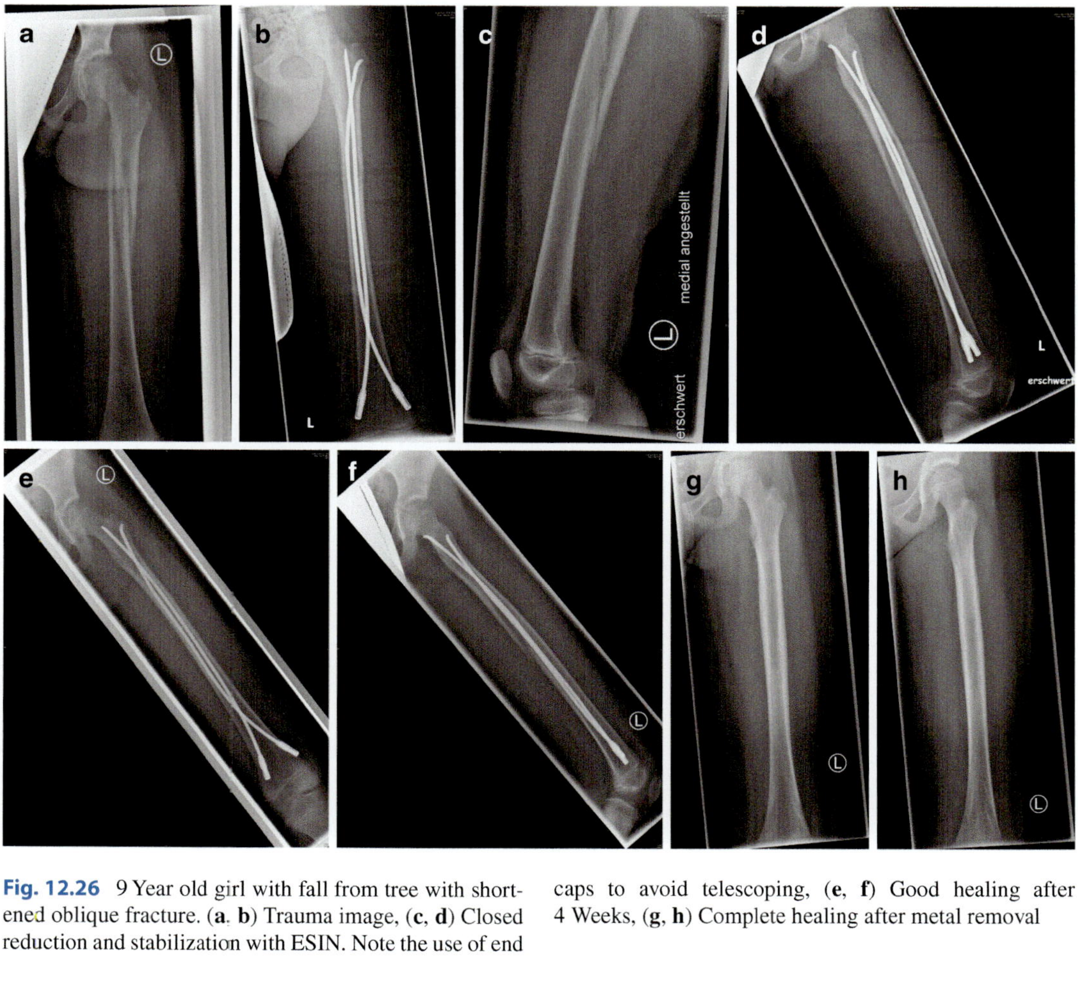

Fig. 12.26 9 Year old girl with fall from tree with shortened oblique fracture. (**a**, **b**) Trauma image, (**c**, **d**) Closed reduction and stabilization with ESIN. Note the use of end caps to avoid telescoping, (**e**, **f**) Good healing after 4 Weeks, (**g**, **h**) Complete healing after metal removal

Compound Femur Fractures

Table 12.4 Complex femoral shaft fractures (Fig. 12.27)

Special features	Approximately 20% of femoral shaft fractures: oblique/spiral fractures with wedge, multifragment fractures, segmental fractures Usually direct trauma, mostly in the middle third	
Diagnostic assessment	X-ray AP (+ lateral) Usually evident displacement with shortening and rotational deformity	
Goals of treatment/limits of correction	Rotation deformity 20° for <3 years, 10° for >3 years Varus 20° for <3 years, 10° for >3 years Valgus to 10° Anteversion 10°/retroversion none Ad latus displacement shaft width for <3 years, to ½ shaft width for >3 years	
Primary treatment	Inpatient admission, analgesia, femoral splint as needed	
Conservative therapy		
Indications	<2 years usually conservative, attention to limits of correction	
Procedure	2 weeks overhead traction +2 weeks hip spica cast	
Follow-up	Loading as tolerated after cast removal, physical therapy if necessary	
X-ray follow-up	Consolidation check at 4 weeks	
Return to sports	Approximately 6 weeks after consolidation	
Operative therapy		
Indications	Surgery is indicted >2 years, usually closed reduction; open reduction is only necessary in exceptional cases	
Procedure	External fixator: Method of choice particularly in polytrauma and for open fractures (Fig. 12.28) Rare: ESIN because of lack of support not always possible (Fig. 12.29) alternative: Fixation of the intramedullary nail with threaded caps or locking screws (Fig. 12.30) Rare: Bridging, biological plate fixation or adolescent lateral locking nail.	
Follow-up	Post-operative depending on fracture type, partial loading for 4–6 weeks until visible callus Physical therapy is usually not necessary, initial gait training as needed	
X-ray follow-up	Position checks post-operative and at 4–6 weeks; at 3–4 week consolidation check	
Hardware removal	At 8–10 weeks for external fixator; at 4–6 months post-operatively for ESIN (after consolidation check)	
Return to sports	Approximately 8 weeks after consolidation	
Complications	Rare: Compartment syndrome, cortical perforation by ESIN, excessive callus formation, pseudobursa/infection at the ESIN entry site, secondary displacement with incorrect implant positioning/size, through telescoping of ESIN, pin infections of external fixator Secondary shortening/rotation deformities in cases of insufficient support	
Growth disturbance	Rare, <10 years lengthening, >10 years shortening	
Follow-up	Twice per year until two years post-trauma With leg-length discrepancy, 1–2 year controls until growth is completed	
Classification	AO: 32-D/4(5).3	LiLa: 3.2.s.4.1–2.

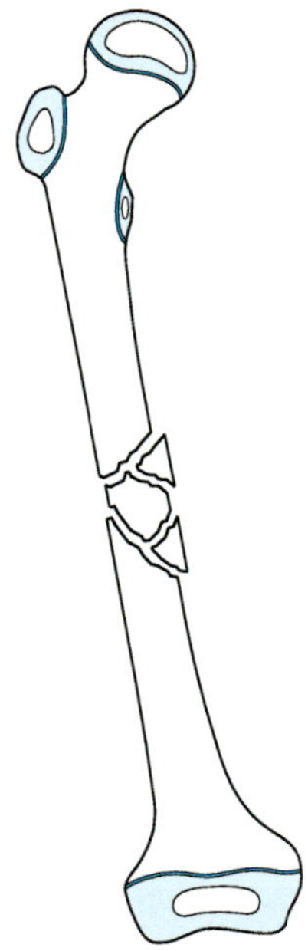

Fig. 12.27 Compound fracture of the femur

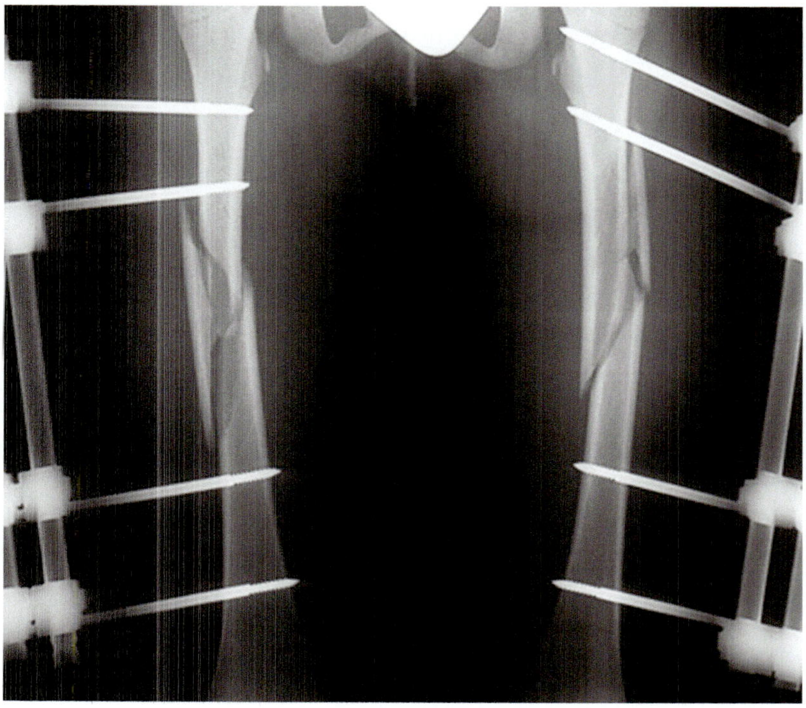

Fig. 12.28 Bilateral femur fracture with wedge fracture and stabilization with external fixateur

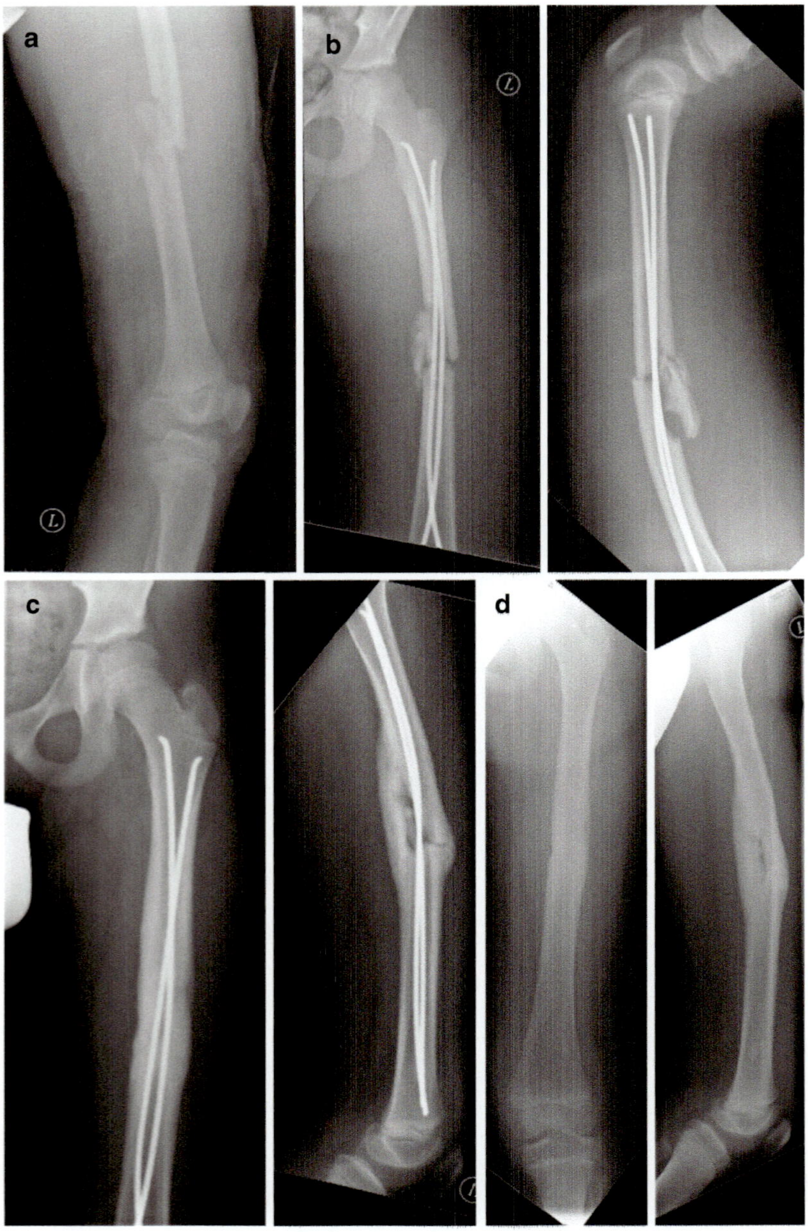

Fig. 12.29 Multi-fragmented femur fracture in a 11 year old boy. (**a**) Trauma image, (**b**) Retrograde ESIN, but not well operated due to too small nails and insufficient reduction, (**c**) Bony healing, (**d**) Femur after metal removal with suboptimal healing which might no more correct in a 11 year old boy

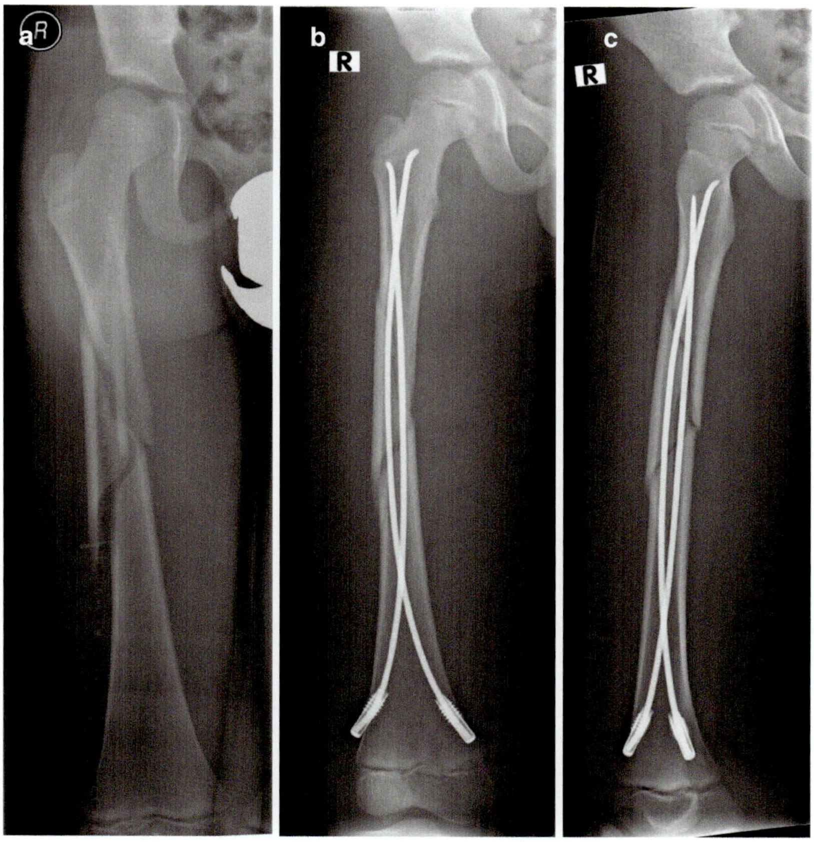

Fig. 12.30 Instable compound fracture of the femur with large wedge fragment in a 7 year old boy. (**a**) Trauma image, (**b**, **c**) Reduction and retrograde ESIN to avoid shortening of the leg

Distal Femur Fractures

Table 12.5 Distal, supracondylar, femoral fractures (Fig. 12.31)

Special features	Rare, extra-articular
Diagnostic assessment	X-ray AP + lateral (femur with hip and knee joints) Angiography if suspected vascular lesion
Goals of treatment/limits of correction	No axial deviation No recurvatum
Primary treatment	Femoral plaster splint, medical analgesia as needed Neurovascular injury: Emergent indication
Conservative therapy	
Indications	Compression fracture and non-displaced supracondylar fracture usually conservative (Figs. 12.32 and 12.33)
Procedure	Femoral cast for 4 weeks
Follow-up	Loading as tolerated after cast removal, physical therapy usually not necessary
X-ray follow-up	Not necessary for compression fractures, clinically: Painless callus For compression fractures consolidation check only at 4 weeks; displaced supracondylar fractures: Position check at 8 days; consolidation check at 4 weeks (without cast)
Return to sports	With symmetrical musculature; approximately 4–6 weeks after consolidation
Operative therapy	
Indications	Unstable displaced fractures, obstructed reduction, concomitant injuries
Procedure	Usually closed reduction under general anesthesia Open reduction in cases of severe displacement, injured soft-tissues, concomitant injuries; neurovascular injuries Antegrade ESIN if possible Descending ESIN if possible, occasionally with short time ext. fixation to control rotational stability (Fig. 12.34) External fixation for definitive treatment (Fig. 12.35) Crossed K-wire fixation, percutaneous plus femoral plaster splint (rather in epiphyseolysis) Alternative: External fixators for soft-tissue damage, polytrauma, "floating knee"; K-wire fixation in small infants (Fig. 12.36) In adolescence: a bridging plate fixing the growth plate for 3 months is possible (Fig. 12.37).
Follow-up	ESIN, external fixator: Free range of motion; partial weight-bearing for approximately 4 weeks K-wire spiking: Femoral cast for 4–5 weeks non-weight-bearing, loading as tolerated after cast removal Physical therapy usually not necessary.
X-ray follow-up	Post-operative position check; consolidation check at 5 weeks without cast
Hardware removal	K-wires: 4–5 weeks post-operatively (after consolidation); outpatient ESIN: 4–6 months post-operatively External fixator: 4–6 weeks post-operatively
Return to sports	With symmetrical musculature; approximately 4–6 weeks after consolidation 4–6 weeks after consolidation
Complications	Vascular lesion after posterior dislocation (femoral vessels) Caution: Additional ligament/meniscus injuries of the knee joint
Growth disturbance	Always femoral overgrowth—discrete leg length increase Growth retardation: Rare
Follow-up	½ year to 2 years Follow-up of leg-length discrepancies and axial deviation X-ray follow-up for axial deviation (to exclude growth plate bridging)
Classification	AO: 33-M/2(3).1–3 LiLa: 3.3.s.2–4.0–2.

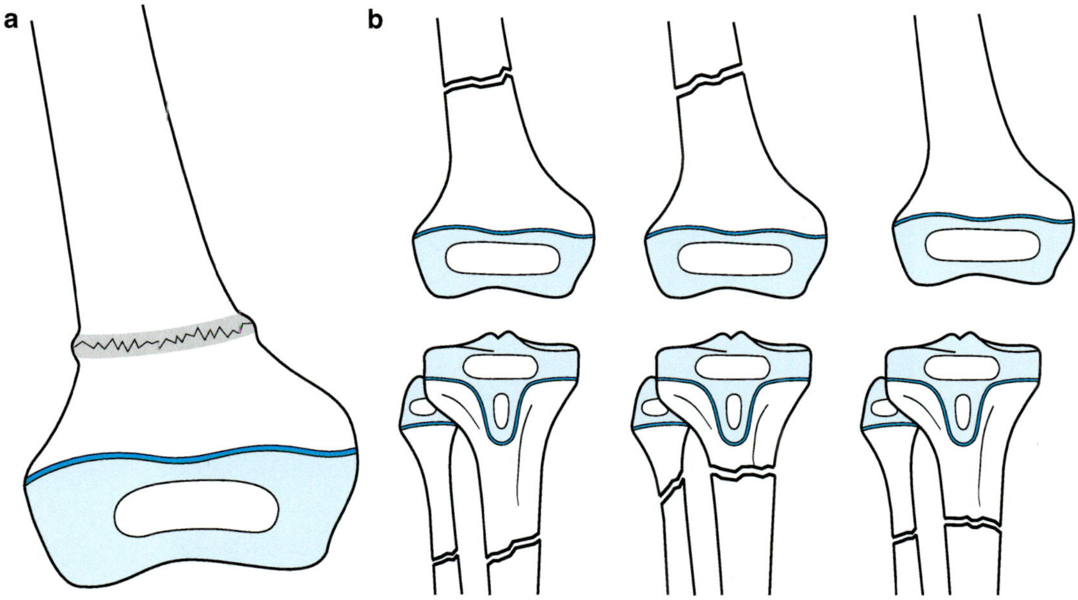

Fig. 12.31 Fractures of the distal femur (**a**) Stable compression fracture (**b**) Transverse fracture

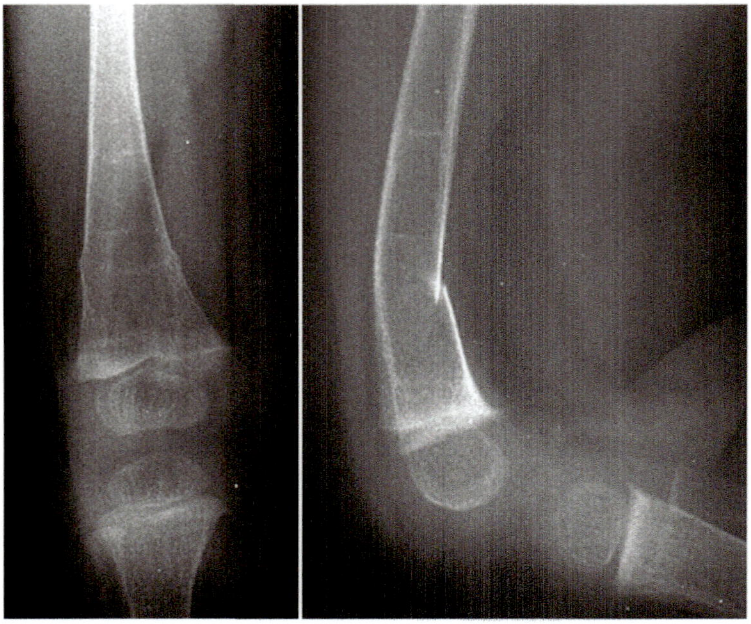

Fig. 12.32 Distal compression fracture of the femur; stable conservative treatment

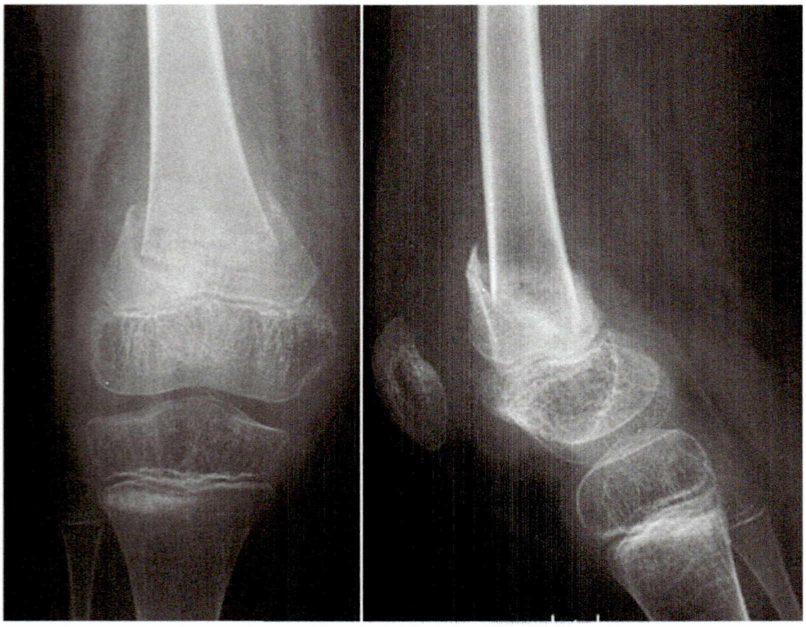

Fig. 12.33 Distal femur fracture with slight displacement. Conservative treatment in the range of tolerance

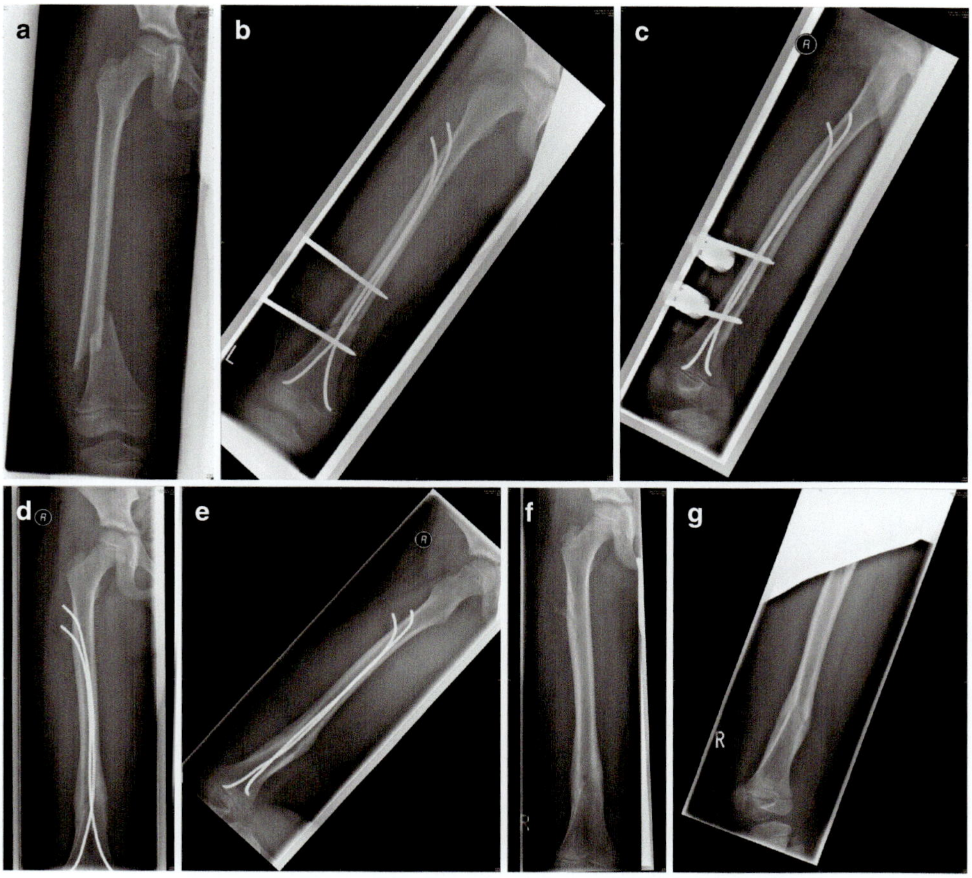

Fig. 12.34 Distal femur fracture of a 7 year old boy after falling in stones. (**a**) Trauma image, (**b**, **c**) Postoperative with ESIN and for 2 weeks ESIN to enhance stability and length (**d**, **e**) Healing with ESIN (**f**, **g**) Final healing in good anatomy

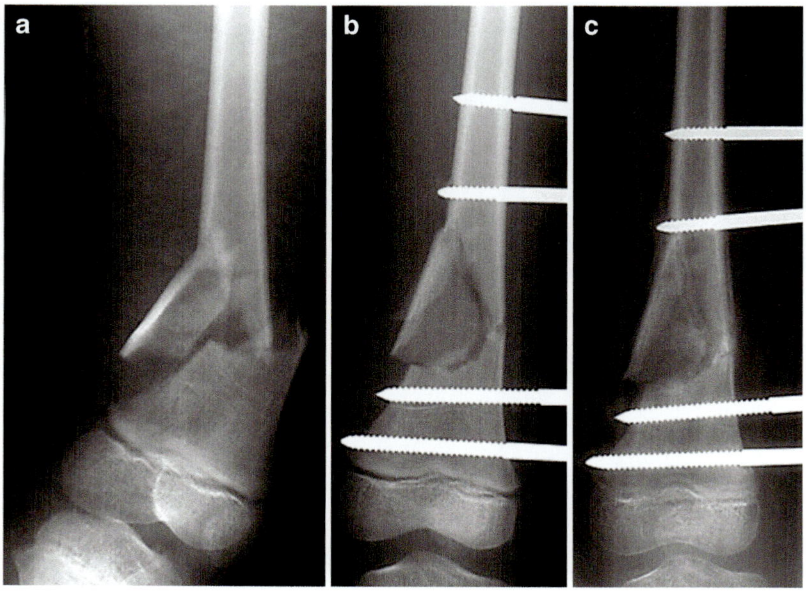

Fig. 12.35 Distal compound fracture of a 9 year old boy. (**a**) Trauma image, (**b**, **c**) Stabilization with Fix. ext.

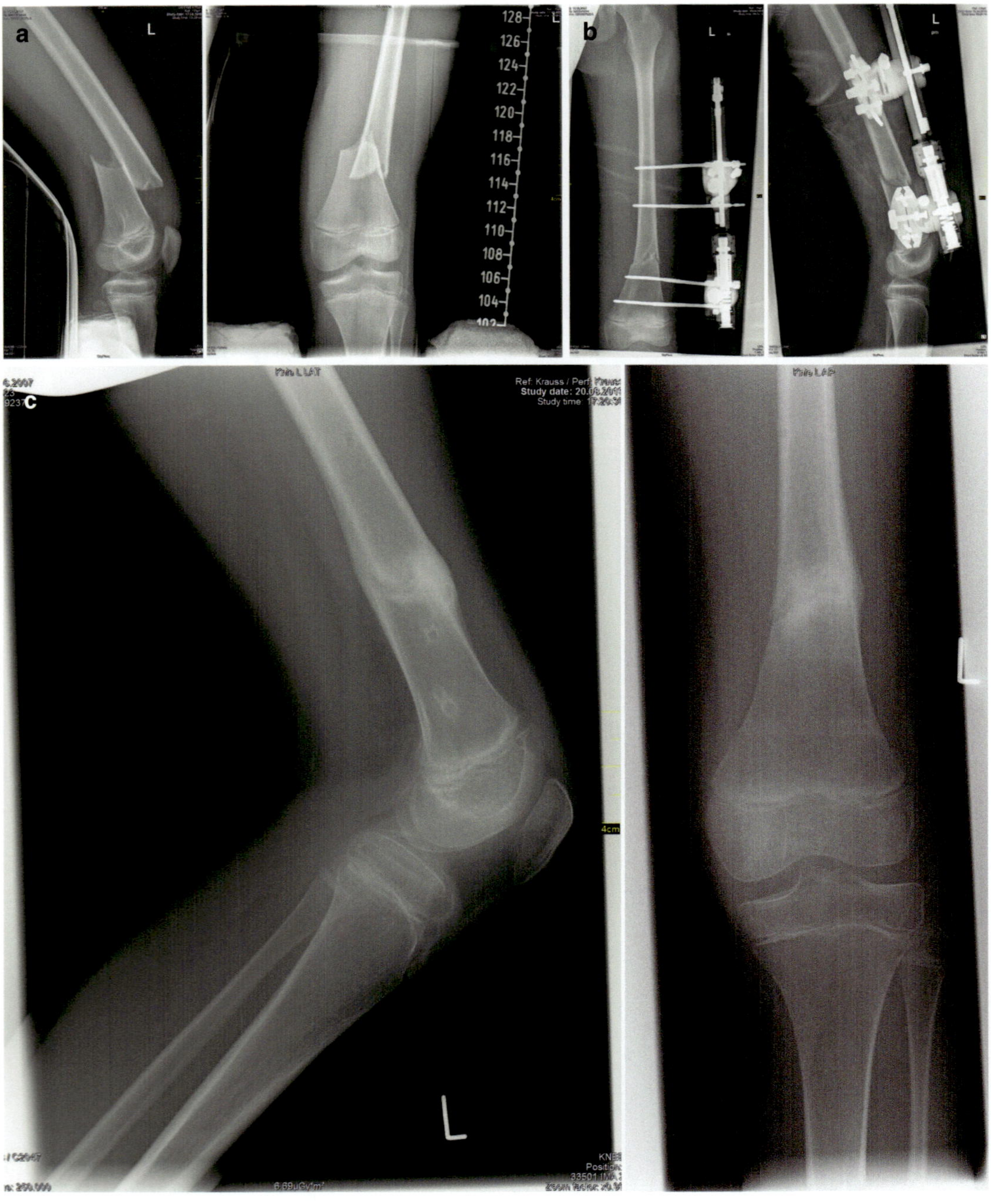

Fig. 12.36 Distal transverse femur fractures in a 12 year old by (a) Trauma image, (b) After reduction and external fixation, (c) After 4 months healing

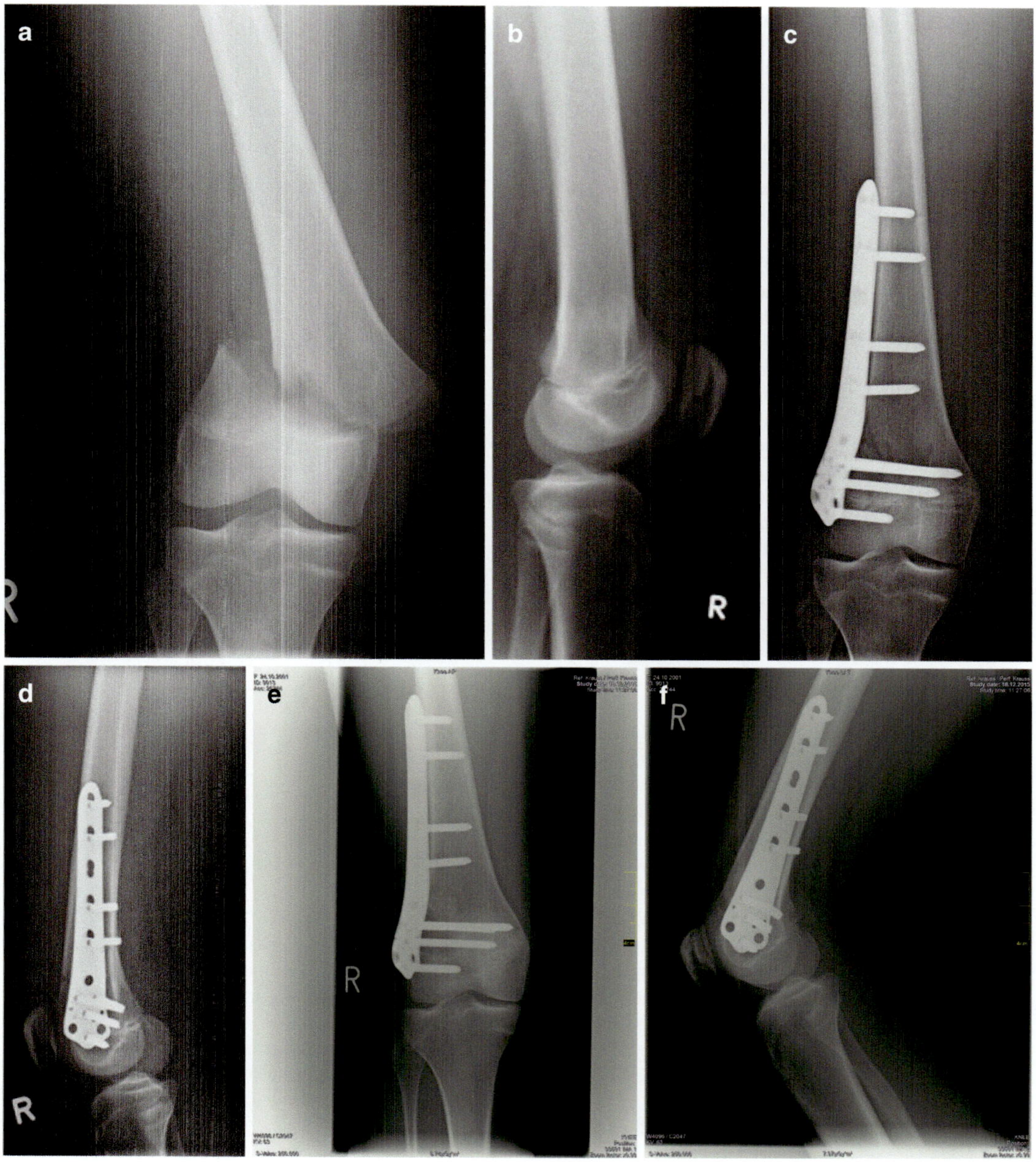

Fig. 12.37 Distal fracture in a 13 year old girl with closing growth plate. (**a**) Trauma image, (**b**, **c**) Stabilization with Plate jumping over the growth plate, (**d**, **e**) Complete healing, however, with closed growth plate now and no impairment, (**f**)

Technical Tipps Femur Fractures

Table 12.6 Technical tips for femur fracture treatment

Technical aspects	Femoral fracture
Conservative therapy	
	Overhead traction Overhead traction with adhesive plaster bandage and elastic wrapping for approximately 3–4 weeks or 2 weeks overhead traction and switch to hip spica cast for another 2 weeks Traction with approximately one third of body weight, buttocks floating distally exact length and rotation checks are impossible and also unnecessary Regular checks of the arrangement are needed Occasional light sedation/analgesia required for placement Can be done if necessary on an outpatient basis, but usually as an inpatient Hip spica cast Fig. 12.38 Goal: Axial alignment, up to 10 mm shortening is tolerable If needed, placement under general anesthesia for reduction After 2 weeks of overhead traction, another 2 weeks in hip spica cast Circular cast from iliac crest extending to and including the foot of the fractured leg and to above the knee of the contralateral leg; alternatively only the pelvic ring Newborns: 90°/90° position of knee and hip Small children: 50°/50° position of knee and hip Minimal abduction to avoid external rotation deformity Adequate freeing of the perineum With the cast, sometimes a wooden support is needed across the anterior aspect of the pelvis/thigh Regular cast checks are necessary
Operative therapy	
Material	ESIN Elastic titanium nail; diameter 2–4 mm (1/3 of the canal diameter) External fixator (various fixator systems available)
Positioning	Supine, draped above the hips, leg freely moveable
Special explanation	Rotation deformity, leg-length discrepancy Secondary displacement ESIN: Irritation/infection (common: Pseudobursa) over the nail end, flexion limitations External fixator: Pin infection
Operative principle	Mostly, retrograde ESIN is the method of choice (Fig. 12.39). For fractures of the distal third of the femur or the distal metaphysis, descending monolateral nail technique is preferable (Fig. 12.40a and 12.40b). Fixation of metaphyseal fractures with nailing is based on other biomechanical principles than those of shaft fracture fixation. Proper internal support must be ensured to stabilize the nail ends and thus, the metaphyseal fragment. The following deviations from standard technique need to be considered. For the descending approach, the monolateral entry sites are subtrochanteric and anterolateral. There is approximately 1–2 cm vertical and 0.5–1 cm lateral separation between them. Skin incisions are sufficiently long to choose. To achieve proper internal tension, i.e., three-point support, one of the nails must be pre-bent to an S-shape so that tension is at the level of the fracture zone. Insert the first pre-shaped nail, then reduce the fracture with the nail and stabilize primarily. Insert the S-shaped nail. After initial contact with the opposing cortex, the nail should be turned 180° and the preload possibly increased. The nail should be advanced to the epiphyseal plate and the nail tips aligned so that they diverge. External fixator 2 (−3) fixator pins each proximally and distally with 2 finger distance to the fracture (Fig. 12.41). The pins are positioned dorsolaterally along the intermuscular septum (muscle preservation), usually two parallel-running connecting rods Avoid overcorrection of length Adequate splitting of the iliotibial band Clinical rotation check intraoperatively Daily pin care by the patient or parent (removal of scabs, shower allowed)
Hardware removal	ESIN At 4–6 months under general anesthesia External fixator After X-ray (with sufficient callus formation at approximately 6–8 weeks), in individual cases also possible as outpatient

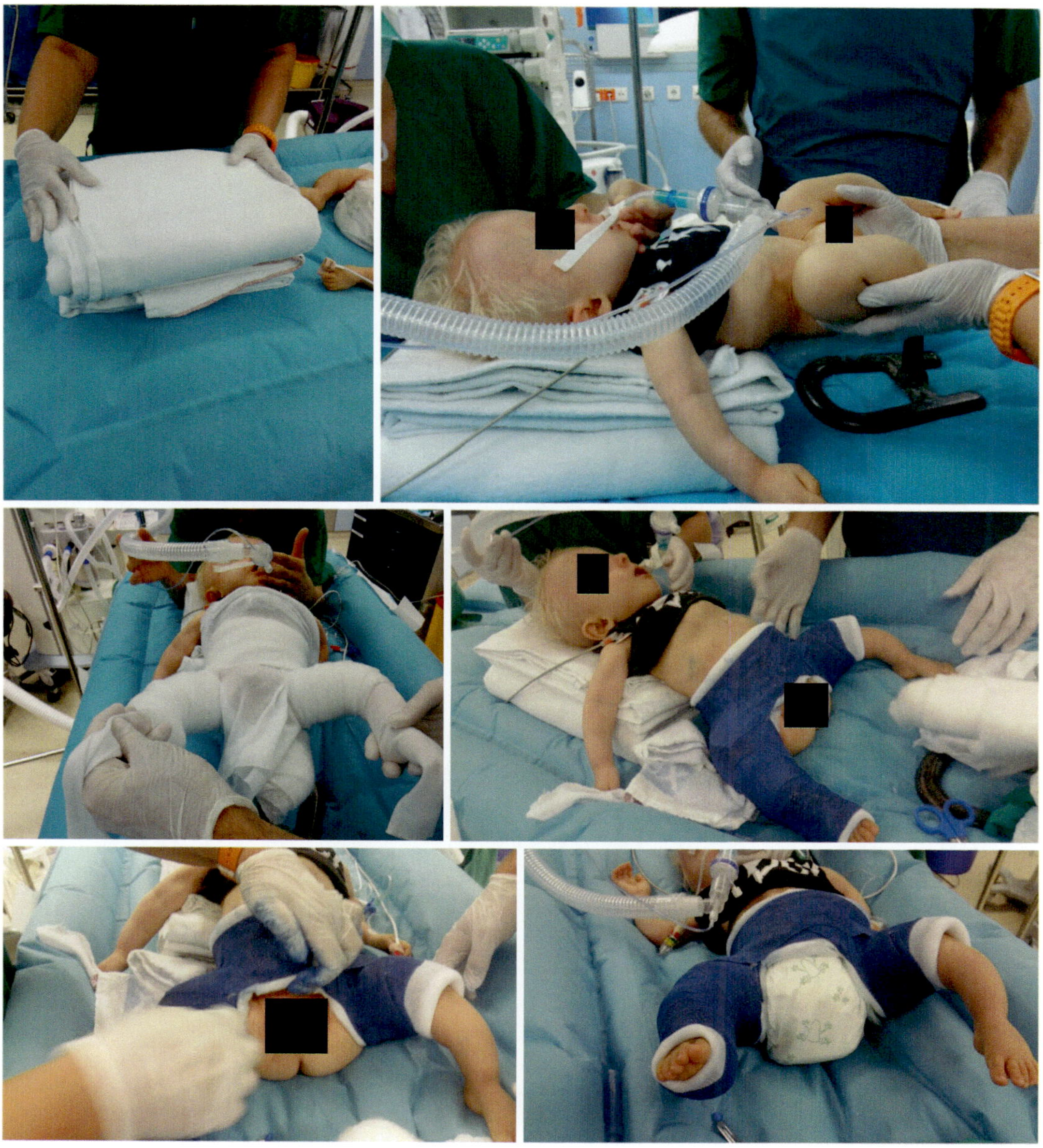

Fig. 12.38 Pelvis-femur cast; hip spika cast image series of procedure: Positioning, dressing, softcast, control of pressure, hygienic aspects

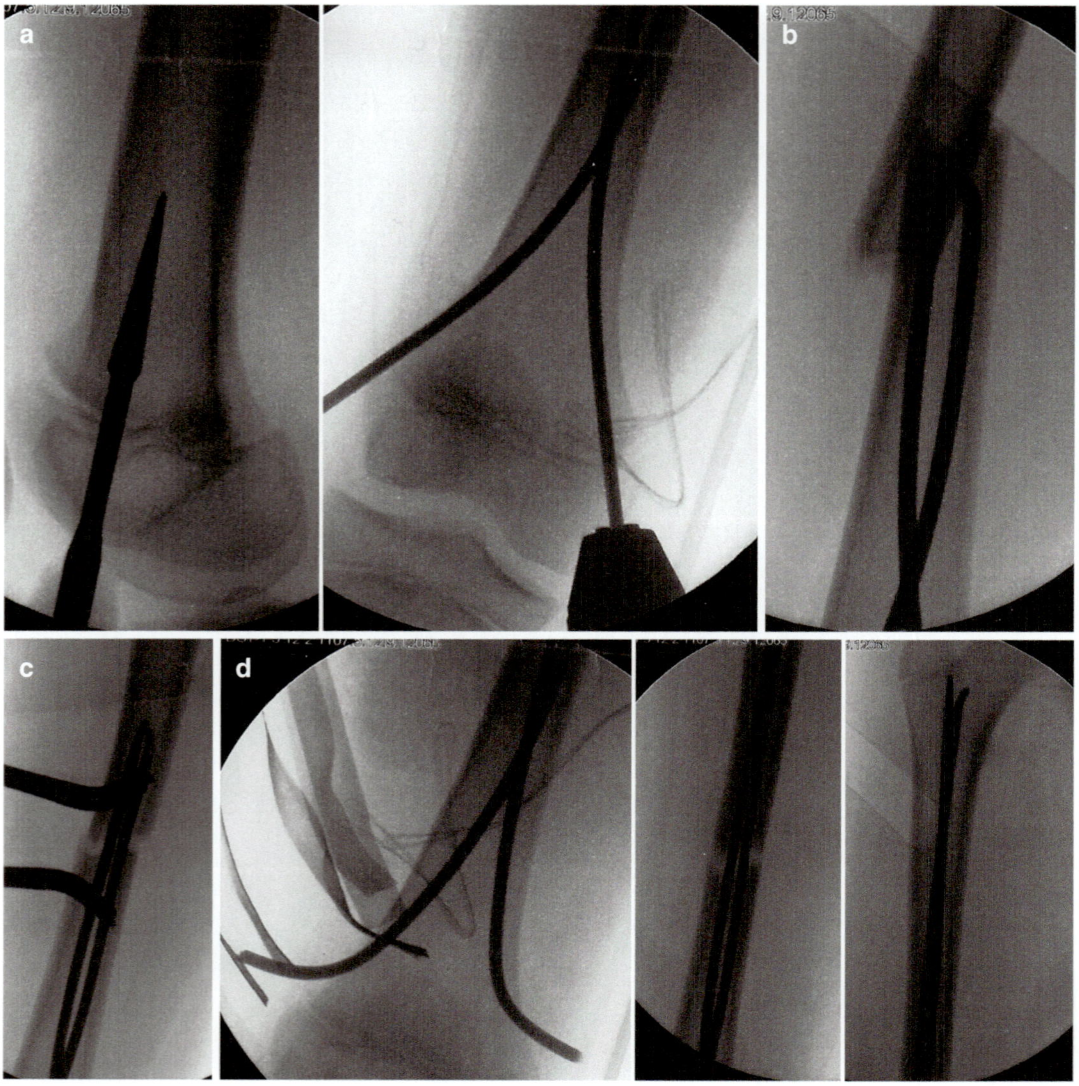

Fig. 12.39 Technique of retrade insertion of ESIN in a spiral fracture of the femur after direct injury (**a**) Insertion point, (**b**) Protrusion of both ESIN, (**c**) Open reduction, if closed reduction is not possible or too high radiation exposure, here with soft tissue in between the fracture ends. (**d**) Final result in 2 views

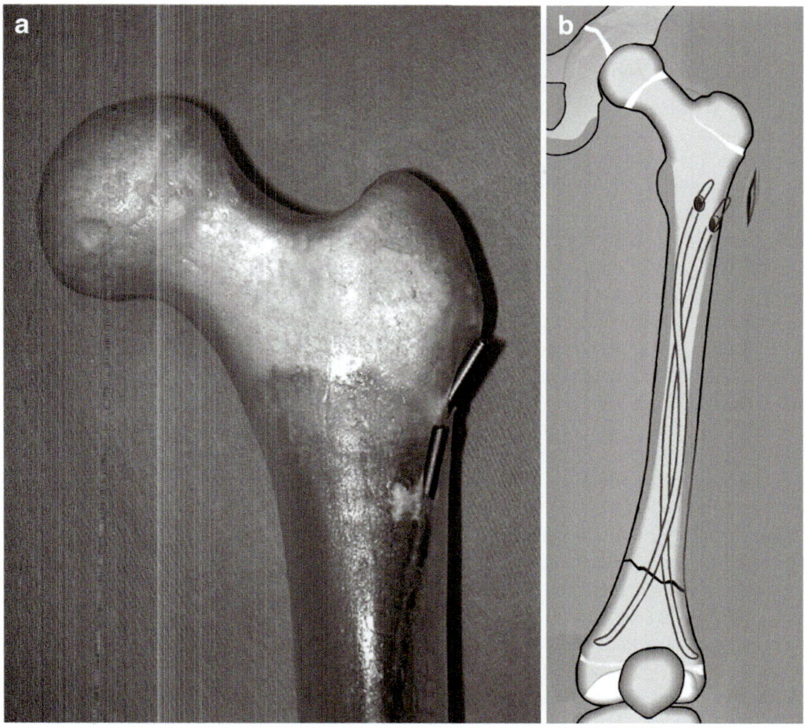

Fig. 12.40 (**a**) Correct position of the entry points on the proximal femur; note the "staggered position." This prevents splitting of the bone. (**b**) Correct positioning of both nails with anterograde technique; note the good tension and contact to the cortex in the distal third

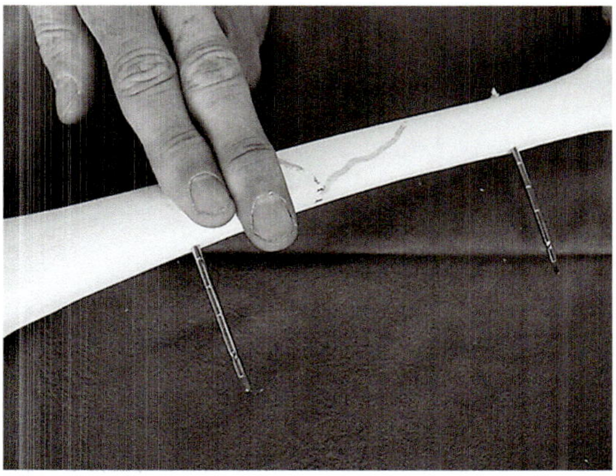

Fig. 12.41 Entry points of the fixator pins, proximal and distal from the fracture! 2 pins prox. And distally in most cases; in proximal femur and older children 3 on both sides might be more stable

Recommended Literature

Dietz HG, Schmittenbecher PP, Illing P (1997) Intramedulläre Osteosynthese im Wachstumsalter. Urban & Schwarzenberg, München

Dietz HG, Schmittenbecher PP, Slongo T, Wilkins KE (2006) Elastic stable intramedullary nailing (ESIN) in children. Thieme

Engström Z, Wolf O, Hailer YD (2020) Epidemiology of pediatric femur fractures in children: the Swedish fracture register. Bmc Musculoskelet Di 21:796

Gordon JE, Manske MC, Lewis TR, O'Donnell JC, Schoenecker PL, Keeler KA (2013) Femoral lengthening over a pediatric femoral nail: results and complications. J Pediatr Orthop 33:730–736

Infante AF, Albert MC, Jennings WB, Lehner JT (2000) Immediate hip Spica casting for femur fractures in pediatric patients. Clin Orthop Relat R 376:106–112

Jakob H, Wyen H, Marzi I (2013) Polytrauma im Kindesalter. Trauma und Berufskrankheit 15:67–74

Joeris A, Bansi G, Knorr P, Lieber J, Schalamon P, Slongo T (2005) ESIN in femur fractures. Eur J Trauma 31:24–32

Kaiser N, Slongo T (2021) Elastisch-stabile intramedulläre Nagelung pertrochantärer Femurfrakturen im Kleinkindesalter (<6 bis 8 Jahre). Oper Orthop Traumatol 33:46–54

Maier M, Marzi I (2008) Die elastisch-stabile Marknagelung der Femurfraktur beim Kind. Oper Orthop Traumatol. https://doi.org/10.1007/s00064-008-1408-6

Metaizeau JP (1988) Ostosynthese chez l'enfant par E.C.M.E.S. Sauramps

Park K-H, Park BK, Oh C-W, Kim D-W, Park H, Park K-B (2020) Overgrowth of the femur after internal fixation in children with femoral shaft fracture—a multicenter study. J Orthop Trauma 34:e90–e95

Rapp M, Kaiser MM, Grauel F, Gielok C, Illing P (2015) Femoral shaft fractures in young children (<5 years of age): operative and non-operative treatments in clinical practice. Eur J Trauma Emerg S 42:719–724

Rapp M, Kraus R, Illing P, Sommerfeldt DW, Kaiser MM (2018) Behandlung der Femurschaftfraktur bei Kindern und Jugendlichen mit einem Körpergewicht ≥50 kg. Unfallchirurg 121:47–57

Schneidmüller D, Kraft C, Bühren V, von Laer L (2014) Wachstumsverhalten nach Oberschenkelschaftfrakturen. Unfallchirurg 117:1099–1104

Strohm PC, Schmittenbecher PP (2011) Fracture stabilization in polytraumatized children. Unfallchirurg 114:323–332

Thompson JD, Buehler KC, Sponseller PD, Gray DW, Black BE, Buckley SL, Griffin PP (1997) Shortening in femoral shaft fractures in children treated with Spica cast. Clin Orthop Relat Res 338:74–78

von Laer L, Kraus R, Linhart WE (2012) Frakturen und Luxationen im Wachstumsalter 6., überarbeitete und erweiterte Auflage 2012 512 S., 1380 Abb., PDF Thieme Verlag. Thieme Verlag

Wani MM, Rashid M, Dar RA, Bashir A, Sultan A, Wani I, Rashid S, O'Sullivan M (2016) Use of external fixator versus flexible intramedullary nailing in closed pediatric femur fractures: comparing results using data from two cohort studies. Eur J Orthop Surg Traumatol 26:223–230

Zeckey C, Monsell F, Jackson M, Mommsen P, Citak M, Krettek C, Omar M (2017) Femoral malrotation after surgical treatment of femoral shaft fractures in children: a retrospective CT-based analysis. Eur J Orthop Surg Traumatol 27:1157–1162

13 Knee

13.1 Physiological Findings

The growth around the knee joint is similar for the distal femur and the proximal tibia, but the lengths grow of the femur is more distally, while the tibia growth is halft on the knee side and half distally (Fig. 13.1). The appearance of the bone in the x-ray is depicted in Fig. 13.2 und the closure of the growth plates is shown in Fig. 13.3. The proximal epiphysis of the tibia shows a proximal and a distal ossification center, which fuse until adolescence. Figure 13.4 shows the typical x-rays around the knee joint in different ages (Figs. 13.4, 13.5, 13.6, and 13.7).

During childhood, the leg axis develops through phases of bow-legs and knock-knees. Infants typically begin with Genu varum, which neutralizes towards the end of the first year as walking begins, transitioning to Genu valgum. Maximal "knock-knees" are seen at the end of the second year. The normal angle is reached around the age of eight, for girls ±7° and boys ±10° (Fig. 13.8). The recurvation of the tibial head is clearly higher birth and flatens slowly from 27° to 4° until the growth plates close (Fig. 13.9).

I. Marzi et al., *Pediatric Skeletal Trauma*, https://doi.org/10.1007/978-3-030-93685-3_13

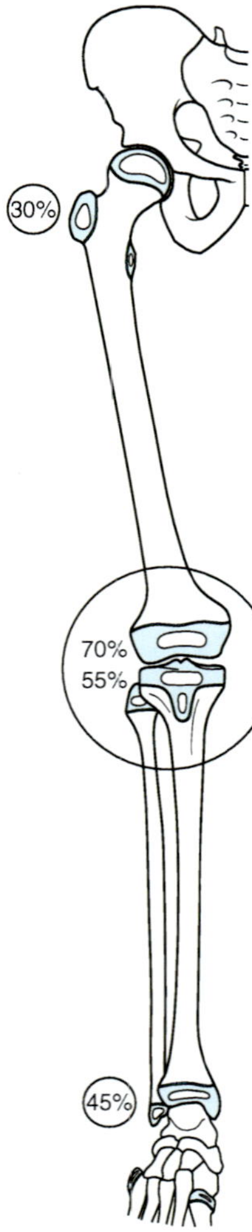

Fig. 13.1 Contribution of epiphyseal plates to longitudinal growth of the lower extremity. Distal femoral epiphysis: –40% of longitudinal growth of the entire leg, –70% of femoral longitudinal growth. Proximal tibial epiphysis: –30% of longitudinal growth of the entire leg, –55% of longitudinal growth of the tibia

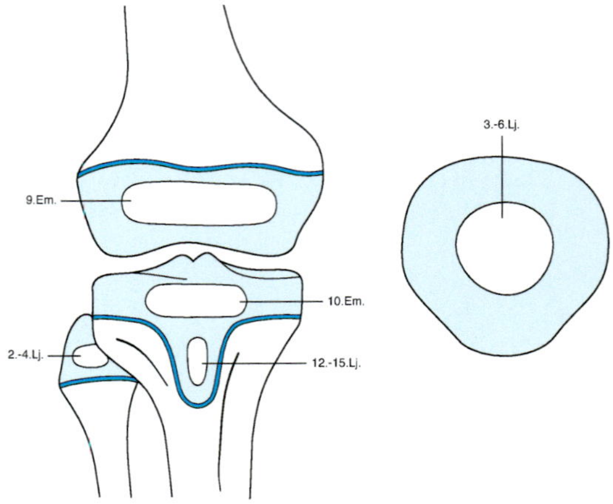

Fig. 13.2 Emergence of the ossification center. *(Lj)* life year; *(Em)* embryonal month

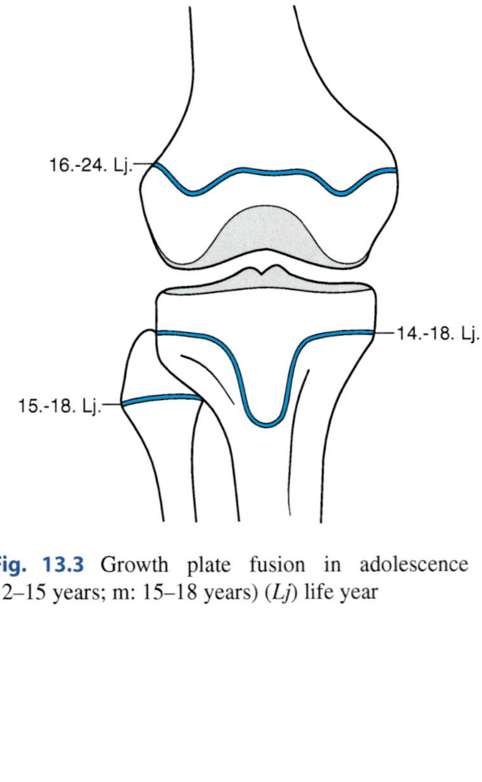

Fig. 13.3 Growth plate fusion in adolescence (f: 12–15 years; m: 15–18 years) *(Lj)* life year

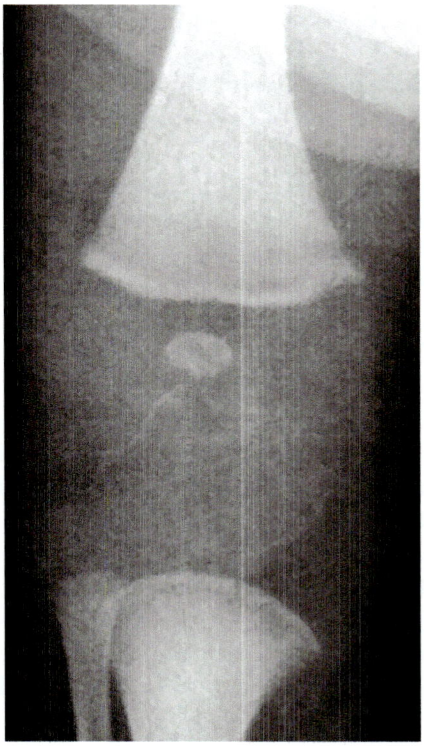

Fig. 13.4 Newborn; visible ossification center of the distal femur

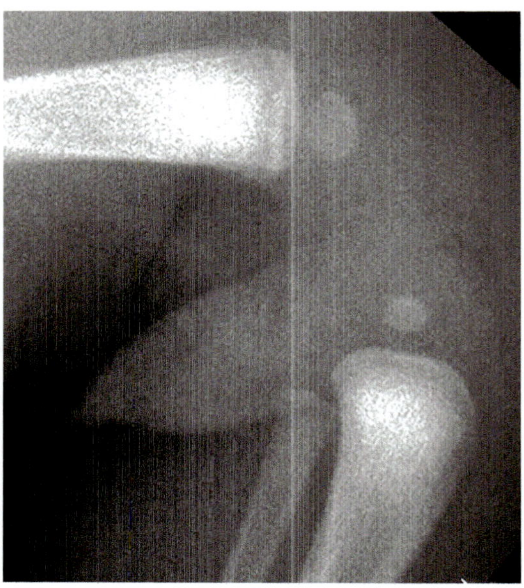

Fig. 13.5 Ossification center at week 2 of life

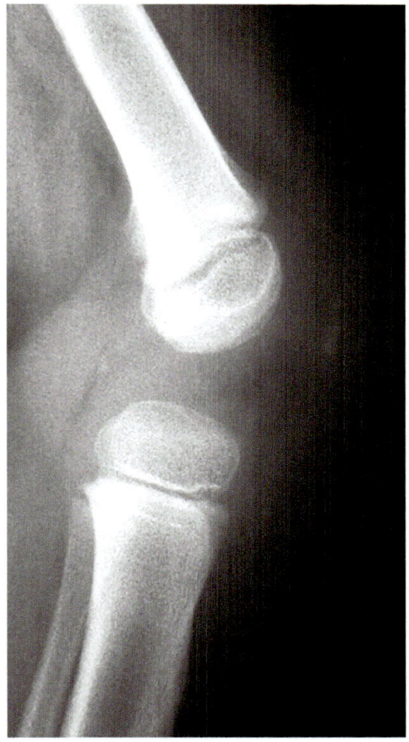

Fig. 13.6 Ossification center at 4 years

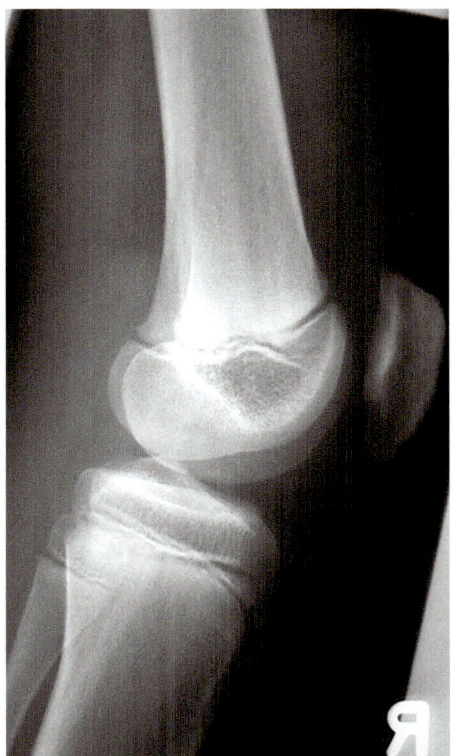

Fig. 13.7 Ossification status at 13 years

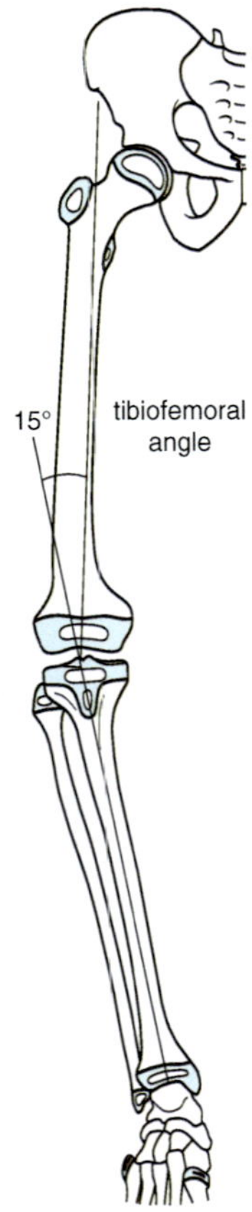

Fig. 13.8 Measurement of the tibiofemoral angle (TFA)

13.2 Fractures around the Knee

Incidence, Mechanism of Injury, and Clinical Presentation

Knee fractures of the distal femur have an incidence of 0.8%, and the proximal tibia, 1.2%. Injuries often occur during athletic activities, but high-speed trauma and falls from a height are also common. Severe injuries like fractures or articular damage are seen less frequently. There are correlations with ligament laxity and flexibility of the developing skeleton. Children have more stable ligaments, and the bulk of traumatic forces act on bone. Thus, osteochondral ligament or apophyseal avulsions are much more common than isolated ligament injuries (Table 13.1).

Diagnosis can be more challenging because of irregular ossification centers and unclear medical history in younger children. In such cases, MRI with or without arthroscopy can be performed in addition to knee radiographs in two planes.

Associated injuries such as articular lesions or vascular damage must be excluded. Of all lower extremity growth plates, the proximal tibia epiphysis is most commonly associated with vascular

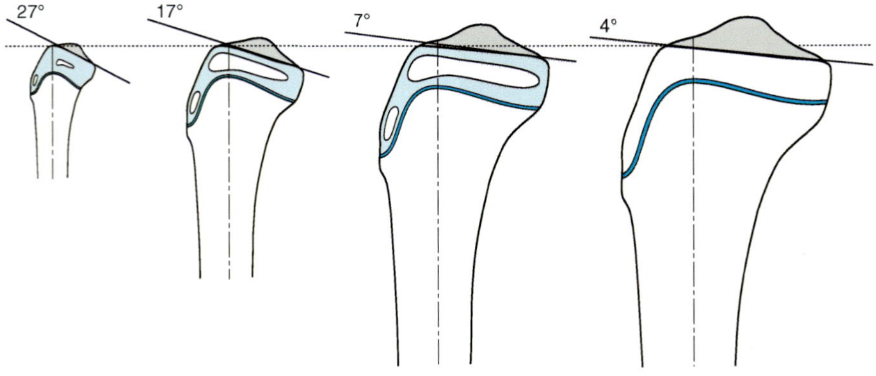

Fig. 13.9 Development in the sagittal plane of the tibial plateau. In the treatment of pediatric tibial plateau injuries, the physiologically increased recurvation of the tibial plateau must be considered; it decreases during development from 27° to 4°

Table 13.1 Fractures around the knee

Distal femur	Salter I/II	Extra-articular
	Salter III/IV	Intra-articular
	Transitional Fractures	Intra-articular
Proximal tibia	Transitional fractures	Intra-articular
	Salter III/IV	Intra-articular
	Salter I/II	Extra-articular
	Tuberosity avulsion	Intra–/extra-articular

injury due to the adjacent trifurcation of the posterior popliteal artery.

If fracture reduction is necessary, it should be performed under general anesthesia. The goal is secure and definitive post-reduction fracture stabilization to prevent secondary displacement and the need for re-reduction. A posterior plaster splint may be sufficient, but an external fixator is useful in certain cases.

However, the likelihood of growth disturbance also decreases with age. Transition fractures occur as the growth plates begin to close, when one portion of the plate is fused and another open. This type of lesion also occurs most frequently in the tibia. When treating transitional fractures, the primary focus should be the anatomical reconstruction of the joint, with less emphasis on risks of growth plate injury and subsequent growth irregularities. Plate-crossing procedures are permitted in these patients since relevant growth has concluded once fusion has begun.

In contrast, growth irregularities must always be expected when the epiphyses are still open. These can also lead to axial malalignment. Overgrowth occurs more or less after every fracture and leads to limb lengthening. The extent depends on the activity and duration of the repair process. Growth inhibition is more likely when the plate itself is injured. Depending on the child's age, premature growth plate fusion can result in considerable leg-length shortening due to the large proportion of longitudinal growth for which the knee-adjacent epiphyses are responsible. In cases of partial inhibition, bridge formation in the growth plate leads to lopsided closure and unequal growth, yielding axial malalignment in different planes. These growth irregularities typically become clinically evident after six months; thus, regular clinical follow up is necessary. If uneven growth is suspected, radiological assessments, including MRI, can be used to determine the extent and pattern of the bridging so that growth plate release or a modulation procedure can be performed, depending on the findings (also see Chap. 20). If the findings are unremarkable, follow up can be discontinued after two years.

Regarding surgical technique, both, percutaneous or open screw fixation works well. Wire fixation is only useful in very young children. Some proximal fractures require additional stabilization with casts or external fixators; plate fixation is rarely indicated, e.g., in cases of metaphyseal flexion fractures or for axial correction while protecting the growth plate.

Epiphyseolysis of the distal femur and treatment options are indicated in Table 13.2.

Epiphyseal and epi-metaphyseal fractures are indicated in Table 13.3.

Epiphyseolysis of the proximal tibia might be more complexe, since the apophysis also has a growth platz, which fuses in time with the proximal tibia growth plate. Injuries are shown in Table 13.4.

Intraartikular fractures of the proximal Tibia occur rarely, but might need operative stabilization in larger gaps and dislocations. Table 13.5 shows the treatement options.

Avulsion Fractures of the tuberositas of the Tibia are more often in older children and prior to the closure of the growth plat. They are classified according to Watson-Jones as extraarticular or intraarticular (Fig. 13.23). The therapeutic, mostly surgical, options are indicated in Table 13.6.

Distal Femur Fractures around the Knee

Table 13.2 Distal femur: epiphyseal disruptions (Fig. 13.10)

Special features	most common fracture of the distal femur; hemarthrosis when there is capsule injury, birth trauma injury; caution: "battered child" syndrome in children <3 years direct trauma; fall from height	
Diagnostic approach	AP and lateral x-ray (femur with hip and knee joints; observe the ratios of the femoral metaphysis to the epiphysis and the femoral to tibial axes!) Angiography: If a vascular injury is suspected Ultrasound if needed: Subperiosteal hematoma	
Treatment goal/limits of correction	Reduction of axial malalignment; <1/5 lateral translation with epiphyseal disruption Complete adjustment of any recurvation in the axis of motion	
Primary treatment	Long-leg plaster splint, medical analgesia as needed, emergency indication: Neurovascular injury and painful displacement	
Conservative treatment		
Indication	Non-displaced fractures (Fig. 13.11)	
Approach	Long-leg cast for 4–5 weeks partial weight-bearing	
Follow up	Weight-bearing as tolerated after cast removal, physical therapy as needed	
Radiological controls	Day 8: Position check; 4 weeks: Consolidation check (cast-free)	
Return to sports	With muscular symmetry; approx. 4–6 weeks after consolidation	
Operative treatment		
Indication	Displaced, painful instability; associated injuries	
Approach	Usually closed reduction; open reduction for severe displacement or entrapped soft tissues Percutaneous crossed K-wire transfixion; screw fixation Alternative: External fixator in cases of soft tissue damage, polytrauma, "floating knee"	
Follow up	K-wire transfixion: Posterior long-leg splint for 4–5 weeks, rolling weight-bearing (Fig. 13.12) Screw fixation: Because of the short lever, long-leg cast 4 weeks; 4 weeks rolling weight-bearing (Fig. 13.13) External fixator: Partial weight-bearing until callus is formed (4 weeks) after cast removal, weight-bearing as tolerated, physical therapy as needed	
Radiological controls	Postoperative position check; at 4 weeks, consolidation check (cast-free)	
Hardware removal	K-wires: 4–5 weeks post-surgery; screws: 12–15 weeks post-surgery; general anesthesia External fixator: 12 weeks post-surgery; can be done as outpatient	
Return to sports	With muscular symmetry; approx. 4–6 weeks after consolidation	
Complications	Vascular lesions with posterior displacement (femoral, popliteal vessels), difficult retention of small metaphyseal fragments Articular damage Uncommon: Peroneal damage; compartment syndrome	
Growth disturbance	Usually overgrowth—discrete leg lengthening Growth inhibition; salter I: 27%	
Follow up	Semi-annually for 2 years Checks for leg-length discrepancy and axial malalignment every 3 months Radiological controls in cases of axial malalignment (exclude growth plate bridging)	
Classification	AO: 33-E/1(2).1–3	LiLa: 3.3.s.1.0–2.

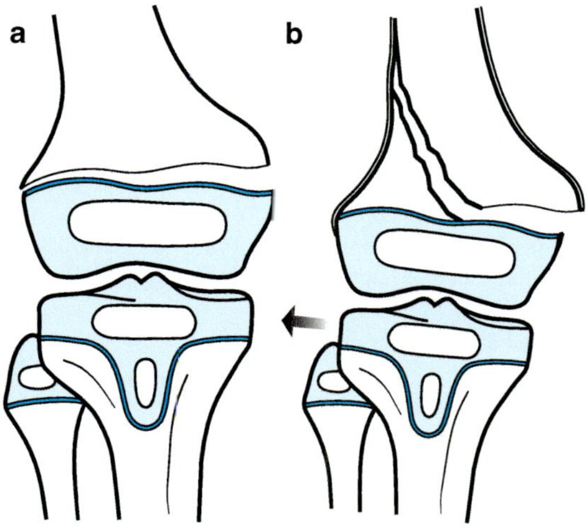

Fig. 13.10 Epiphyseolysis of the distal femur (**a**) Salter-Harris I; (**b**) Salter-Harris II

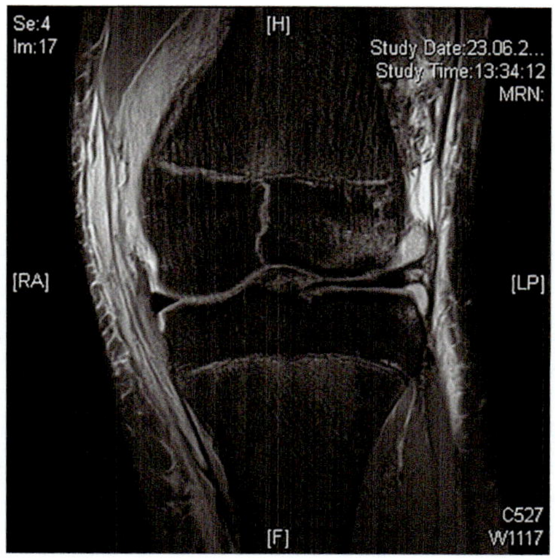

Fig. 13.11 Epiphyseal fracture of the distal femur. Only a gap in MRI, therefore conservative therapy

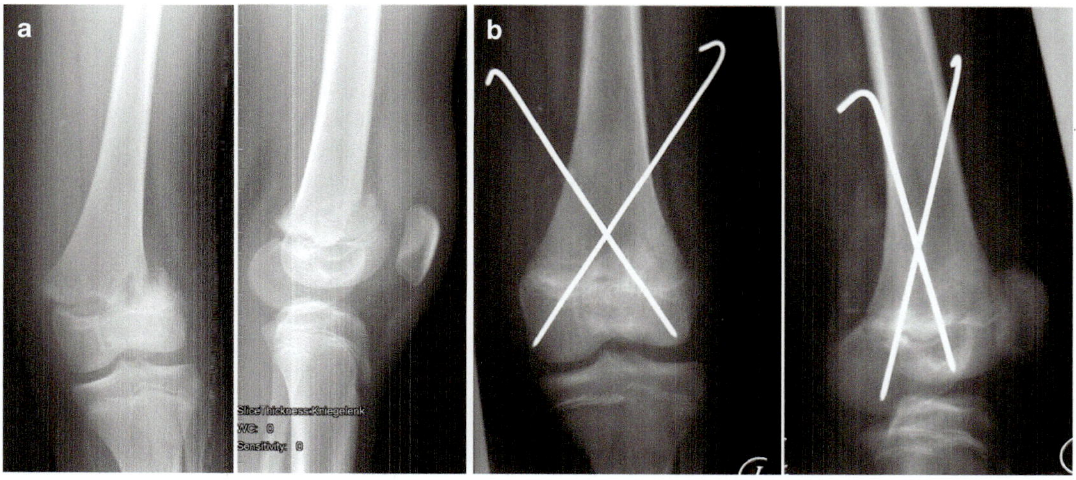

Fig. 13.12 Salter-Harris-II-fracture of the distal femur in a 10 year old girl. (**a**) Trauma image, (**b**) After reduction and K-wire fixation

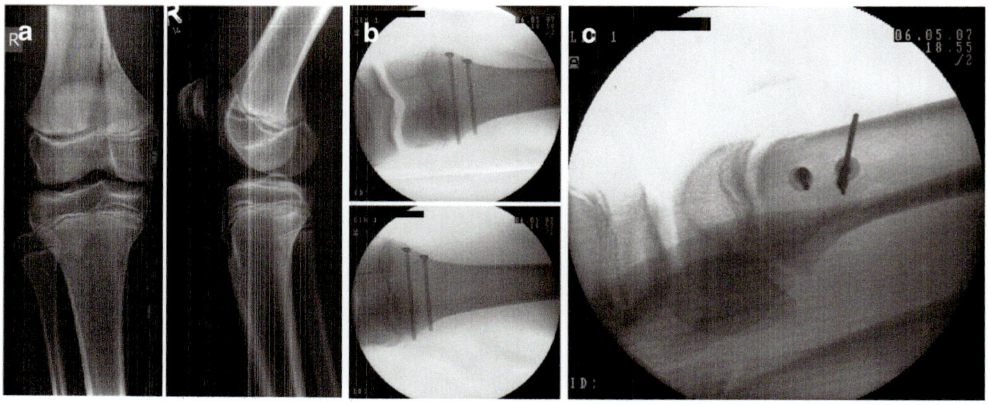

Fig. 13.13 Salter-Harris-II-fracture of the distal femur in a 14 year old boy with a big metaphyseal wedge. (**a**) Trauma image, (**b**, **c**) Intraoperative images with reduction, cannulated lag screws over K-wires

Table 13.3 Distal femur: epiphyseal and epi-metaphyseal fractures (Fig. 13.14)

Special features	Intra-articular; severe trauma; often direct
Diagnostic approach	AP and lateral x-rays (femur with hip and knee joints) Angiography: If a vascular injury is suspected MRI if needed; differential diagnosis: Ligament injury
Treatment goal/limits of correction	No axial malalignment; displacement <2 mm Congruent joint surfaces without a step, osteoarthritis prevention
Primary treatment	Long-leg plaster splint, medical analgesia if needed, if needed, joint aspiration for hemarthrosis Emergency indication: Neurovascular injury; massive hemarthrosis
Conservative treatment	
Indication	Conservative treatment only with minimal fracture dehiscence (<2 mm); usually not possible
Approach	Long-leg cast for 4–5 weeks
Follow up	Weight-bearing as tolerated after cast removal, physical therapy as needed
Radiological controls	Day 8: Position check; 5 weeks: Consolidation check (cast-free)
Return to sports	With muscular symmetry; approx. 4–6 weeks after consolidation
Operative treatment	
Indication	Direct reduction usually necessary → joint reconstruction!; arthroscopic support if neededreduction and screw fixation or open approach
Approach	Crossed K-wire transfixion; screw fixation (Figs. 13.15 and 13.16)
Follow up	Screw fixation according to fragment size Free mobility, 4–5 weeks rolling weight-bearing; motor splint K-wire transfixion: Small fragments with posterior long-leg plaster splint for 4–5 weeks Weight-bearing as tolerated after cast removal, physical therapy as needed
Radiological controls	Postoperative position check; at 5 weeks, consolidation check (cast-free)
Hardware removal	K-wires 5 weeks post-surgery; screws 4–6 months post-surgery
Return to sports	With muscular symmetry; approx. 4–6 weeks after consolidation
Complications	Vascular lesions with posterior displacement (femoral, popliteal vessels), postoperative hemarthrosis; limited mobility Uncommon: Peroneal damage; compartment syndrome Articular damage; associated ligament injuries reported in up to 38%
Growth disturbance	Overgrowth—discrete leg lengthening Growth inhibition; salter IV: High risk (leg-length discrepancy: 25–56%, axial malalignment: 33–83%)
Follow up	Semi-annually for 2 years Controls of leg-length discrepancies and axial malalignment every 3 months Radiological controls in cases of axial malalignment (exclude growth plate bridging)
Classification	AO: 33-E/3(4).1–3 LiLa: 3.3.a.1–5.0-2.

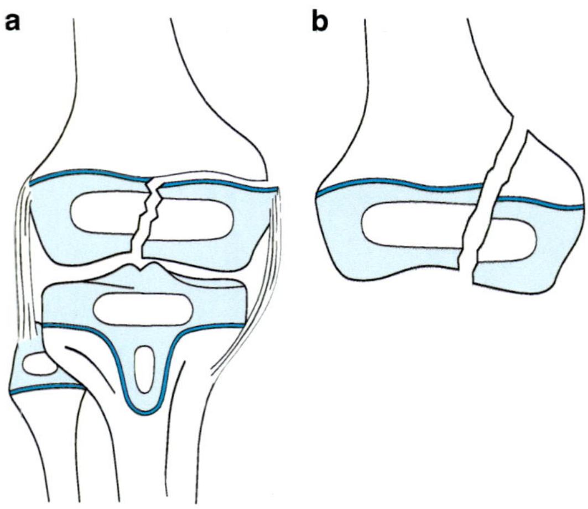

Fig. 13.14 (**a**, **b**) Distale femur. A epiphyseal and transepi-metaphysyseal fracture

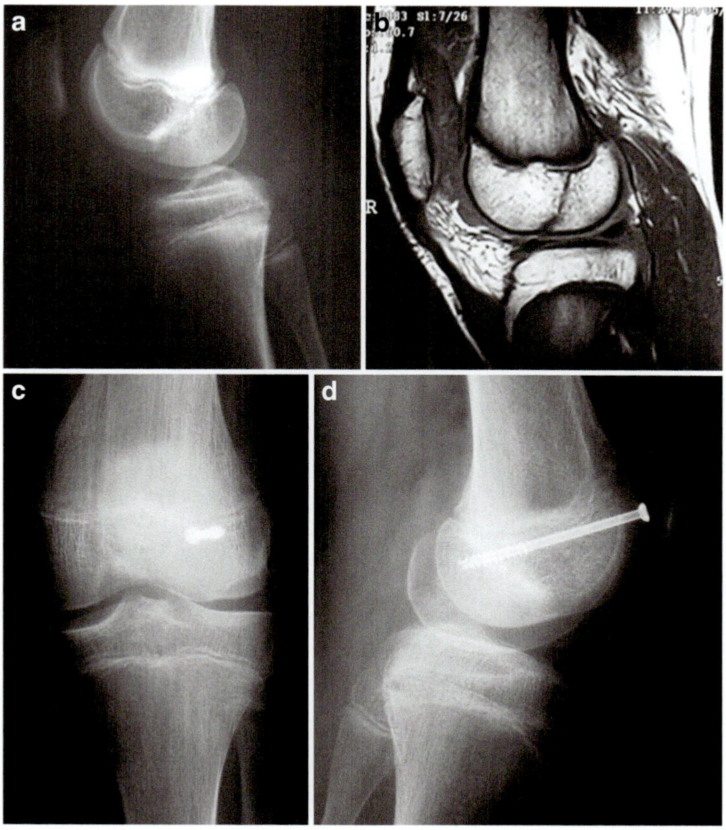

Fig. 13.15 Fracture of the distal epiphysis of the femur of a 13 year old by. (**a**) Trauma x-ray, (**b**) MRI, (**c**, **d**) Arthroskopic controlled lag screw osteosynthesis with cannulated screw

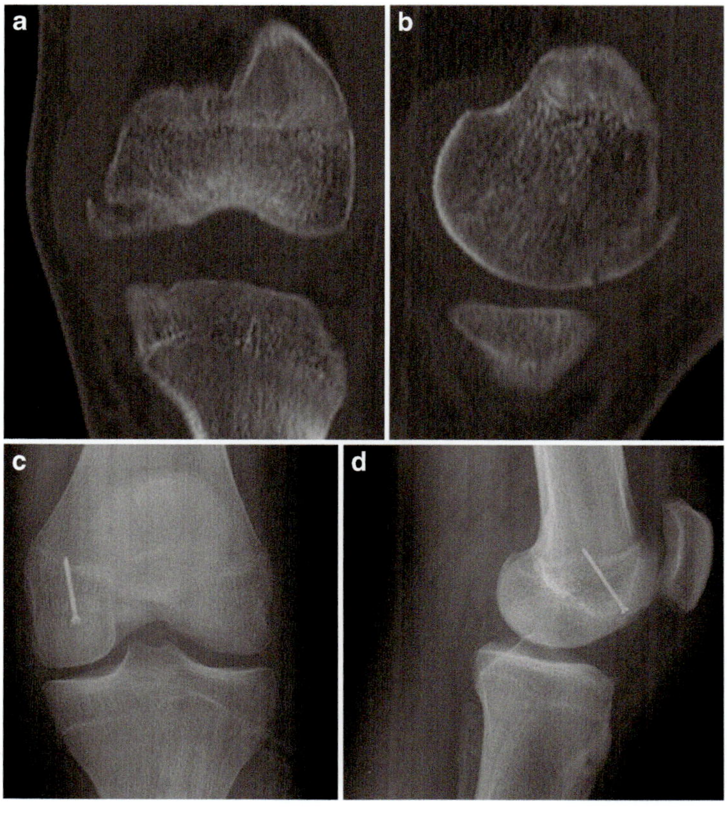

Fig. 13.16 Osteochondral fracture of the medial condyle of the distal femur after a motobike accident in an adolescent boy. (**a**, **b**) CT scan due to hemarthros withour clear fracture x-ray. (**c**, **d**) Postoperative arthroscopic assisted reduction and screw osteosynthesis

Proximal Tibia Fractures around the Knee

Table 13.4 Proximal tibia: epiphyseal disruptions (Fig. 13.17)

Special features	Salter I	
Diagnostic approach	AP and lateral x-rays, MRI if optional (unclear fracture; suspected ligament injury) Suspected vascular injury: Doppler ultrasound/angiography	
Treatment goal/limits of correction	Joint alignemrent and reconstruction	
Primary treatment	Long-leg plaster splint, medical analgesia if needed, joint aspiration for hemarthrosis if needed	
Conservative treatment		
Indication	Stable, non-displaced fractures, generally conservative	
Approach	Long-leg cast for 5 weeks	
Follow up	After cast removal, weight-bearing as tolerated; physical therapy if needed	
Radiological controls	1 week; consolidation check	
Return to sports	With muscular symmetry; approx. 4–6 weeks after consolidation	
Operative treatment		
Indication	Instability, displacement	
Approach	Closed reduction and K-wire fixation in children with open growth plates Fig. 13.18 Closed reduction and stable screw fixation over the epiphyseal line in adolescents, when closure of the growth plate can almost be expected (Fig. 13.19)	
Follow up	Long-leg cast 4–5 weeks; functional after cast removal; physical therapy as needed	
Radiological controls	At 1 week; consolidation check at 4–5 weeks	
Hardware removal	At 4–5 weeks	
Return to sports	With muscular symmetry; approx. 4–6 weeks after consolidation	
Complications	Vascular injury (popliteal artery) → compartment syndrome Associated ligament injuries Associated fracture of the proximal/distal fibula	
Growth disturbance	Rare	
Follow up	Weekly until free function; then semi-annually for 3-years Checks for leg-length discrepancy and axial malalignment every 3 months Radiological controls in cases of axial malalignment (exclude growth plate bridging)	
Classification	AO: 41-E/1(2).1–3	LiLa: 4.1.s.1.0–2.

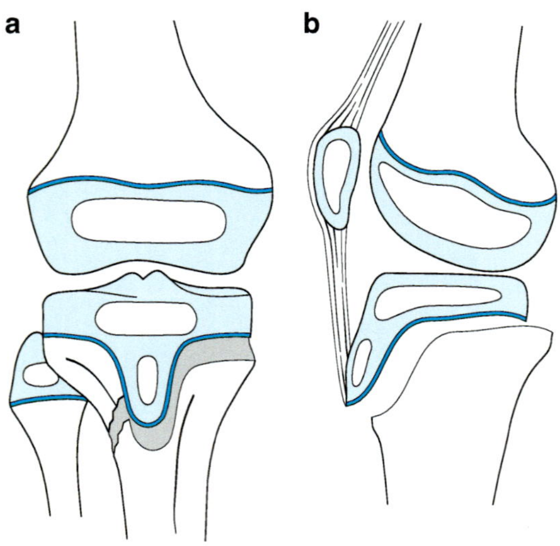

Fig. 13.17 Proximal tibia: Epiphyseolysis. Note the course of the growth plate of the proximal tibia. (**a**) A.P. view and (**b**) lateral view

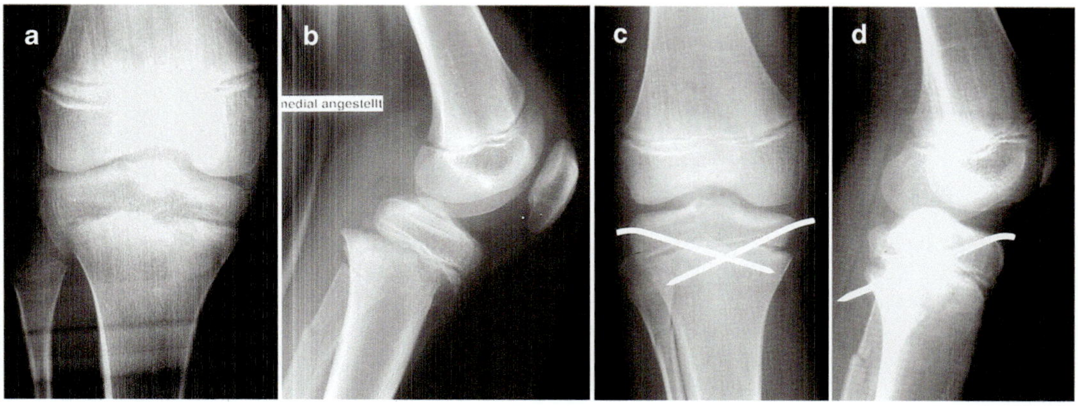

Fig. 13.18 Epiphyseolysis of the proximal tibia of a 14 year old boy (Salter-Harris-II). (**a**, **b**) Trauma image, (**c**, **d**) Crossed K-wire fixation after reduction

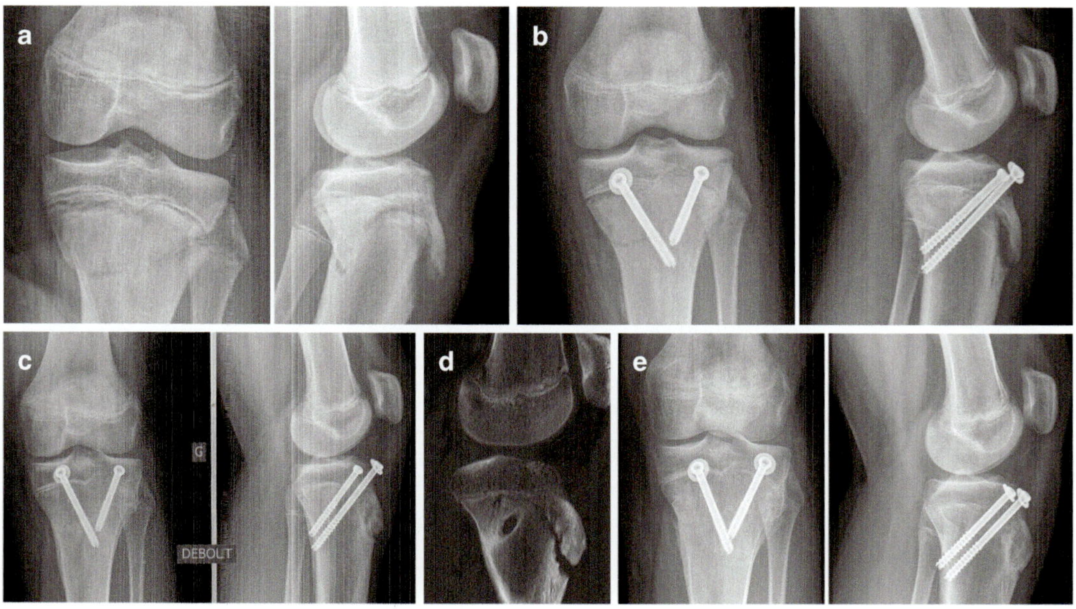

Fig. 13.19 Epiphysiolysis oft he proximal tibia with metaphyseal wedge in a 13 year old boy after fall on the knee. (**a**) Trauma image, (**b**) 3 Weeks postoperative, (**c**) 3 Months with healing, (**d**) After metal removal and new trauma with fracture 4 months after first trauma, (**e**) Healing 4 months after re-osteosynthesis

Table 13.5 Proximal tibia: epiphyseal and epi-metaphyseal fractures (Fig. 13.20)

Special features	Rare; intra-articular; direct trauma, hyperextension especially in adolescents
Diagnostic approach	AP and lateral x-rays, arthroscopy if needed MRI if needed (unclear fracture course; suspected ligament injury) Doppler ultrasound/angiography for suspected vascular injury
Treatment goal/limits of correction	Joint reconstruction Displacement <2 mm
Primary treatment	Long-leg plaster splint, medical analgesia if needed, If needed, joint aspiration for hemarthrosis
Conservative treatment	
Indication	Non-displaced fractures, displacement <2 mm (Fig. 13.21)
Approach	Long-leg cast for 5 weeks, rolling weight-bearing
Follow up	Functional: Weight-bearing as tolerated Physical therapy as needed
Radiological controls	Position check at 7 days, consolidation check at 5 weeks
Return to sports	With muscular symmetry; approx. 4–6 weeks after consolidation
Operative treatment	
Indication	Displacement >2 mm; associated injuries, pronounced hemarthrosis
Approach	Usually open reduction (joint reconstruction), screw fixation (Fig. 13.22)
Follow up	Rolling weight-bearing for 5 weeks, free mobility
Radiological controls	Postoperative position check; consolidation check 5 weeks post-surgery
Hardware removal	12 weeks post-surgery
Return to sports	With muscular symmetry; approx. 4–6 weeks after consolidation
Complications	Pronounced hemarthrosis; limited mobility
Growth disturbance	Inhibitory growth irregularities with axial malalignment possible <12 years; follow up checks
Follow up	Weekly until free function; then semi-annually for 2 years Checks for leg-length discrepancy and axial malalignment every 3 months Radiological controls in cases of axial malalignment (exclude growth plate bridging)
Classification	AO: 41-E/3(4).1–3 LiLa: 4.1.a.1–5.0-2.

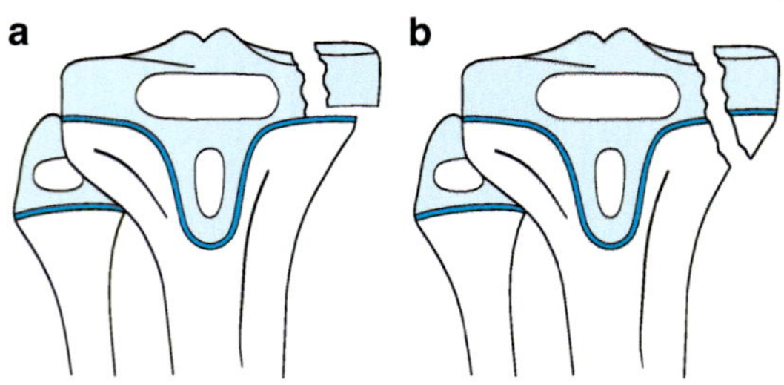

Fig. 13.20 Proximal tibia (**a**) Epiphyseal (Salter-Harris III), (**b**) Epi-metaphyseal fracture (Salter-Harris IV)

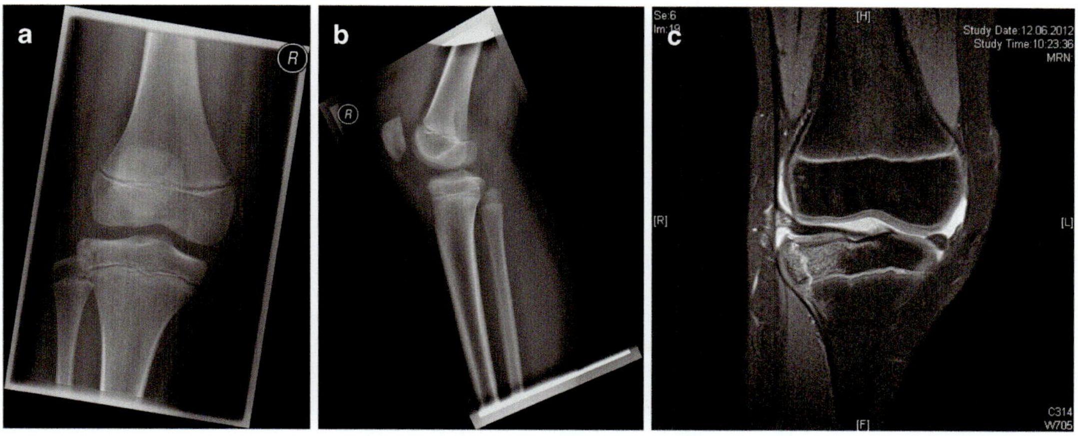

Fig. 13.21 Proximal epiphyseal fracture of the tibia, Type Salter-Harris IV (Aitken 3). (**a**, **b**) X-ray, (**c**) MRI

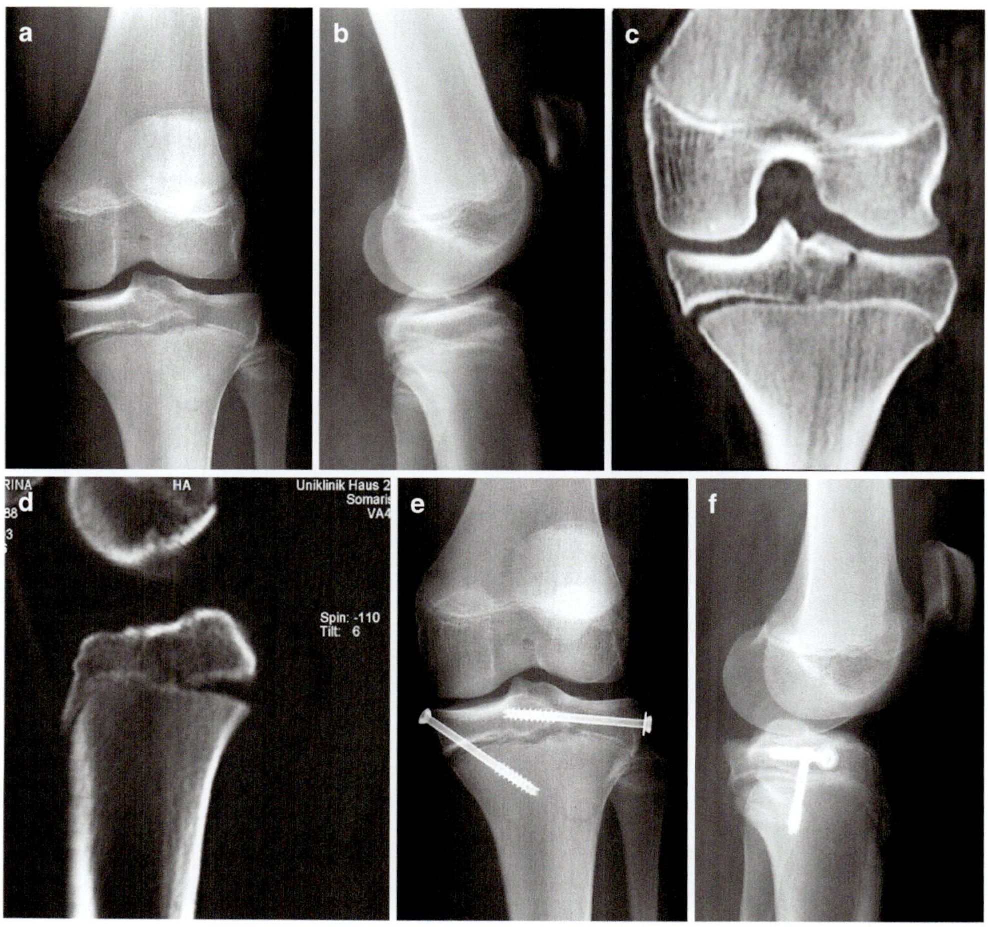

Fig. 13.22 Transition fracture of the proximal tibia of a 14 year old girl after school sports. (**a**, **b**) Trauma image, (**c**, **d**) CT scan, (**e**, **f**) Lag screw osteosynthesis. In this case crossing the growth plate is possible due to started closure of the growth plate

Proximal Tibial Avulsion Fractures

Table 13.6 Tibial tuberosity avulsion

Special features	Extra and intra-articular; especially in male adolescents Possible correlation with Osgood-Schlatter disease Watson-Jones Classification (Fig. 13.23): I—extra-articular II—extra-articular III—intra-articular	
Diagnostic approach	AP and lateral x-rays Clinical: Local hematoma, hemarthrosis; limited extension Arthroscopy as needed	
Treatment goal/limits of correction	Functional reconstruction Displacement <5 mm	
Primary treatment	Long-leg plaster splint, medical analgesia if needed	
Conservative treatment		
Indication	Types I, II: Non-displaced fractures, displacement <5 mm	
Approach	Long-leg cast for 6 weeks, rolling weight-bearing	
Follow up	Functional: Weight-bearing as tolerated	
Radiological controls	Consolidation check at 6 weeks	
Return to sports	With muscular symmetry; approx. 4–6 weeks after consolidation	
Operative treatment		
Indication	Type II and III fractures with displacement >5 mm; joint involvement; associated soft-tissue injury (Fig. 13.24)	
Approach	Open reduction, screw fixation, usually in adolescents so possible to cross the growth plate (Fig. 13.25) Type III: With screw fixation (Fig. 13.26) or tension band wiring If needed, arthroscopy or open ligament and joint reconstruction or suture of the patellar tendon might be necessary (Fig. 13.27) Soft-tissue reconstruction	
Follow up	Rolling weight-bearing for 6 weeks, free mobility In cases of soft-tissue reconstruction: Long-leg splint until wound healing	
Radiological controls	Postoperative position check; consolidation check 6 weeks post-surgery	
Hardware removal	12 weeks post-surgery	
Return to sports	With muscular symmetry; approx. 4–6 weeks after consolidation	
Complications	Results are good after anatomical reduction, growth plate closure possible (most are fully grown) Meniscus lesions	
Growth disturbance	Rare (since most are adolescents)	
Follow up	Weekly until free function; then semi-annually for 3-years Controls for leg-length discrepancies and axial malalignment Radiological controls in cases of axial malalignment (exclude growth plate bridging)	
Classification	AO: 41-E/7.1–3	LiLa: 4.1.a.5.1–2.

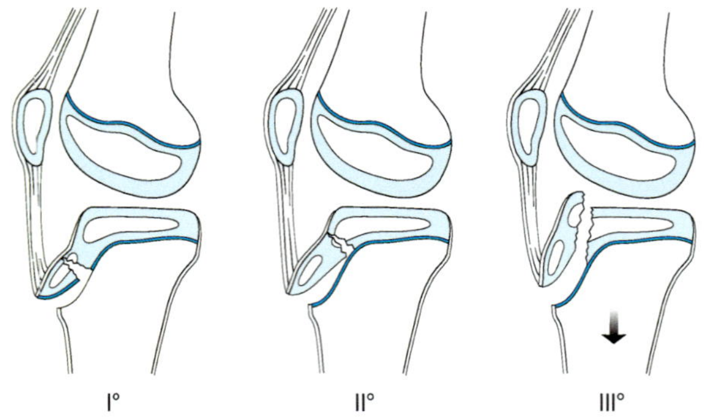

Fig. 13.23 Types of avulsion fractures of the tuberositas tibiae

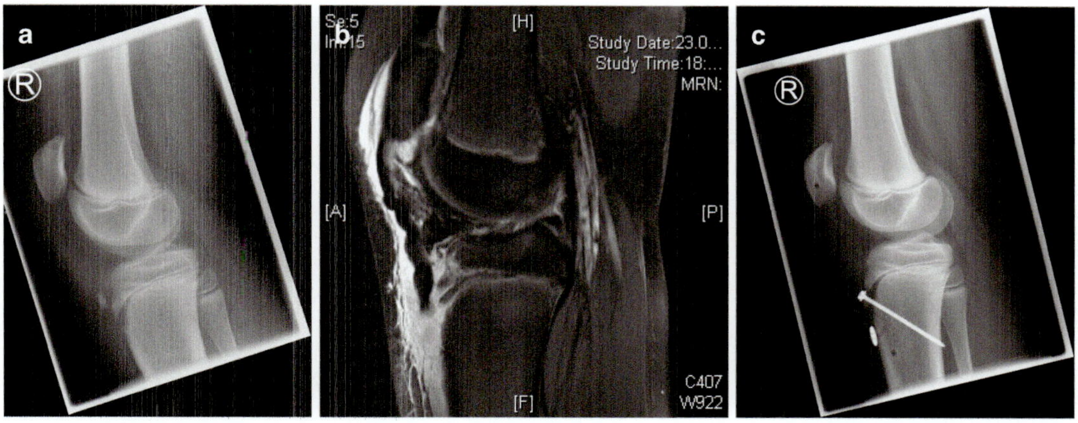

Fig. 13.24 Type I avulsion of the tuberositas tibia with the patella ligament. (**a**) X-ray, (**b**) MRI, (**c**) X-ray after refixation with screw and suture

Fig. 13.25 Large avulsion fracture Type II/III of the proximal tuberositas tibia with line into the epiphysis in 14 year old girl. (**a**, **b**) Trauma image, (**c**, **d**) After reduction and fixation with 4 cannulated lag screws

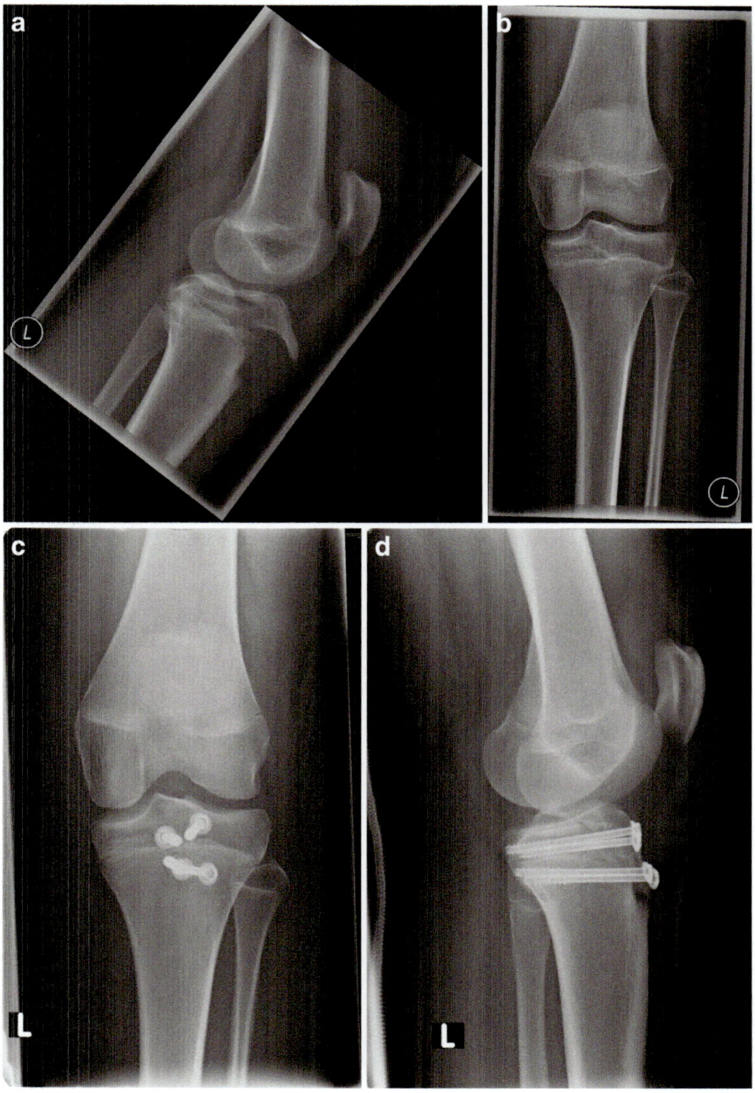

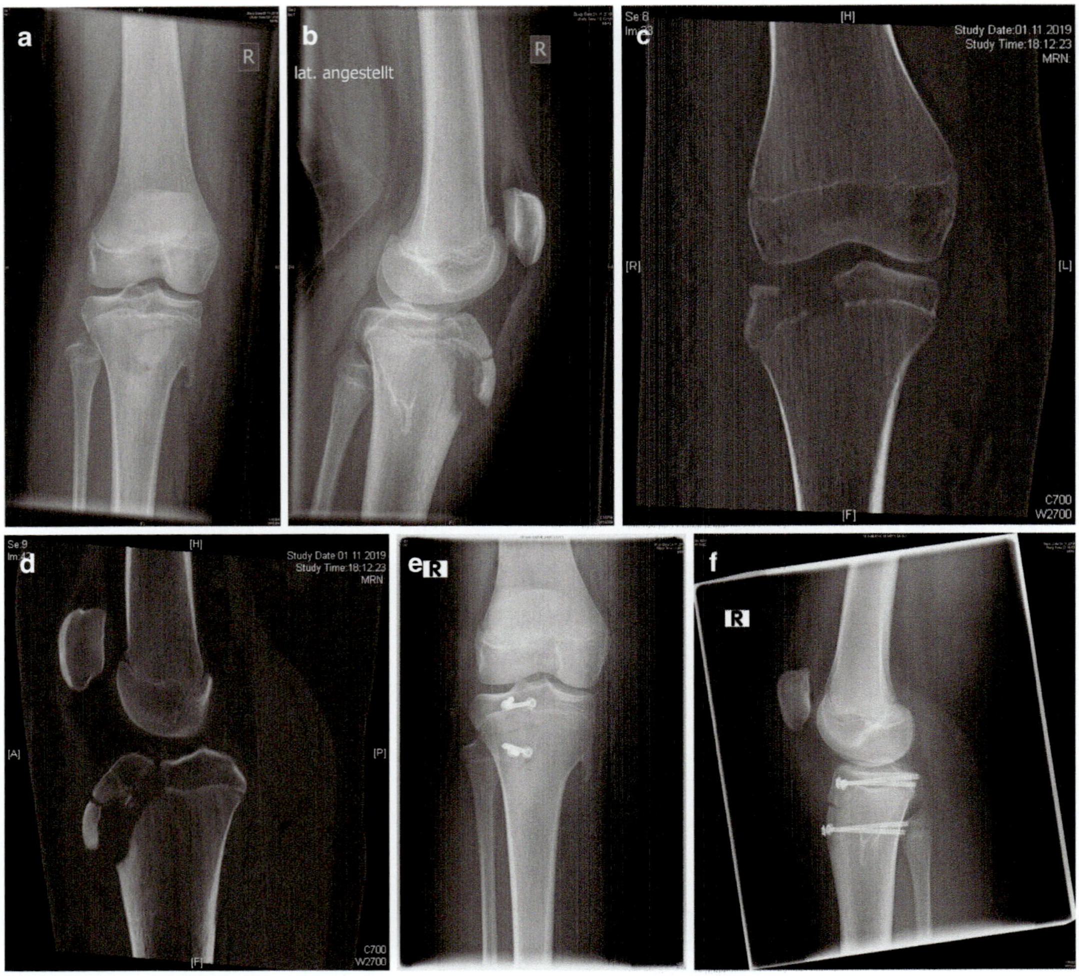

Fig. 13.26 Large avulsion fracture Type III of the proximal tuberositas tibia with large gap of the epiphysis in the 14 year old girl. (**a**, **b**) Trauma image, (**c**, **d**) CT scan, (**e**, **f**) After reduction and screw osteosynthesis

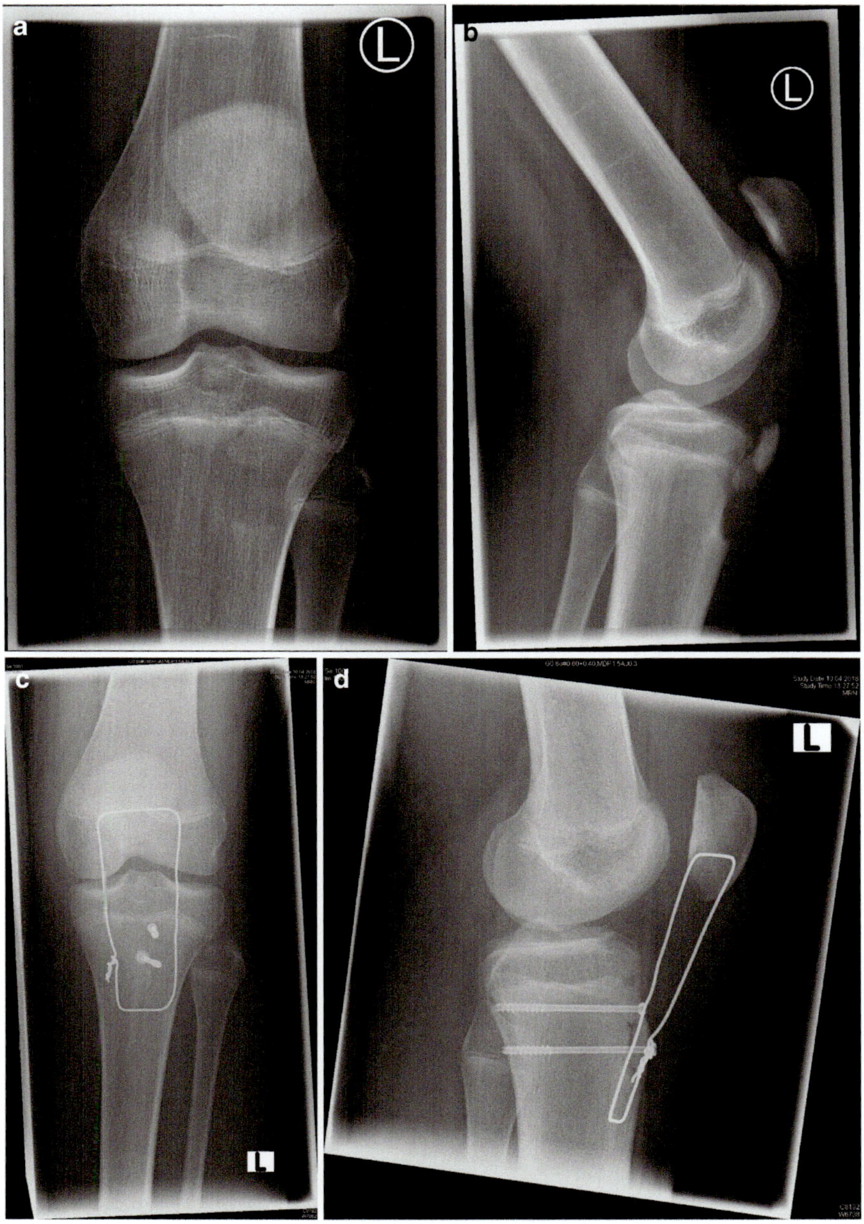

Fig. 13.27 15 Year old boy with bony and intraligamentous patallar tendon avulsion fracture, (**a**, **b**) Trauma image, (**c**, **d**) Refixation of bony avulsion with 2 screws and suture of tendon, secured with McLaughlin Cerclage

Reconstruction of the fractures around the knee joint should be closed, if possible and fixation with percutaneous screws is often possible (Table 13.7). Alternatives are K-wire fixation needing an additional cast or external fixateur.

The surgical treatment of proximal Tibial fractures is usually performed by closed reduction and screw or crossed K-wire osteosynthesis (Table 13.8). In joint fractures or ligamentous avulsion fractures open reconstruction is necessary and rarely an arthroscopic view of the knee joint is required.

Table 13.7 Technical aspects—fractures of the distal femur

Closed reduction/casting technique	Anterior displacement: reduction in flexion, immobilization in flexion (20–30°) Posterior displacement: reduction in extension; immobilization in extension
General material	Fluoroscopy Arthroscopy (option)
Positioning	Supine; free but draped leg; foldable foot section (optional arthroscopy and/or epiphyseal reduction usually in knee flexion). Fluoroscopy in two planes Prone position for vascular injury
Approach	Open reduction: Approach from the side of the metaphyseal fragment Vascular injury: Posteromedial approach
Special clarification	Growth disturbances; leg-length discrepancies, axial malalignment Compartment syndrome
Operative principle	Crossed K-wire transfixion Fig. 13.28 Material: K-wires, diameter 1.6–2.0 mm From medial and lateral, percutaneous → hardware removal possible without extra general anesthesia In cases of small fragments, crossing of the growth plate is acceptable; as vertically as possible to minimize damage Cross-point proximal to the fracture → rotational stability Screw fixation Fig. 13.29 Material: Cancellous screws with short threads, titanium; cannulated if needed (e.g., 4.5 mm) Stab incision on the side of the metaphyseal fragment External fixator (additional, instead of cast) Material: Rod fixator (e.g., monotube) Pin position: Lateral femur (posterior to the insertion of the vastus lateralis muscle) Distal pin → at least 1 cm from the epiphyseal plate Pin distance to fracture: 2 finger-widths Descending ESIN
Hardware removal	K-wires: Outpatient if needed, if left percutaneous ESIN/screws/external fixator: General anesthesia
Other special features	None

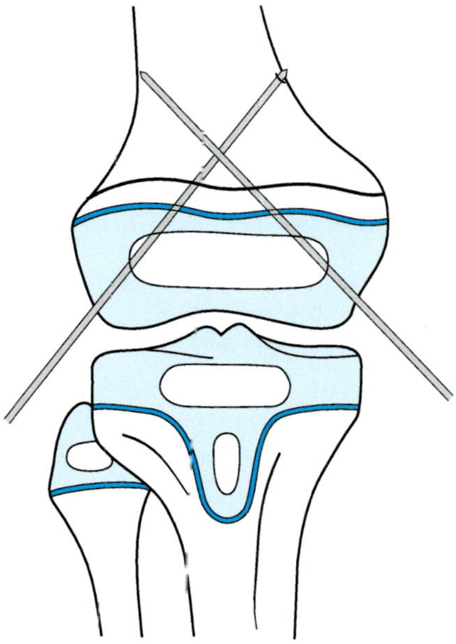

Fig. 13.28 Crossed K-wire osteosynthesis after reduction of distal femur epiphyseolysis

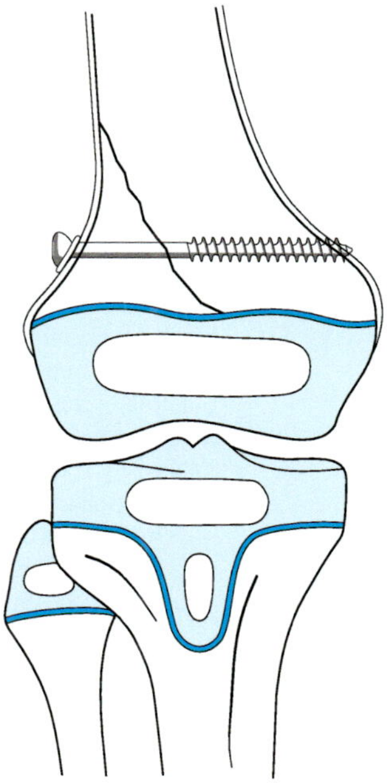

Fig. 13.29 Screw osteosynthesis (Salter-Harris I) injury of the distal femur. Note the screw metaphyseal parallel andabove the growth plate

Table 13.8 Technical aspects fractures of the proximal tibia

General Material	Fluoroscopy Arthroscopy option
Positioning	Supine position; free draped leg; foldable foot section (arthroscopy) Fluoroscopy in two planes
Special clarification	Growth disturbances; leg-length discrepancies, axial malalignment Vascular injury → compartment syndrome Peroneal nerve lesion
Operative principle	Screw fixation (Fig. 13.30) Material: Cannulated, self-tapping cancellous screws with short threads, titanium; washer 3.5–5 mm if needed Fracture of the proximal tibia: Closed reduction and fixation via stab incision; open reduction preferably through an anterolateral approach Tuberosity fracture:Midline incision (slightly medial to the patellar tendon) → reduction in extension → if needed, 2 screws for rotational stability (Fig. 13.31) → adolescent injury → growth plate can be crossed Avulsion of the patella ligament needs to be fixed by sutures or ancors (Fig. 13.27)
Hardware removal	Screws under general anesthesia K-wires as outpatient
Other special features	None

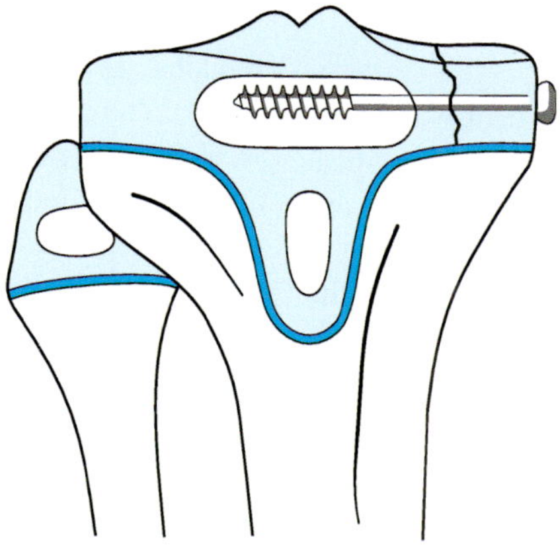

Fig. 13.30 Compression osteosynthesis of a distal Salter-Harris-II fracture of the proximal tibial epiphysis. The screws run parallel to the epiphyseal line

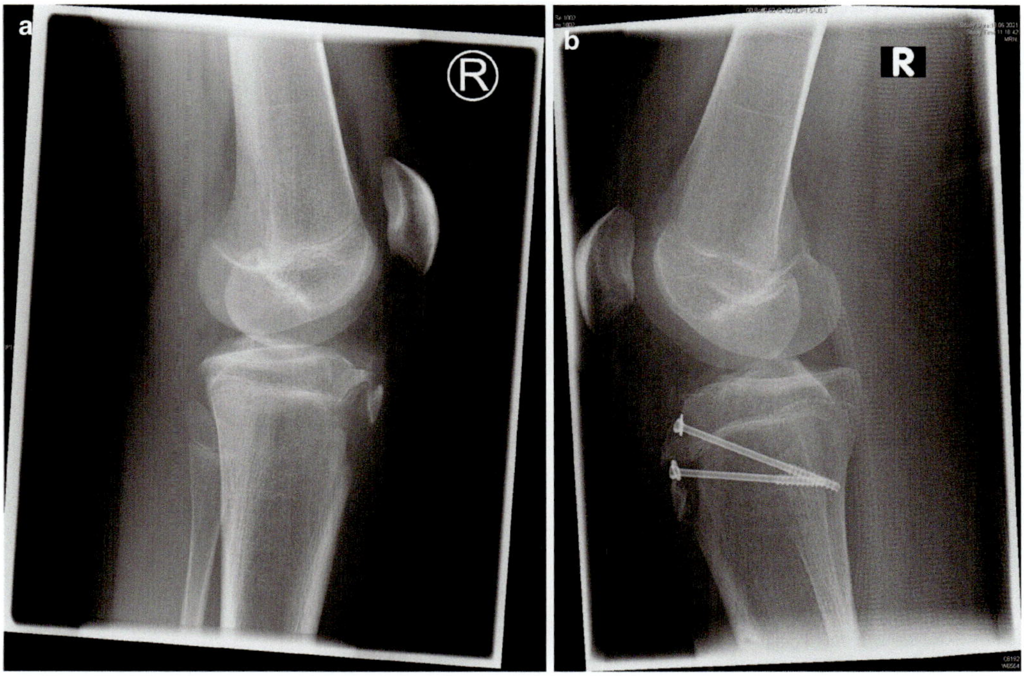

Fig. 13.31 Avulsion fracture of the tuberorsitas tibia Type I. (**a**) Trauma image, (**b**) X-ray after screw fixation

13.3 Patellar Injuries

In most cases, an ossification center emerges between ages 3 and 6 years. Additional ossification centers appear in 30% of cases. These can fuse with the remaining patella over the course of growth or result in a bipartite patella. A bipartite patella is an ossification variant that generally remains asymptomatic (Figs. 13.32a, b and 13.33). The chondral connection to the patella is a weak point for compression and shearing forces, and avulsion fractures occur rarely. In most cases, no specific treatment is needed; in rare cases, resection of the bony fragment is necessary.

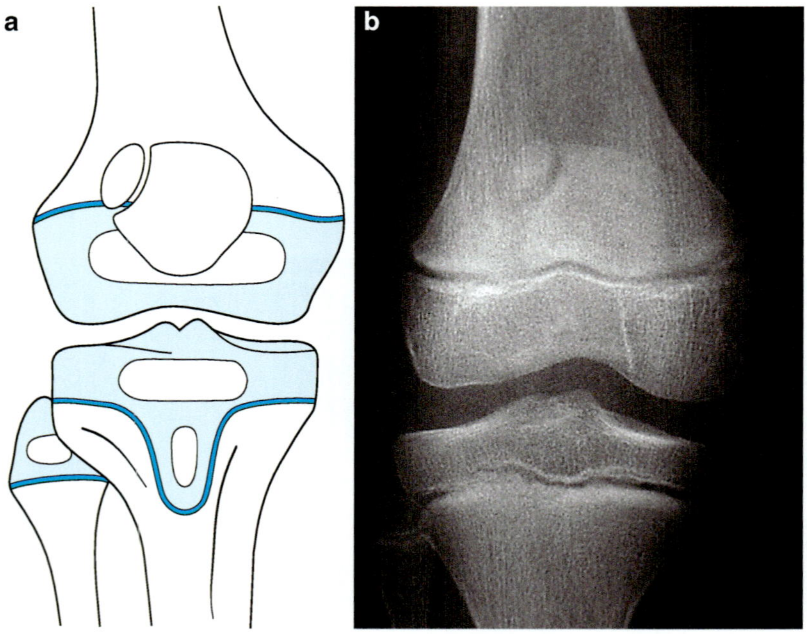

Fig. 13.32 Patella bipartita, most often form. (**a**) Scheme, (**b**) X-ray

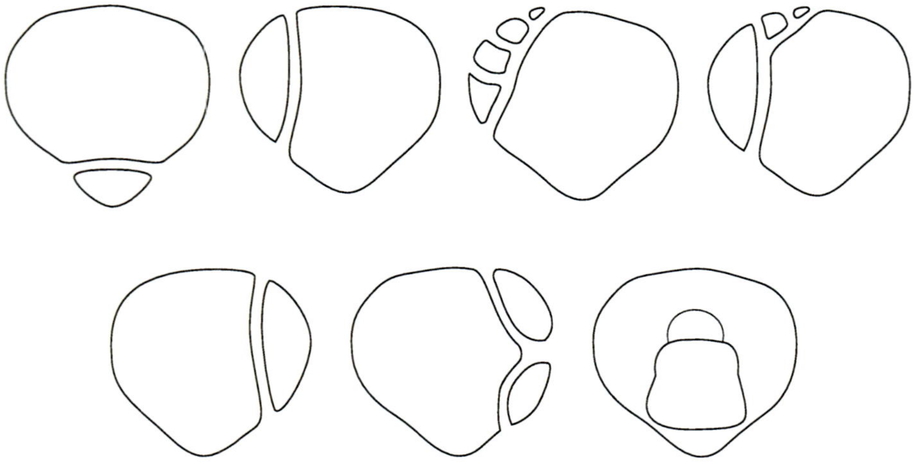

Fig. 13.33 Patella bipartita, rare forms

Patella Fracture

The incidence of patella fractures is 1%. Fractures around the patella are much less common in children than adults. The pediatric knee joint is more flexible because of lax ligaments and the bone remaining sheathed in cartilage. There is a distinction between longitudinal and transverse fractures, and similar as in adults longitudinal undisplaced fractures do not need always surgical treatment (Fig. 13.34). However, this must be differentiated from a bipartite patella. Displaced fractures and most transverse fracture need a functional stable osteosynthesis, either by tension band wiring (Fig. 13.35) or screw osteosynthesis (Fig. 13.36). A particular pattern of patella fractures in children are osteochondral avulsion fragments with the patella ligament together, the so called typical sleeve fracture. They are sometimes recognized only by a small bony shell at the inferior patellar pole (Fig. 13.37) When the patellar tendon is insufficient, an MRI should be performed to exclude an injury requiring surgery (Fig. 13.38). In adults, hemarthrosis usually indicates an ACL rupture. In children, however, with unremarkable radiographic findings, hemarthrosis more commonly indicates an osteochondral fracture, capsular ligament injury, or patellar dislocation.

The treatment options for patella fractures and avulsion fractures are indicated in Table 13.9.

The technical options for refixation of a patella fracture are indicated in Table 13.10.

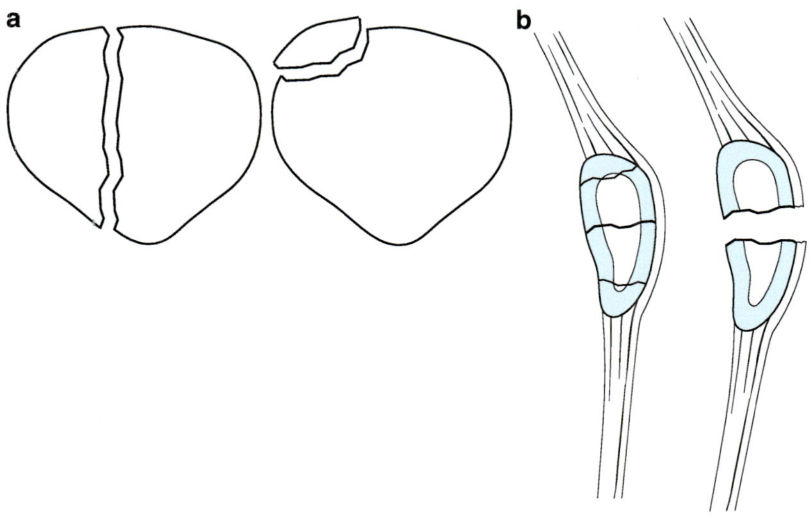

Fig. 13.34 Fracture of the patella. (**a**) horizontal view, (**b**) lateral view

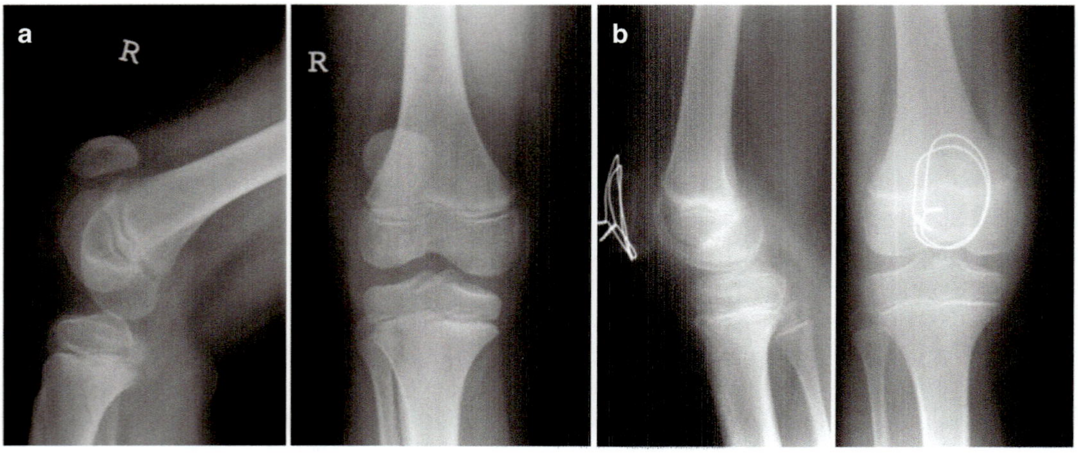

Fig. 13.35 Displaced patella fracture. (**a**) X-ray, (**b**) Reduction and cerclage

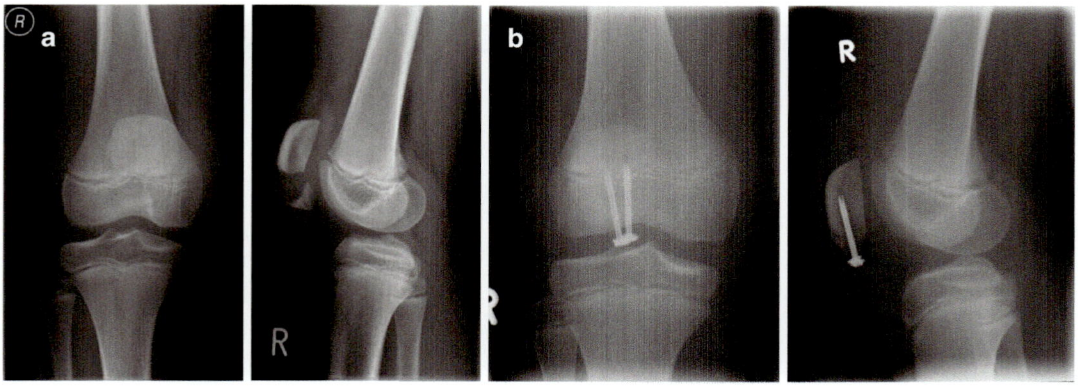

Fig. 13.36 Transverse fracture of the lower patella, (**a**) Trauma image, (**b**) After reduction and screw fixation

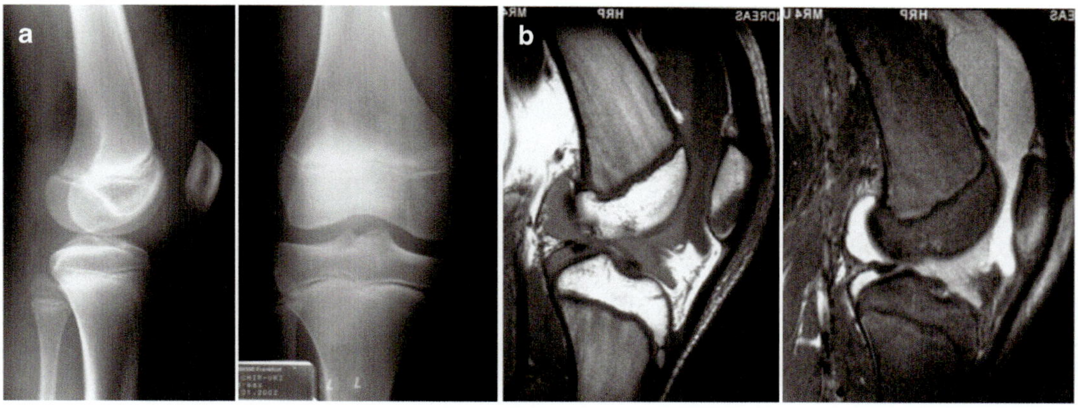

Fig. 13.37 Sleeve-fracture of the patealla of a 11 year old boy. (**a**) Trauma image with small bony lesion of the inferior end, (**b**) MRI of the avulsion of the patella tendon

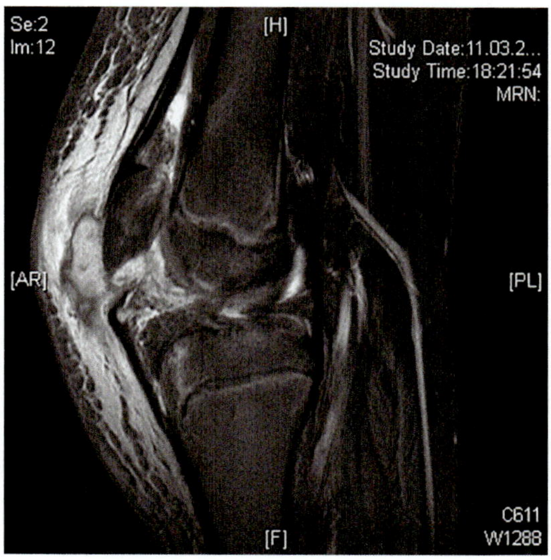

Fig. 13.38 Sleeve fracture of the proximal patellar tendon at the distal patella pole

Table 13.9 Patalla fracture

Special features	Rare; direct trauma, especially in adolescents Osteochondral fracture, especially post-patellar dislocation Sleeve fracture: osteochondral avulsion fracture; especially ages 8–12 years, abrupt quadriceps exertion (e.g., high jump)
Diagnostic approach	AP and lateral x-rays, axial patella in vertical fracture MRI in hemarthros recommended, if reason not evident Arthroscopy when therapeutic measures are expected
Treatment goal/limits of correction	Joint congruence, reconstruction of the extensor apparatus
Primary treatment	Long-leg plaster splint or orthosis, analgesia If needed, joint aspiration for hemarthrosis Emergency indication: Displaced fractures
Conservative treatment	
Indication	Non-displaced fractures (see Fig. Above, MRI, preserved extensors), especially vertical fractures (<2 mm) (Fig. 13.39)
Approach	Long-leg cast or orthosis for 4 weeks with rolling weight-bearing
Follow up	After cast removal, 2 weeks rolling weight-bearing, then weight-bearing as tolerated; physical therapy as needed
Radiological controls	At 5 weeks cast-free
Return to sports	Free function and muscular symmetry; at approx. 3 months
Operative treatment	
Indication	Displaced fractures
Approach	Transverse fractures: Open reduction and tension-band fixation or screw fixation (Fig. 13.40) Vertical fractures: Arthroscopically-assisted screw fixation, possibly open Sleeve fracture: Transosseous fixation suture if needed.) (Fig. 13.41) Osteochondral fracture: Refixation with resorbable materials or removal of small fragments
Follow up	Tension band: Exercise stability; rolling weight-bearing for 5 weeks, then weight-bearing as tolerated; possible physical therapy Usually knee orthosis, possibly long-leg cast for 4 weeks
Radiological controls	5 weeks post-surgery, cast-free
Hardware removal	6 months post-surgery
Return to sports	Free function and muscular symmetry; at approx. 3 months
Complications	Joint step = pre-arthritis Non-union; fixation avulsion, patella Alta
Growth disturbance	None
Follow up	Weekly until free function

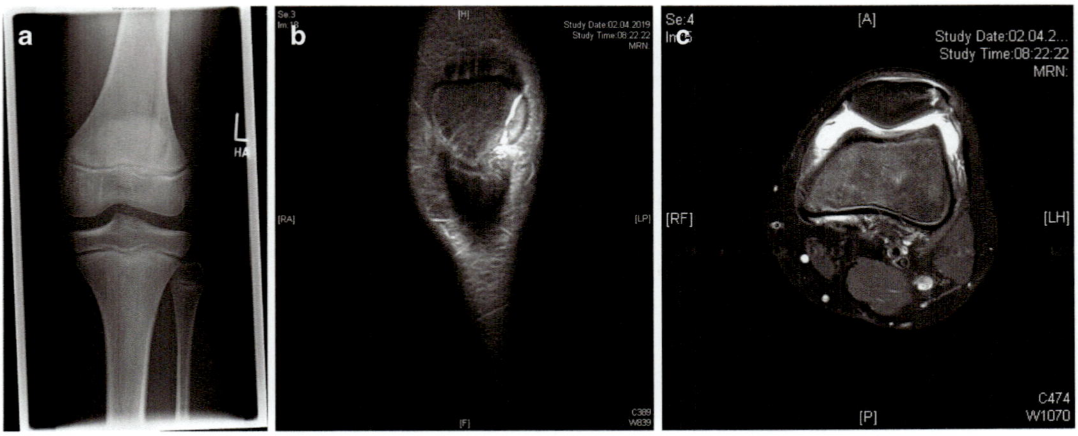

Fig. 13.39 Longitudinal fracture of the patella. (**a**) X-ray, (**b**, **c**) MRI view

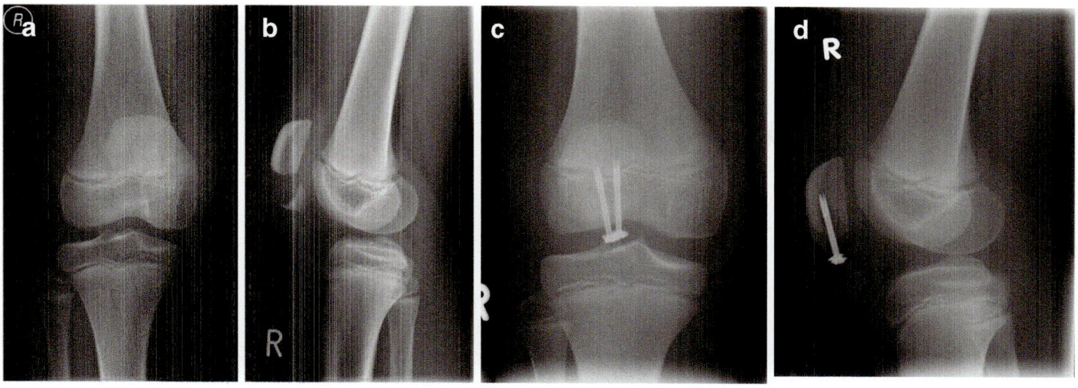

Fig. 13.40 Transversal fracture of the distal patella. (**a**, **b**) Trauma image, (**c**, **d**) Screw fixation after open reduction

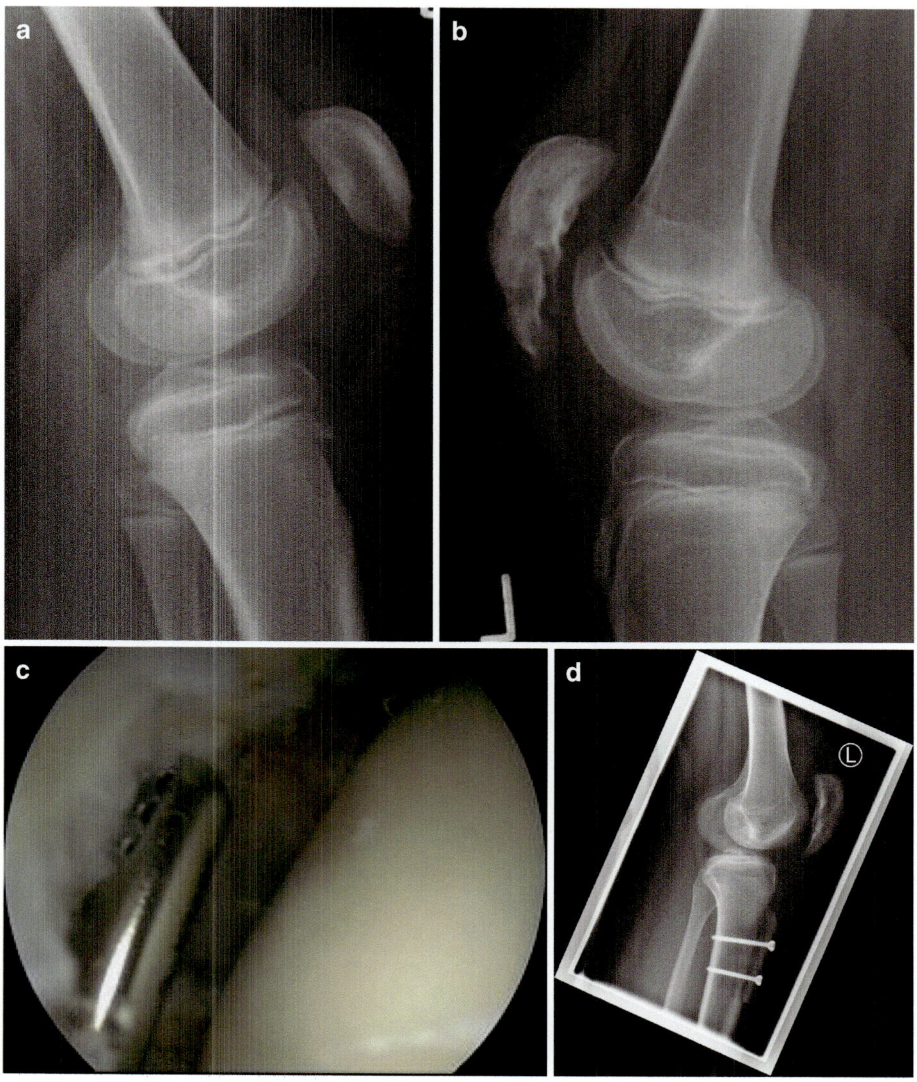

Fig. 13.41 Sleeve fracture with secondary post-traumatic deformity, (**a**) Fracture pattern, (**b**) Deformity from patellar ligament tension, (**c**) Arthroscopic findings with osteophyte ablation, (**d**) Release with Fulkerson osteotomy

Table 13.10 Patella fracture—technical aspects

General material	Fluoroscopy
Positioning	Supine position; knee roll (knee in approx. 20° flexion) Thigh tourniquet
Approach	Transverse approach or straight anterior approach Reduction in extension
Special clarification	Pre-arthritis Non-union Material failure Secondary fixation loosening Sensory deficits (especially with a transverse incision)
Operative principle	Screw fixation Small fragment cancellous screws, diameter 3.5–4.5 mm, if needed cannulated with short threads Indication: Vertical fracture Fig. 13.42; pole fracture Figs. 13.43 and 13.44 Palpatory control of the joint surface; no steps accepted Tension band Material: K-wire, diameter 1.6 mm; cerclage wire 1.25 mm, semi-circular hollow needle Not crossed (equatorial cerclage) and/or crossed (tension band) (Fig. 13.45) Palpatory control of the joint surface Parallel K-wires, relatively posterior Passing the cerclage wire under the K-wires and the tendon, tensioning the wires (fluoroscopic controls)
	Transosseous fixation suture with 1.0 PDS Resorbable bone pins Screw fixation (Fig. 13.46) Fibrin glue
Hardware removal	6 months post-surgery
Other special features	None

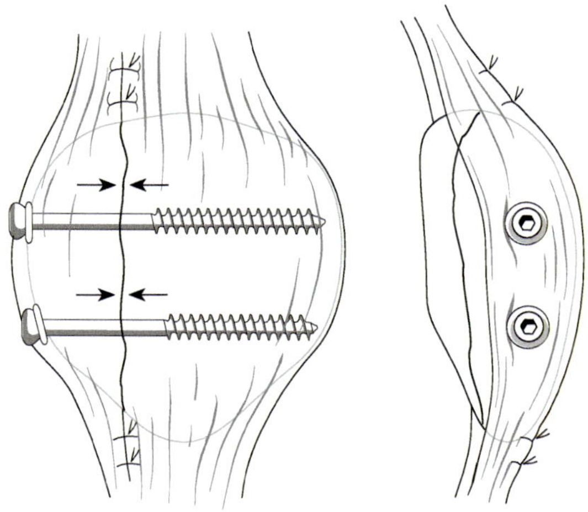

Fig. 13.42 Screw osteosynthesis of vertical fracture of the patella

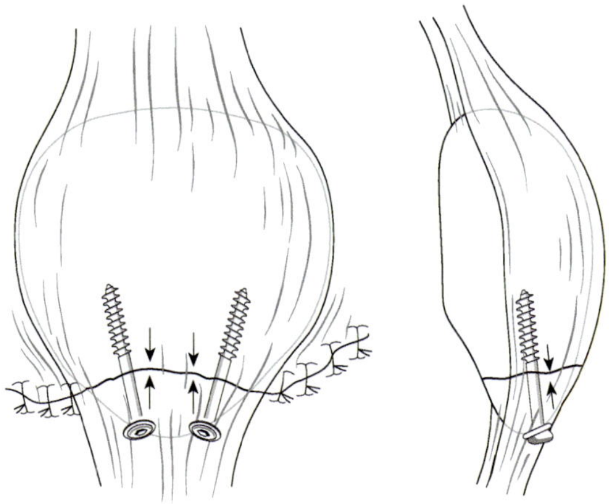

Fig. 13.43 Screw osteosynthesis of a transverse fracture of the patealla, eventually with additional suture

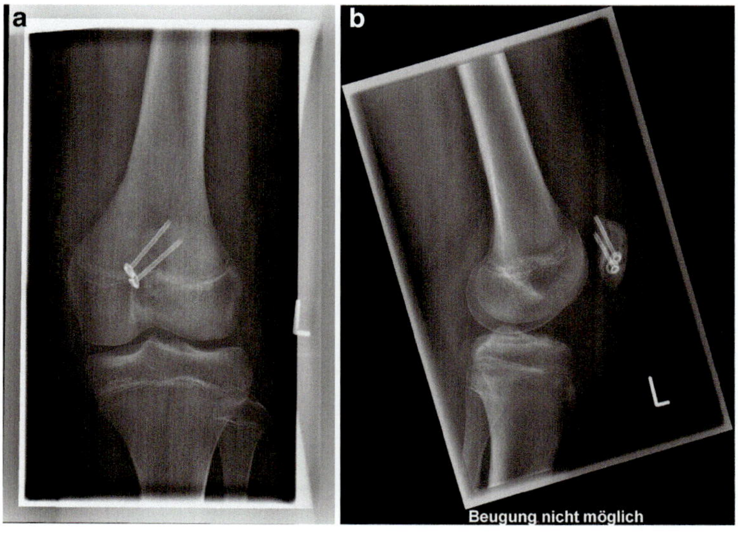

Fig. 13.44 Longitudinal patella fracture, fixation with 2 crews. (a) ap view, (b) lateral view

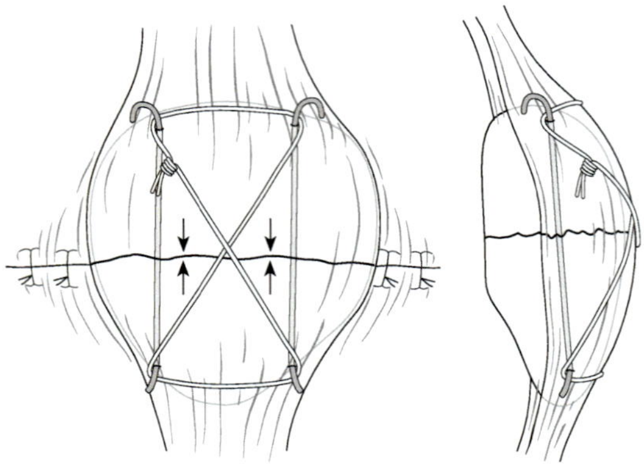

Fig. 13.45 Tension band wiring of oblique fracture of the patella

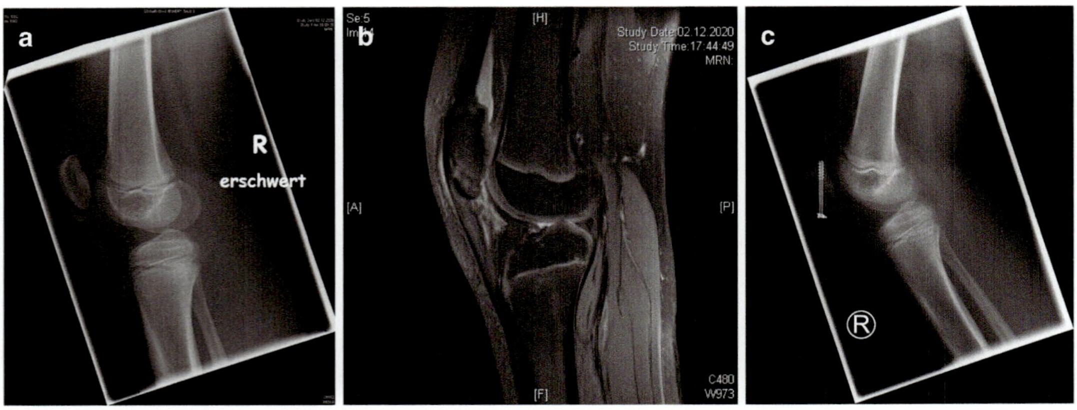

Fig. 13.46 Sleeve fracture of the patella with small bony fragment (**a**) X-ray, (**b**) MRI, (**c**) Refixation with screw and suture

Patellar Dislocation

Uneven static and dynamic forces on the patella (evident by an increased Q-angle; Fig. 13.47a) can result in lateralization within the femoropatellar groove (Fig. 13.47b) and eventually, patellar dislocation. About 90% of these are traumatic dislocations, individual events or chronic recurrences resulting from secondary capsular instability. The incidence of dislocation is approximately 7–49 per 100,000, of which around 11% show musculoskeletal symptoms. The incidence increases to 100 per 100,000 in children aged 9–15 years, with girls more commonly affected.

Patellofemoral (PF) instability is expressed not only through patellar dislocation but through subluxation and general instability. Other nontraumatic causes are much more challenging to correct (Table 13.11).

In normal physiology and balanced biomechanics, the patella is lateralized in extension and is engaged through the soft tissues; the medial patellofemoral ligament (MPFL) is taut. With 15–30° flexion, the ligament is relatively relaxed. It builds a high level of tension between 45 and 100°. With physiological tracking, bony engagement begins between 20 and 40° and increases until about 100°, supported by active stabilizers from around 60°. During normal patellar tracking, this leads to patellar medialization from the lateral, then re-lateralization distally.

When the stabilizers are disrupted, the biomechanics are altered, and PF instability results.

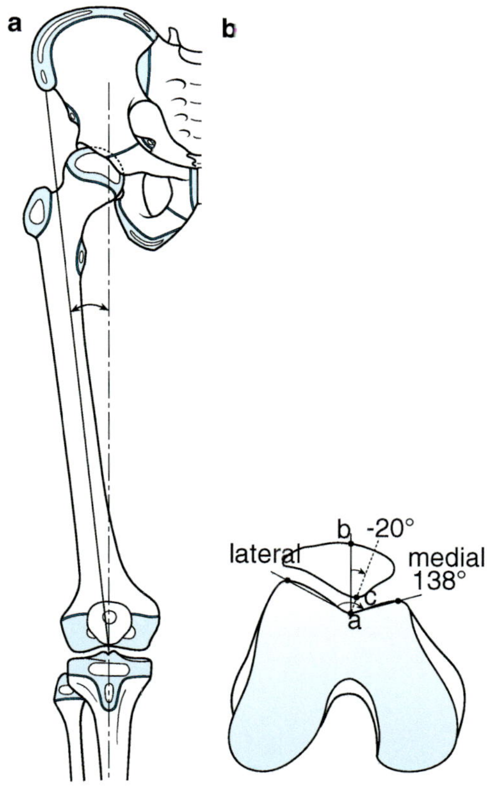

Fig. 13.47 (**a**) Q-angle: quadriceps force vector = increased with chronic patellar dislocation; Normal values: m = 8–10°; f = 10–15°, Merchant congruence determination of femoropatellar tracking; *Sulcus angle:* The angle of the trochlear groove, Normal value: 138°. (**b**) *Congruence angle:* (1) Line between the patellar apex and deepest point of the groove. (2) Line between the posterior patellar edge and deepest point of the groove. Normal values: −6 to −16°, > 0: angle lies lateral to congruence line, >+16°: frequent patellar dislocation

The fundamental factors predisposing for instability or dislocation are:

- Contralateral dislocation

Static Factors

- Lateral condyle hypoplasia
- Patellar or Trochlear dysplasia
- Axial malalignment (Genu valgum),
- Torsional deformity (Coxa valga with antetorsion, AT angle, CCD angle, TT angle)
- Patella alta

Table 13.11 Sub-classification of patellar dislocations

Congenital dislocation:	Dislocation at birth and extensor apparatus shifted laterally
Habitual dislocation:	Generally chronic, due to congenital malformation of kneecap stabilizers
Traumatic dislocation (90%):	Single incidence or recurrent chronic due to secondary instability of the capsule ligament apparatus
Neurogenic dislocation:	e.g., in quadriplegia, the abnormal force of the vastus lateralis muscle

Active Stabilizers

- vastus medialis muscle insufficiency/injury

Passive Stabilizers

- medial capsule-ligament insufficiency/injury
- pathological TTTG (tibial tuberosity trochlear groove distance)
- increased patellar tilt
- contracture of the lateral capsule structures and the vastus lateralis muscle

The diagnosis is not always easy to make because there is usually spontaneous patellar reduction at the injury scene. A targeted history and immediate clinical examination are essential for classifying the dislocation (Table 13.12).

There are various radiological parameters; however, these can only be correctly used with a completely ossified patella (Blumensaat; Insall and Salvati) (Fig. 13.48). On clinical examination, traumatic dislocation usually leads to tenderness over the medial retinaculum, medial patella, or lateral femoral condyle, depending on the mechanism of injury, with a positive apprehension test (pain when mimicking the dislocation mechanism). Associated injuries such as soft-tissue damage and osteochondral fractures must always be considered. Children with generalized joint hyperlaxity are at lower risk for accompanying intra-articular injuries.

MRI offers valuable information regarding associated injuries that influence outcome and treatment, e.g., associated osteochondral fracture or MPFL injury with ligamentous tears or avulsions of the patella or medial femoral condyle

Table 13.12 Patellar dislocation classification

Type I: traumatic dislocation	Rare; associated osteochondral fractures and soft-tissue damage	Treatment: conservative without associated injury; surgical with associated injury
Type II: Chronic dislocation chronic recurrent/habitual: Congenital or acquired	Especially in adolescent girls; cause: Femoropatellar groove dysplasia, extensor apparatus insufficiency, valgus leg axis (increased Q-angle); common non-specific chronic knee pain	Treatment: Primary conservative (muscle building), operative secondary to persistent complaints
Type III: Habitual dislocation (congenital)	Especially in hyperactive children; attention deficit disorder; several and arbitrary dislocations per day, generally asymptomatic, no associated injuries	Treatment: Conservative

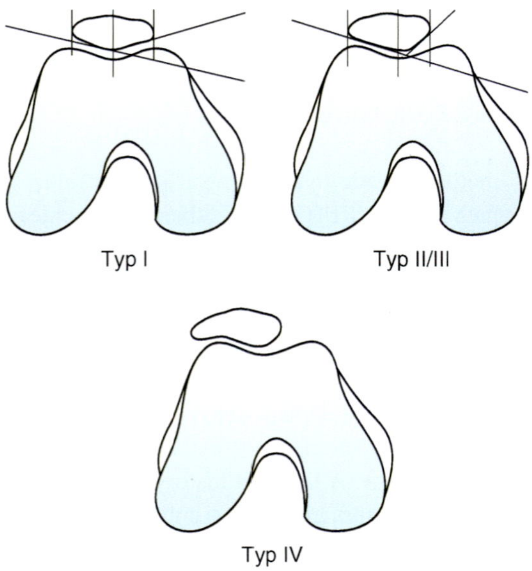

Fig. 13.48 Patella luxation and forms of patella

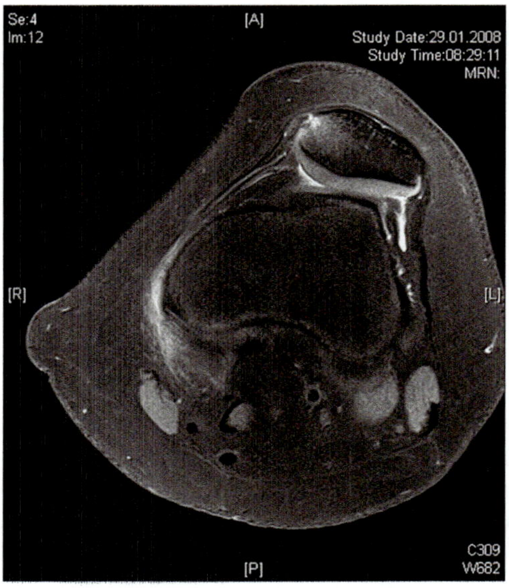

Fig. 13.49 Rupture of the medial retinaculum on the patellar side of the patellofemoral ligament (MPFL) of a 13 year old boy. Here, the suture or doubling of the medial ligament close to the patella is necessary

(Figs. 13.49, 13.50, and 13.51). Primary arthroscopy can also be useful when there is massive hemarthrosis. Joint aspiration showing beads of fat on the blood gives clear evidence of an osteochondral injury. In cases of primary dislocation without associated injury, conservative treatment is indicated with strengthening of the oblique head of the vastus medialis (quadriceps) muscle to improve patellar tracking. However, the rate of re-dislocation after conservative treatment is cited in the literature as 15–63% without risk factors and up to 88% when risk factors are present.

Risk Factors:

- trochlear dysplasia
- immature skeleton
- CDI > 1.45
- contralateral dislocation

In contrast, the re-dislocation rate is 7–25% after operative treatment.

In cases of chronically recurring patellar dislocations, axial and rotational assessments and measurement of predisposing factors are necessary along with detailed history, clinical examination, and operative reports (when applicable) because subsequent treatment will be based on all of this information. Above all, patellar deviation from physiological tracking (maltracking) must be evaluated.

The following parameters and aspects should be noted as indicated in Table 13.13.

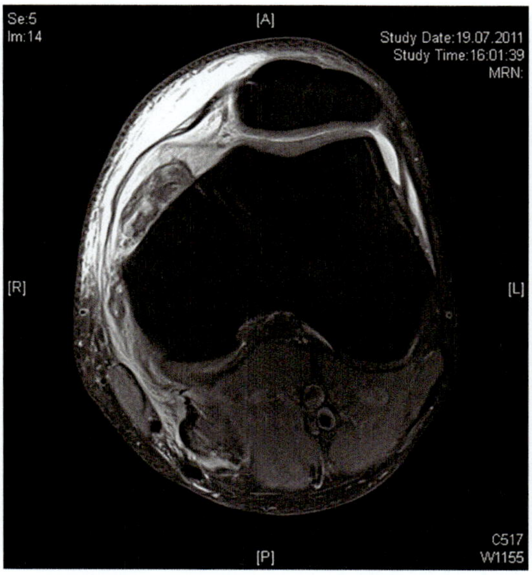

Fig. 13.50 MRI of a typical MPFL rupture of a 15 year old boy. Here, the MPFL is ruptured from the medial femur (Tuberculum adduktorium) and without tension. Refixation at the femur necessary

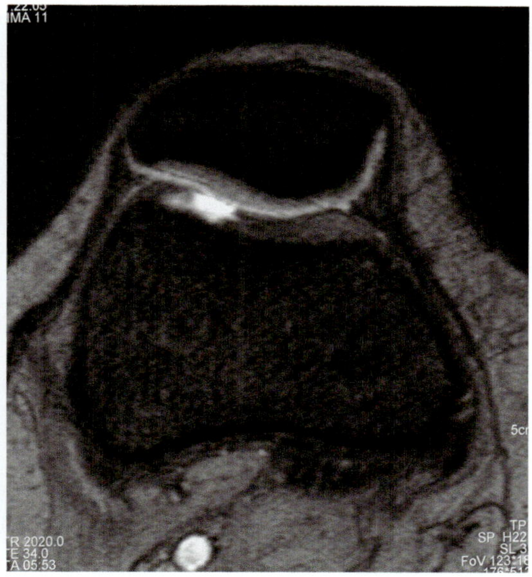

Fig. 13.51 Osteochondral flake after patella luxation of the cartilage of the femur behind the patella

There are many operative treatment methods, which can be divided roughly into soft-tissue restraining and bony procedures. Ultimately, the operative approach is selected based on assessments of the lesions and risk factors.

Corrective procedures for chronic dislocations with patellar maltracking should be approached according to pathology. Individual analysis of the often complex pathology must be considered along with patient age, remaining growth, and growth plates. The need for correction, possibly with a combination of techniques, should also be discussed. For example, when there is MPFL rupture and insufficiency, MPFL reconstruction is obvious. If the TT-TG distance is over 20 mm, a soft-tissue or bony tibial tuberosity transfer can be added if needed. Valgus deformity plays a special role in patellar dislocation, and bony correction (growth modulation or corrective osteotomy) should be considered. When there is more than 20–30° femoral anteversion or more than 40° external rotation of the tibia, derotation osteotomy is more likely indicated. Patella alta is usually corrected with a bony tibial tuberosity transfer. For this procedure, the biomechanical effects are relevant, particularly contact pressure, which needs to be balanced with anteriorization. Correction for pronounced trochlear/patellar dysplasia is rarely performed in children and adolescents (Tables 13.14 and 13.15).

Table 13.13 Checklist patellar dislocation

• Fractures, chondral lesions/avulsions, loose bodies
• MPFL lesions, retinacular lesions
• Trochlear dysplasia (e.g., facet asymmetry, sulcus depth)
• Patellar elevation (e.g., Caton Deschamps index)
• Torsional deformities of the femur or tibia (AT angle, CCD angle, TT angle)
• Leg axis deformity (especially valgus)

Table 13.14 Patellar dislocation—diagnostic and indications

Special features	Type I: traumatic Type II: chronic habitual: especially in adolescent girls; femoropatellar dysplasia, Genu valgum, extensor insufficiency Type III: habitual: voluntary, painless dislocations (!), often with neuromuscular disease Patellar shapes according to Wiberg: Type I/II: symmetrical/asymmetrical = physiological Type III: severe asymmetry/alpine hunter's cap deformity = pathological
Diagnostic approach	Usually spontaneous reduction X-rays of the knee in two planes + axial patella (post-reduction); in toddlers, ultrasound due to predominant cartilage For recurrent dislocations: Axial images (assessment of patellar shape and trochlear dysplasia) When there is a clinically remarkable axis: Whole leg standing images to check the axis, with supplemental torsion angle MRI if needed (Fig. 13.52) With persistent effusion: Arthroscopy Primary dislocation without arthroscopy: MRI (intra-articular, especially cartilage, MPFL, and TT-TG assessment)
Treatment goal/limits of correction	Joint congruence Prevention of re-dislocation
Primary treatment	Immediate reduction through knee extension (if this does not work, flexion of the hip joint with extended knee) Long-leg plaster splint, medical analgesia if needed If needed, joint aspiration for hemarthrosis
Conservative treatment	
Indication	Habitual: Primarily conservative No associated osteochondral injuries
Approach	Long-leg cast or orthosis for 3 weeks with weight-bearing as tolerated
Follow up	Functional; muscle building (quadriceps muscle), physical therapy
Radiological controls	None
Return to sports	With muscular symmetry and asymptomatic knee; at approx. 6 weeks, if needed wearing a brace for sports
Operative treatment	
Indication	Associated osteochondral injuries; recurrent dislocations; unsuccessful conservative treatment, subacute, congenital pathology, MPFL rupture
Approach	Primary: Diagnostic arthroscopy and refixation/removal of osteochondral flakes via mini-arthrotomy, MPFL repair (important medial stabilizer) close to the patella (Fig. 13.53); bony refixation as needed, plication of the medial retinaculum (Fig. 13.54) Secondary: Arthroscopic or open procedure and reconstructive techniques (MPFL reconstruction with gracilis/semitendinosus tendon or quadriceps strips, soft-tissue or bony tibial tuberosity transfer) or deformity correction (growth modulation, varying/torsion-correcting rotational osteotomy, bony tibial tuberosity transfer)
Follow up	6 weeks of orthosis, with 2 weeks each of 30°, 60°, and 90° flexion; 2 weeks partial weight-bearing, full weight-bearing on standing, and then transition to full weight-bearing Passive mobility Physical therapy, somatic muscle building, initially passive
Radiological controls	6 weeks after the bony procedure, none for soft-tissue procedures
Hardware removal	With straight leg axes, post-consolidation
Return to sports	Free function, muscular symmetry; at approx. 12 weeks
Complications/associated injuries	Rupture of the medial retinaculum; rupture of the medial patellofemoral ligament (MPFL); osteochondral flake (medial patella/lateral femoral condyle) Re-dislocation; chondromalacia patellae (CMP) with suboptimal patellar tracking also within the trochlear groove; persistent instability of the trochlear groove
Growth disturbance	Possible in interventions near the growth plates (e.g., temporary epiphysiodesis for axial correction)
Follow up	Every 3 weeks until free function and symptom-free

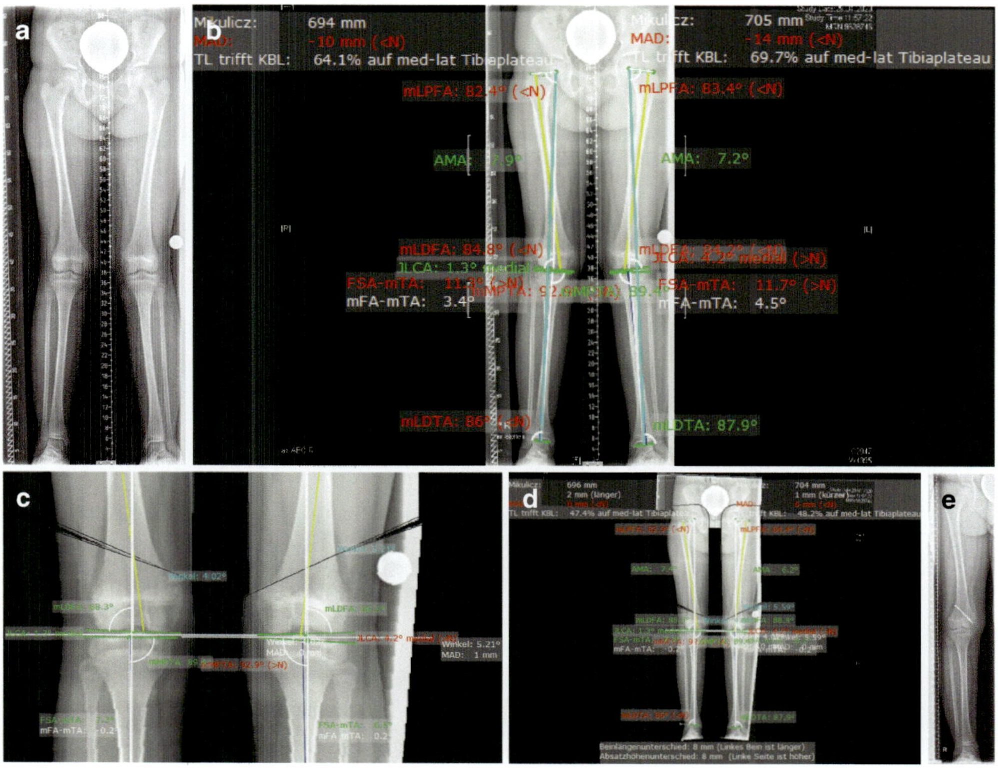

Fig. 13.52 Valgus deformity and correction. (**a**) X-ray of standing patient of both sides. (**b–d**) Measurement of axis, deviation and planning of correction. (**e**) Epiphyseodesis of the medial growth plate with a screw

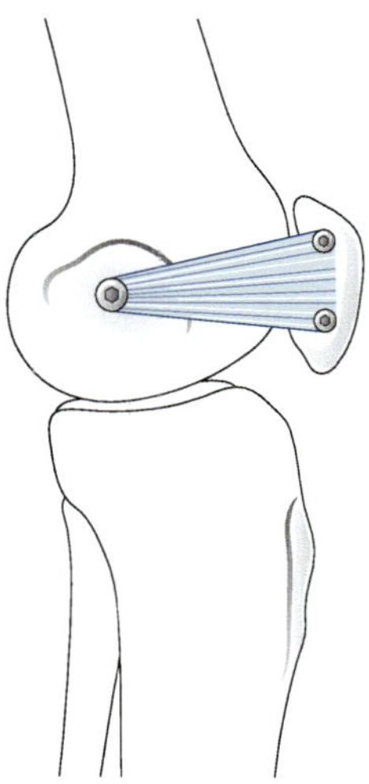

Fig. 13.53 Refixation of MPFL at the tuberculum adductorium of the medial femur with a cork-bio-screw in anatomical position. After arthroscopy to exclude intraarticular osteochondral lesions, direct appraoch to the rupture site. Exposition of the ruptured MPFL and refixation with bio-cork-screws and suture of the MPFL. Ideal position is important to have a good alignment of the patella

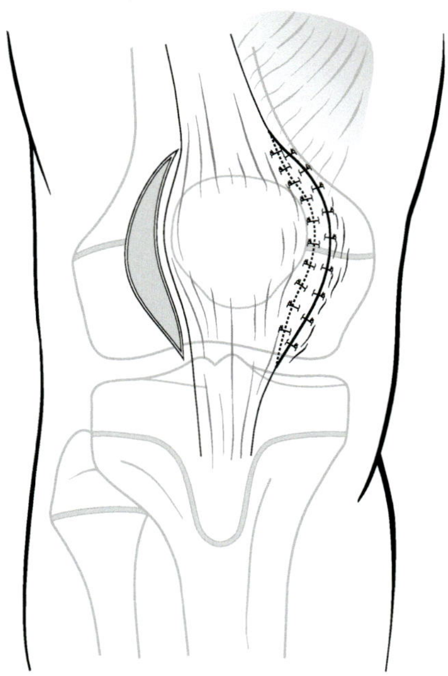

Fig. 13.54 Doubling of the medial retinaculum (lateral release is only in few cases recommended)

Table 13.15 Patellar dislocation—technical aspects

Positioning	Supine position; free draped leg; foldable foot section (arthroscopy) Open: supine position; knee roll (knee in approx. 20° flexion) Thigh tourniquet
Approach	Caution: Infrapatellar branches of the saphenous nerve (medial over the pes anserinus)
Special clarification	With flakes: Pre-arthritis Re-dislocation Lesion of cutaneous nerves → pre-patellar numbness post-surgery Overcorrection Non-union
Operative principle	Diagnostic arthroscopy In flexion: Inspection of the loading surface of the patella on the trochlear groove; in cases of minimal lateralization and recurrent patellar dislocation, medial plication or suture of the capsule-ligament apparatus is sufficient, a lateral release is performed only when there is persistent patellar tilt, observation and removal of adhesions and folds Osteochondral flakes Reduction and fixation with screws, transfixion suture, resorbable pins, fibrin glue Restraining procedures Soft-tissue procedures → optimization of the extensor mechanism and passive patellar tracking – MPFL reconstruction with gracilis/semitendinosus tendon or Fig. 13.55 – MPFL reconstruction with quadriceps strips (Lenschow modification) – Tibial tuberosity transfer if needed (roux-Goldthwait modification) Lateral release Contraindication: Severe femoropatellar dysplasia Extra-synovial vertical splitting of the lateral capsule If needed, resection of 1 cm wide strip of capsule to avoid scar readaptation Medial plication Reconstruction of the medial retinaculum and capsular plication *Open:* Approach through a medial skin incision, incision of the medial retinaculum and doubling (Fig. 13.54) *Arthroscopic:* 1. Anterolateral approach 2. Stab incision for the cannula along the medial patellar rim holding the periosteum 3. Stab incision; subcutaneous spreading and advancing an eyelet 3–6 cm medially 4. Incision with a second cannula through the suture loop with loop 5. Binding of the skin bridge between the cannulae 6. Grasp the thread through the suture loop from the medial incision 7. Withdraw the loop (second cannula) in the subcutaneous tissues 8. Withdraw the eyelet and knot in extension (knot lies subcutaneously under the skin incision) 9. Depending on the extent: 3–5 repetitions Alternative 1. Insert both cannulae 2. Draw the suture (PDS 2/0) through both cannulae with the suture eyelet 3. Knots on the capsule after splitting of the soft-tissue bridge between the cannulae
	Bony interventions Centralizing the patella in the groove and medialization of the quadriceps muscle traction Tuberosity transfer according to Elmslie and Trillat Fig. 13.56 Material: K-wire 2 mm; cancellous screws 6.5 mm; cortical screws 5 mm; washer Contraindication: Open growth plates, genu valgum >10° Approach: Lateral parapatellar incision Tuberosity anteromedialization, lateral release and medial capsular plication if needed Subperiosteal exposure of the tuberosity to 5 cm distal Breaking point: 3.2 mm transverse drill canal, approx. 4 cm distal to the tuberosity beneath the cortex (protecting the attachment of the patellar tendon) Osteotomy sloped mildly to medial → with simultaneous anteriorization Fixation with 2 cancellous screws introduced proximally and 1 cortical screw placed distally
Hardware removal	Screws: At 6 months
Other special features	None

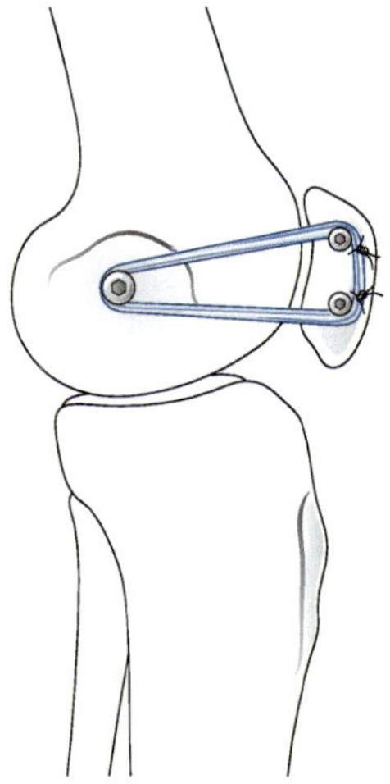

Fig. 13.55 In chronic luxation situation and after exclusion of other reasons for patella luxation a secondary MPFL plastic can be performed. The gracilis tendon is taken from the medial tibial head with a tendon stripper. Approach between the tuberculum adductorium and the medial patella. V-Type fixation of the gracilis tendon on the medial patella border with suture anchor and fixation at the rotation point at the femur, which should be controlled by lateral x-ray

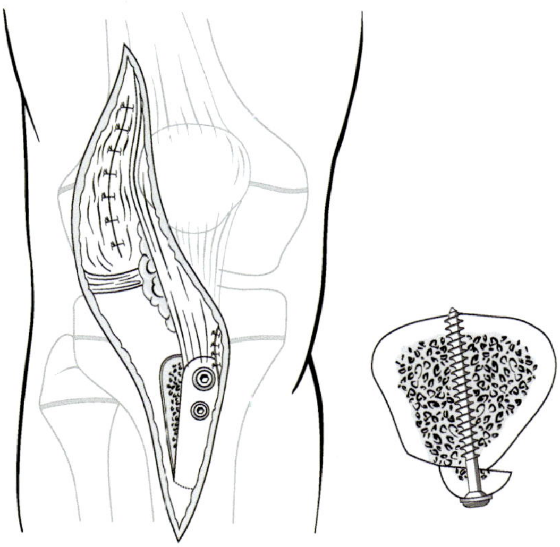

Fig. 13.56 Elmslie and Trillat procedure

13.4 Pediatric Knee Ligament Injuries

Isolated ligament injuries are much less common than osteochondral injuries in children because of higher ligament stability. Thus, epiphyseal or bony ligament avulsion injuries are more common than ligament ruptures when growth plates are wide open. With advancing age, the general hyperlaxity of the capsule-ligament structures decreases, and the bony structures (apophyses) increase in stability, and thus, the incidence of ligament ruptures increases. Because of increasing sports activities, sometimes because of insufficient training, ligamentous injuries are becoming more common even in children under ten years, especially anterior cruciate ligament (ACL) injuries. When there is instability with buckling or "giving way," cruciate ligament replacement at a young age has been found to prevent secondary knee damage.

When the growth plates remain wide open, the clinical diagnosis of ligament injury is more challenging, as there is individual variability in plate gapping ability. A bony avulsion can often be detected radiologically. Hemarthrosis indicates articular knee injury, and in adolescent children, when there is no fracture, it is a relatively clear indication of an ACL rupture. In girls, on the other hand, patellar dislocation is most likely, with hemarthrosis caused by capsule or retinacular tears. In boys, hemarthrosis is most often caused by ACL rupture or traumatic meniscus injury. Diagnosis can usually be made in children without purely diagnostic arthroscopy through careful clinical examination and MRI. Arthroscopic intervention is generally necessary for massive hemarthrosis, osteochondral fragments, cruciate ligament, or meniscus injuries, just as in patellar dislocation.

Although rare, when there is knee pain and instability in younger children without adequate trauma, growth-related abnormalities such as cruciate aplasia or Osgood-Schlatter disease must be considered.

Approach to joint effusion/hemarthrosis:

- X-rays in two planes: epiphyseal disruption, eminence or collateral ligament avulsions
- MRI: to exclude articular knee damage (cruciate ligaments, meniscus, osteochondral flake, patellar dislocation with MPFL lesion) (Fig. 13.57)
- Joint aspiration: exceptionally, in cases of severe pain

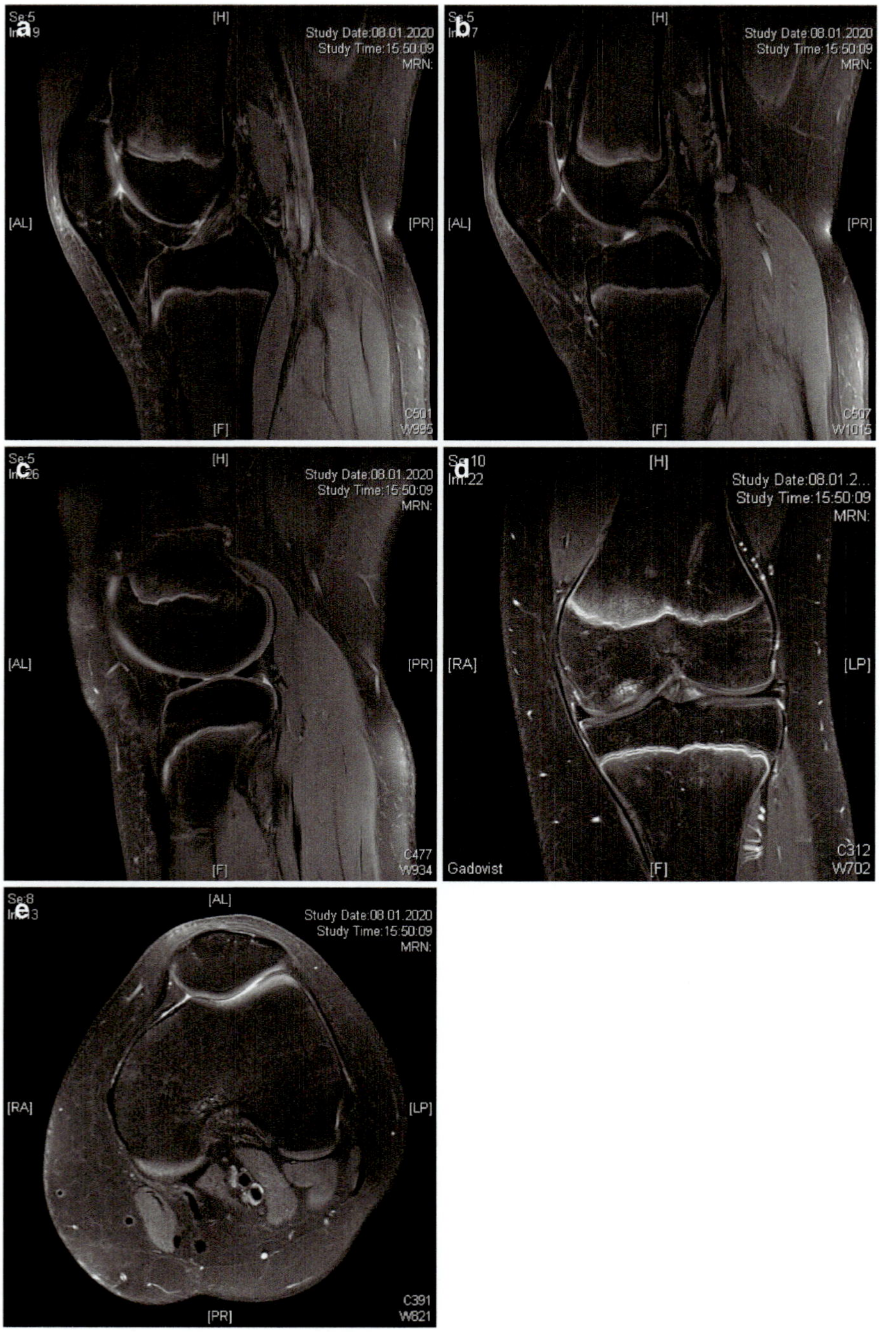

Fig. 13.57 12 Year old girl with patella dislocation. MRI with typical anatomy of a child, (**a**–**e**) various MRI views

– Arthroscopy: for massive hemarthrosis, signs of entrapment, instability, loose joint bodies on radiology, patellar fractures and dislocations, and x-ray or MRI findings indicating a need for surgery

Intercondylar Eminence (Tibial Spine) Avulsion Fractures

There are age-dependent differences in ACL injuries. Below the age of 12, there are essentially bony avulsions (eminence fracture). Over 12, ligamentous ruptures are more common.

Intercondylar eminence fracture is the most common epiphyseal fracture of the proximal tibia. This is intra-articular but does not affect the epiphyseal plate. Classification is based on the degree of displacement, according to Meyers and McKeever. (Figure 13.58 Eminentia-intercondylaris-Ausriss:EinteilungnachMeyers und McKeever).

The treatement of avulsion fractures of the anterior cruciate from the Tibia depend on the classification:

– Grade I non-displaced fracture

Conservative Treatment

– Grade II hanging fracture

Closed reduction and fixation, under arthroscopic control, retro—or antegrade.

– Grade III displaced fracture

Arthroscopic reduction and fixation with pull-out suture or screws; open refixation in exceptional cases.

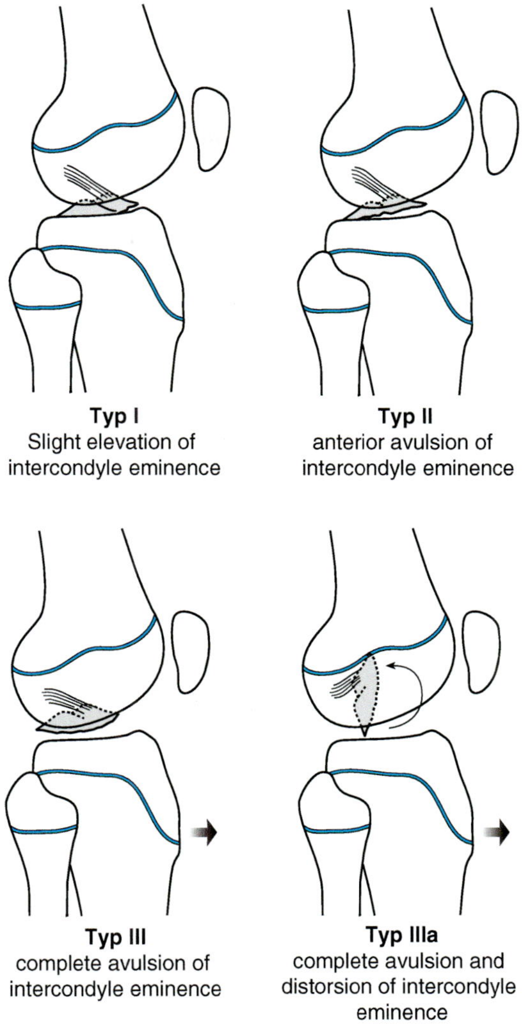

Fig. 13.58 Intercondylar eminence avulsion: Meyers and McKeever classification

Starting with grade II, operative reduction and fixation can be necessary. In grades II and III, the anterior horns of the menisci must be inspected, as a displaced bony fragment would lie above them (Table 13.16). These can become entrapped or present obstacles to reduction. The technical

Table 13.16 Intercondylar eminence avulsion/bony ACL avulsion

Special features	With hemarthrosis, consider ACL avulsion Most common epiphyseal fracture of the tibia Meyers and McKeever Classification	
Diagnostic approach	Clinical: Hemarthrosis, instability AP and lateral x-rays knee Primary arthroscopy If needed, MRI to assess associated injuries	
Treatment goal/limits of correction	Ligament stability, prevent long-term consequences (meniscus lesion, cartilage damage) Treatment of associated injuries	
Primary treatment	Long-leg plaster splint in extension, medical analgesia as needed, thromboprophylaxis as needed If needed, joint aspiration for hemarthrosis (pain reduction)	
Conservative treatment		
Indication	Non-displaced ligament avulsions, grades I (Fig. 13.59), **rarely grade II**	
Approach	Long-leg cast in extension for 3 weeks, then in 10° flexion for another 3 weeks with full weight-bearing	
Follow up	Mobilization as tolerated, muscle building (quadriceps muscle) Physical therapy	
Radiological controls	Position control at 1 week; consolidation check at 6 weeks	
Return to sports	Free function, muscular symmetry; at approx. 12 weeks	
Operative treatment		
Indication	Displaced, unstable ligament avulsions, grades II (Fig. 13.60) and III (Fig. 13.61); associated injuries	
Approach	Arthroscopy, arthroscopic reduction and fixation with repair, screws, or with K-wires	
Follow up	According to method; usually long-leg cast or brace for 6 weeks with weight-bearing as tolerated After cast removal: Muscle building (quadriceps muscle) Physical therapy	
Radiological controls	Post-operative position control; 6 weeks post-surgery	
Hardware removal	At 12 weeks	
Return to sports	Free function, muscular symmetry; at approx. 12 weeks	
Complications/ associated injuries	Meniscus, collateral ligament, cartilage lesions Premature osteoarthritis with persistent instability	
Growth disturbance	Rare	
Follow up	Weekly until free function	
Classification	AO: 41-E/7.1–3	LiLa: 4.1.a.5.0–2.

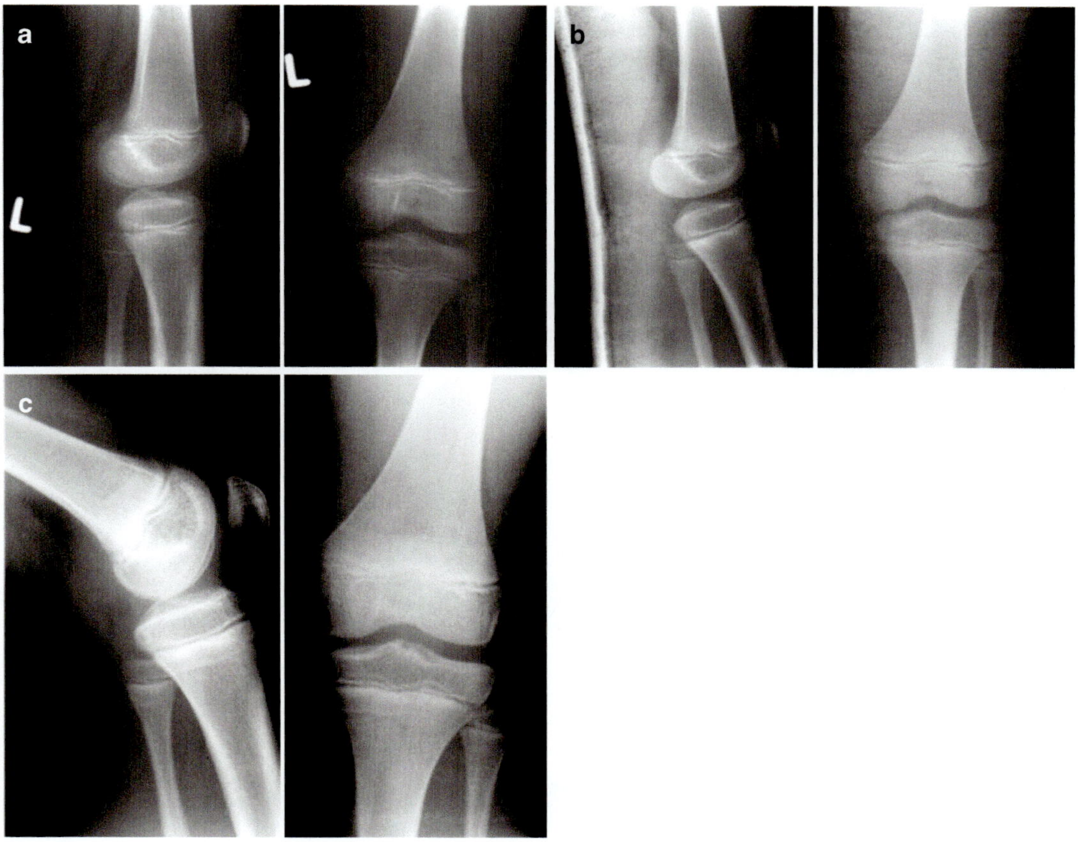

Fig. 13.59 Bony avulsion fracture of the ACL Type I according to Meyers and McKeever. (**a**) Trauma image, (**b**) Conservative treatment in extension tutor cast, (**c**) Good healing

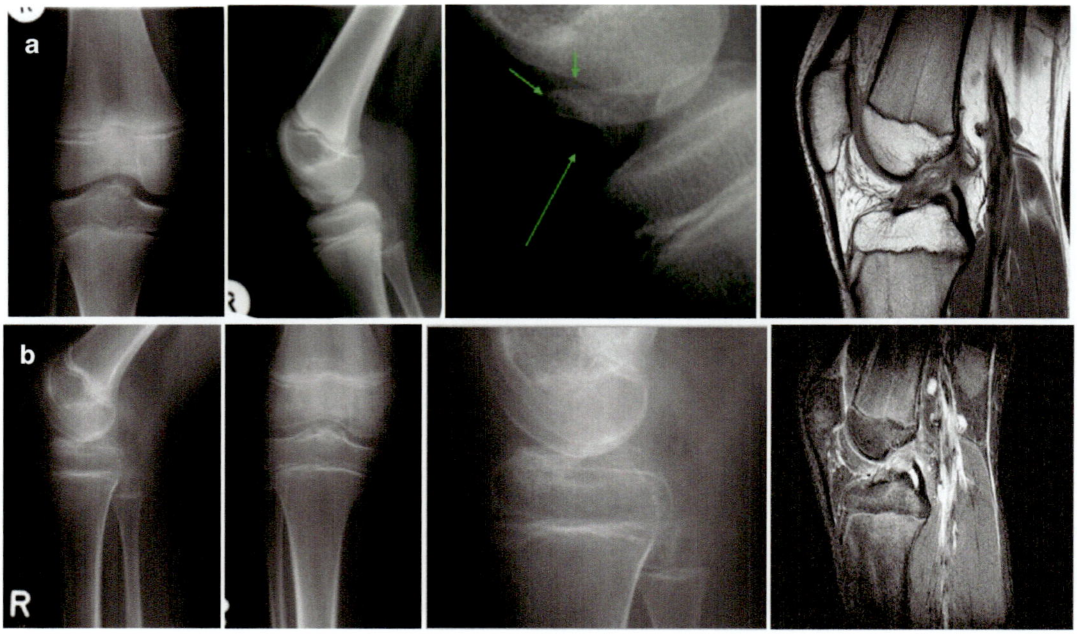

Fig. 13.60 Bony avulsion fracture of the ACL at the tibia, type II acc. to Meyers and McKeever. (**a**) Trauma image, (**b**) Healing after arthroscopic repair with extension suture

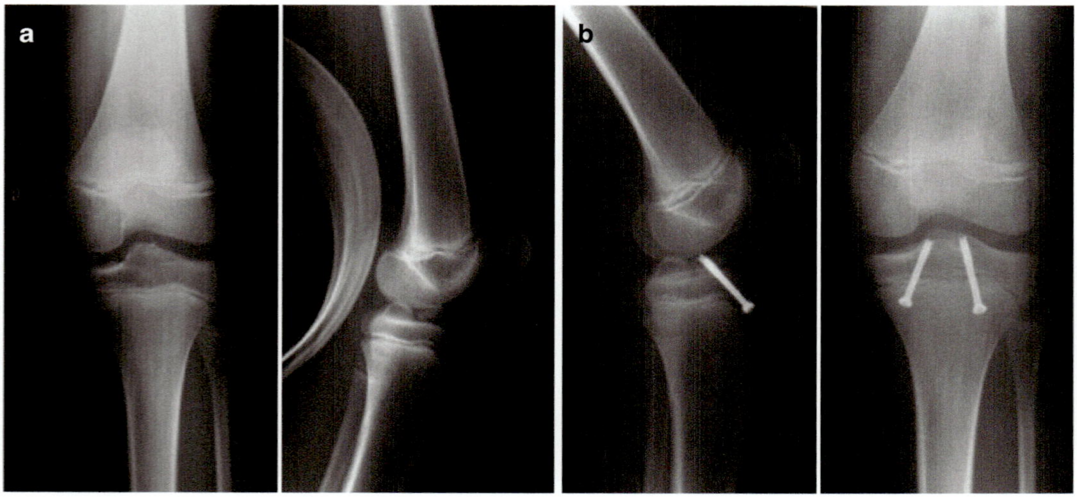

Fig. 13.61 Avulsion fracture Type III acc. To Meyers and McKeever. (**a**) Truama image, (**b**) Retrograde screw fixation after reduction within the epiphysis under arthroskopic view

options for surgical treatment are shown in Tables 13.17 and 13.18 and all options are followed by a tutor cast or a knee brace without limitations.

Knee ligament stability should be followed until growth is completed to confirm enduring stability. Secondary ACL insufficiency can be observed after bony refixation and healing.

Ligamentous Cruciate Ligament Lesions

Isolated ligamentous cruciate ligament injuries occur most frequently in adolescents but are increasingly observed in children under ten years. This may be the result of increased participation in aggressive sports activities or also because of improved diagnostic approaches, especially MRI (Fig. 13.62) In 50% of cases, there are associated injuries requiring treatment.

Treatment of cruciate ligament injuries has been discussed for years. Because of the high rate of meniscus lesions after pediatric ACL injuries (approximately 50% at one year), prompt ligament reconstruction is currently recommended. In the current literature, operative replacement is recommended for all complete ACL ruptures with instability (buckling) due to the increased rate of instability-related meniscus and cartilage lesions, and thus, the risk of premature osteoarthritis. No relevant growth disorders have been evident due to drilling through the growth plates in the child-adapted operative technique and tendon replacement surgery. Overall, the results are good post-ACL reconstruction. However, the number of children under the age of twelve is low in most studies (Table 13.17).

In children with extensive growth to come (<12 years), ligamentous ACL repair is still recommended by some authors. This is an attempt to regain a stable ligament through scar formation. Results vary according to study but appear unsatisfactory overall. Secure healing and stability are assured in these cases when good transosseous fixation is possible. Otherwise, replacement should be performed.

Injuries to the posterior cruciate ligament (PCL) are rare and are mainly found in knee subluxations/dislocations. Clinical stability testing and MRI generally lead to the diagnosis. Results of conservatively-treated PCL ruptures are generally good. In these cases, distal ligament ruptures have a slightly better healing tendency than proximal avulsions.

Re-fixation of the posterior tibial attachment of a PCL with bony avulsion should be considered through an open approach when there is fragment displacement.

If the ligament is completely torn with dehiscence, semitendinosus tendon reconstruction restores stability. This is done partly arthroscopically for the femoral fixation, with an extra posterior approach to adjust for the course of the growth plate. The same approach is recommended for persistent posterior instability after ligamentous or conservative therapy.

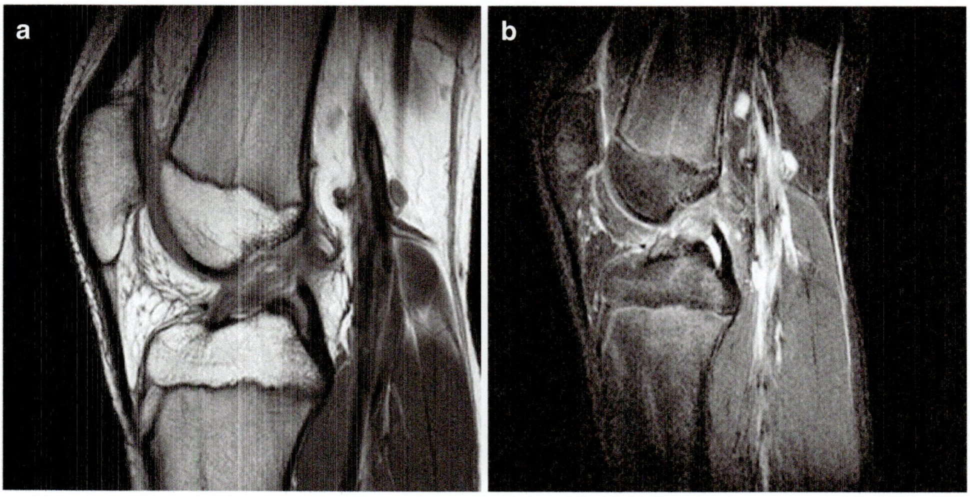

Fig. 13.62 (**a**, **b**) Intraligamentous rupture of the anterior cruciate ligament MRI

Table 13.17 Ligamentous ACL tear (Fig. 13.63)

Special features	especially in adolescents >12 years
Diagnostic approach	Clinical: Hemarthrosis, instability AP and lateral x-rays knee MRI to confirm the diagnosis (Fig. 13.64) Arthroscopy (Fig. 13.65)
Treatment goal/limits of correction	Ligament stability, prevent long-term consequences (meniscus lesion, cartilage damage) Treatment of associated injuries
Primary treatment	Long-leg plaster splint in extension, medical analgesia as needed, thromboprophylaxis as neededif needed, joint aspiration for hemarthrosis
Conservative treatment	
Indication	Isolated ACL rupture, children <12 years, no buckling (controversial because of potential for consequent damage in cases of instability)
Approach	Functional
Follow up	Mobilization as tolerated, muscle building (quadriceps muscle) Physical therapy
Radiological controls	None
Return to sports	Free function, muscular symmetry; at approx. 12 weeks
Operative treatment	
Indication	Complete rupture (especially >12 years) Symptomatic instability (buckling, recurrent effusion, pain) Associated injuries
Approach	ACL replacement with semitendinosus tendon; steep drill canal with short growth plate crossing; drill canal and tendon same diameter; fixation outside the growth plate (e.g., bioresorbable screws) Alternative: Ligament repair and bony refixation with bracing
Follow up	According to operative method: Generally, brace without movement restrictions under partial weight-bearing for 4 weeks, then gradual increased loading Mobilization as tolerated, muscle building (quadriceps muscle) Physical therapy
Radiological controls	Postoperative
Hardware removal	If needed at 6 months Usually biodegradable fixation materials (e.g., interference screws)
Return to sports	Free function, muscular symmetry
Complications/associated injuries	Meniscus, collateral ligament, cartilage lesions Premature osteoarthritis with persistent instability
Growth disturbance	Rare; if so, then mostly iatrogenic
Follow up	Weekly until free function; discharge when free of symptoms after 1.5 years and follow up when growth is completed

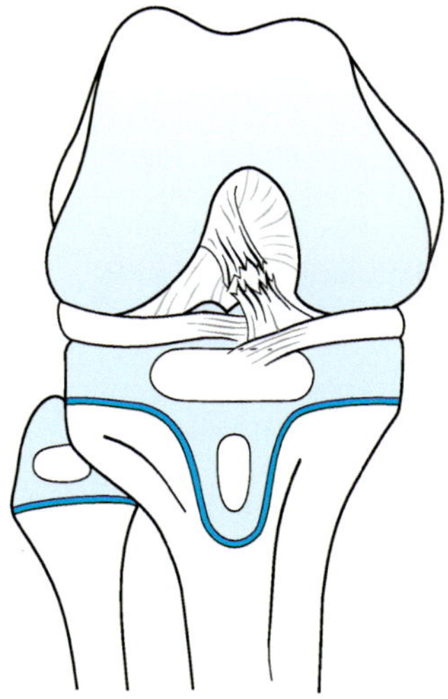

Fig. 13.63 Intraligamentous rupture of the anterior cruciate ligament

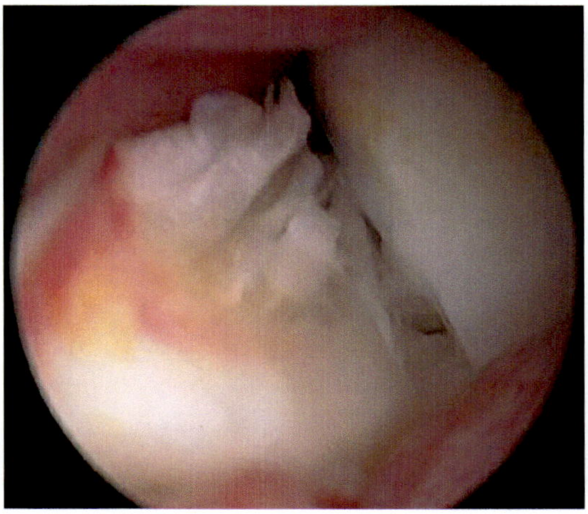

Fig. 13.64 Acute traumatic rupture of the ACL—arthroscopic view

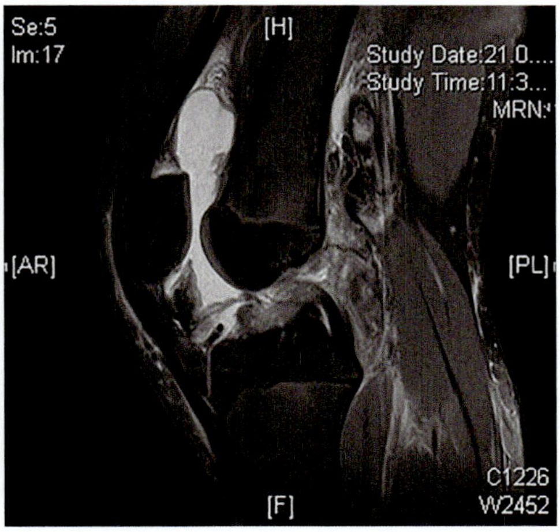

Fig. 13.65 Acute traumatic rupture for the ACL in MRI, see large intraarticular hematoma

Table 13.18 Technical options for bony ligament avulsion and intraligamentous ACL rupture

General Material	Fluoroscopy Arthroscopy option
Positioning	Supine position; free draped leg; foldable foot section (arthroscopy) Enable simultaneous fluoroscopy; thigh tourniquet
Approach	Arthroscopy Open approach: Mini-arthrotomy medial to the patella
Special clarification	Chronic instability (premature osteoarthritis) Functional limitation Growth irregularities with growth plate fusion Sensory disturbance in region of the infrapatellar nerve
Operative principle	Bony avulsion: Screw fixation Material: Cannulated cancellous screws with short threads 3.5–4.5 mm washer Retrograde course (Fig. 13.66) Retrograde Eminentiaverschraubung : From distal to proximal, also possible through the epiphysis with the indicated screw length Anterograde course: From proximal to distal (problem with hardware removal, mostly arthroscopic) Approach: Anterograde: Higher medial approach (in 80° flexion) Bony avulsion: Transosseous suture Material: PDS (strength 0) For small fragments or multi-fragmentation Positioning arthroscopic with targeting device; suture through mini-arthrotomy or arthroscopic Figure 13.67 Bony avulsion: K-wire fixation Material: 1.4 mm K-wires, crossed percutaneously in small children ACL reconstruction, semitendinosus technique Variety of different techniques Basic principle to protect growth plates (Figs. 13.68, 13.69, and 13.70) Alternative A (most widely used): Transepiphyseal drill canals; during fixation, important to watch that no bone or foreign material is brought to the level of the growth plate and that a steep canal with the same width as the graft is placed (preventing bridging callus), only the tendon (graft) crosses the growth plate, to date no major growth disorders have been reported Alternative B: Epiphyseal drill canals while protecting the plates Fig. 13.71 Alternative C: Metaphyseal drill canals, the graft is guided around the growth plate
Hardware removal	Wires and screws under anesthesia

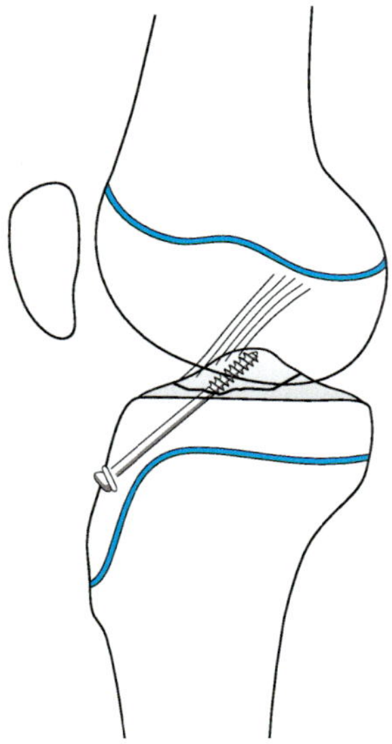

Fig. 13.66 Retrograde screw fixation with lag screw; under arthroscopic and radiologic view

Fig. 13.67 8 Year old girl with bony avulsion and intraligamentous tears, (**a**, **b**) Trauma image, (**c**, **d**) Antegrade screw from arthroscopic view and extension suture with button within the epiphysis

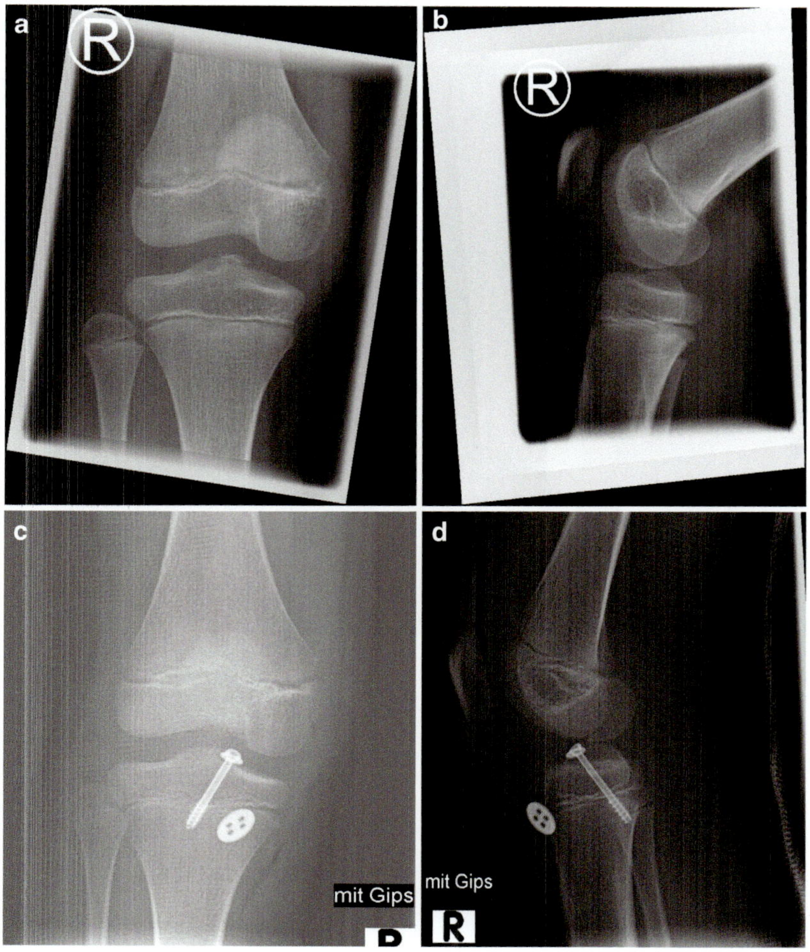

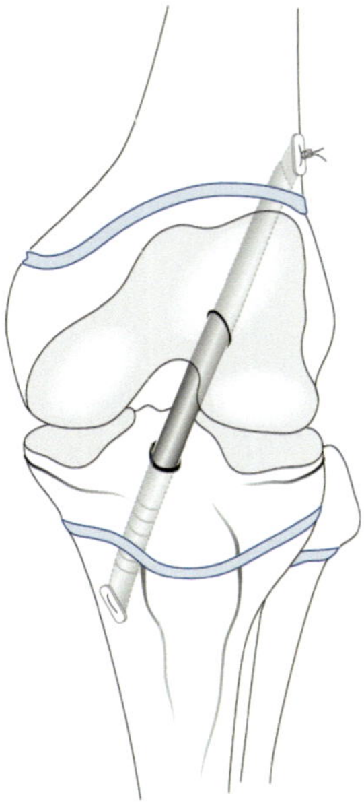

Fig. 13.68 Transepiphyseal drill holes; in children steep and central in order not to injure the growing line

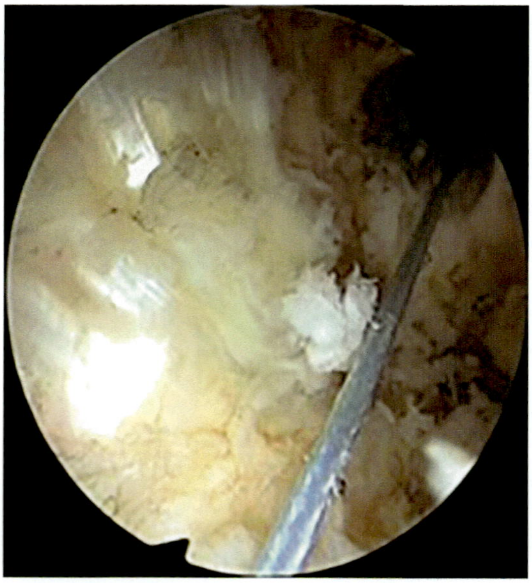

Fig. 13.69 Arthroscopic line of ACL—Replacement. Note on the left side the posterior cruciate, on at 1 o Clock the femoral canal and the shuttle suture

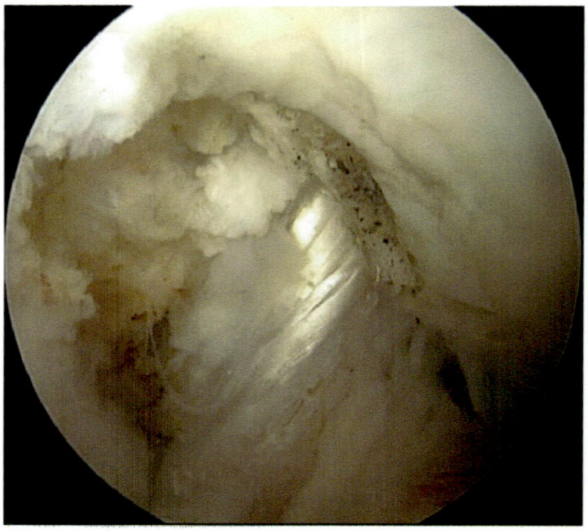

Fig. 13.70 Arthroscopic replacement with semitendinosus tendon visible with femoral insertion of a 14 year old girl

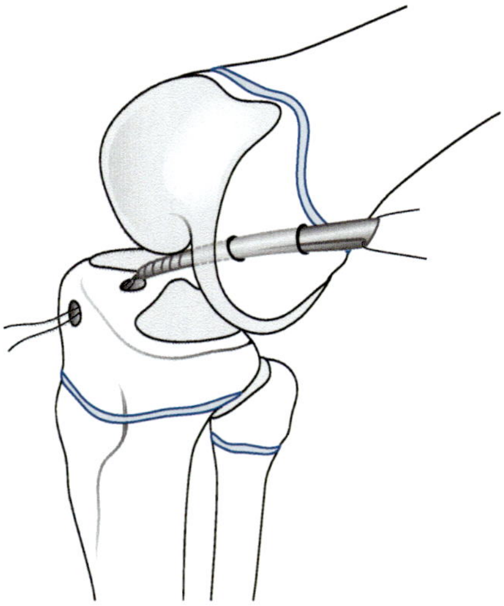

Fig. 13.71 Intra-epiphyseal drill canals without crossing the growth plates

Femoral Collateral Ligament Avulsions

The collateral ligaments consist of longer fibers along the femoral metaphysis and shorter fibers along the femoral epiphysis. Both areas can yield bony avulsions (Fig. 13.72), for detailed diagnostics, an MRI is necessary (Fig. 13.73). The injuries can be classified according to Hughston with pediatric adaptions (Table 13.19).

Conservative treatment is possible in most cases. Only when there is massive instability (especially of the lateral collateral ligament, posterolateral joint area) is repair necessary. In these cases, there are often associated intraarticular injuries that require surgery anyway (Table 13.20).

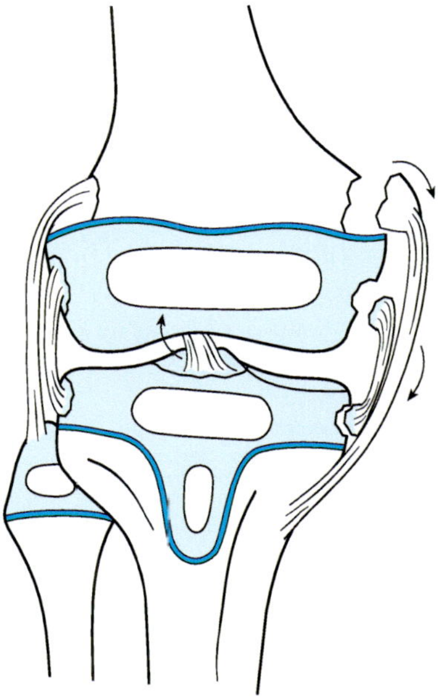

Fig. 13.72 Bony avulsion fractures around the knee joint

As in adults, the stabilizing structures on the lateral side are:

- Fibular collateral ligament
- Popliteus musculotendinous complex
- Popliteofibular ligament
- Popliteomeniscal fascicles
- Anterolateral ligament
- Biceps femoris muscle complex
- Fascia lata

On the medial side, stability issues alongside the medial collateral ligament, meniscus, and anterior cruciate ligament must be assessed and targeted for treatment to avoid complex problems.

Stabilizing structures on the medial side are:

- Semimembranosus complex
- Posterior oblique ligament
- Popliteal oblique ligament
- Posteromedial joint capsule with the posterior horn of the medial meniscus

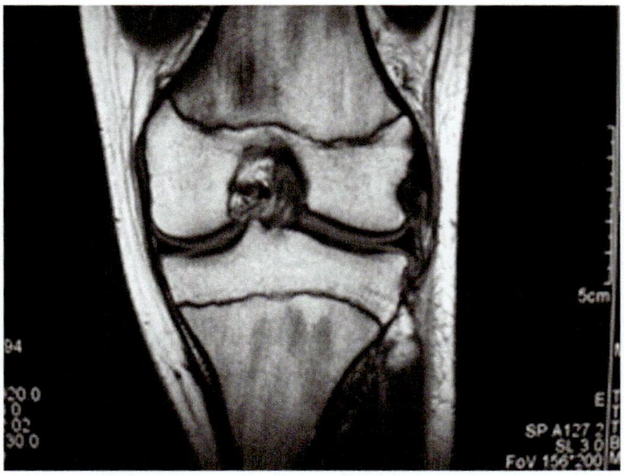

Fig. 13.73 Rupture of the lateral collateral ligament in MRI

Table 13.19 Collateral ligament instability: modified Hughston classification

Grade I	No instability, minimal ligament distortion, mild tenderness to palpation	Conservative treatment; early functional
Grade II	No instability, mid-grade ligament distortion, severe tenderness	Conservative treatment; early functional, if needed splint or orthosis
Grade III	Instability + to +++, complete ligament rupture	Exclude articular knee injuries: Arthroscopy; isolated rupture: Conservative treatment, orthosis

Table 13.20 Femoral collateral ligament avulsion/collateral ligament rupture (adapted Hughston classification)

Special features	Rare; especially with wide open growth plates Metaphyseal and epiphyseal avulsions Pure ligament injuries: especially >12 years			
Diagnostic approach	Clinical instability (contralateral comparison!) X-ray: Knee in two planes MRI for suspected epiphyseal injury and articular knee damage Arthroscopy for suspected articular knee damage			
Treatment goal/limits of correction	Ligament stability			
Primary treatment	Long-leg plaster splint, medical analgesia if needed			
Conservative treatment				
Indication	Generally conservative treatment Non-displaced ligament avulsions			
Approach	Ligamentous rupture: According to instability: Grade I+ till grade II+: Early functional, tape; Grade II+ till grade III+: Knee brace, weight-bearing as tolerated Ligament avulsion: Long-leg cast for 4 weeks with weight-bearing as tolerated			
Follow up	Mobilization as tolerated, muscle building (quadriceps muscle)			
Radiological controls	At 4 weeks			
Return to sports	Free function, muscular symmetry; at approx. 4 weeks			
Operative treatment				
Indication	Displaced, unstable ligament avulsions (especially lateral collateral ligament) (ligamentous rupture: Instability grade III)			
Approach	Arthroscopy: Diagnostic → exclude associated injuries Bony avulsion: Open reduction and screw fixation Ligamentous lesion: Ligament repair			
Follow up	Knee orthosis for 4 weeks with weight-bearing as tolerated Mobilization as tolerated, muscle building (quadriceps muscle)			
Radiological controls	Postoperative, consolidation check at 4–6 weeks			
Hardware removal	At 6 months			
Return to sports	Free function, muscular symmetry; at approx. 4 weeks			
Complications/associated injuries	With grade III+ instability and most associated injuries (meniscus lesion, cruciate rupture)			
Growth disturbance	Metaphyseal avulsions: Growth inhibition possible (through healing bridge formation → axial malalignment)			
Follow up	Weekly until free function; then semi-annually for 2 years Controls for leg-length discrepancies and axial malalignment Radiological controls in cases of axial malalignment (exclude growth plate bridging)			
Classification	AO: 33-E/7.1–3	33-M/7.1–3	LiLa: 3.3.s.5.0–2	3.3.a.5.0–2.

13.5 Meniscus Injuries

The incidence of meniscus lesions is lower in children than adults, with approximately 2.5%. The lateral meniscus is more mobile than the medial meniscus, which is fused with the capsule and the medial collateral ligament. This makes the medial meniscus more susceptible to injury. The increased rate of lateral meniscus lesions in children is attributed to the higher prevalence of discoid meniscus on this side. Most common are longitudinal ruptures of the posterior horn; bucket-handle tears typically begin appearing in adolescence (Table 13.21).

Vascular supply of the menisci decreases during growth with increasing load. However, vascularization of the edges enables spontaneous healing of incomplete meniscal ruptures in children.

Clinical examination is very important for diagnosis with various tests, although it can be difficult depending on age. MRI is currently a standard diagnostic procedure. Figure 13.74 shows Stoller's grading for meniscal injuries on MRI, with only grade III having clinical relevance (Fig. 13.75).

The goal of treatment is meniscus preservation through refixation and repair Fig. 13.76). If preservation is impossible, the smallest possible partial resection should be carried out. Total meniscectomy leads to significantly increased rates of osteoarthritis in the long term. Meniscus transplants should thus be considered in children or at a young age (Fig. 13.77).

Discoid meniscus is rare (29/1300 meniscectomies) (Fig. 13.78); the incidence is 0.4%, with a higher incidence in Asian children.

The etiology of discoid meniscus is not yet definitely understood. It occurs typically in the lateral compartment and is usually asymptomatic or only becomes symptomatic in adulthood. However, it is more susceptible to injury and can become symptomatic after rupture. Patients usually complain of clicking with movement, as well as chronic pain and recurrent knee effusions. On clinical examination, there is often a palpable click, blocking, intra-articular effusion, quadriceps atrophy, positive meniscus sign, and (usually lateral) joint line tenderness to palpation. Diagnostic imaging includes conventional radiography in two planes, with the AP showing possible lateral joint space widening, bulging of the lateral tibial plateau, flattening of the lateral femoral condyle, hypoplasia of the intercondylar eminence, and elevation of the fibular head. On MRI, thickness > 5 mm between the anterior and posterior horns on sagittal cuts indicates discoid meniscus. Imaging of unstable variants is difficult, but non-macroscopically evident meniscal lesions can be visualized.

Surgery is indicated only in symptomatic cases; a painless click should be observed to start. The goal is partial meniscectomy of the ruptured portion if needed with repair and refixation.

Watanabe Classification:

- Type I complete discoid meniscus, normal fixation along the posterior capsule, complete coverage of the tibial plateau
- Type II incomplete discoid meniscus, normal fixation along the posterior capsule, 80–100% coverage of the tibial plateau.
- Type III Wrisberg ligament, abnormal posterior fixation, posterior fixation through the meniscofemoral ligament

Type III is particularly unstable and thus, results in more symptoms. The instability leads to the typical movement-dependent clicking.

Unstable forms are often found in complete discoid menisci and are more common in younger children.

Table 13.21 Meniscus lesions

Special features	Rare; types of tear: flap tear, radial tear, bucket-handle tear Sometimes associated with discoid meniscus
Diagnostic approach	Clinical: Click phenomenon, blocking, chronic knee pain, propensity for swelling, Positive meniscus sign X-rays of the knee in two planes MRI (Fig. 13.79) Arthroscopy
Treatment goal/limits of correction	Meniscus preservation as much as possible, prevention of premature osteoarthritis
Primary treatment	Symptomatic; if needed immobilization, unloading
Conservative treatment	
Indication	Stable discoid menisci; asymptomatic clicking; minimal grade tears
Approach	Functional; observation
Follow up	Not necessary
Radiological controls	Not necessary
Return to sports	2 weeks
Operative treatment	
Indication	Symptoms (effusion, pain, blocking)
Approach	Arthroscopy; refixation with repair, partial meniscus resection
Follow up	Partial resection: Free mobility, partial weight-bearing for 2 weeks Refixation (generally posterior horn): Max. Flexion 70° for 4 weeks (orthosis), Partial weight-bearing for 6 weeks
Radiological controls	Not necessary
Hardware removal	Not necessary
Return to sports	With muscular symmetry; symptom-free; at approx. 6 weeks, with repair at 12 weeks
Complications/associated injuries	Premature osteoarthritis, re-rupture post-repair
Growth disturbance	None
Follow up	Every 2 weeks until free function

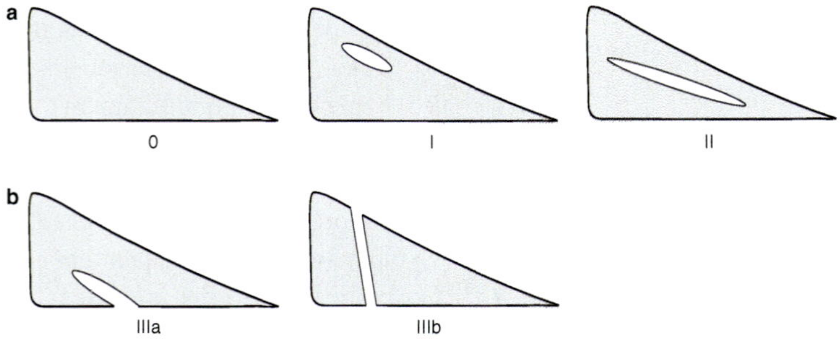

Fig. 13.74 Stoller grades of meniscus lesions on MRI. 0: homogeneous black meniscus, I: round signal, without reaching the superior or inferior surfaces, II: linear signal, without reaching the superior or inferior joint surfaces, III: linear signal, reaching the surface; (**a**) One surface, (**b**) Both surfaces

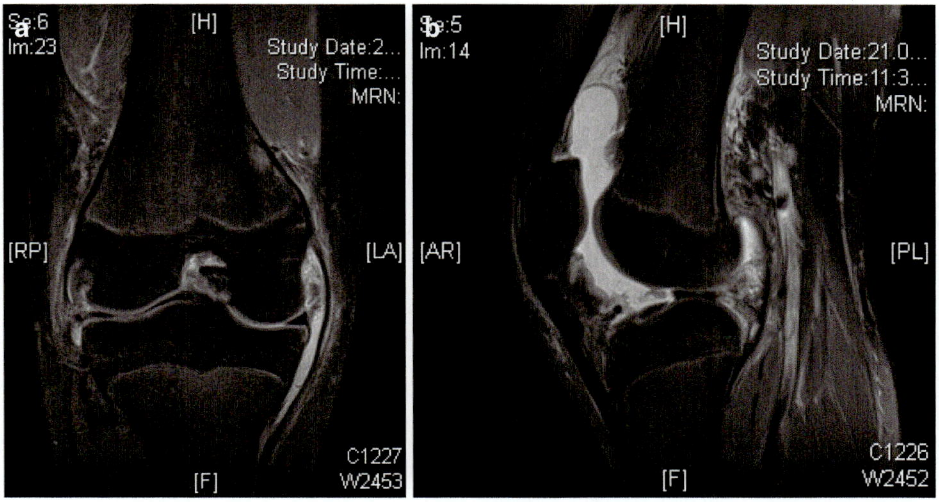

Fig. 13.75 Bucket handle rupture of the lateral meniscus in a 14 year old boy, (**a**) A.P. view in MRI, (**b**) Lateral view in MRI

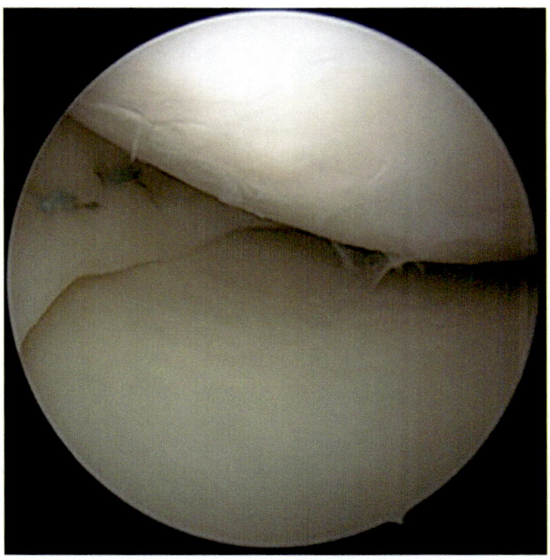

Fig. 13.76 Arthroscopic suture of a meniscus—all inside technique

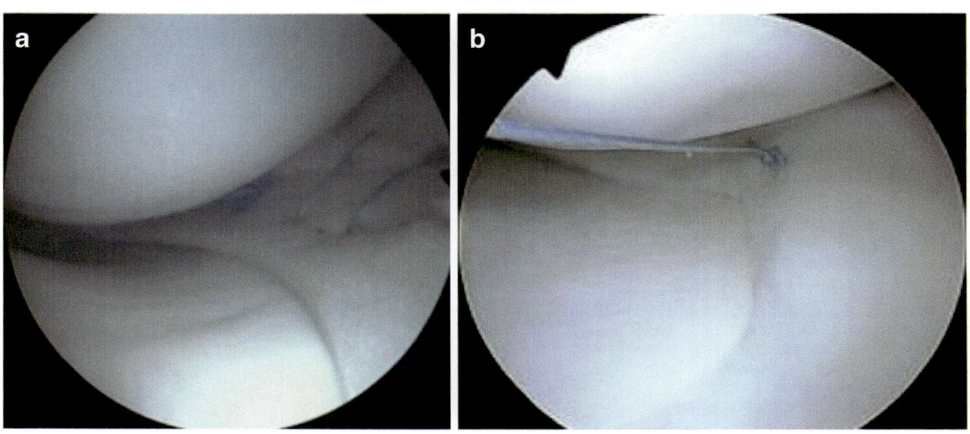

Fig. 13.77 Artificial meniscus replacement, fixation with sutures (**a**, **b**)

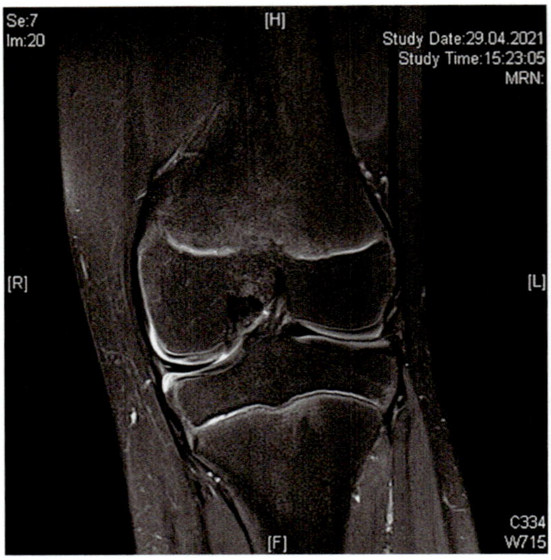

Fig. 13.78 Discoid meniscus

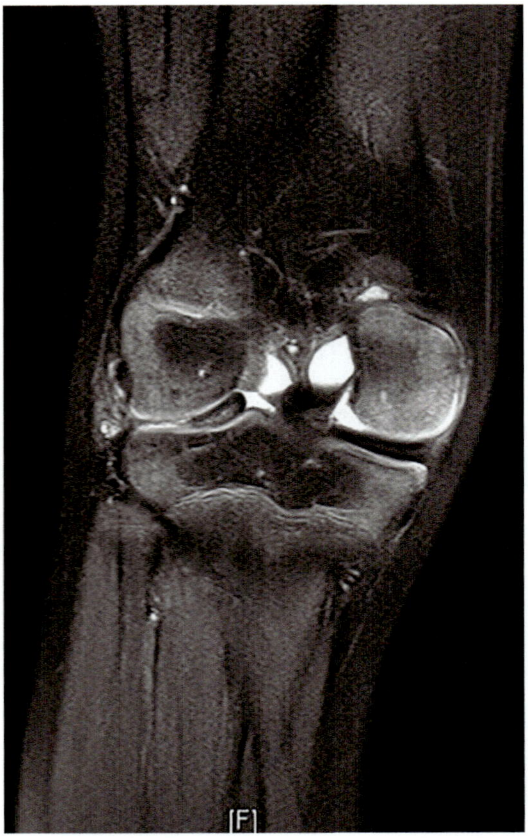

Fig. 13.79 Bucket-Handle rupture of the meniscus

Recommended Literature

Agatstein L, Skaggs AW, Brown MJ, Friel N, Haus B (2019) Patellar stabilization procedures in the pediatric population: incidence and demographics. Orthop J Sports Med 7:2325967119S00127

Ahn JH, Shim JS, Chan H, Oh WH (2001) Discoid laterla mensicus in children: clinical manifestations and morphology. J Pediatr Orthop 21:812–816

Beck A, Kinzl L, Rüter A, Strecker W (2001) Frakturen mit Beteiligung der distalen Femurepiphyse. Unfallchirurg 104:611–616

Dietz HG, Schmittenbecher PP, Illing P (2001) Intramedulläre Osteosynthese im Wachstumsalter. Urban & Schwarzenberg, München

Green NE, Swiotkowski MF (1998) Skeletal trauma in children, 2nd edn. Saunders, Philadelphia

Kaivers P, Busch T, Lies A (2003) Die Ausrißfraktur (sleeve fracture) des oberen Patellapols beim Kind. Unfallchirurg 106:676–679

Kremer L, Voth M, Marzi I (2017) Fractures of the lower extremities in childhood: part 1: fractures of the thigh and in the proximity of the knee. Der Chirurg; Zeitschrift für alle Gebiete der operativen Medizen 85:451–412

Marzi I (2016) Kindertraumatologie, 3rd edn. Springer, Berlin

Meyers MH, FM MK (1959) Fracture of the intercondylar eminence of the tibia. JBJS Am 41:209–222

Mortensen SO, Stausholm AM, Thorninger R (2019) Screw osteosynthesis of transverse fracture of the patella in children. World J Pediatric Surg 2:e000014

Nelitz M, Wagner D (2020) Instabile Patella bei Kindern und Jugendlichen. Arthroskopie 33:428–432

Ogden JA, Tross RB, Murphy MJ (1980) Fractures of the tibial tuberosity in adolescents. JBJS 62(A):205–215

Petersen W, Benedetto KP (2013) Different techniques for replacement of the anterior cruciate ligament. Arthroskopie 26:6–11

Reuter DS, Mellerowicz H (2016) Avulsionsverletzungen der proximalen Tibia. Der Orthopäde 45:226–232

Schlichte LM, Sidharthan S, Green DW, Parikh SN (2019) Pediatric management of recurrent patellar instability. Sports Med Arthrosc 27:171–180

Schneidmüller D, Maier M, Mack M, Straub R, Marzi I (2005) Therapeutische Relevanz der Magnetresonanztomographie bei Gelenkverletzungen im Kindesalter. Unfallchirurg 108:537–543

Seil R, Frosch KH, Becker R (2015) Kreuzbandverletzungen im Wachstumsalter. SFA Stifung 27:1–32

Sellnow L, Maier M, Schneidmüller D, Mack M, Marzi I (2009) Diagnostische Wertigkeit der MRT nach Patellaluxation im Kindes- und Jugendalter. päd 1–6

Senekovic V, Veselko M (2003) Anterograde arthroscopic fixation of avulsion fractures of the tibial eminence with a cannulated screw: five-years results. Arthroscopy 19:54–61

Sidharthan S, Wang G, Schlichte LM, Fulkerson JP, Green DW (2020) Medial patellofemoral ligament reconstruction in skeletally immature patients. Jbjs Essent Surg. Techniques 10:e0110.1-3

Vogt B, Schiedel F, Rödl R (2014) Guided growth in children and adolescents. Orthopade 43:267–284

Ziebarth K, Kolp D, Kohl S, Slongo T (2013) Anterior cruciate ligament injuries in children and adolescents: a review of the recent literature. Euro J Pediatr Surg: official journal of Austrian Association of Pediatric Surgery [et al] = Zeitschrift für Kinderchirurgie 23:464–469

Tibia and Fibula

14

14.1 Physiological Findings

Fascial Compartments of the Lower Leg

The lower leg has four distinct compartments (Fig. 14.1) which may develop in principal a compartment syndrome after injuries. The clinical signs are of the lower leg are swelling, hematoma, strong tension, reduction in blood perfusion, loss of sensomototory functions. Therefore, a dedicated clinical assessment of the lower leg is warranted ftre any injury and early signs of a compartment syndrome shall be noted. If there is any doubt about a compartment syndrome, the surgical decompression of all four (!) compartments has to be performed immediately in order to rescue the soft tissue and the lower leg. Also, the deep posterior compartment is the most difficult to assess but is very important as well. The four compartments are listed in Table 14.1.

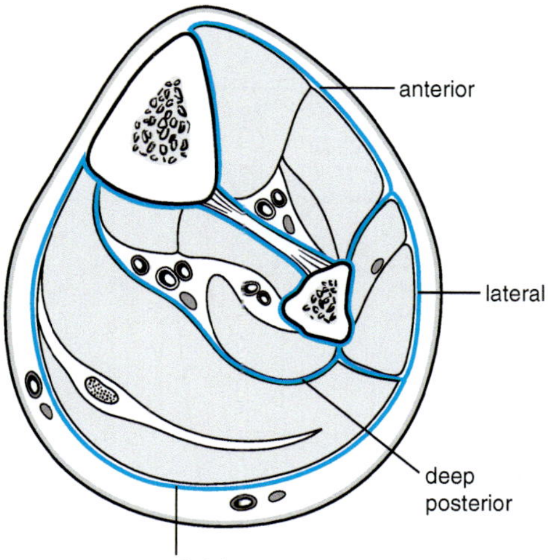

Fig. 14.1 Fascial compartments of the lower leg

Table 14.1 Compartments of the lower leg

Compartment	Muscles/Vessels/Nerves
Anterior	– Extensor digitorum longus muscle – Extensor hallucis longus muscle – Tibialis anterior muscle – Anterior tibial artery – Deep peroneal (fibular) nerve
Lateral	– Peroneus (fibularis) muscles, longus and brevis – Superficial peroneal (fibular) nerve
Superficial posterior	– Soleus muscle – Gastrocnemius muscle
Deep posterior	– Flexor digitorum longus muscle – Flexor hallucis longus muscle – Tibialis posterior muscle – Posterior tibial artery – Peroneal (fibular) artery – Tibial nerve

I. Marzi et al., *Pediatric Skeletal Trauma*, https://doi.org/10.1007/978-3-030-93685-3_14

14.2 Fractures of the Tibial Shaft

Incidence, Mechanism of Injury, and Clinical Presentation

The incidence of lower leg fractures is 5.8%. They are among the most common lower extremity injuries. 70% of cases are isolated tibia fractures, and 30% are complete lower leg fractures, tibia and fibula.

Fractures of the Proximal Metaphysis The peak age for these injuries is between 3 and 6 years. 50% of cases involve an associated fracture of the proximal fibula (especially greenstick fractures). There are two very different types of fractures: the mostly unproblematic compression fractures and bowing fractures. Compression fractures are usually non-displaced, and they occur most often in small children with good potential with correction. Thus, axial and growth disturbances are uncommon.

Metaphyseal bowing fractures are less frequent but more problematic because of the potential late consequences. The mechanism of injury is a lateral-acting force with an extended knee joint, which produces a metaphyseal bowing fracture of the tibial metaphysis with a partially intact periosteal tube laterally (greenstick fracture). This results in a more or less pronounced valgus malalignment, which is not always evident on the initial x-ray. When an isolated medial fracture gap is visible on conventional AP x-ray, a valgus deformity is present. If this displacement is left in place, the valgus angulation can increase, resulting in a Genu valgum (knock-knee) deformity. A valgus deformity can develop even when fractures are well-reduced. This type of deformity will usually develop within the first year of trauma. The cause is still debated in the literature. Possible etiologies include increased blood flow to the medial side of the proximal tibia, a blocking effect of the still-intact fibula, asymmetrical overgrowth of the medial tibial epiphysis, incomplete reduction of the fracture, loss of the stabilizing effect of the pes anserinus, or impacted soft tissues (pes anserinus, medial collateral ligament) in the medial fracture gap. Parents need to be educated about the potential for this growth disorder and clinical controls are indicated.

In cases of an asymptomatic post-traumatic valgus deformity, corrective osteotomy should only be carried out once growth is completed, as spontaneous correction can still occur. However, growth modulation is advisable in some instances of disabling valgus misalignment if there is a risk of recurrence. The magnitude of deviation is measured with the epiphyseal angle; both leg axes should be available for treatment planning (Fig. 14.2).

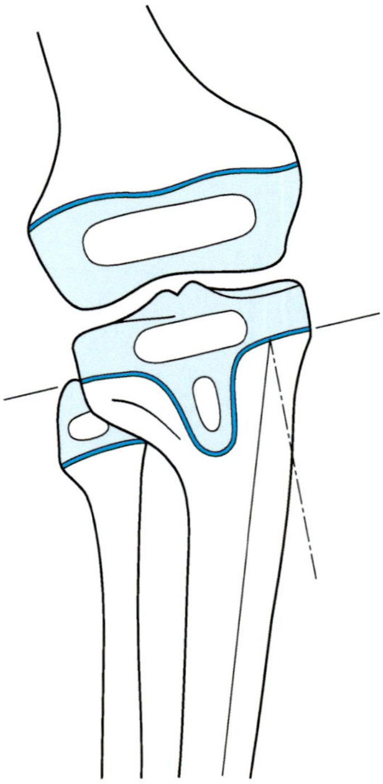

Fig. 14.2 Epiphyseal angle

The pattern of lower leg shaft injuries varies according to child age. In small children with insufficient bone stability, there are more non-displaced, isolated tibial torsion fractures with the fracture line sometimes barely visible. Direct trauma-induced transverse fractures of the tibia alone or in combination with the fibula become increasingly common in 6 to 10-year-olds. Sports-related injuries are more prevalent in adolescents, often leading to oblique fractures of the distal third (Fig. 14.3).

The second most common injury in battered child syndrome is to the tibia –26% of all abused children have tibia fractures—and this must be investigated in suspicious cases.

Overgrowth can occur after any lower leg fractures and, depending on the child's age and the need for remodeling, it can result in up to 1 cm of leg lengthening. The course of healing for isolated tibia fractures tends to increase varus deformity (50–60%) due to the surrounding muscular forces and the blocking effect of the uninjured fibula. In principle, axial misalignment can correct spontaneously in children <10 years. However, because of the long remodeling phase required, with extended growth activity and the potential for leg-length discrepancy, it should not be accepted. Rotational deformity does not correct spontaneously. Thus, adequate reduction must be ensured to prevent knee or ankle joint problems. Physiological rotation must also be considered. Physiological external rotation is usually 10–15°, with the second metatarsal ray projecting onto the extension of the tibial axis.

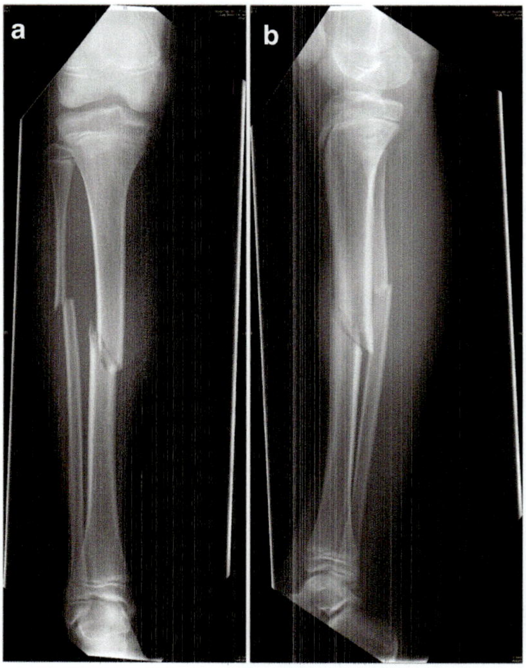

Fig. 14.3 Fracture of the diaphyseal tibia, short, oblique in a 14 year old boy

Corrective treatment for residual deformity should be performed no sooner than one year post-trauma in patients with symptoms and not until the conclusion of growth (if at all) in patients without symptoms.

Isolated Fractures of the Tibial Shaft Isolated undisplaced tibial shaft fractures are considered stable and can therefore be treated conservatively if there is no shortening to promote varus deformity (Fig. 14.4). In cases of shortening, an external fixator will restore length with the intact fibula and lead to a perfect healing in general.

Combined Fractures of the Tibia/Fibula Shaft In combined shaft fractures, the fibula's blocking effect does not occur, and a valgus deformity is more likely to develop because of the muscles pulling anterolaterally. Management differs for stable injuries, in which the fragments of a transverse tibial fracture are still in contact, from that for unstable oblique fractures or completely displaced fractures. Minimally or non-displaced, stable fractures can be managed conservatively in a long-leg cast. Unstable fractures, long oblique fractures, combined lower leg fractures, multi-fragment fractures, or angulation

>10°, are usually surgically stabilized (Fig. 14.5). In these cases a compartment syndrome needs to be detected and controlled early on (Fig. 14.6) Our experience is that children treated operatively often become pain-free more quickly than those treated conservatively. Children also have better function after mobilization-stable treatment than after several weeks of long-leg cast immobilization.

Fixation of tibial shaft fractures is achieved primarily with elastic stable intramedullary nail (ESIN) or external fixator. Plate fixation is usually not used in children and reserved for particular indications. The risks, advantages, and disadvantages of each method need to be discussed in detail with the patient and the parents so that a treatment decision can be made together according to individual needs.

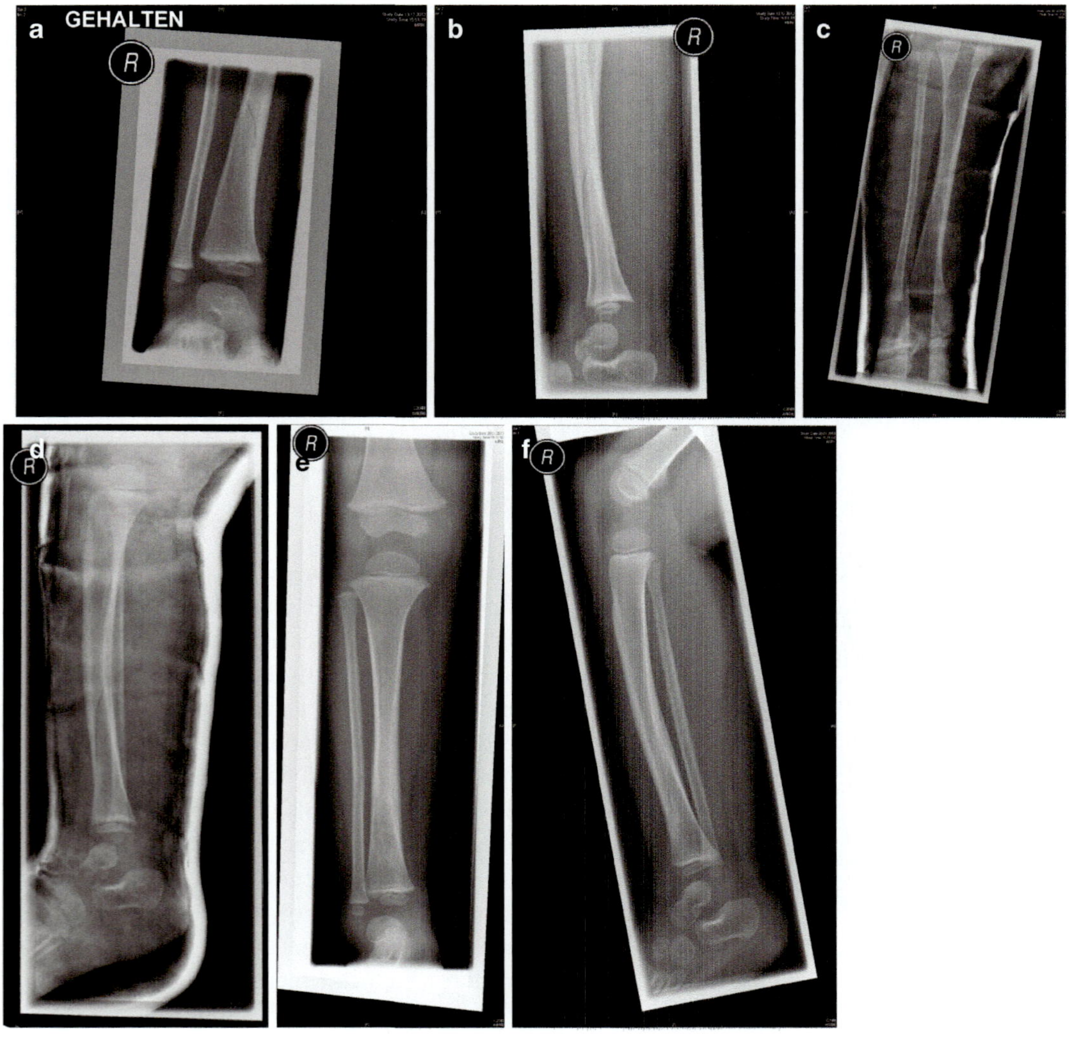

Fig. 14.4 Tibiaschaft fracture, undisplaced, (**a**, **b**) Trauma image, (**c**, **d**) Treatment in a cast, (**e**, **f**) Complete anatomical healing

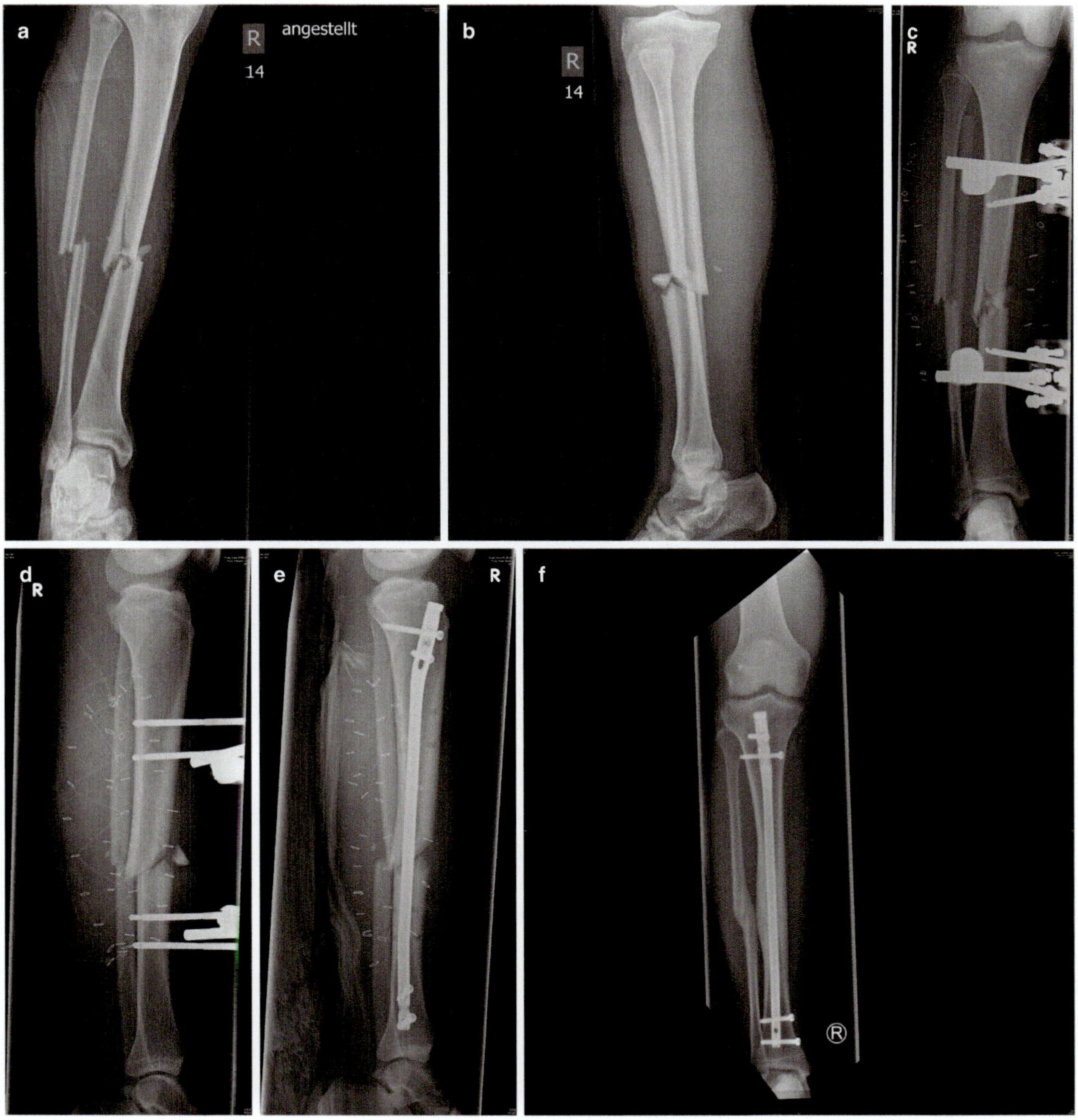

Fig. 14.5 Instable displaced lower leg fracture of a 16 year old boy with compartment syndrome. (**a**, **b**) Trauma image, (**c**, **d**) Primary fixation with external fixateur. (**e**) Intramedullary nailing after 1 week and removal of external fixateur (**f**) Complete healing prior to metal removal

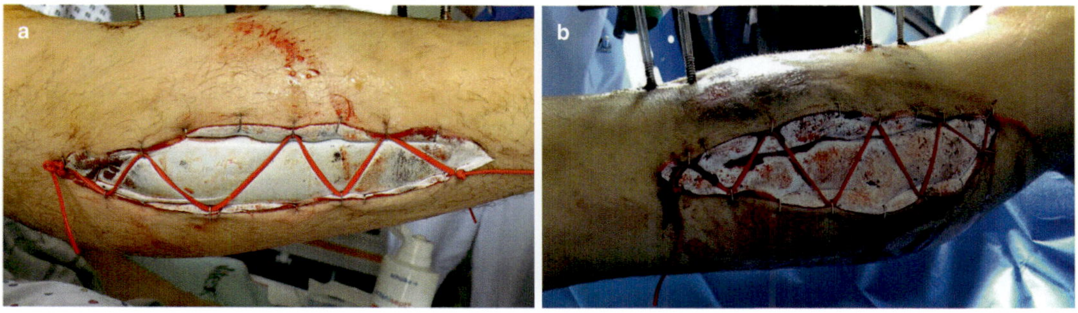

Fig. 14.6 Lower leg after decompression of a compartment syndrome. (**a**) Lateral side, (**b**) Medial side (case of Fig. 14.5)

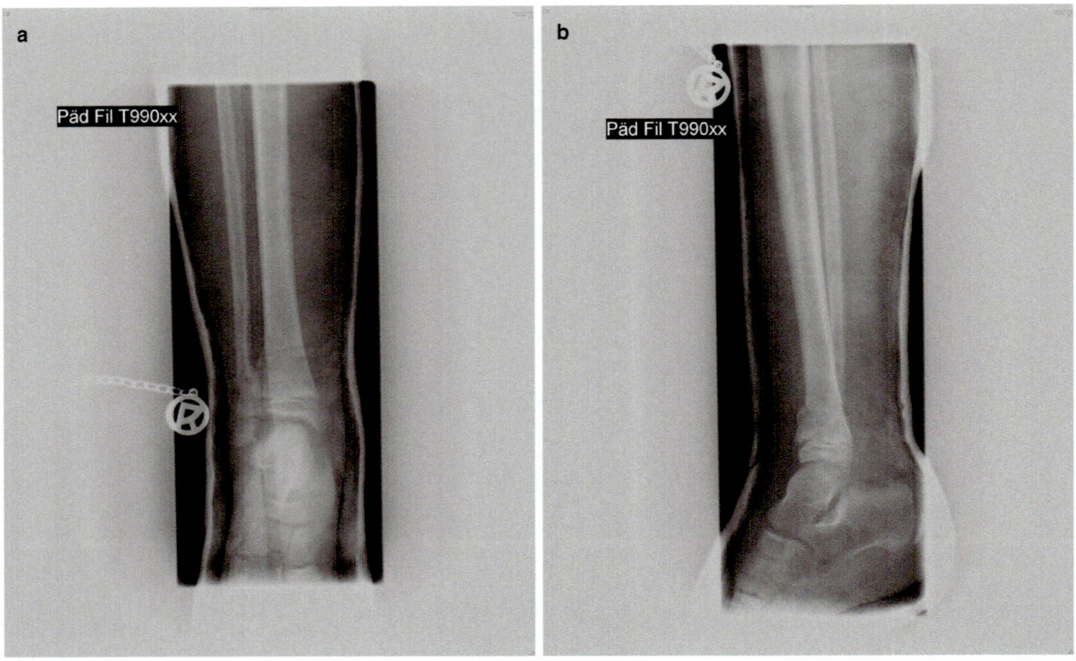

Fig. 14.7 Fracture of the distal femur and tibia. The axis needs to be controlled in the cast. (**a**) A.P. view und (**b**) lateral view

Fractures of the Distal Tibial Metaphysis These fractures are differentiated into compression and bowing fracture types. Compression fractures are generally uncomplicated and often occur in the context of bicycle spoke injuries. Bowing fractures are possible after all distortion trauma. There is often a recurvation deformity. If the angulation is not corrected, partial stimulation of the nearby growth plate can induce overgrowth as occurs with the proximal metaphysis. However, this area has good potential for correction; angulation up to 10° can remodel in children up to ten years of age (Fig. 14.7).

Isolated Fibula Fracture This fracture is uncommon and usually the result of direct impact trauma (Fig. 14.8). There is often an associated injury to the distal tibial epiphysis.

Open Fractures The tibia is more commonly affected. Approximately 9% of all tibia fractures are open; most are caused by high-speed trauma. The classification is based on Gustillo and Anderson. Treatment is carried out according to the same principles of adult surgery: rapid, thorough surgical wound debridement, systemic antibiotic therapy, and stabilization of the fracture, usually using an external fixator with a planned second-look procedure. Compared to adults, children have better soft-tissue healing overall, and bone defects can be partially filled via the periosteal reaction. Nevertheless, there is a risk of delayed fracture healing (16%) or non-union (7.5%) as well as infection (superficial: 8%, deep: 3%) or compartment syndrome (4%).

Compartment Syndrome Compartment syndrome can develop after any lower leg fracture. Normal tissue pressure is 0 mmHg. When pressure increases continuously to over approximately 30 mmHg, there is irreversible muscle damage of the affected compartment (after approximately 4–5 hours). Typical symptoms are excessive pain increasing with movement and

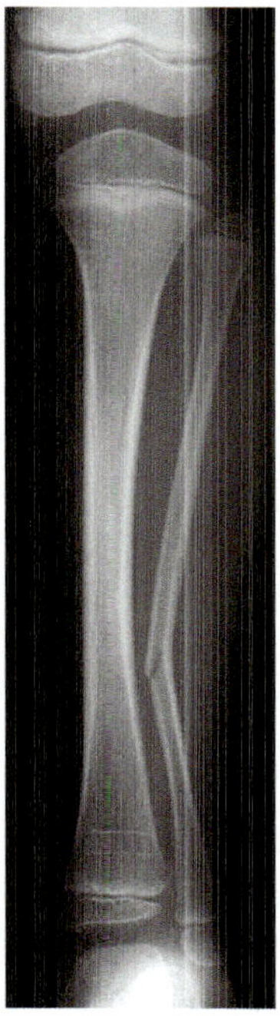

Fig. 14.8 Isolated fibular fracture, flexion fracture, here with tibial bowing

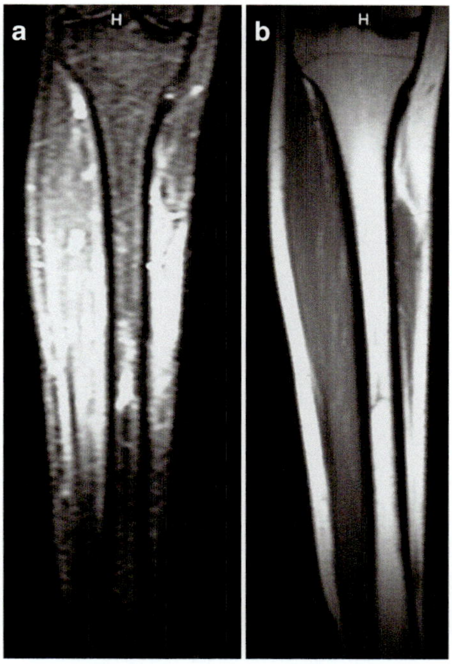

Fig. 14.9 Stress fracture of the tibial shaft. (**a**) Bone marrow edema (**b**) Fracture line

sensorimotor deficits, along with severe soft-tissue swelling and muscle rigidity. When there is increased pressure in the posterior compartment, patients complain of severe pain on passive toe mobilization, plantar hyperesthesia, and toe flexor weakness. As a late consequence, ischemic muscle (Volkmann's) contracture can result in claw toes and reduced ankle mobility. In impending compartment syndrome, all constricting bandages should be removed, and anti-swelling measures such as elevation and cooling should be carried out immediately. If symptoms persist, fasciotomy must be performed in short time.

Stress Fracture The tibia is a common location for stress reactions and stress fractures. These mainly affect adolescents, often with a history of increased loading (from sports practice, training changes). The symptoms are non-specific, exercise-dependent pain, sometimes with swelling and signs of inflammation. The initial x-ray is often unremarkable; the periosteal reaction is only visible over time. The diagnosis is usually made with an accurate history and clinical findings. MRI can confirm the diagnosis, especially in the early stages, and it can exclude other potential conditions on the differential like osteomyelitis and malignancy (e.g., Ewing's sarcoma) when the diagnosis is unclear. Typically, the T2-weighted, fat-suppressed images show a diffuse signal increase from bone marrow edema and periosteal thickening. If needed, the fracture gap may be visible on T1-weighted images (Fig. 14.9). The patient and parents must first be educated about the problem. Treatment for a stress reaction consists of reducing or avoiding the inciting strain, with temporary relief via forearm crutches if necessary. As soon as the patient is symptom-free, loading (sports) can be gradually resumed. A complete fracture can usually be treated conservatively with plaster cast immobilization.

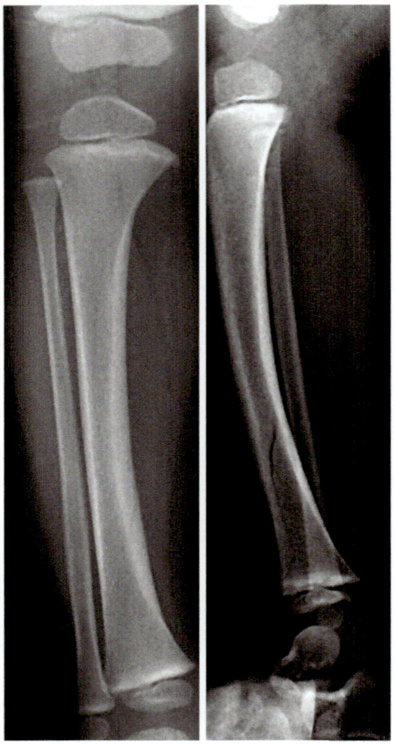

Fig. 14.10 Toddler's fracture

Toddler's Fracture A special form of an isolated spiral tibia fracture with a very small fracture line (Fig. 14.10). The etiology is rotational trauma with a fixed foot, especially in small children (<3 years), associated with a stress reaction from the extra load of the child just beginning to walk. Most of these cases are recognized when the child suddenly favors one leg without an observed trauma. The diagnosis is commonly made in retrospect since primary radiographs are often normal. After 10–14 days, periosteal callus formation is noticeable and indicates the presence of fracture. Treatment is always conservative in a long-leg cast for approximately four weeks, with a good prognosis. The fracture is healed, when the child starts to stand on his own.

Floating Knee A floating knee results from ipsilateral femur and tibia fractures (Figs. 14.11 and 14.12). Most of these are the result of high-speed trauma. Operative stabilization is recommended for both fractures to offer better treatment options and more rapid mobilization of pediatric polytrauma patients. There are often concomitant injuries to the knee ligaments or meniscus.

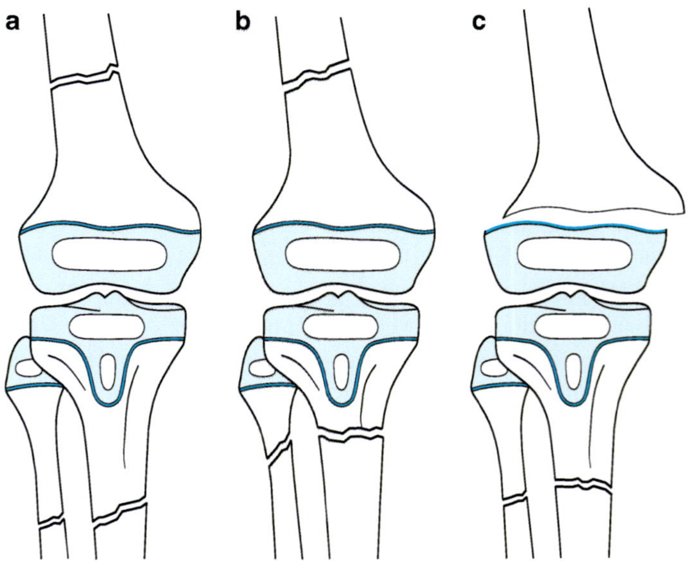

Fig. 14.11 Floating knee. (**a**) Diaphyseal fractures (**b**) Diaphyseal + metaphyseal fracture (**c**) Diaphyseal + epiphyseal fracture

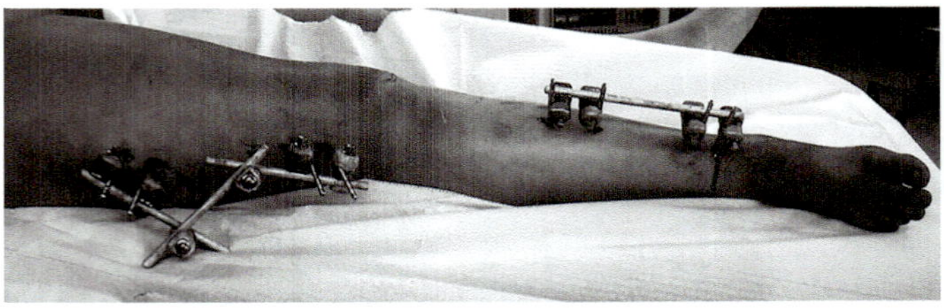

Fig. 14.12 Polytrauma after a traffic accident (11-year-old girl). Floating knee type A, primary stabilization with external fixator

Classification

Lower leg fracture types and etiologies (modified from Rockwood and Wilkins 2001) are listed in Table 14.2. For specific pediatric classifications see Chap. 20.

The fracture types of the proximal tibial metaphysis are indicated in Table 14.3.

Diagnostic and Procedure to treat isolated fractures of the Tibia are indicated in Table 14.4.

The treatment concepts of complete lower leg fractures are indicated in Table 14.5.

Fractures of the distal tibia might be treated conservatively or operatively, depending from the stability and displacement (Table 14.6).

Specific technical aspects of the treatment of the lower leg are indicated in Table 14.7.

Table 14.2 Fracture patterns of the lower leg

Proximal Tibial metaphysis		
Distal Tibial metaphysis		
Diaphyseal fractures	Isolated tibia fracture	Traumatic stress fracture
	Isolated fibular fracture	Traumatic stress fracture
	Combined lower leg fracture	
Special fractures	Toddler's fracture; Floating knee	

Fractures of the Proximal Tibia

Table 14.3 Fractures of the proximal tibial metaphysis (Fig. 14.13)

Special features	Especially young children (<8 years) Compression fracture: uncomplicated Bowing fracture: valgus risk
Diagnostic approach	Radiology: AP and lateral (including knee) x-ray (Fig. 14.14) Oblique views as needed (to better assess fracture gap)
Treatment goal/limits of correction	No angulation, especially no valgus (epiphyseal angle 0°), no rotational deformity Compression of the medial fracture line (!) to prevent medial overgrowth
Primary treatment	Long-leg plaster splint, analgesia
Conservative treatment	
Indication	Usually conservative
Approach	<10° valgus: Long-leg plaster circular cast in extension and under varus stress → day 8: Cast wedging (medial compression!) >10° valgus; side-to-side shift: Closed reduction and long-leg cast → day 8: Cast wedging
Follow up	Weight-bearing as tolerated, physical therapy if needed
Radiological controls	Day 8: Position control (wedging for angulation); consolidation control: At 4–6 weeks
Return to sports	With unlimited function, symmetrical muscle ratios (approx. 4 weeks post-consolidation)
Operative treatment	
Indication	Obstacle to reduction, associated injuries, open fractures; >10° valgus
Approach	Closed reduction, open only if needed Compression over medial external fixator to avoid valgus deformity development alternatively short compression plate fixation (3.5 mm) (Fig. 14.15—Evtl. Neu)
Follow up	Partial weight-bearing (rolling) for 4 weeks, then weight-bearing as tolerated
Radiological controls	Postoperative position check; 6 weeks post-surgery: Consolidation check
Hardware removal	With verified consolidation: External fixator: At approx. 8 weeks; plates: 4–6 months
Return to sports	With unlimited function, symmetrical muscle ratios (approx. 4 weeks post-consolidation)
Complications	Axial misalignment (genu valgum) (Fig. 14.16) Compartment syndrome
Growth disturbance	Stimulative growth disturbances (leg-lengthening, partial: Valgus deformity)
Follow up	Weekly until unlimited function; every 6–12 months for clinical leg-length and angulation checks up to 2 years post-trauma
Classification	AO: 41-M/2(3).1–3 LiLa: 4.1.s.2–4.0-2.

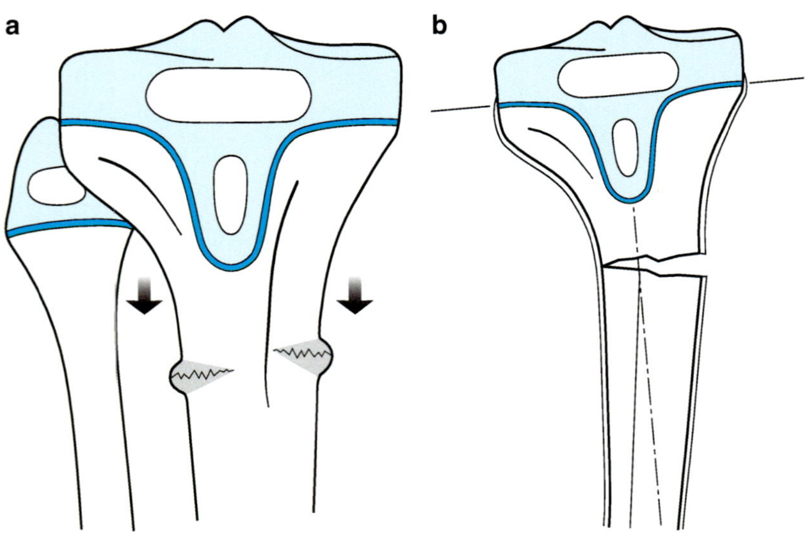

Fig. 14.13 Fracture of the proximal tibial metaphysis. (**a**) Compression fracture, (**b**) Bowing fracture

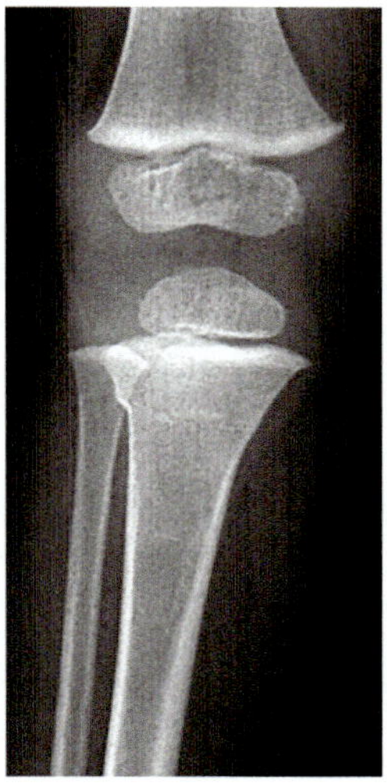

Fig. 14.14 Proximal compression fracture of the tibia

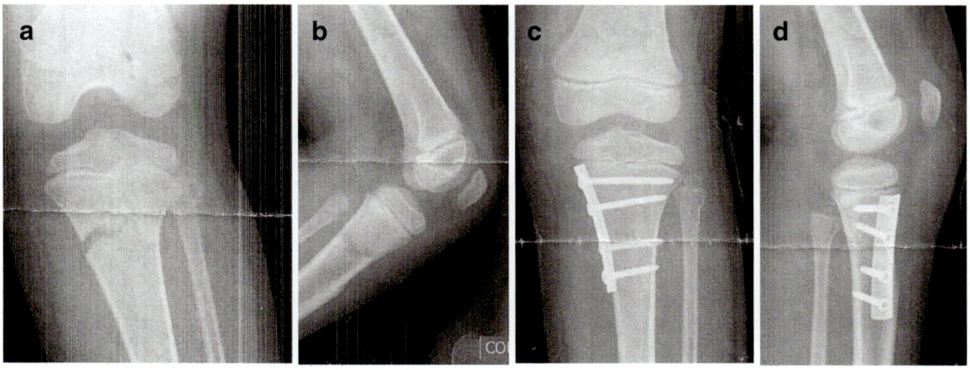

Fig. 14.15 Proximal tibia fracture with valgus deformity in a girl. (**a**, **b**) Trauma image. (**c**, **d**) Medial compression with plate

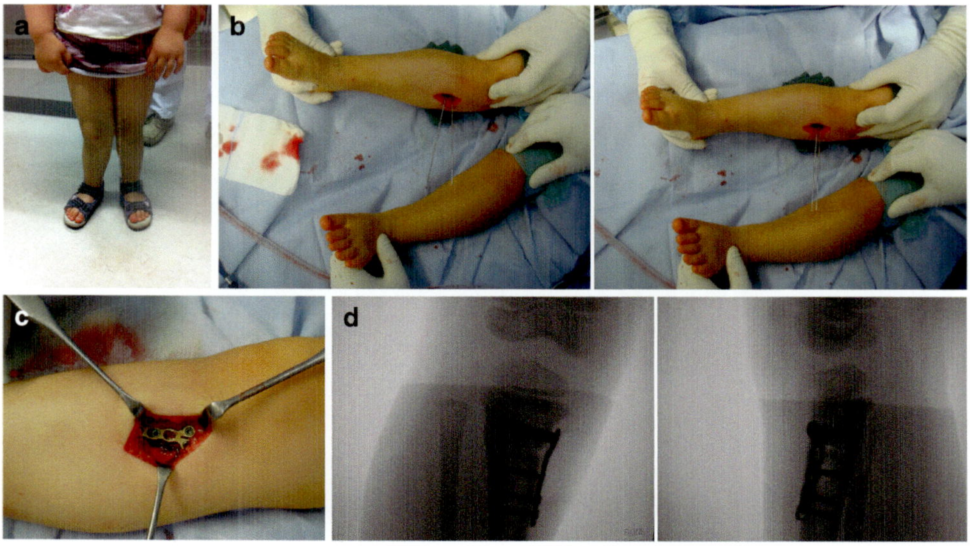

Fig. 14.16 Posttraumatic valgus deformity of a 3 year old girl. (**a**) Clinical deformity, (**b**) Intraoperative correction with K-wire orientation, (**c**) Intraoperative medial plate osteosynthesis (**d**) Postoperative x-ray with correction A.P. view and lateral view

Fractures of the Tibia Shaft

Table 14.4 Isolated fracture of the tibial shaft (Fig. 14.17)

Special features	Most common fracture of the lower extremity Special form: Toddler's Fracture (stress fracture in toddlers)
Diagnostic approach	Radiology: AP and lateral (including adjacent joints) (Fig. 14.18)
Treatment goal/limits of correction	<10 years: Varus: Up to 5°, valgus: 0°, re/antecurvation: 10°, no rotational deformity
Primary treatment	Long-leg plaster splint, analgesia
Conservative treatment	
Indication	Closed oblique and transverse tibial fractures without significant shortening
Approach	Closed long-leg cast for 4–6 weeks with partial (rolling) weight-bearing (Fig. 14.19) With angulation: Wedging on day 8
Follow up	Weight-bearing as tolerated; physical therapy as needed
Radiological controls	Day 8: Position check (cast wedging for angulation; in cases of primary angulation, wedging and then x-ray); consolidation check at 4–6 weeks
Return to sports	With unlimited function, symmetrical muscle ratios (approx. 4 weeks post-consolidation)
Operative treatment	
Indication	Displaced fractures (shaft, shortening, rotation), open fractures, (impending) compartment syndrome, polytrauma Relative: Transverse fractures (slower healing, often significant hematomas in cases of direct trauma)
Approach	External fixator (direct correction of tibia with a stable fibula) (Fig. 14.20) ESIN (risk of varus deformity when tibia fragment telescoping occurs with a stable fibula!) (Fig. 14.21)
Follow up	Partial (rolling) weight-bearing for 4 weeks, then weight-bearing as tolerated
Radiological controls	Postoperative position check; 6 weeks post-surgery: Consolidation check
Hardware removal	With verified consolidation: External fixator: At approx. 8 weeks; ESIN: At 3–4 months
Return to sports	With unlimited function, symmetrical muscle ratios (approx. 4 weeks post-consolidation)
Complications	Angulation (especially varus deformity) Compartment syndrome
Growth disturbance	Stimulative growth disturbances (leg lengthening to 1 cm)
Follow up	Weekly until unlimited function; every 6–12 months for clinical leg-length and angulation checks up to 2 years post-trauma
Classification	AO: 42-D/1–5.1–3 LiLa: 4.2.s.2–4.0-2.

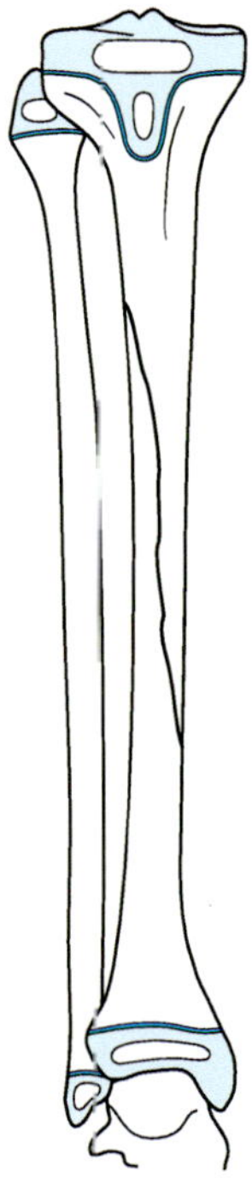

Fig. 14.17 Isolated tibial shaft fracture

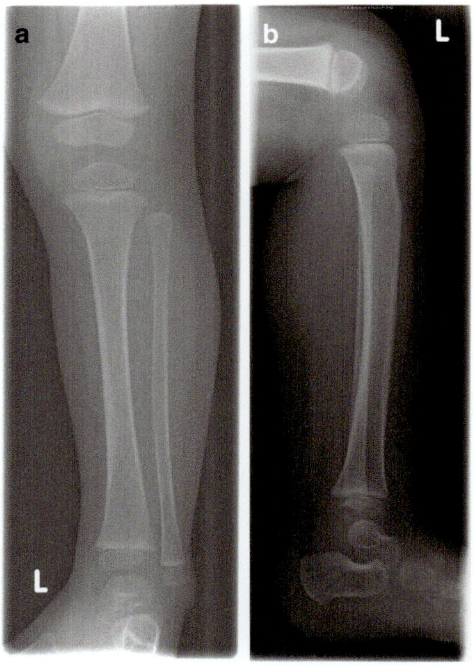

Fig. 14.18 Toddlers fracture of a 2 year old child. Conservative treatment in cast. (a) A.P. view. (b) lateral view

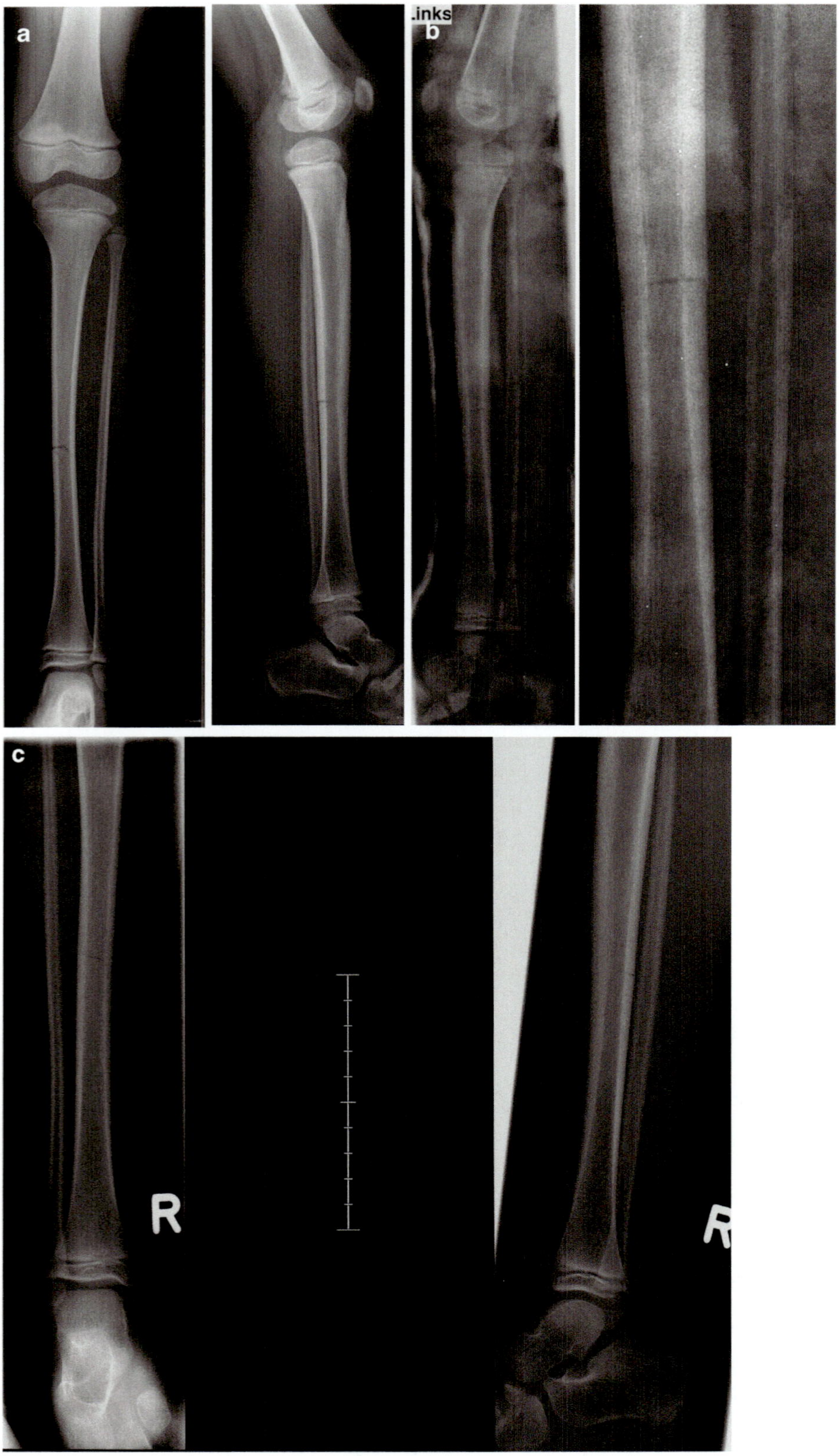

Fig. 14.19 Non-displaced isolated tibial shaft fracture of a 9 year old boy with conservative treatment. (a) Trauma images, (b) Conservative treatment with cast, (c) Bony healing

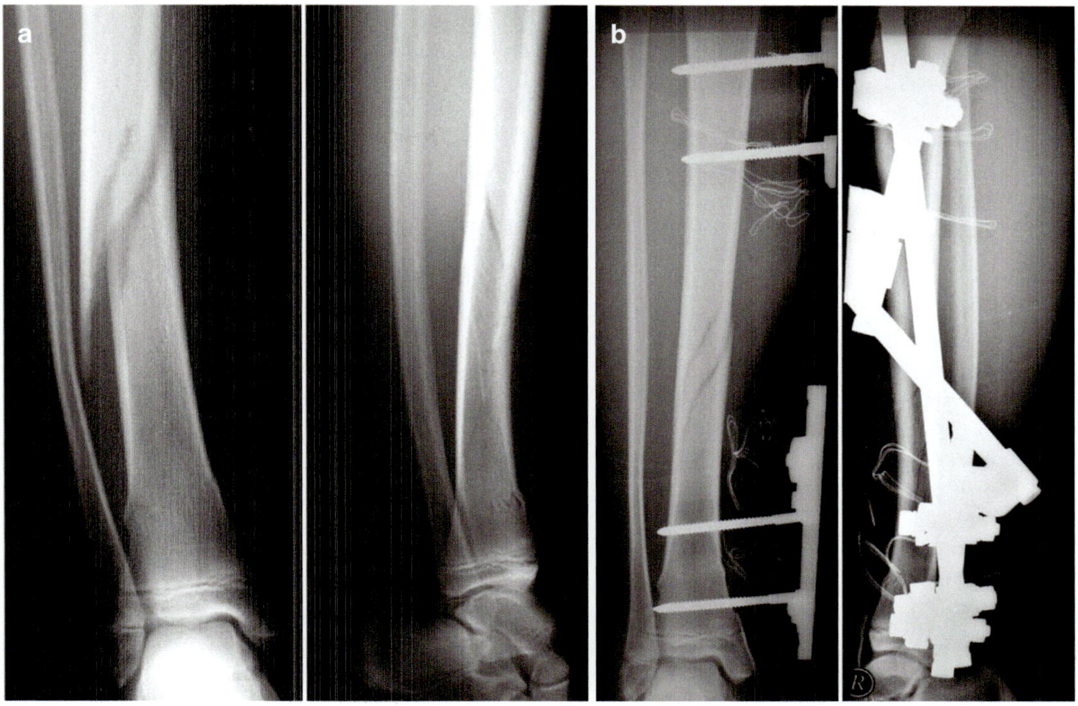

Fig. 14.20 Tibial shaft spiral fracture and compression fracture of the tibia in a 14 year old boy. (**a**) Trauma image, (**b**) Reduction and stabilization with eternal fixateur of the tibia

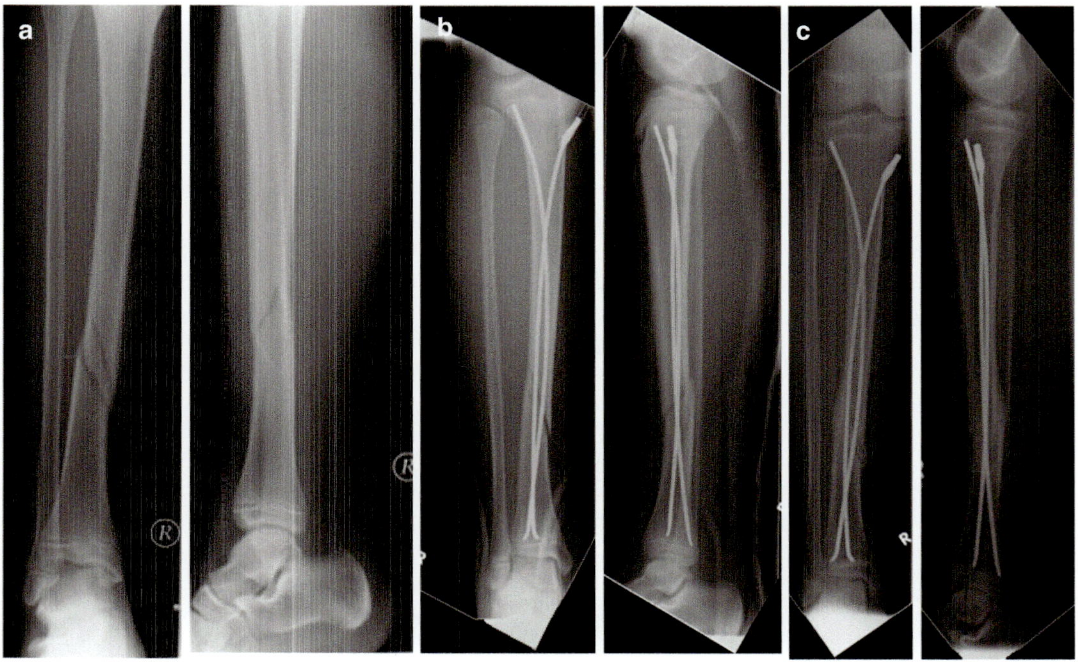

Fig. 14.21 Oblique fracture of the lower leg with bowing of the fibula in a 13 year old boy. (**a**) Trauma image, (**b**) Stabilization with ESIN including endcap to ovoid telescoping, (**c**) Bony healing

Table 14.5 Combined fractures of the tibia/fibula shaft (Fig. 14.22)

Special features	Attention to open fractures; soft tissue management is critical	
Diagnostic approach	Radiology: AP and lateral x-rays (including adjacent joints)	
Treatment goal/limits of correction	<10 years: Varus: Up to 5°, valgus: 0°, re/antecurvation: 10°, no rotational deformity	
Primary treatment	Long-leg plaster splint, analgesia, sterile covering for open fractures	
Conservative treatment		
Indication	Relative: Stable non-displaced leg fractures (14.22 conservatively treated undisplaced lower leg fracture neu)	
Approach	Long-leg circular cast for 4–6 weeks, partial (rolling) weight-bearing	
Follow up	Weight-bearing as tolerated, physical therapy if needed	
Radiological controls	Day 8: Position check (wedging for angulation); consolidation check: At 4–6 weeks	
Return to sports	With unlimited function, symmetrical muscle ratios (approx. 4 weeks post-consolidation)	
Operative treatment		
Indication	Usually all combined lower leg fractures Especially unstable fractures, open fractures, (impending) compartment syndrome, polytrauma	
Approach	External fixator (compartment syndrome, open fractures, long oblique fractures, multi-fragment fractures) (Fig. 14.23) ESIN. At best in transverse and short oblique fractures (Fig. 14.24) also possible in open fractures, if there is good soft-tissue management possible	
Follow up	Partial (rolling) weight-bearing for 4 weeks, then weight-bearing as tolerated	
Radiological controls	Postoperative position check; 6 weeks post-surgery: Consolidation check	
Hardware removal	With verified consolidation: External fixator: At approx. 8 weeks, ESIN: At 3–4 months	
Return to sports	With unlimited function, symmetrical muscle ratios (approx. 4 weeks post-consolidation)	
Complications	Angulation (especially valgus deformity) Compartment syndrome	
Growth disturbance	Stimulative growth disturbances (leg lengthening to 1 cm)	
Follow up	Weekly until unlimited function; every 6–12 months for clinical leg-length and angulation checks up to 2 years post-trauma	
Classification	AO: 42-D/1–5.1–3	LiLa: 4.2.s.2–4.0-2.

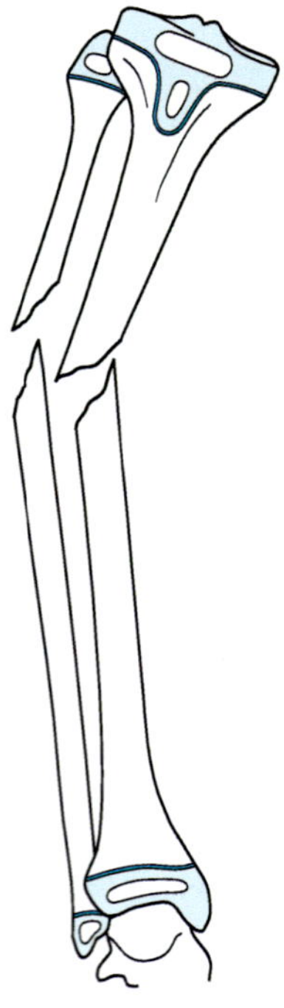

Fig. 14.22 Complete lower leg fracture

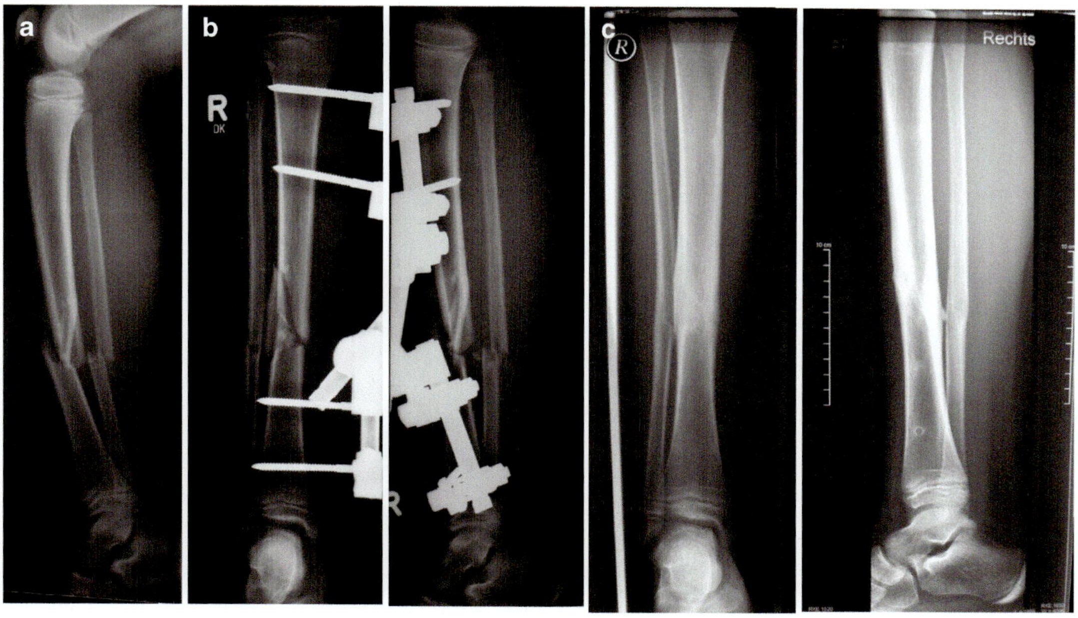

Fig. 14.23 Lower leg fracture of a 9 year old boy. (**a**) Trauma image, (**b**) Postoperative with external fixateur, (**c**) Healing

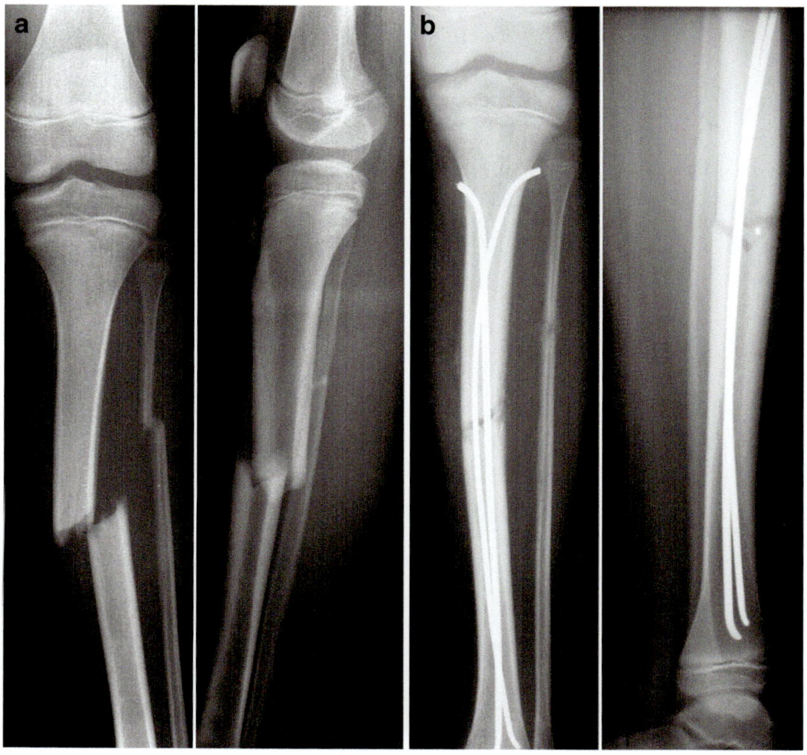

Fig. 14.24 Complete lower leg fracture after traffic accident of a 12 year old boy. (**a**) Trauma image, (**b**) Stabilization with ESIN

Fractures of the Distal Tibia

Table 14.6 Fractures of the distal tibial metaphysis (Fig. 14.25)

Special features	Differentiating torus from bowing fractures of the metaphysis is difficult in individual cases
Diagnostic approach	Radiology: AP and lateral (including the ankle)
Treatment goal/limits of correction	Varus: 5°, valgus: 10°, re/antecurvation 10°, no rotational deformity
Primary treatment	Long-leg plaster splint, analgesia (Fig. 14.26)
Conservative treatment	
Indication	Usually conservative (Fig. 14.27)
Approach	Short-leg cast for 4 weeks with weight-bearing as tolerated Angulation <10°: Day 8: Cast wedging (Fig. 14.28) Angulation >10°: Primary reduction With recurvation deformity: Cast in equinus position
Follow up	No specific follow up
Radiological controls	Day 8: Position check (cast wedging for angulation); consolidation check: At 4–6 weeks (cast-free)
Return to sports	With unlimited function, symmetrical muscle ratios (approx. 4 weeks post-consolidation)
Operative treatment	
Indication	Reduction obstacle, severely displaced fractures, open fractures
Approach	Crossed K-wires, percutaneous; post-surgery: Short-leg plaster splint External fixator in individual cases with or without K-wire fixation (Fig. 14.29) ESIN with correct positioning of the nails (bending anteriorly, tips to the dorsal side) (Fig. 14.30 NEW ESIN distale tibia)
Follow up	Partial (rolling) weight-bearing for 4 weeks, then weight-bearing as tolerated
Radiological controls	Postoperative position check; 6 weeks post-surgery: Consolidation check (cast-free)
Hardware removal	With verified consolidation: External fixator: After approx. 8 weeks, K-wires: At 4–6 weeks (outpatient)
Return to sports	With unlimited function, symmetrical muscle ratios (approx. 4 weeks post-consolidation)
Complications	Axial deviation (especially recurvatum) Compartment syndrome Adhesion of the flexor hallucis longus tendon after conservative therapy → PT
Growth disturbance	Partially stimulative growth disturbances → usually without clinical relevance Partially inhibitory growth disturbance, rare
Follow up	Weekly until unlimited function; every 6–12 months for clinical leg-length and angulation checks up to 2 years post-trauma
Classification	AO: 43-M/2(3).1–3 LiLa: 4.3.s.2–4.0-2.

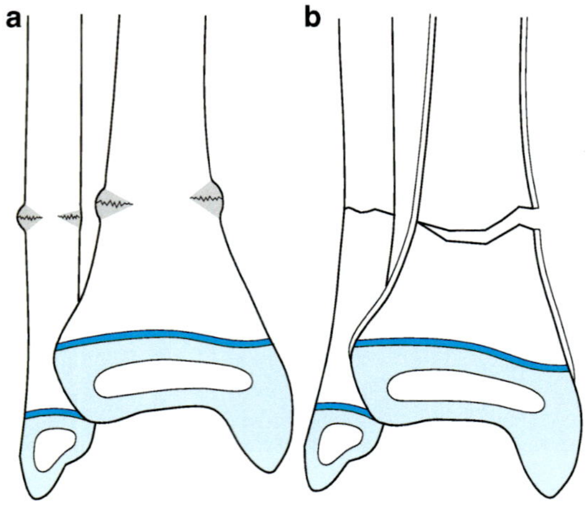

Fig. 14.25 Fracture of the distal metaphysis. (**a**) Compression fracture, (**b**) Bowing fracture

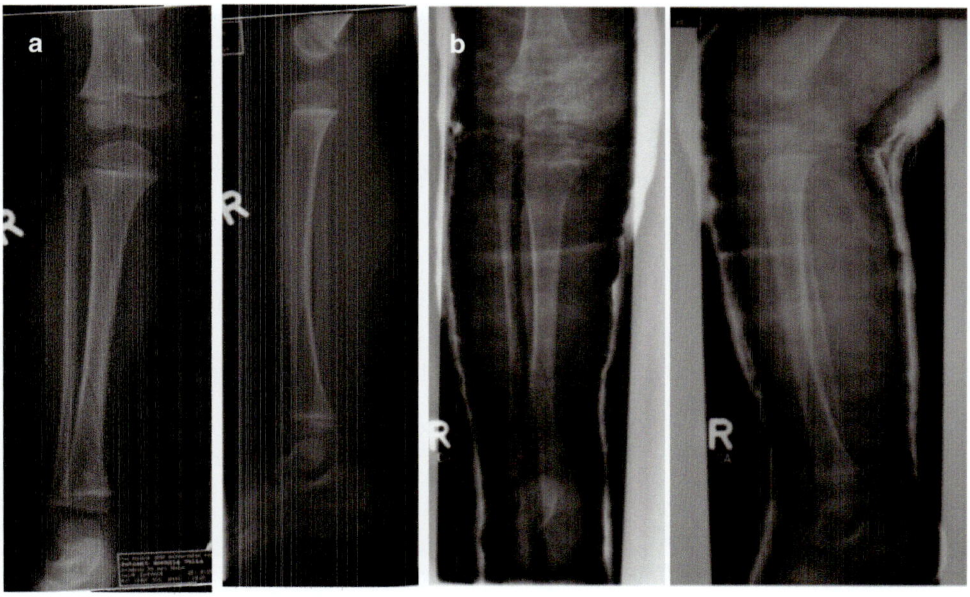

Fig. 14.26 Distal undisplaced spiral fracture of the tibia. (**a**) Trauma image, (**b**) With conservative treatment in a cast

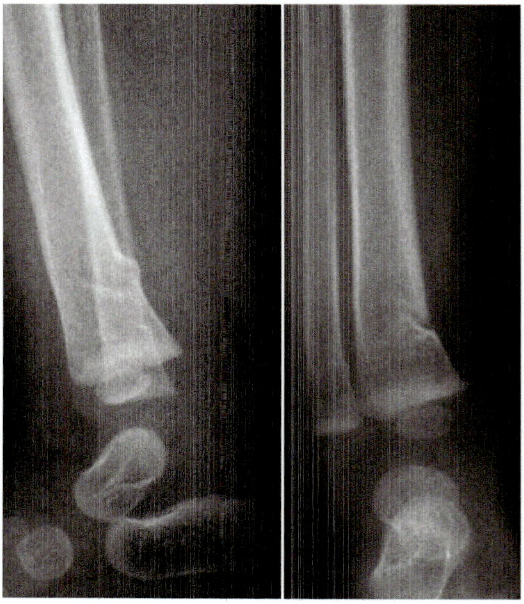

Fig. 14.27 Compression fracture of the distal tibia and fibula of a small child. Conservative treatment in cast for 3–4 weeks

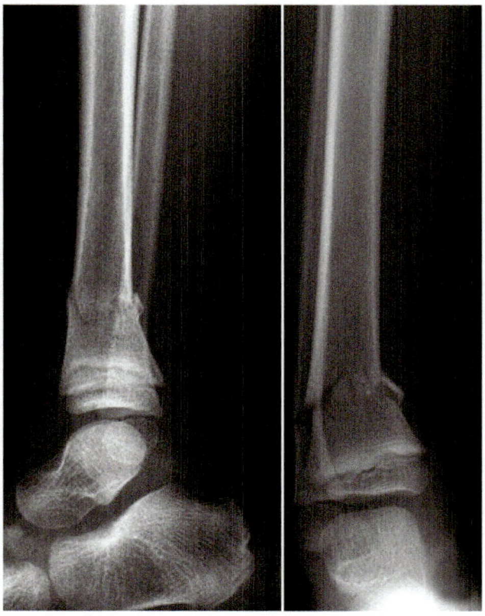

Fig. 14.28 Slightly displaced distal fracture of tibia and fibula in a small child. Conservative treatment for 3–4 weeks in a cast

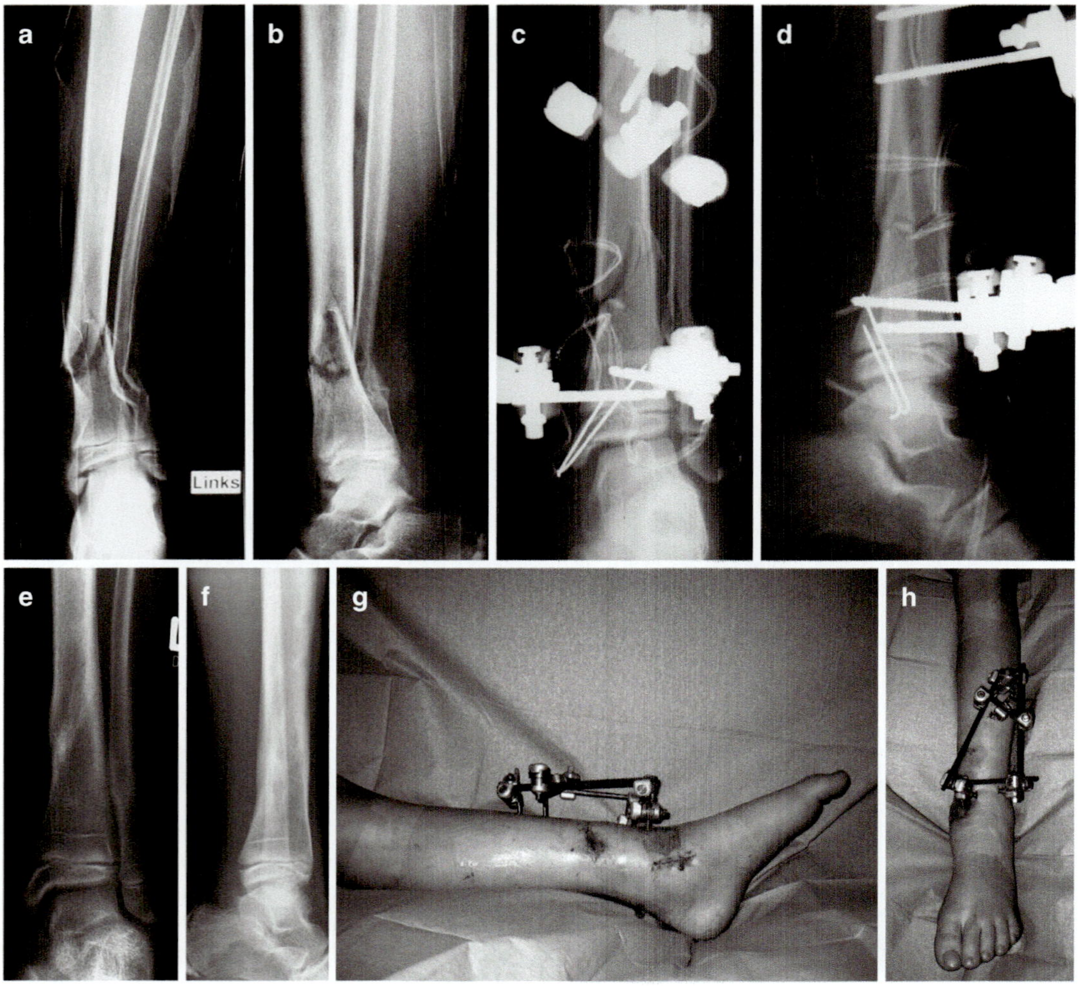

Fig. 14.29 Lower leg metaphyseal fracture third degree, boy, 10 years, skateboarding accident. (**a**, **b**) Trauma images: open fracture grade 3 of the medial malleolus and the distal tibia, bending of the fibula. (**c**, **d**, **g**, **h**) Stabilization with external fixator and K-wire transfixion. (**e**, **f**) X-ray control 1 year post-surgery

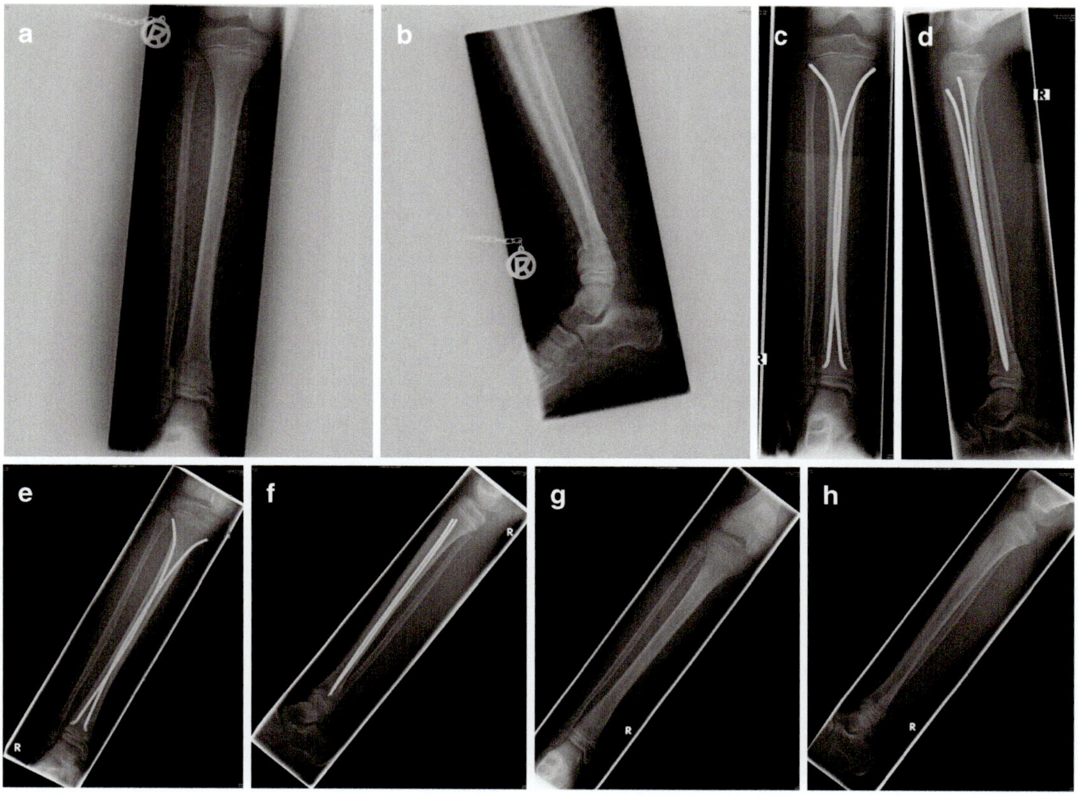

Fig. 14.30 (**a**, **b**) Increasing dislocation of the distal lower leg fracture (Fig. 14.7) in x-ray control. (**c**, **d**) Operative correction and stabilization with ESIN, (**e**, **f**) Healing in correct position, (**g**, **h**) Consolidation after metal removal

Technical Aspects

Table 14.7 Technical aspects lower leg

Material	ESIN elastic intramedullary nail → Usually titanium → Diameter: 2.5–4 mm (1/3 of the medullary canal diameter) External fixator Various fixator systems available Image intensifier
Positioning	Supine Drape for freely movable leg
Operative principle	External fixator (proximal metaphysis) (Fig. 14.31) Caution: Apophyseal plate of the tibial tuberosity Medial compression with the external fixator is practical and possible External fixator (shaft) (Fig. 14.32) Caution: Apophyseal plate of the tibial tuberosity 2 fingers distance from the fracture No pins through the fracture gap ESIN: Leg shaft fracture (Fig. 14.33) Because the tibia has a triangular cross-section, special care must be taken when placing nails. The eccentric position of the tibia related to the muscles surrounding it has an unfavorable influence on the ESIN biomechanics. The tibia is nailed from proximal. Technique for the tibia differs from the femur in the following ways. Determine the nail entry point: Nail entry points are medial and lateral to the tibial tuberosity. Make incisions: Make a 2–3 cm skin incision above each planned entry point from proximal. Note: When perforating the cortex, take care not to injure the proximal tibial epiphyseal plate or the tibial apophysis. Check the position of the nail tips. The nails tend to move posteriorly because of the medullary canal's triangular shape; this can lead to recurvation. Before the nails are definitively inserted, turn the tips of both nails slightly toward posterior to achieve the physiological antecurvation of the tibia. Approximate the fracture fragments as much as possible to avoid fixation in a distracted position. Shorten nails: Keep the nail ends short and bend only minimally because of the limited soft-tissue cover.
Compartment division	Bilateral incisions: 1. Anterolateral incision: Lateral and anterior compartments2. Posteromedial incision: Posterior compartments Unilateral incision: Parafibular incision along the entire fibular length 1. Lateral compartment: Caution: The superficial peroneal nerve runs in the distal tibial third through the intermuscular septum into the extensor compartment 2. Subcutaneous dissection toward anterior and longitudinal division (caution: Superficial peroneal (fibular) nerve in the distal third). 3. Superficial posterior compartment: Subcutaneous dissection toward posterior and longitudinal splitting of the fascia 4. Deep posterior compartment: Approach between the peroneal muscles and the triceps surae, with longitudinal splitting of the fascia (caution: Tibial artery, vein, nerve) Skin closure with synthetic skin replacement (e.g., epigard, syspurderm) Secondary closure or split-thickness skin graft at 5–8 days
Hardware removal	ESIN: At 4–6 months External fixator: At approx. 8 weeks

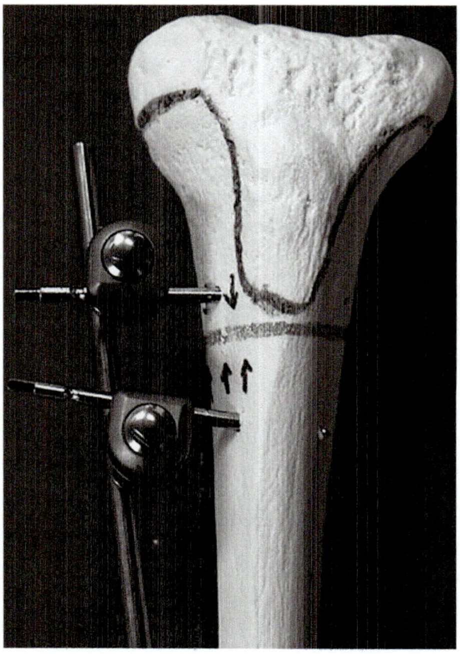

Fig. 14.31 External fixateur to compress the medial proximal tibia metaphysis; model assembly

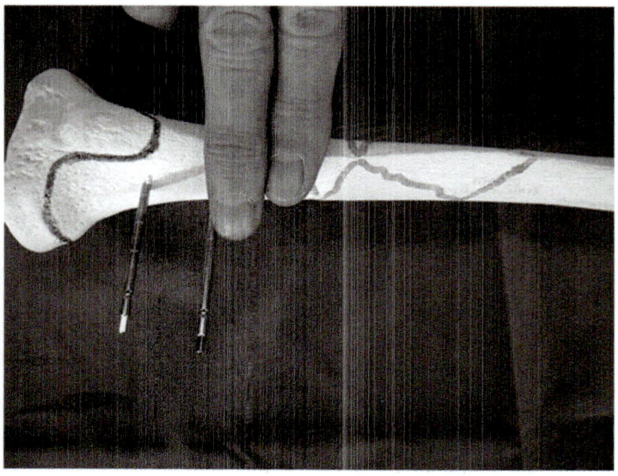

Fig. 14.32 External fixateur to stabilize compound fractures of the tibia shaft; model assembly

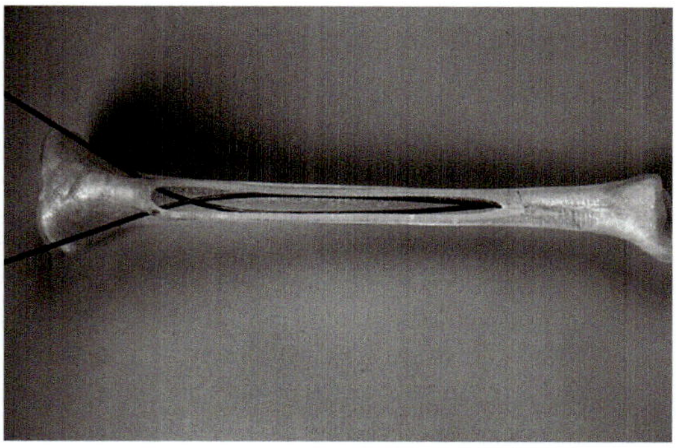

Fig. 14.33 Principles of ESIN for the tibia. Because of the tibia's triangular shape, the anterolateral and medial entry points on the proximal tibia lead to "posterior glide" of the nails

Recommended Literature

Andreacchio A, Marengo L, Canavese F, Pedretti L, Memeo A (2016 Sep) Comparison between external fixation and elastic stable intramedullary nailing for the treatment of femoral shaft fractures in children younger than 8 years of age. J Pediatr Orthop B 25(5):471–477

Andreacchio A, Alberghina F, Marengo L, Canavese F (2019 Apr) Pediatric tibia and femur fractures in patients weighing more than 50 kg (110 lb): mini-review on current treatment options and outcome. Musculoskelet Surg 103(1):23–30

Arslan H, Kapukaya A, Kesemenli C, Subasi M, Kayikci C (2003) Floating knee in children. J Pediatr Orthop 23:458–463

Ganesan RP, Anbu S, Palaniappan M, Kolundan K, Kannan K, Subramaniankarunanithi S (2017) Elastic stable intramedullary nailing of femoral and tibial shaft fractures in children. J Evol Med Dent Sci 5:5196–5201

Giertych BF, Hosseinzadeh P, Milbrandt TA, Muchow R, Noonan K (2019) Lower extremity fractures in children: how to avoid pitfalls and manage complications. Instr Course Lect 68:427–442

Green NE (1983) Tibia Valga caused by assymmetrical overgrowth following a nondisplaced fracture of the proximal tibial metaphysis. J Pediatr Orthop 3:235–237

Jubel A, Andermahr J, Isenberg J, Schiffer G, Prokop A, Rehm KE (2004) Erfahrungen mit der elastisch stabilen intramedullären Nagelung (ESIN) diaphysärer Frakturen im Kindesalter. Orthopade 33:928–935

Kremer L, Voth M, Marzi I (2017) Fractures of the lower extremities in childhood: part 1: fractures of the thigh and in the proximity of the knee. Der Chirurg; Zeitschrift für alle Gebiete der operativen Medizin 85:451–412

Liu H, Wang H, Shao B, Lu H, Zhang S, Ou L et al (2019 Sep) Epidemiological evaluation of traumatic lower limb fractures in children: variation with age, gender, time, and etiology. Medicine (Baltimore) 98(38):e17123

Marengo L, Paonessa M, Andreacchio A, Dimeglio A, Potenza A, Canavese F (2015) Displaced tibia shaft fractures in children treated by elastic stable intramedullary nailing: results and complications in children weighing 50 kg (110 lb) or more. Eur J Orthop Surg Traumatol 26:311–317

Pandya NK (2016 Jun) Flexible intramedullary nailing of unstable and/or open tibia shaft fractures in the pediatric population. J Pediatr Orthop 36(Suppl 1):S19–S23

Patel NK, Horstman J, Kuester V, Sambandam S, Mounasamy V (2018 Sep) Pediatric Tibial shaft fractures. Indian J Orthop 52(5):522–528

Reuter DS, Mellerowicz H (2016) Avulsionsverletzungen der proximalen Tibia. Orthopade 45:226–232

Rickert KD, Hosseinzadeh P, Edmonds EW (2018 Sep) What's new in pediatric Orthopaedic trauma: the lower extremity. J Pediatr Orthop 38(8):e434–e439

Schmidt AH, Finkemeier CG, Tornetta P 3rd (2003) Treatment of closed tibial fractures. Instr Course Lect 52:607–622

Siegmeth A, Wruhs O, Vecsei V (1998) External fixation of lower limb fractures in children. Eur J Pediatr Surg 8:35–41

Slongo TF (2005) Complications and failures of the ESIN technique. Injury 36:S78–S85

Slongo T (2020 Dec) Technique and biomechanics of Kirschner wire osteosynthesis in children. Oper Orthop Traumatol 32(6):509–529

Stenroos A, Puhakka J, Nietosvaara Y, Kosola J (2020 Dec) Treatment of closed tibia shaft fractures in children: a systematic review and meta-analysis. Eur J Pediatr Surg 30(6):483–489

Till H, Huttl B, Knorr P, Dietz HG (2000) Elastic stable intramedullary nailing (ESIN) provides good long-term results in pediatric long-bone fractures. Eur J Pediatr Surg 10:319–322

Tuten HR, Keeler KA, Gabos PG, Zionts LE, MacKenzie WG (1999) Posttraumatic tibia Valga in children. A long term follow up note. JBJS Am 81:799–810

Ankle Joint

15

15.1 Physiological Findings

Accessory bones are common, most notably between the ages of seven and ten, and may merge with secondary ossification centers (Fig. 15.1). Most common are the os trigonum (Fig. 15.2), the subfibular bone (Fig. 15.3) or isolated ossification centers (Fig. 15.4). These ossification centers should be differentiated from older ligatmentous avulsions, in particular in adolescents. Fibular ossicle: isolated ossification center lateral to the distal fibular metaphysis. The distal fibula epiphysis might be slightly displace to the medial side. They are frequently considered potential bony avulsion injuries during differential diagnosis, but this is uncommon and only relevant in the case of sharp-edged fragments.

The epiphyseal plates can have irregular borders and isolated ossification centers occur medial or lateral of the malleoli. The ossification centers appear at different ages and fuse at defined time points (Fig. 15.5).

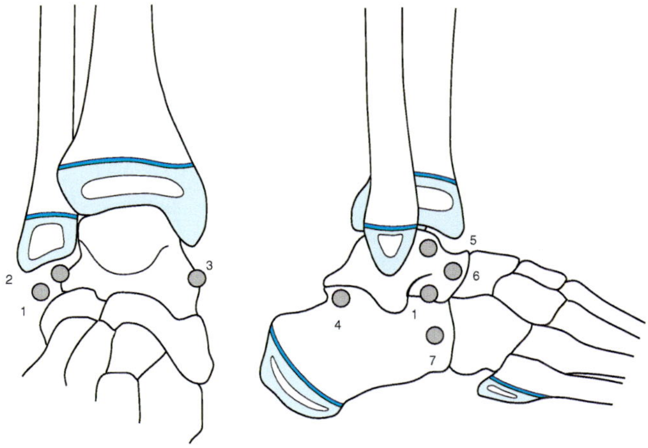

Fig. 15.1 Accessory ossification centers (1) Os tibiale externum, (2) Talus accessorius, (3) Talus secundarius, (4) Os trigonum, (5) Os talotibiale, (6) Os supratalare, (7) Calcaneus secundarius

I. Marzi et al., *Pediatric Skeletal Trauma*, https://doi.org/10.1007/978-3-030-93685-3_15

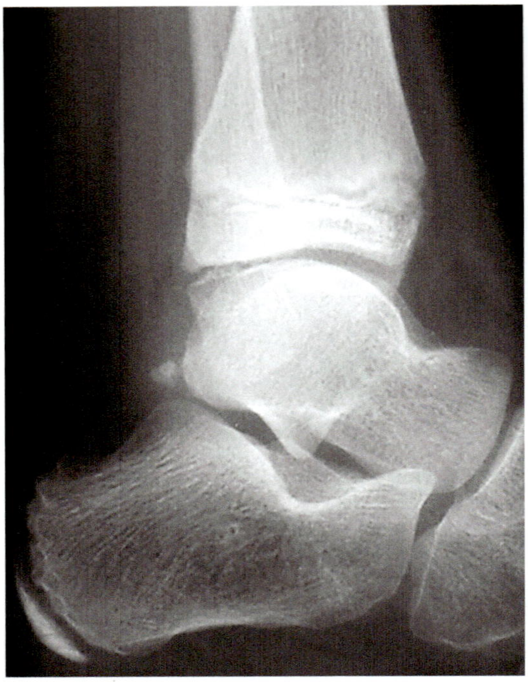

Fig. 15.2 Os trigonum (10 years)

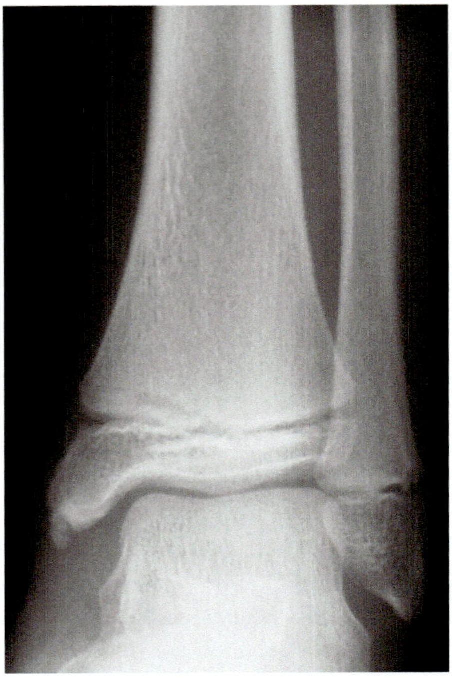

Fig. 15.4 Isolated ossification center of the medial malleolus (10 years)

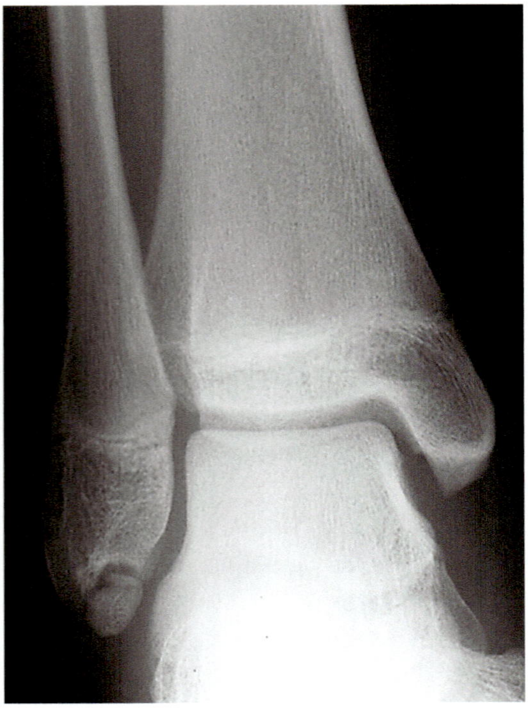

Fig. 15.3 Os subfibulare (15 years)

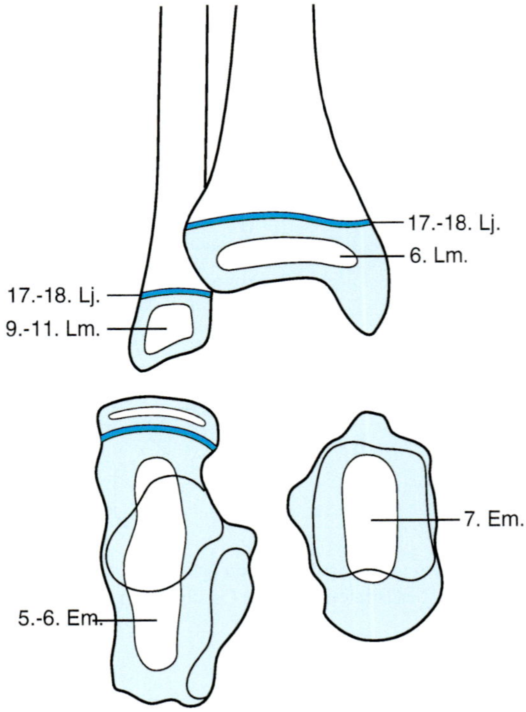

Fig. 15.5 Ossification centers around of the ankle and hindfoot. (*Lj*) life year, (*Em*) embryonal month, (*Lm*) life month

15.2 Distal Tibia Fractures

Incidence, Mechanism of Injury, and Clinical Presentation

The incidence of distal tibial fractures is 4.9%.

Ankle distortion is one of the most common musculoskeletal traumas. In adults, it generally leads to ligament complex injuries. During childhood, it leads to avulsions and growth plate fractures because the ligaments are more stable than the osteochondral structures.

The most commonly used fracture classifications are those of Salter and Harris and Aitken for growth plate injuries. In wide-open growth plates, the fracture line is usually medial, outside the loading region of the ankle, and almost always perpendicular to the plate. Salter-Harris II injuries are the most common, with Salter-Harris III and IV injuries significantly less prevalent. Marked displacement and instability in Salter-Harris II injuries must be reduced and usually held with K-wires. However, these are shaft fractures without direct joint involvement. In the treatment of small children, the potential for remodeling plays an important role. In contrast, Salter-Harris III and IV are intraarticular injuries with joint widening or even step-offs in addition to the growth plate involvement. As in adults, such fractures with disruption of the joint cartilage must be anatomically reduced with compression and screw fixation. Displacement around 2 mm can be tolerated, in particular gaps. Step-offs should not exceed 2 mm.

From about 12 years, the growth plates begin to fuse - in girls sooner than boys - starting along the medial tibia (Fig. 15.6). When trauma occurs, the fracture course and injury pattern change, leading to "transition fractures" on the way to adulthood. Shearing force disrupts partially-open epiphyses by moving through the closed portion towards the joint. The older the child, the more fused the growth plate, and thus, the more lateral and anterior the epiphyseal fracture will be. This is called a "twoplane" or Tilleaux fracture. It corresponds functionally to a bony rupture of the anterior syndesmosis with participation of the ankle joint.

Depending on the force involved, a dorsal metaphyseal wedge can break off, similar to a posterior Volkmann triangle in adults. This is called a triplane fracture. If the metaphyseal fracture ends within the growth plate, it is called a triplane I fracture. If it passes through the posterior epiphysis, it is a triplane II fracture. Gross displacement is uncommon; however, gaps are

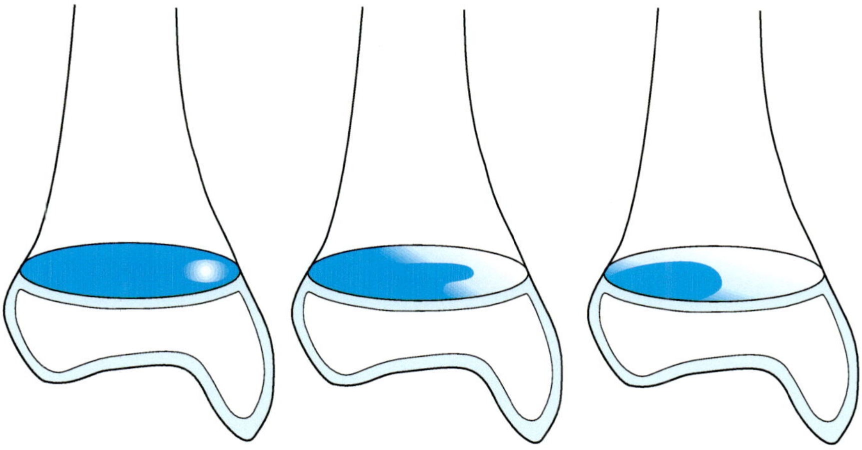

Fig. 15.6 Distal tibial growth plate closure: Starts anteromedially, continuous towards posterior, finishes anterolateral

often evident. Although transition fractures show characteristic patterns according to age, MRI or CT imaging can be used in individual cases when better information is needed for operative planning. In contrast to Salter type fractures, growth disturbances are unlikely since the children are older and the growth plate has begun to fuse; the growth phase is ending. Anatomical reduction of the articular fracture is still critical because the fracture line runs through the ankle loading region. Gaps or step-offs up to 2 mm can be tolerated.

One growth disturbance that does occur is partial epiphyseal closure of the distal tibia. If this is suspected over follow-up, MRI can show potential bone bridges and assist with further treatment planning. However, those corrections are mandatory and not always successful (see Chap. 20).

Fractures of the Distal Fibula Fractures of the distal fibula occur mostly after supination trauma, combined with Salter I or II fractures of the distal tibia. In most cases, reduction and fixation of the tibia fracture achieve stable fibular reduction, and individual fixation is rarely necessary. Any residual bending of the fibula can be left if the ankle is in good position with an intact syndesmosis because it will correct with growth. Isolated fibular fractures are rare and generally minimally displaced; thus, conservative therapy in a short-leg cast should be sufficient (Fig. 15.7).

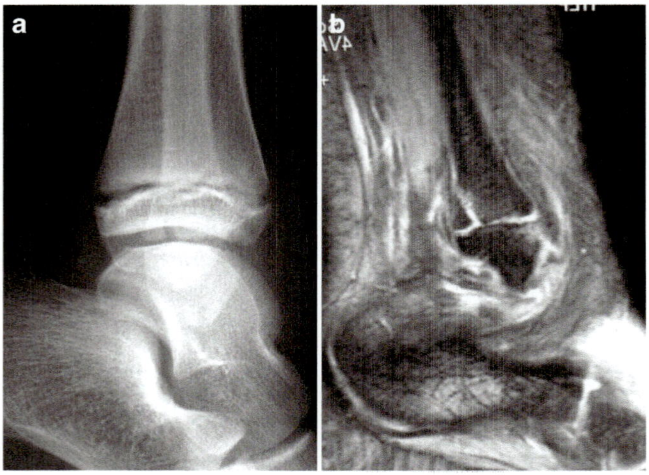

Fig. 15.7 Isolated Salter II injury of the distal fibula. (**a**) X-ray, (**b**) MRI

Classifications

The Harris growth arrest line, a radiopaque line occurring due to bony insult, can be used to record any post-traumatic growth disturbances. It typically runs parallel to the growth plate. The prognosis of ankle fractures depends on child age, trauma severity, localization and type of fracture, extent of displacement, and correct anatomical reduction. As long as the growth plate is open (Fig. 15.8), the most common classifications are Aitken or Salter and Harris (Table 15.1). The classification of transition fractures begins when the growth plates begin to fuse (Table 15.1).

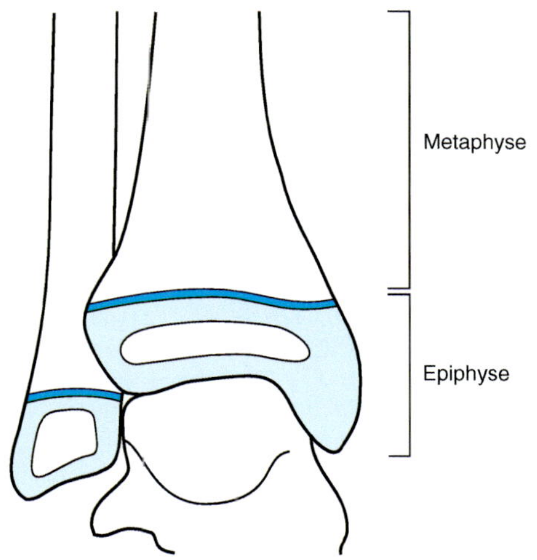

Fig. 15.8 Growth plate pattern along the distal leg

Epiphyseal disruptions of type Salter-Harris-I take place only if the epiphyseal line is open, without additional bony fragment (Fig. 15.9) as indicated in Table 15.2.

Epiphyseal disruptions of type Salter-Harris-II take place only if the epiphyseal line is open, but with an, additional bony fragment (Fig. 15.13) as indicated in Table 15.3.

Epiphyseal fracture of type Salter-Harris III take place only if the epiphyseal line is still open (Table 15.4) and the fracture only affects the epiphysis (Fig. 15.18) as indicated in Table 15.5.

Epiphyseal disruptions of type Salter-Harris IV (Aitken 3) take place only if the epiphyseal line is still open, but with an, additional bony fragment (Fig. 15.22) as indicated in Table 15.5.

Table 15.1 Classifications of distal tibial fractures

 Aitken 1	Salter-Harris I Salter-Harris II	Lesion of the metaphyseal portion of the growth plate
Aitken 2 Aitken 3	Salter-Harris III Salter-Harris IV	Lesion of the epiphyseal portion of the growth plate
Twoplane		Epiphyseal fracture with partial fusion
Triplane I Triplane II		Epi-metaphyseal fracture in partial plate closure

15.3 Epiphysiolysis and Epiphyseal Fractures of the Distal Tibia

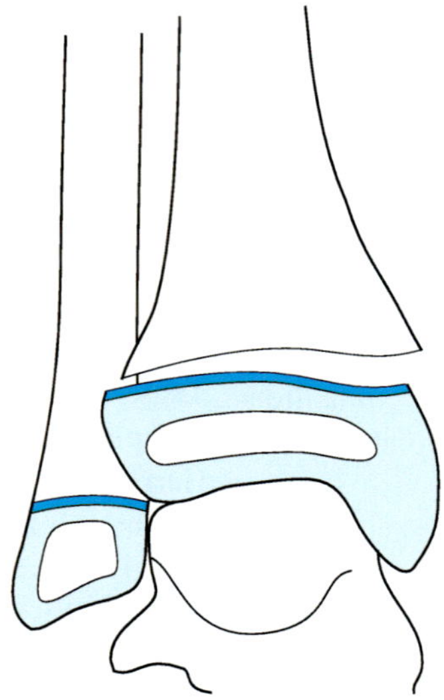

Fig. 15.9 Epihyseolysis type Salter-Harris-I

Table 15.2 Epiphyseal disruptions of the distal tibia type Salter-Harris I or Aitken 1

Special features	Uncommon; particularly >10 years	
Diagnostic approach	AP and lateral x-rays; often not initially evident radiographically. x-ray control for persistent complaints: Widening of the growth plate, metaphyseal densification, callus over the clinical course	
Treatment goal/limits of correction	<10 years: 20° retro or anteversion, 20° varus/valgus, side-to-side: ¼ shaft width (>10 years: Axial alignment no rotation deformity no residual misalignment once the growth plate has begun to fuse	
Primary treatment	Short-leg plaster splint, medical analgesia as needed	
Conservative treatment		
Indication	Generally conservative, observance of correction limits	
Approach	4 weeks short-leg cast, increase weight-bearing after 2 weeks (Fig. 15.10)	
Follow up	Weight-bearing as tolerated after cast removal; physical therapy usually not necessary	
X-ray controls	8th day position control; 4-week consolidation check (cast-free)	
Return to sports	Approx. 4 weeks after consolidation	
Operative treatment		
Indication	Generally closed reduction; open reduction in cases of severe displacement, soft-tissue involvement	
Approach	Closed reduction under general anesthesia and knee flexed to 90° (muscle relaxation) With soft resistance: Crossed K-wire transfixion (Figs. 15.11 and 15.12)	
Follow up	4 weeks short-leg cast, non-weight-bearing weight-bearing as tolerated after cast removal, physical therapy is generally not necessary	
X-ray controls	Postoperative position control; 4-week consolidation check (cast-free)	
Hardware removal	4 weeks post-surgery (after consolidation)	
Return to sports	Approx. 4 weeks after consolidation	
Complications	Rare: Compartment syndrome, flexor hallucis longus tendon adhesion	
Growth disturbance	Approx. 15% premature growth plate fusion (rarely with serious consequences, since most are >10 years)	
Follow up	Every six months for two years Check for rear foot axis asymmetry and leg-length differences	
Classification	AO: 43-E/1.1.-3	LiLa: 4.3.s.1.0–2.

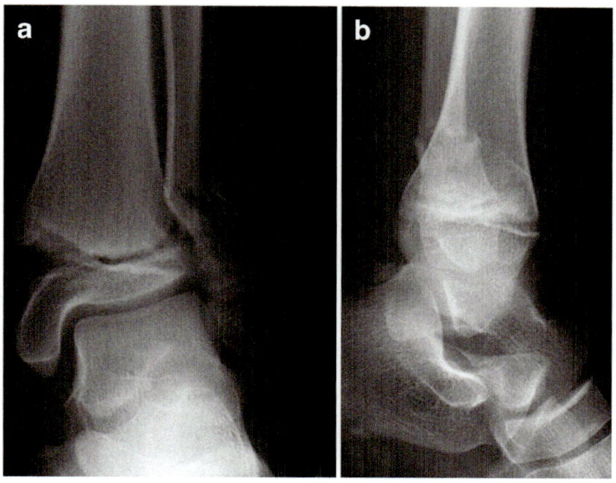

Fig. 15.10 Epihyseolysis of the distal tibia, type Salter-Harris-I, with bowing fracture of the fibula. (**a**) A.P. view, (**b**) lateral view

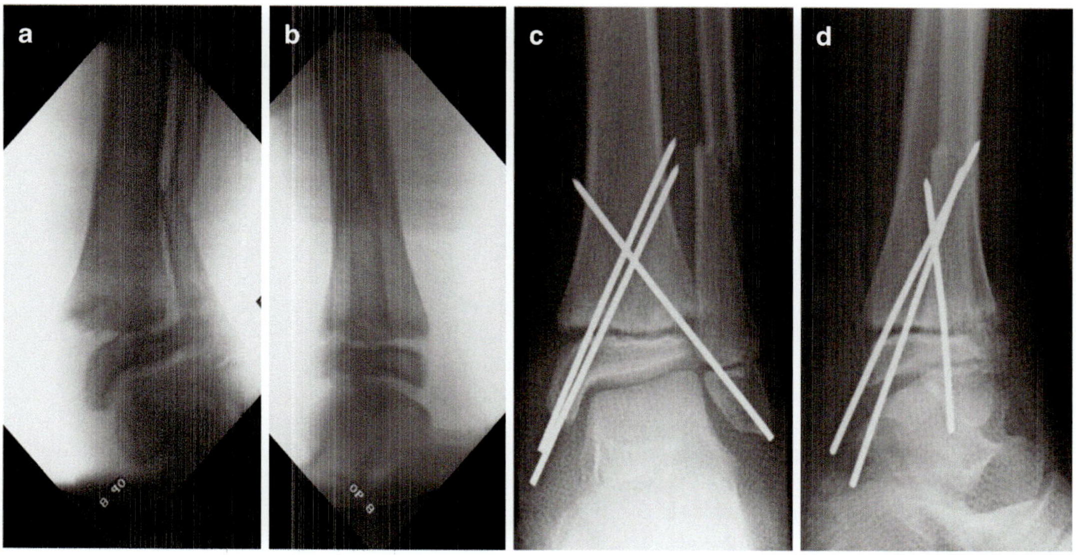

Fig. 15.11 Salter I fracture, boy, 10 years, recreational trauma. (**a**, **b**) Trauma images. (**c**, **d**) K-wire fixation after reduction

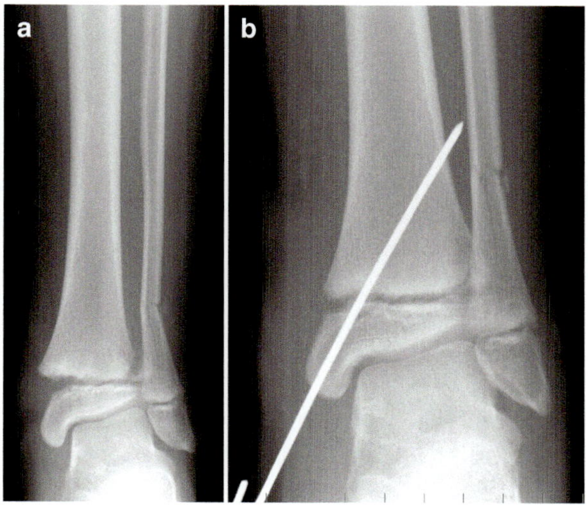

Fig. 15.12 Epihyseolysis of the distal tibia, type Salter-Harris-II with additional fracture of the fibula. (**a**) Trauma image, (**b**) K-wire fixation and 4 weeks lower leg cast. The fibula does not need to be addressed

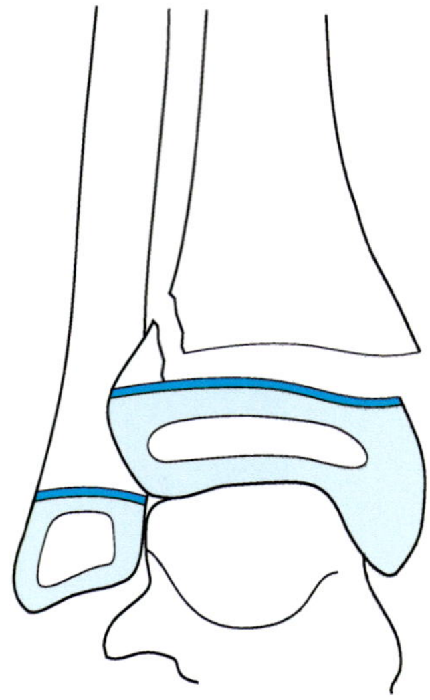

Fig. 15.13 Epiphyseal disruption with metaphyseal wedge fragment (type Salter-Harris II)

Table 15.3 Epiphyseal disruptions with metaphyseal wedge type Salter-Harris II or Aitken 1

Special features	Most common injury; supination trauma
Diagnostic approach	AP and lateral x-rays, oblique views as needed
Treatment goal/limits of correction	No rotation deformity <10 years: 10° retro or anteversion, 10° varus/valgus, side-to-side misalignment >10 years: Axial alignment No residual misalignment once the growth plate has begun to fuse
Primary treatment	Short-leg cast, medical analgesia as needed
Conservative treatment	
Indication	Generally conservative, observance of correction limits
Approach	4 weeks in ankle cast, non-weight-bearing; cast wedging on eighth day as needed
Follow up	Weight-bearing as tolerated after cast removal, physical therapy is generally not necessary
X-ray controls	8th day position control; 4-week consolidation check (cast-free)
Return to sports	Approx. 4 weeks after consolidation
Operative treatment	
Indication	Generally closed reduction; open reduction in cases of severe displacement, soft-tissue involvement
Approach	Closed reduction under general anesthesia and knee flexed to 90° (muscle relaxation) Depending on the size of the metaphyseal fragment and patient age: K-wire fixation (Figs. 15.14 and 15.15) or screw fixation (Figs. 15.16 and 15.17).
Follow up	4 weeks short-leg cast, non-weight-bearing weight-bearing as tolerated after cast removal, physical therapy is generally not necessary
X-ray controls	Postoperative position control; 4-week consolidation check (cast-free)
Hardware removal	K-wires 4 weeks post-surgery; screws 12 weeks post-surgery (after consolidation)
Return to sports	Approx. 4 weeks after consolidation
Complications	Nerve or tendon irritation from approach
Growth disturbance	Approx. 15% premature growth plate closure (rarely with serious consequences, since most are >10 years)
Follow up	Every six months for two years Check for rear foot axis asymmetry and leg-length differences
Classification	AO: 43-E/2.1–3 LiLa: 4.3.s.1.0–2.

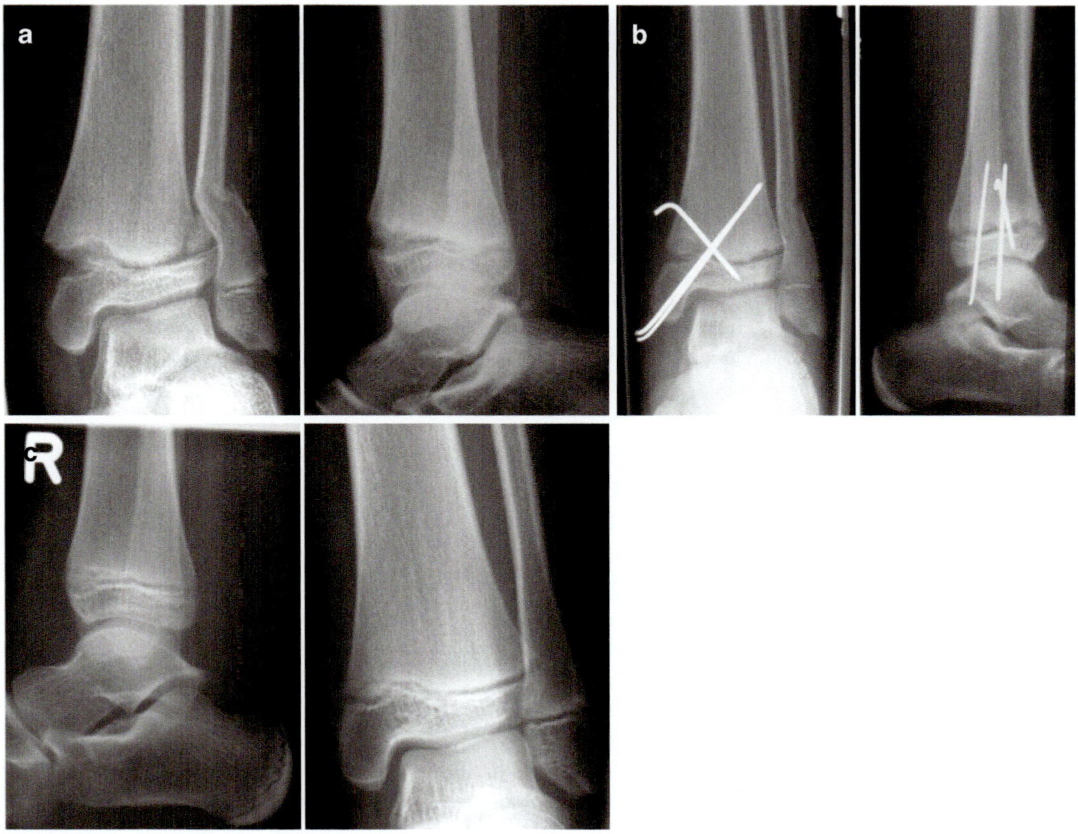

Fig. 15.14 Salter-Harris II fracture of the distal tibia with a metaphyseal wedge and bowing of the fibula in a 11 year old boy. (**a**) Trauma image, (**b**) Closed reduction and K-wire transfixation of the tibia; the fibula does not need to be fixed only together with the tibia with a lower leg cast. (**c**) Bony anatomical healing of tibia and fibula

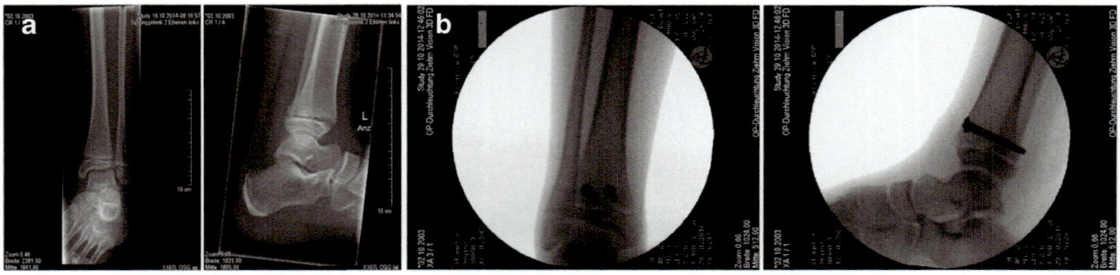

Fig. 15.15 Argely displaced Salter-Harris II fracture of the distal tibia with a small metaphyseal wedge and a displaced bowing fracture of the fibula in a 12 year old boy after bicycle fall. (**a**) Trauma image, (**b**) Closed reduction and percutaneous K-wire stabilization of the tibia. The fibula is redressed but does not need a separate fixation

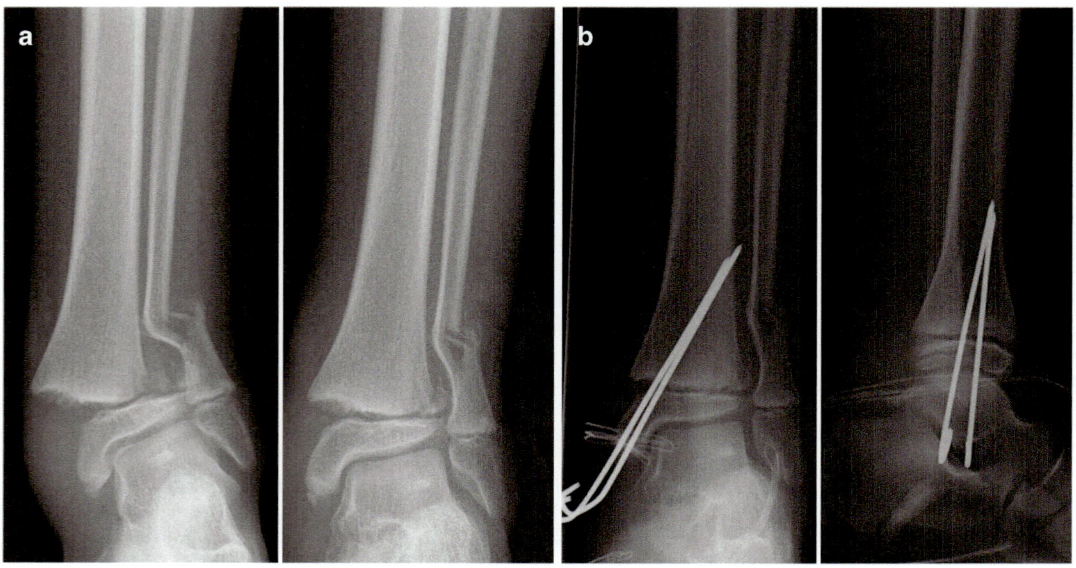

Fig. 15.16 Salter-Harris II fracture of the distal tibia with a displaced metaphyseal wedge in a 11 year old girl. (**a**) Trauma image, (**b**) Closed reduction and cannulated percutaneous screw fixation from anterior to posterior after closed reduction

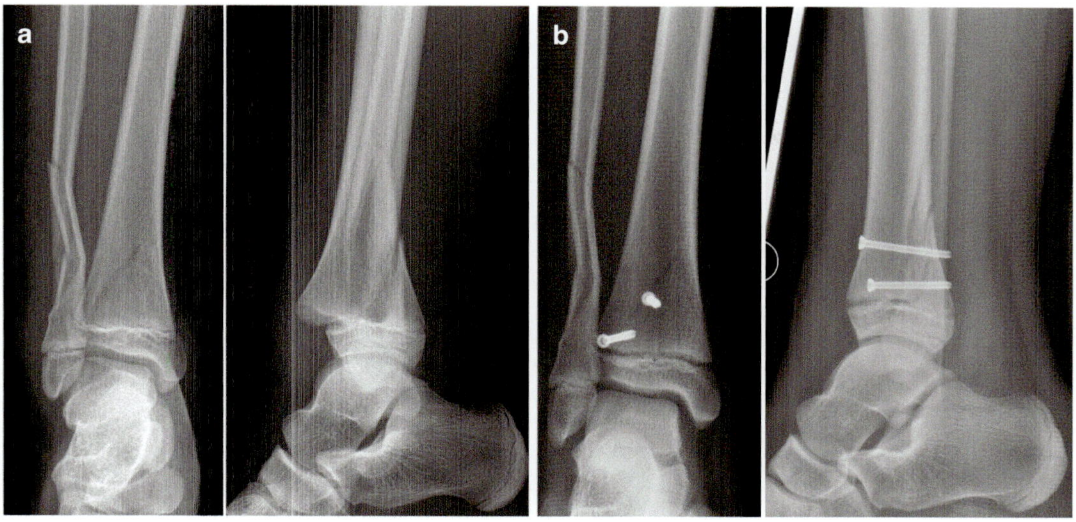

Fig. 15.17 Salter-Harris II fracture of the distal tibia with a large and displaced metaphyseal wedge in a 12 year old girl after fall in school sports. (**a**) Trauma image, (**b**) Closed reduction and cannulated percutaneous screw fixation from anterior to posterior after closed reduction and leaving the fibula in the cast (from Auner and Marzi 2013, Springer)

Table 15.4 Epiphyseal fractures of the distal tibia (Salter-Harris III or Aitken 2)

Special features	Especially <10 years, distortion trauma (supination and inversion) If growth plates are still open (<10 years), the medial epiphysis is typically affected (Fracture line outside of the loading zone)
Diagnostic approach	AP and lateral x-rays, oblique AP view as needed in exceptional cases, MRI to visualize fracture pattern and joint congruity
Limits of correction	Fracture gap <2 mm
Primary treatment	Short-leg plaster splint, medical analgesia as needed
Conservative treatment	
Indication	Fracture gap <2 mm (Fig. 15.19)
Approach	Plaster splint for approx. 5 days then circular cast for 4 weeks, partial weight-bearing (rolling)
Follow up	Weight-bearing as tolerated after cast removal, physical therapy is generally not necessary
X-ray controls	8th day position control; 4-week consolidation check (cast-free)
Return to sports	Approx. 4 weeks after consolidation
Operative treatment	
Indication	Fracture displacement >2 mm
Approach	Open reduction; possible closed reduction with minimal displacement Screw fixation (Figs. 15.20 and 15.21) For small fragments K-wires are possible
Follow up	4 weeks non-weight-bearing; with stable fixation cast immobilization is not necessary, otherwise 4 weeks short-leg cast, non-weight-bearing Weight-bearing as tolerated after cast removal, physical therapy is generally not necessary
X-ray controls	Postoperative position control, 4-week consolidation check (cast-free)
Hardware removal	At 12 weeks
Return to sports	Approx. 4 weeks after consolidation
Complications	Associated injury: Posterior metaphyseal fragment; epiphyseal disruption of the distal fibula; lateral ligament ruptures
Growth disturbance	20% premature growth plate fusion, especially after displaced fractures
Follow up	Every six months for two years Check for rear foot axis asymmetry and leg-length differences
Classification	AO: 43-E/3.1–3 LiLa: 4.3.a.1.0–2.

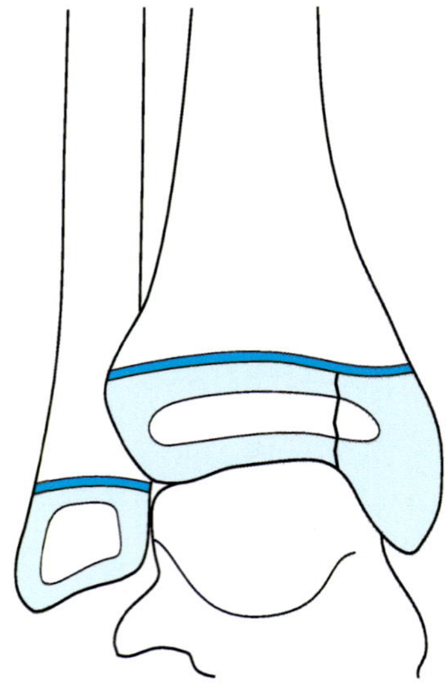

Fig. 15.18 Epiphyseal fracture of the distal tibia type Salter-Harris III or Aitken 2

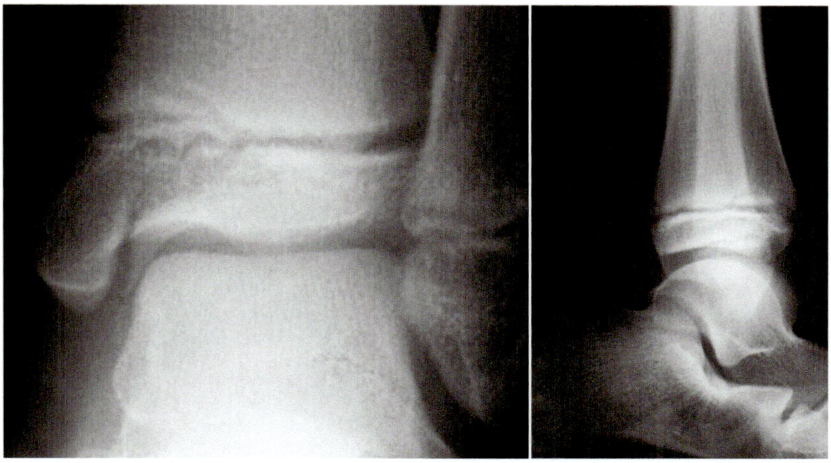

Fig. 15.19 Epiphyseal fracture of the distal tibia type Salter-Harris III or Aitken 2 without relevant dislocation

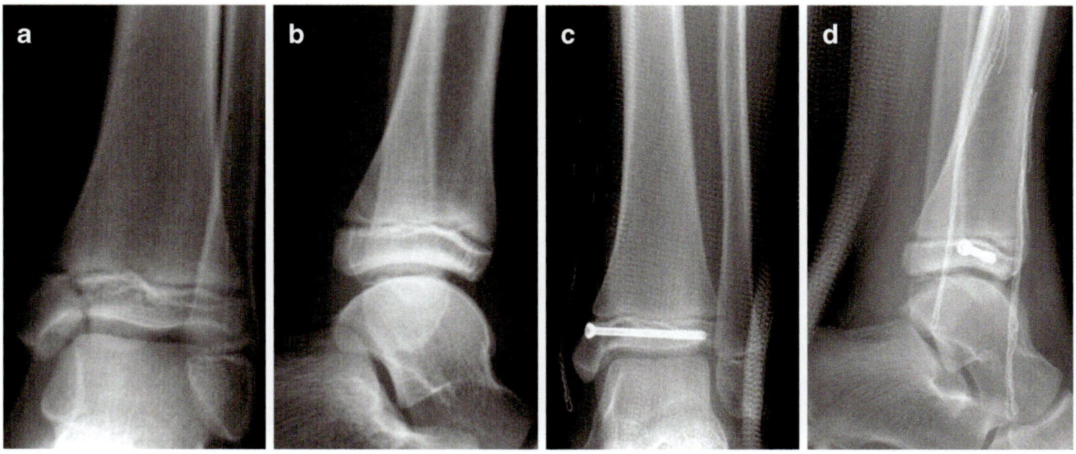

Fig. 15.20 Salter III fracture, girl, 12 years. (**a**, **b**) Trauma image, (**c**, **d**) Screw fixation—percutaneous

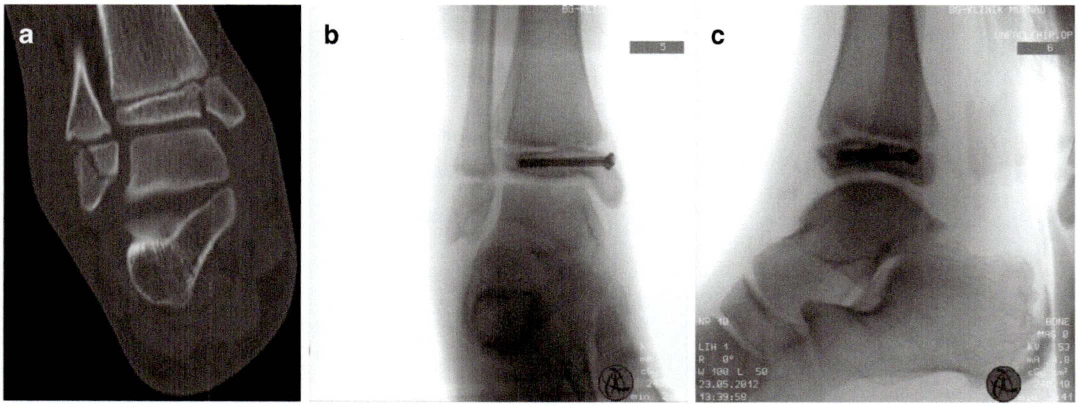

Fig. 15.21 Salter-Harris III (Aitken 2) fracture of the distal tibia epiphysis (**a**) CDT scan, (**b**, **c**) Postoperative after closed reduction and cannulated screw fixation parallel to the growth line. It is important not to touch the growth line or the joint cartilage!

Table 15.5 Epi-metaphyseal fractures type Salter-Harris IV and Aitken 3

Special features	Especially <10 years, distortion trauma (supination and inversion) If growth plates are still open (<10 years), the medial epiphysis is typically affected (Fracture line outside of the loading zone)	
Diagnostic approach	AP and lateral x-rays, oblique AP view as needed (Fig. 15.23) MRI in unclear cases, to visualize complex fractures	
Limits of correction	Fracture gap <2 mm	
Primary treatment	Short-leg plaster splint, medical analgesia as needed	
Conservative treatment		
Indication	Fracture gap <2 mm	
Approach	Plaster splint for approx. 5 days then circular cast for 4 weeks, partial weight-bearing (rolling)	
Follow up	Weight-bearing as tolerated after cast removal, Physical therapy is generally not necessary	
X-ray controls	8th day position control; 4-week consolidation check (cast-free)	
Return to sports	Approx. 4 weeks after consolidation	
Operative treatment		
Indication	Fracture displacement >2 mm, shortening of the medial malleolus and incongruence	
Approach	Closed or open reduction Screw fixation if possible (Fig. 15.24) If needed, K-wires for small fragments	
Follow up	4 weeks partial weight-bearing (rolling) with stable screw fixation, temporary short-leg plaster splint for swelling/pain, not absolutely necessary For K-wire fixation, 4 weeks plaster immobilization and non–/partial (rolling) weight-bearing Weight-bearing as tolerated after cast removal, physical therapy is generally not necessary	
X-ray controls	Postoperative position control, 4-week consolidation check (cast-free)	
Hardware removal	At 12 weeks	
Return to sports	Approx. 4 weeks after consolidation	
Complications	Unstable fixation leads to joint incongruity	
Growth disturbance	Up to 20% premature growth plate fusion, especially after displaced fractures	
Follow up	Every six months for two years Check for rear foot axis asymmetry and leg-length differences	
Classification	AO: 43-E/4.1–3	LiLa: 4.3.a.2.0–2.

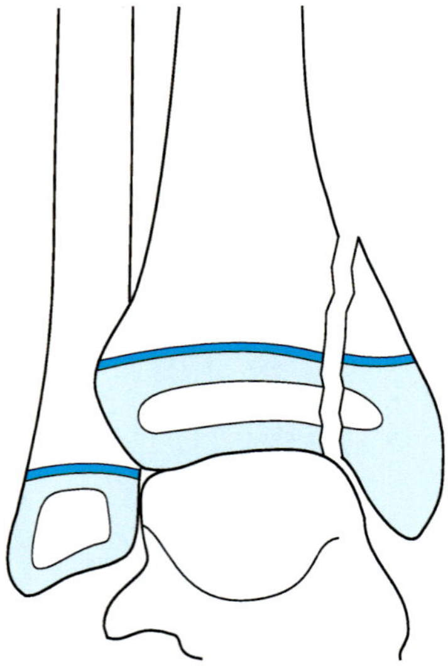

Fig. 15.22 Epiphyseal fracture of the distal tibia, type Salter-Harris II and Aitken 3

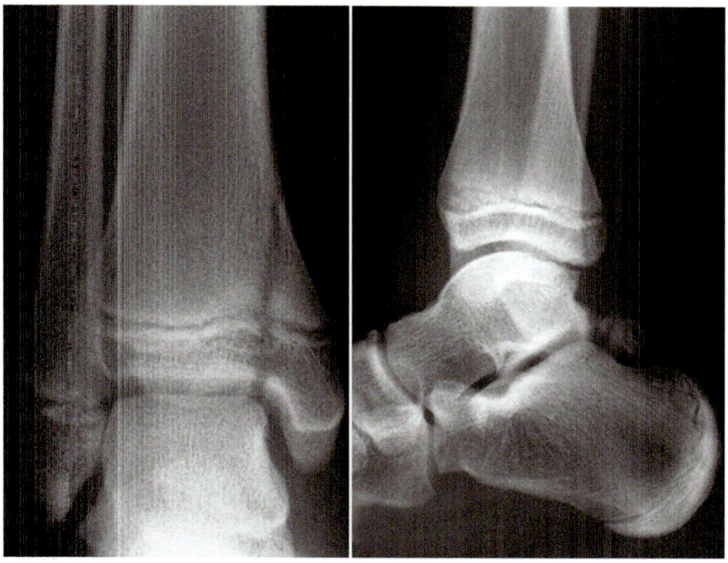

Fig. 15.23 X-ray of a typical Salter-Harris IV fracture (or Aitken 3) at the medial side of the distal tibia

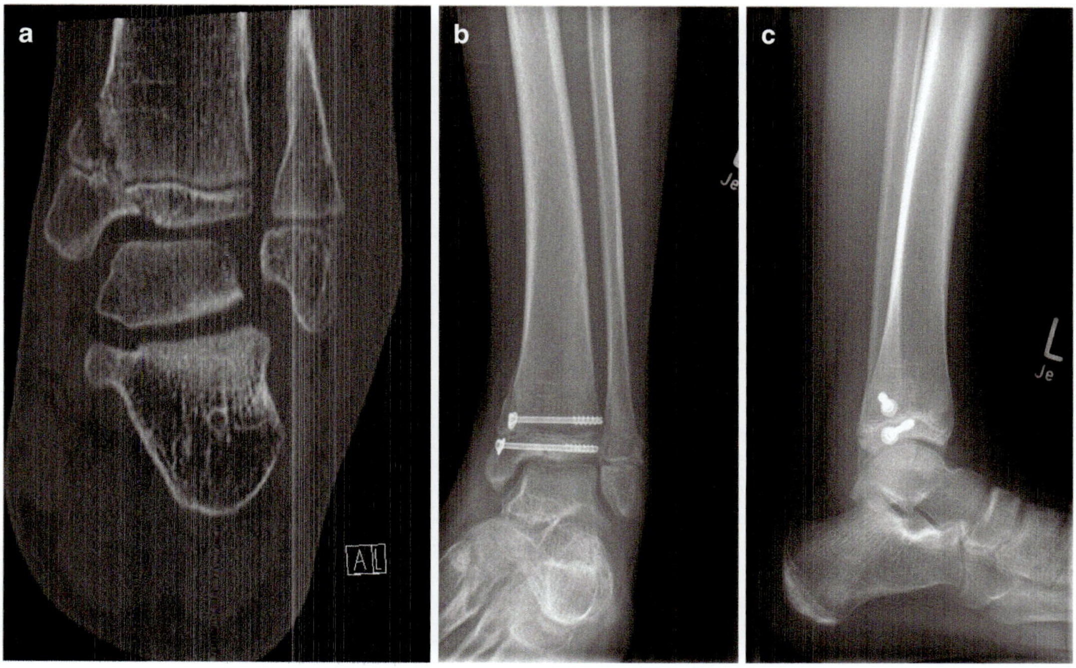

Fig. 15.24 Salter-Harris IV injury of a girl. (**a**) CT scan, (**b**, **c**) Osteosynthesis with 2 parallel screws above and below the epiphyseal line under protection of the growth line

15.4 Transitional Fractures

The transitional fractures are defined once the growth plate begins to close. This is at the distal tibia at the medial side extending in a circle line to the anterior edge of the tibia. Thus, transitional fractures medially are at the beginning of the closure of the growth plate and fractures at the anterior lateral side just prior completion of the growth plate. Neithertheless, from the beginning of the closure of the growth plate, the growth seems to stop at this side of the bone. According to the epiphyseal fractures, a fracture within the epiphysis (corresponding a Salter-Harris III or Aitken 2 fractures) are called twoplane fractures (Fig. 15.25). Table 15.6 shows the facts of a Twoplane transitional fractue.

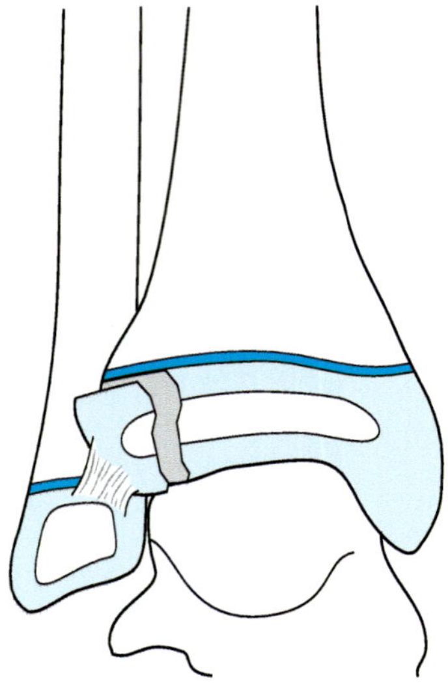

Fig. 15.25 Transition fracture only in the epiphysis-twoplane fracture

Table 15.6 Transition fractures—twoplane

Special features	Fracture line within the loading zone → anatomical reduction needed for Tilleaux fracture
Diagnostic approach	AP and lateral x-rays, oblique AP view as needed Exceptional cases: MRI or CT for preoperative planning
Limits of correction	Displacement <2 mm
Primary treatment	Short-leg plaster splint, medical analgesia as needed
Conservative treatment	
Indication	Displacement <2 mm
Approach	Plaster splint for approx. 5 days then circular cast for 6 weeks, partial weight-bearing (rolling)
Follow up	Weight-bearing as tolerated after cast removal, physical therapy is generally not necessary
X-ray controls	8th day position control; 6-week consolidation check (cast-free)
Return to sports	Approx. 4 weeks after consolidation
Operative treatment	
Indication	Displacement >2 mm
Approach	Anatomical reduction and screw fixation – closed reduction (rather medial and central fractures) (Fig. 15.26) or – open reduction (rather lateral fractures) (Figs. 15.27 and 15.28)
Follow up	4 weeks non-weight-bearing; with stable fixation cast immobilization is not necessary, otherwise 4 weeks short-leg cast, weight-bearing as tolerated after cast removal, physical therapy is generally not necessary
X-ray controls	Postoperative position control, 6-week consolidation check (cast-free)
Hardware removal	At 12 weeks
Return to sports	Approx. 4 weeks after consolidation if symptom-free
Complications	Potential premature arthritis in cases of joint incongruity
Growth disturbance	None, because growth plates are beginning to fuse
Follow up	Quarterly: Functional assessments until unlimited function
Classification	AO: 43-E/5.1–3 LiLa: 4.3.a.3.0–2.

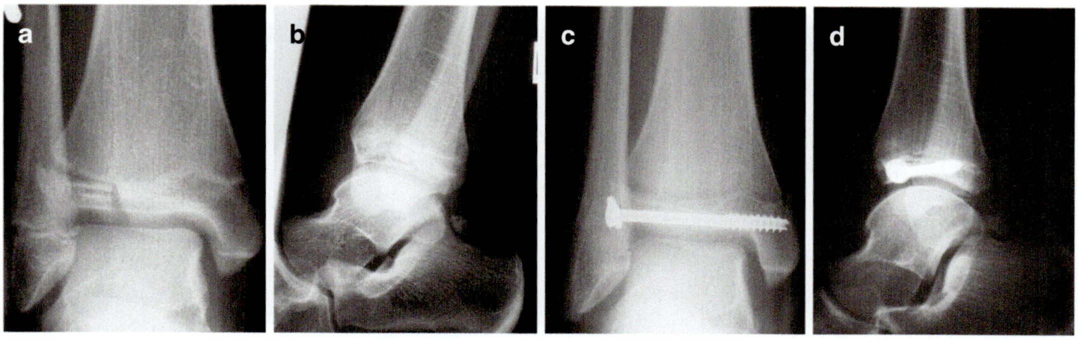

Fig. 15.26 Twoplane fracture, girl, 13 years, injury during physical education class. (**a**, **b**) Trauma images. (**c**, **d**) Screw fixation, parallel to the epiphyseal line in order to close the fracture gap. This is often possible in a closed approach

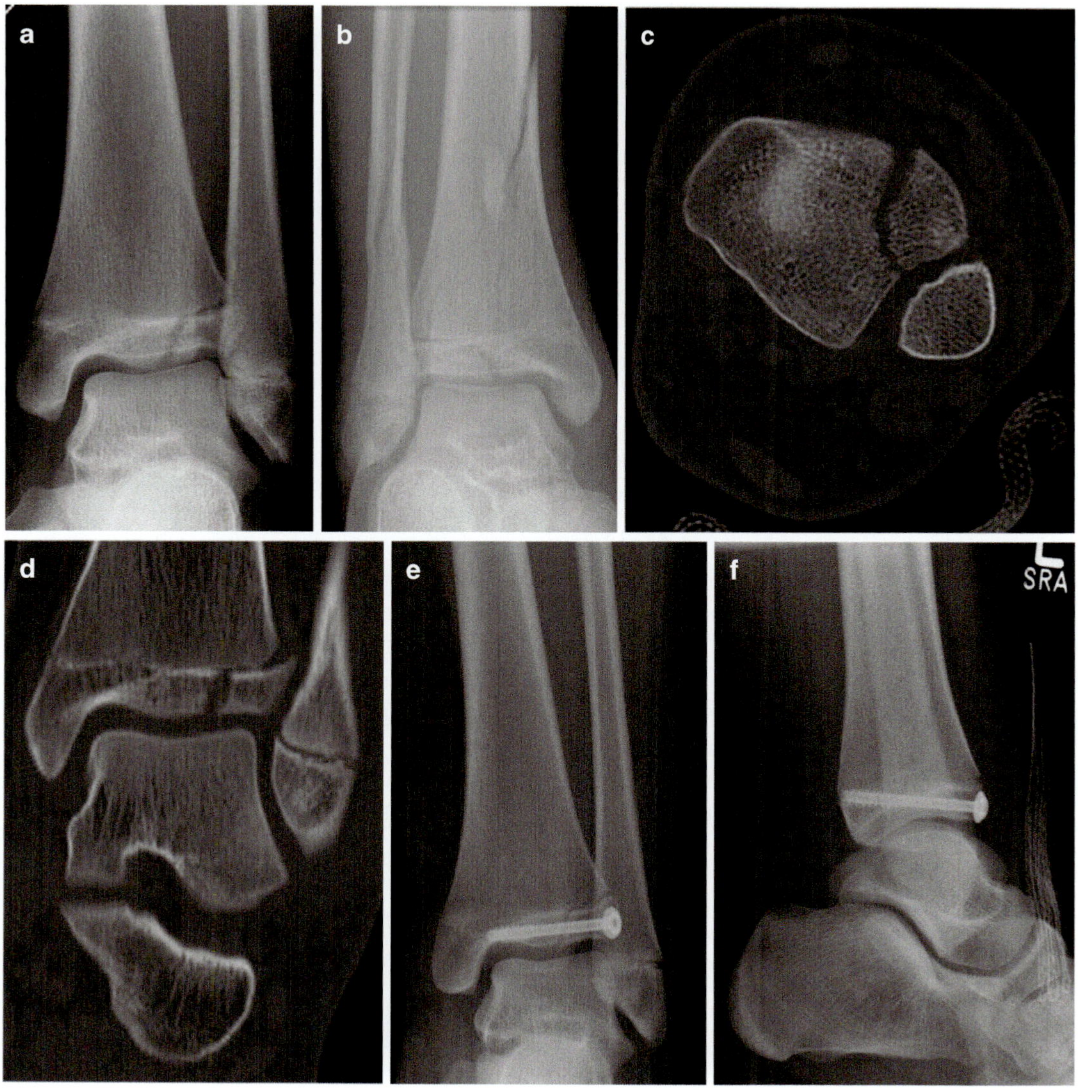

Fig. 15.27 Twoplane fracture of the distal tibia after jump from a 1 m board of a 12 year olds girl. (**a**, **b**) Trauma images, (**c**, **d**) CT scan transversal and coronar view. (**e**, **f**) X-ray after open reduction under view and lag-screw fixation (from Auner and Marzi 2013 Springer)

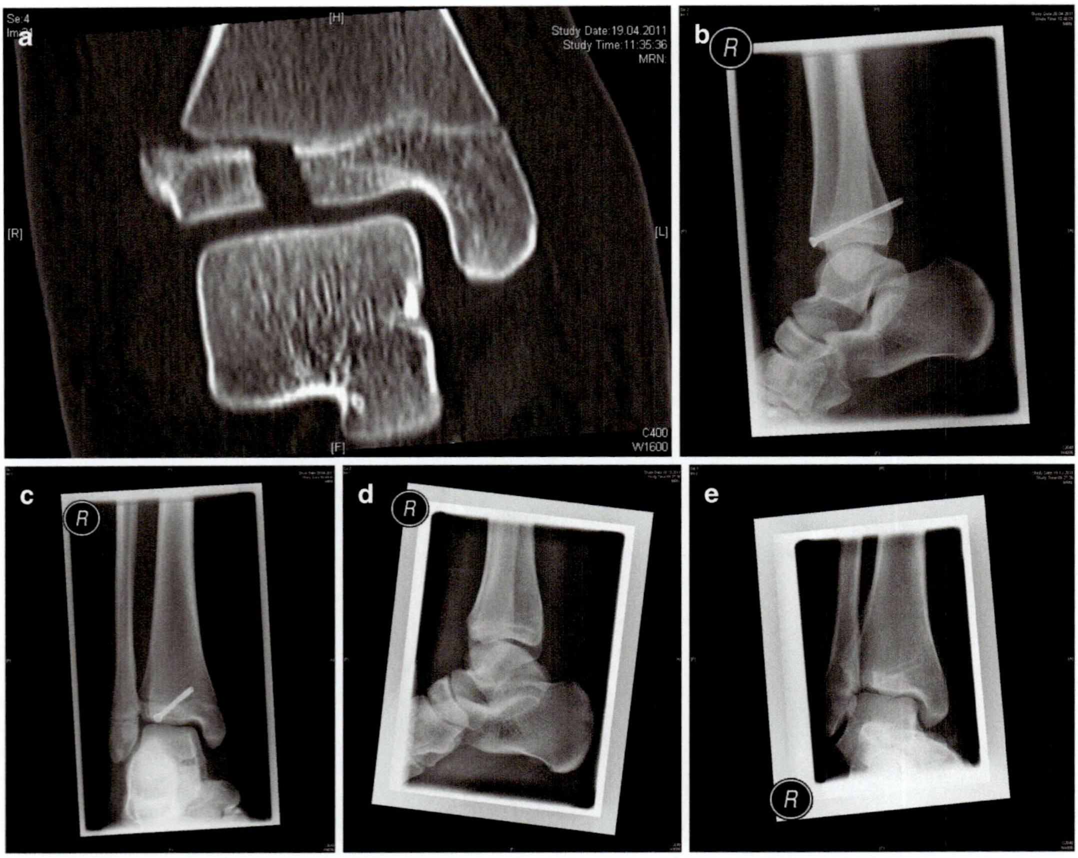

Fig. 15.28 Twoplane fracture with large displacement in a 12 year old girl. (**a**) CT image showing the articular fracture and the already closed growth plate medial, (**b**, **c**) Open reduction and screw fixation. Due to the mostly closed growth plate an oblique screw passing the epiphyseal line is the best choice and possible. (**d**, **e**) X-ray of complete healing after metal removal. Note the completely closed epiphyseal growth plate now

Transitional fracture can also have a metaphyseal fragment. Two types are differentiated: Triplane I fractures with a fracture in the epiphysis and a metaphyseal fracture ending at the growth line (Fig. 15.29). Triplane II fracture with a fracture of the epiphysis and a metaphyseal fracture, however, this metaphyseal fracture line crosses the epiphyseal line (Fig. 15.30). Thus, in the Triplane II fractures at least 2 fracture lines are in the joint cartilage, sometimes the fractures are even more complex. Figure 15.31 shows 3-D printings of the transitional fractures for better understanding.

Transitional Fractures of the Triplane Type are indicated in Table 15.7.

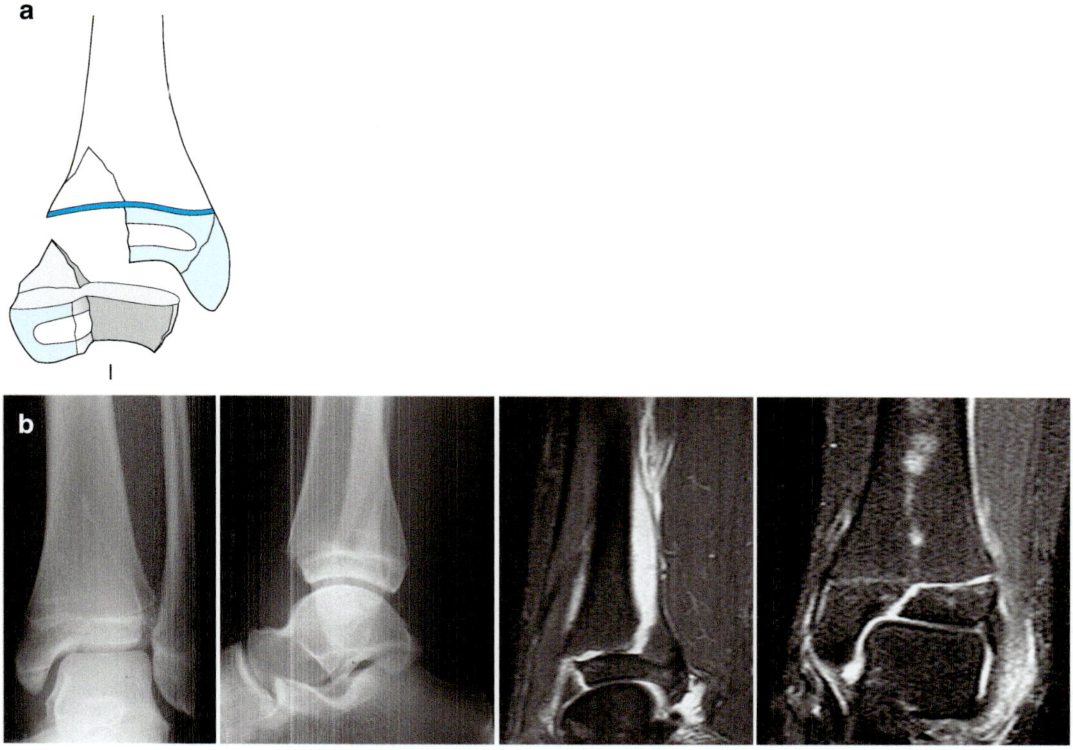

Fig. 15.29 Triplane I fracture with a fracture line in the epiphysis in the A.P. view and a fracture line above the epiphyseal line in the lateral views. (**a**) Scheme (**b**) X-ray and MRI

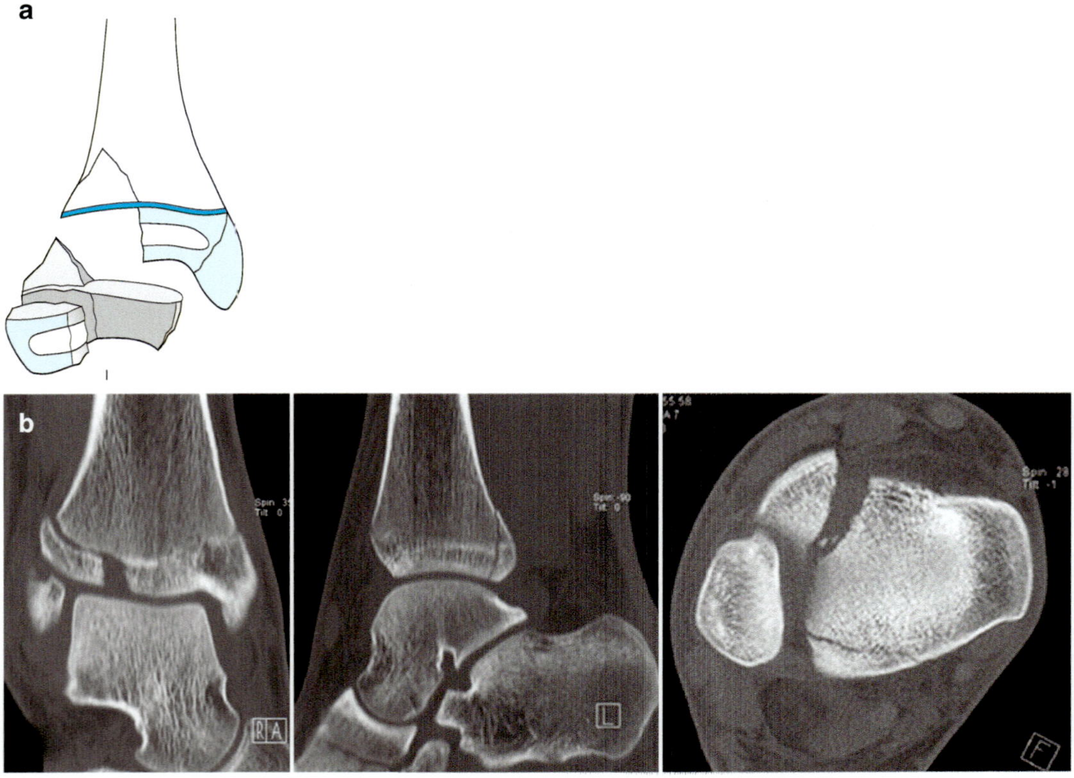

Fig. 15.30 Triplane II fracture with a fracture line in the epiphysis in the A.P. view and a fracture line crossing the epiphyseal line in the lateral view of the CT. (**a**) Scheme, (**b**) CT-scan A.P. view. Lateral and transversal

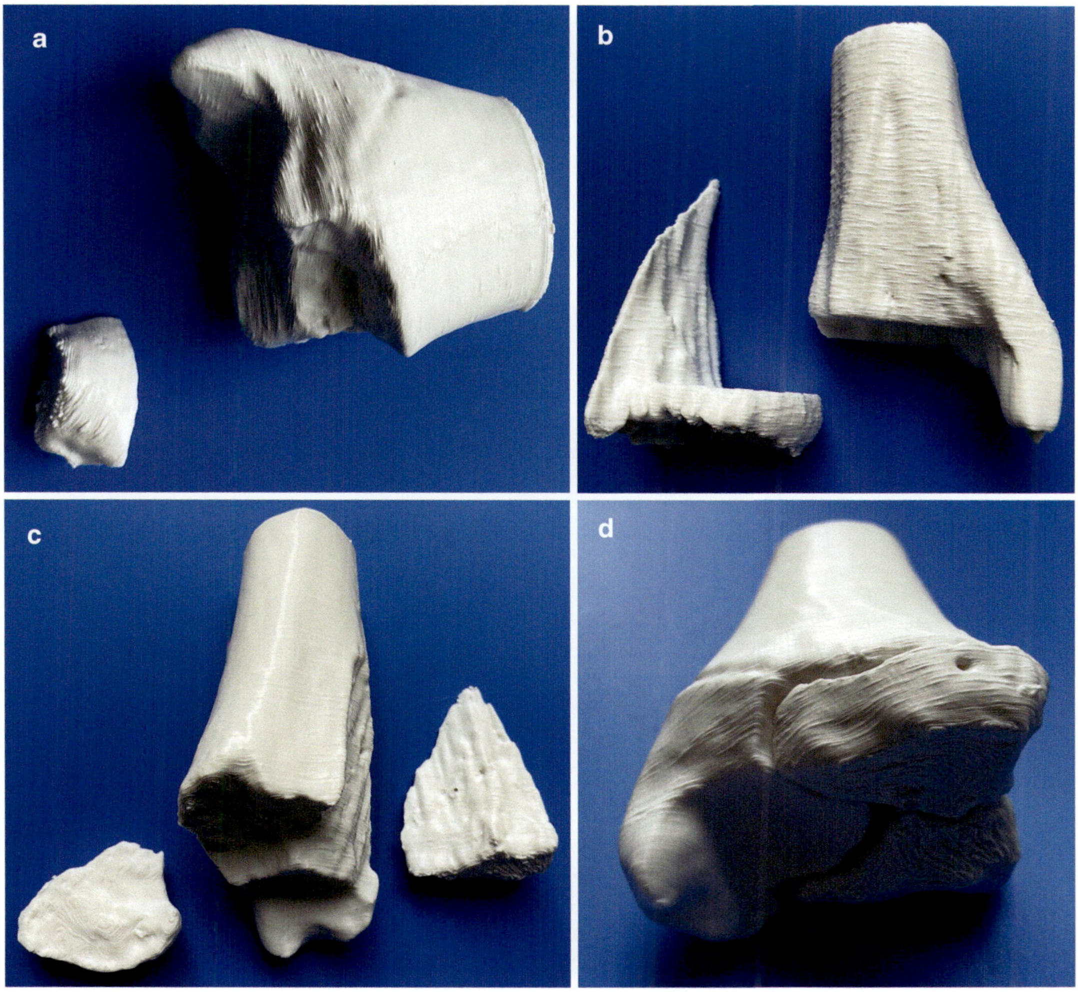

Fig. 15.31 3 D printing of transitional fractures. (**a**) Twoplane fracture, (**b**) Triplane I fracture, (**c**, **d**) Triplane II fracture

Table 15.7 Transitional fracture—Triplane Type I and Type II

Special features	Triplane I: associated posterior metaphyseal fracture Triplane II: posterior fracture line runs through the metaphysis and epiphysis fracture line within the loading zone → exact reduction necessary	
Diagnostic approach	AP and lateral x-rays, oblique AP view as needed If needed, MRI or CT to visualize fracture course and preoperative planning	
Limits of correction	Displacement <2 mm	
Primary treatment	Short-leg plaster splint, medical analgesia as needed	
Conservative treatment		
Indication	Displacement <2 mm	
Approach	Plaster splint for approximately 5 days, then circular cast for 4–6 weeks, partial weight-bearing (rolling)	
Follow up	Weight-bearing as tolerated after cast removal, physical therapy is generally not necessary	
X-ray controls	8th day position control; 6-week consolidation check (cast-free)	
Return to sports	Approx. 4 weeks after consolidation	
Operative treatment		
Indication	Displacement >2 mm	
Approach	Open reduction and screw fixation (Figs. 15.32, 15.33, and 15.34).	
Follow up	4 weeks non-weight-bearing; with stable fixation cast immobilization is not necessary, otherwise 4–5 weeks short-leg cast, non-weight-bearing Weight-bearing as tolerated after cast removal, physical therapy is generally not necessary	
X-ray controls	Postoperative position control, 6-week consolidation check (cast-free)	
Hardware removal	At 12 weeks	
Return to sports	Approx. 4 weeks after consolidation if symptom-free	
Complications	Potential premature arthritis in cases of joint incongruity	
Growth disturbance	None, because growth plates are beginning to fuse	
Follow up	Quarterly: Functional assessments until unlimited function	
Classification	AO: 43-E/6.1–3	LiLa: 4.3.a.4.0–2.

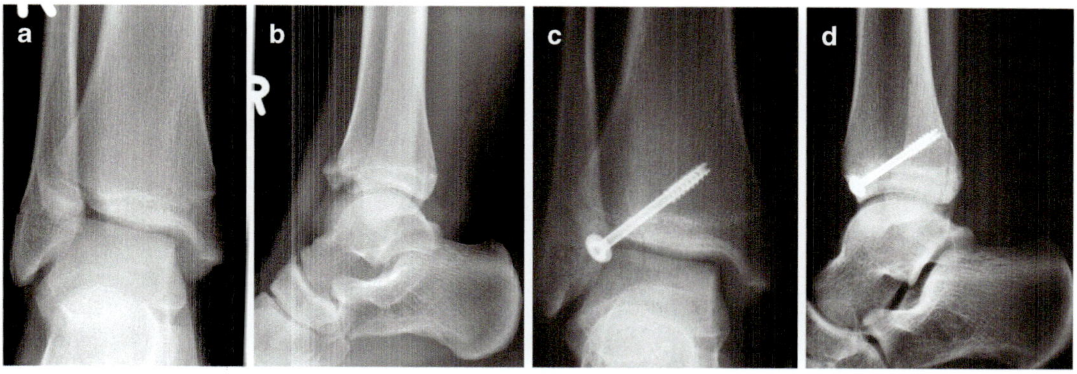

Fig. 15.32 Triplane II fracture with displaced twoplane component and undisplaced metaphyseal fractures line across the growth plate. (**a**, **b**) Trauma image, (**c**, **d**) Screw osteosynthesis across the epiphyseal line from lateral. This is only allowed in transitional fractures!

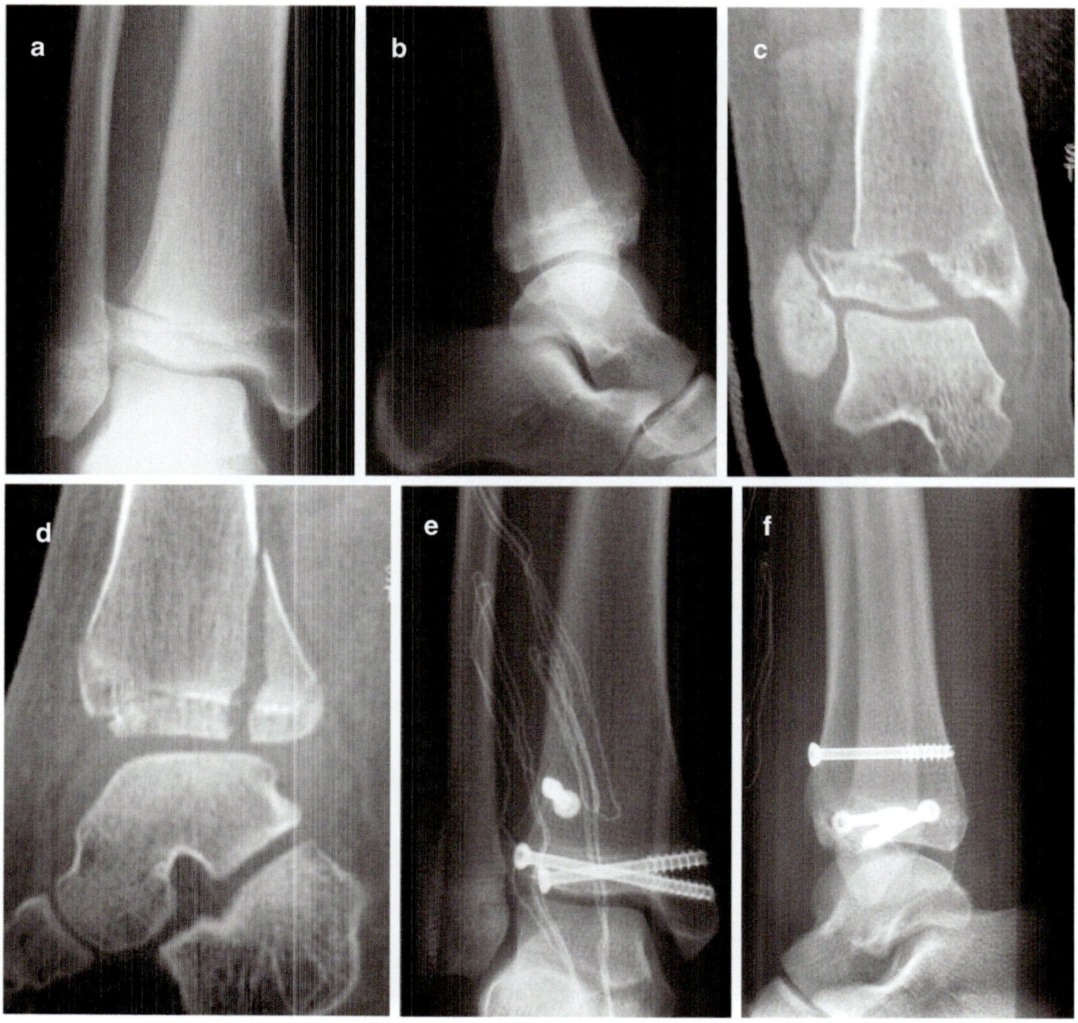

Fig. 15.33 Triplane II fracture, girl, 13 years. (**a–d**) Trauma images. (**e**, **f**) Screw fixation with fixation of the metaphyseal fracture

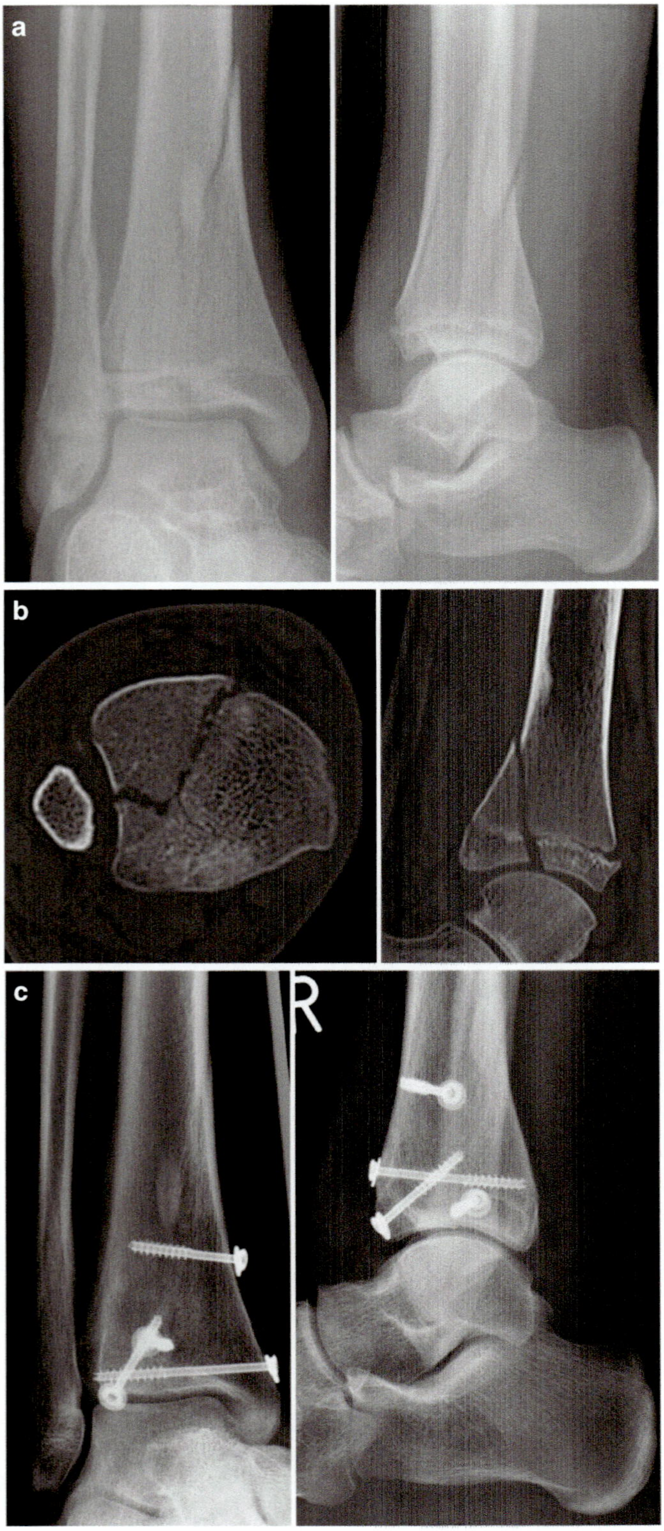

Fig. 15.34 Triplane II fracture, boy, 15 years. (**a**) X-ray, (**b**) CT scan, (**c**) Healing after multiple screw osteosynthesis of the various fragments and final closure of the growth plate. (From Auner and Marzi, Springer 2013)

15.5 Ankle Distortion Trauma

Incidence, Mechanism of Injury, and Clinical Presentation

The incidence of ankle distortion trauma is approximately 10–15%.

Lateral ligament ruptures are usually unproblematic and can be treated conservatively (Table 15.8). Under the age of ten, injuries are typically cartilaginous or bony, affecting the fibula. Ligament ruptures are much more common in older children, like adults. Two-thirds of cases involve the anterior talofibular ligament. The calcaneofibular ligament is concomitantly ruptured in 20% of these cases (Fig. 15.35). The diagnosis is usually made from a combination of history and the typical clinical presentation of swelling and tenderness, with or without hematoma, over the affected ligaments. A single conventional radiograph is performed to rule out osteochondral injuries. Further imaging such as MRI or stress images are primarily reserved for exceptional cases because they do not affect care.

Treatment of isolated ligament injuries is always primarily conservative with anti-swelling measures, non-weight-bearing, and elastic bandages as needed. Approximately 10% of cases yield a long-term outcome of persistent instability, regardless of implementation of conservative management or primary ligament repair, even in adults. Thus, primary repair is generally not indicated. If symptoms persist for longer than one week or the ligaments are ruptured (hematoma), the ankle can be stabilized with an orthosis and otherwise followed functionally. In some cases, physical therapy with muscle strengthening (especially the peroneal muscles) and coordination training (proprioception) is useful.

Bony ligament tears are also treated conservatively through immobilization in a short-leg plaster splint. Conservative management yields satisfactory results in over 90% of ligament injuries. Increased lateral gapping (calcaneofibular ligament) and/or anterior talar translation (anterior drawer sign; talofibular ligament) on contralateral comparison indicates chronic instability. In these cases, instability can be verified with stress images. Pathological radiological measurements are increased lateral gapping of ≥10° and anterior talar translation of ≥10 mm compared to the unaffected side. Ligament repair is indicated only when symptoms persist (recurrent swelling, instability, pain) despite intensive proprioceptive training over more than three months.

The primary surgical treatment of choice is anatomical ligament reconstruction, when the ligament stumps can be sewn together. This method achieves good long-term results overall with exceptions for long-term instability and conditions of general hyperlaxity. A periosteal flap is a common modification of ligament reconstruction (Fig. 15.36). Reconstruction is the primary method of choice because it is technically simple to perform, has few complications, and yields better long-term results. Tenodesis and ligament grafts are recommended alternatives. However, these cannot restore normal anatomy and inevitably lead to altered ankle mechanics. Thus, these approaches are not regularly used in childhood.

Concomitant osteochondral fractures (flake fractures) of the talus occur rarely and may need operative fixation depending on size. Associated growth plate disruptions of the distal fibula are also uncommon and can be treated conservatively with cast immobilization for three weeks after reduction. Isolated syndesmosis ruptures occur occasionally and can be temporarily fixed with a screw, as in adults. However, in adolescents, bony syndesmotic avulsions are more common (transition fractures: the anterolateral fragment corresponds to a bony syndesmosis tear) and are fixed with a compression screw. In these cases, with intact ligaments, an additional syndesmotic screw is not necessary.

Table 15.8 Lateral ligament injuries of the ankle joint

Special features	Most common ankle injury Typically, from supination trauma <12 years mostly bony, also cartilaginous ligament injuries >12 years intra-ligamentous ruptures chronic instability: rare
Diagnostic approach	AP and lateral x-rays If needed, MRI (exclude osteochondral injury, assess syndesmosis) (Fig. 15.37). Chronic instability: Stress functional images, clinically increased lateral gapping, increased anterior talar translation
Limits of correction	Lack of symptoms; no chronic instability (pain, recurrent supination trauma, recurrent swelling)
Primary treatment	Anti-swelling measures, as needed short-leg plaster splint, medical analgesia
Conservative treatment	
Indication	Almost always conservative
Approach	Ligament complex rupture: "RICE" (rest, ice, compression, elevate), elastic bandage; non-weight-bearing Bony avulsion: Short-leg plaster splint for 4 weeks
Follow up	Orthosis as needed (e.g., air cast), physical therapy for persistent instability (proprioception training)
X-ray controls	Not necessary
Return to sports	Approx. 4–6 weeks after injury if symptom-free
Operative treatment	
Indication Talar flake fractures	Repeat injury; gross instability (all three lateral ligaments); re-rupture after ligament repair; treatment-resistant chronic instability
Approach	Ligament repair, with periosteal flap reinforcement when tissue is lacking and tenodesis with peroneal brevis tendon only as a last resort Talar flake fracture: Refixation with fibrin glue and resorbable pins
Follow up	6 weeks short-leg cast with full weight-bearing, with flake fracture partial weight-bearing
X-ray controls	Not necessary
Hardware removal	Not necessary
Return to sports	Approx. 4 weeks after cast removal if symptom-free with muscular symmetry
Complications	10% chronic instability (conservative/operative treatment) Talar flake fracture → Osteochondrosis dissecans
Growth disturbance	None
Follow up	4 weeks after return to sports, quarterly follow-up until symptom-free
Classification	AO: 43-E/7.1–3 LiLa: 4.3.a.5.0–2.F.

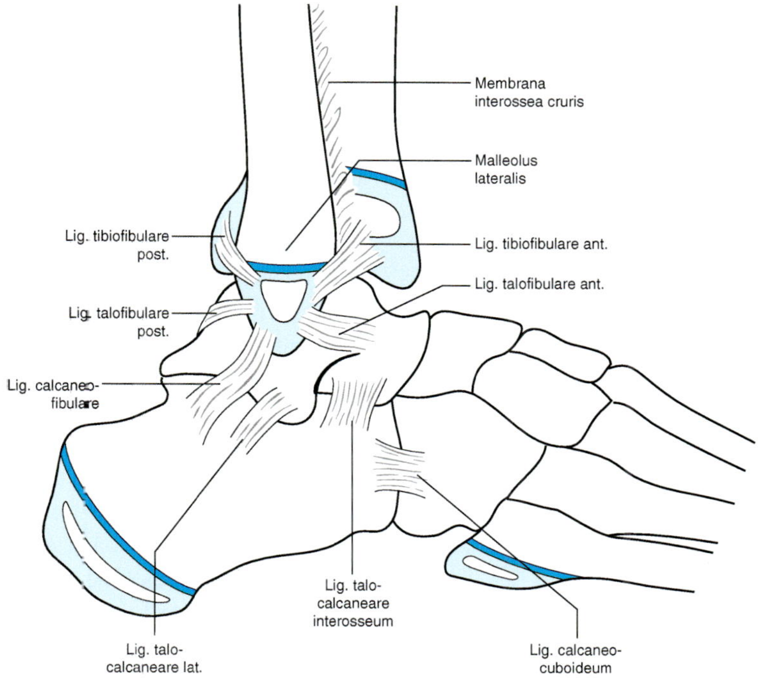

Fig. 15.35 Lateral ligament complex of the ankle

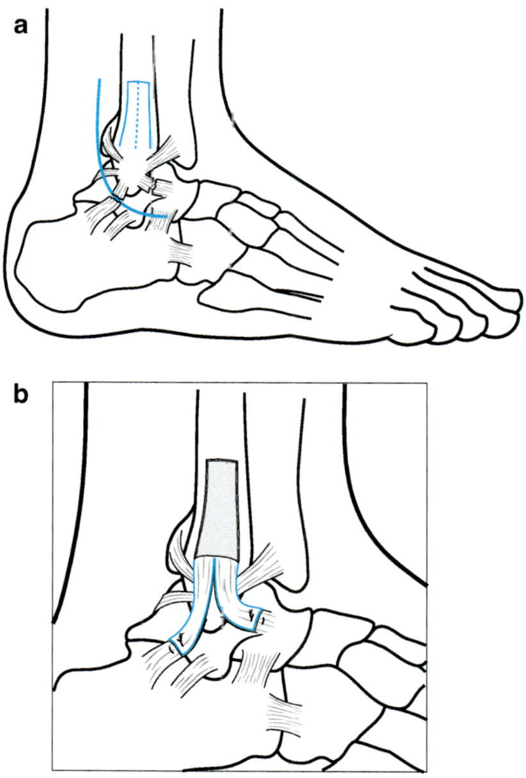

Fig. 15.36 Reconstruction of the lateral ankle joint instability with a periosteol flap. (**a**) Incision and preparation, (**b**) Enhancement of the fibular ligaments with the flap

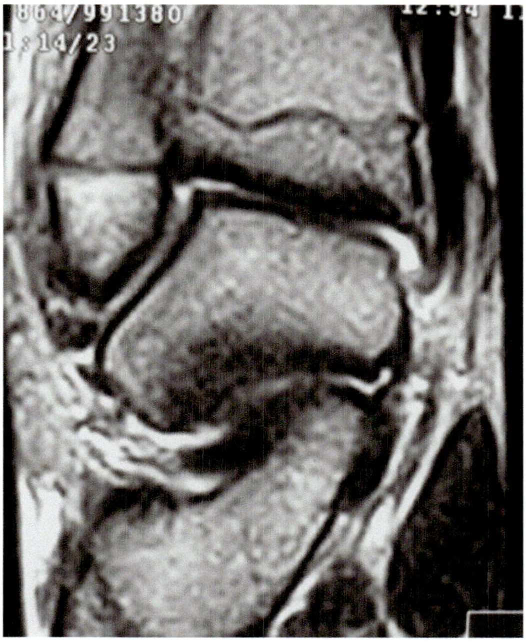

Fig. 15.37 MRI of lateral ligamentous rupture of the ankle joint

15.6 Osteochondritis Dissecans of the Talus

Incidence, Mechanism of Injury, and Clinical Presentation

Osteochondritis dissecans (OCD) is aseptic necrosis of the subchondral bone, mostly affecting the medial talus (85%). The incidence is 0.09%, with clusters in the 10–20 and 20–30 age ranges. Etiological factors are still under discussion. Along with trauma and microtrauma, vascular, genetic, endogenous, and bacterial factors are suspected contributors. Many authors consider trauma as the primary etiology. After that, clusters of OCD are seen in ball sports participants with repetitive microtraumas (basketball, football, etc.).

The course is progressive and has been internationally classified, e.g., according to Berndt and Harty (Fig. 15.38).

The initial symptom is pain. In the fragment stages, there can be sensations of blocking and instability. The current diagnostic approach includes MRI, which provides information regarding the vitality of the fragment and condition of the cartilage. However, MRI findings do not correlate with symptom severity.

Treatment depends on the stage (Fig. 15.38 and Table 15.9). The goals are to revitalize the area and to prevent progression (fragment accumulation) and arthritis. Any residual cartilage damage is a pre-arthritic deformity. Treatment principles are load reduction, marrow revitalization, and fragment refixation. In Stages I and II, first-line therapy is conservative, especially during childhood. The operative strategy for early stages is to revitalize using retrograde or antegrade drilling. For small defects <7 mm, debridement and additional bone marrow stimulation methods (e.g., drilling) are performed. For larger lesions, reconstruction is attempted with similar methods used in the knee, e.g., with microfracturing and bone-cartilage grafts. In cases of large and central defects, debridement with cancellous bone graft and a covering membrane might be necessary, or with medial malleolar osteotomy. Because of the growth risks of osteotomy, this is preferably left to adolescents. There are isolated reports of good results from

1. Initial stadium 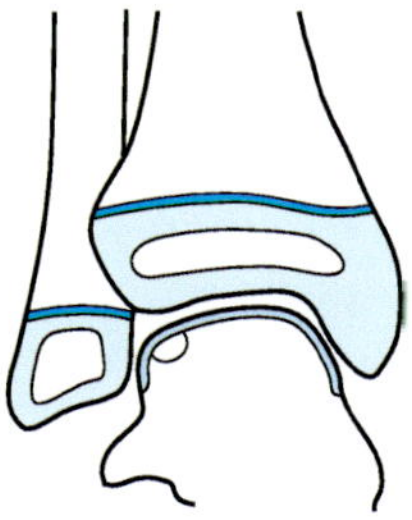	subchondral osteonecrosis; cartilage intact; regeneration possible	conservative treatment
2. Demarcation 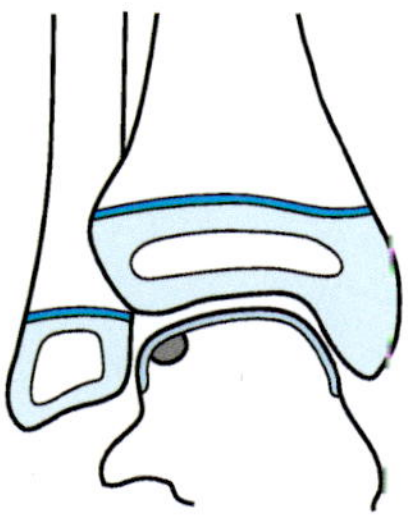	Sclerotic demarcation of necrosis; cartilage intact; regeneration unlikely	painless; conservative; symptomatic: conservative for 6-12 Wo, in case of persistence: operative
3. Dissect in place 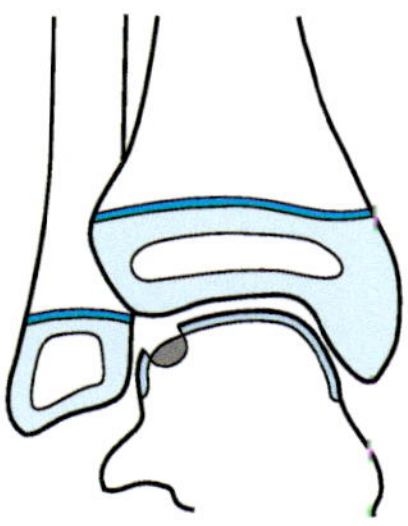	Fragmentation, loss of integrity with surrounding healthy tissue	operative therapy
4. Free dissect 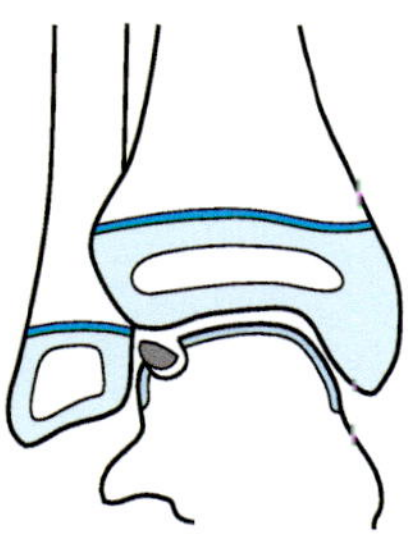	free joint body	operative therapy

Fig. 15.38 Berndt and Harty classification of osteochondritis dissecans

Table 15.9 Osteochondritis dissecans of the talus (Fig. 15.39)

Special features	Common in the second decade Athletes (recurrent microtraumas, supination injuries) Mostly medial talar shoulder		
Diagnostic approach	AP and lateral, oblique x-rays MRI (stage determination, with contrast: Vitality determination) (Fig. 15.40) Arthroscopy if needed		
Limits of correction	Stage I	subchondral necrosis	conservative
	Stage II	subchondral sclerosis	conservative/operative
	Stage III	in situ lesion	operative
	Stage IV	displaced fragment	operative
Primary treatment	–		
Conservative treatment			
Indication	Stage I Stage II - therapeutic trial 6–12 weeks		
Approach	Non-weight-bearing with crutches, break from sports, NSAIDs as needed		
Follow up	Physical therapy: Proprioception training		
X-ray controls	MRI control every 3 months if clinical symptoms persist		
Return to sports	When symptom-free		
Operative treatment			
Indication	Persistent complaints in Stage II Stage III, Stage IV		
Approach	Retrograde drilling (stage III) (Fig. 15.41) Retrograde debridement and cancellous bone graft (stage II/III with intact cartilage) Antegrade drilling, microfracturing (Stage II/III) Antegrade debridement, cancellous bone graft and refixation (stage III with lost integrity to surroundings; stage IV with intact cartilage surface) Antegrade debridement, curettage, resection (Stage IV with cartilage damage) Defect <7 mm: Debridement and drilling Defect >7 mm: Cartilage reconstruction		
Follow up	8–12 weeks non-weight-bearing		
X-ray controls	MRI controls every 3 months (with contrast: Revascularization?)		
Hardware removal	Not necessary		
Return to sports	When symptom-free		
Complications	Arthritis		
Growth disturbance	Pre-arthritis		
Follow up	Every 3 months until symptom-free		

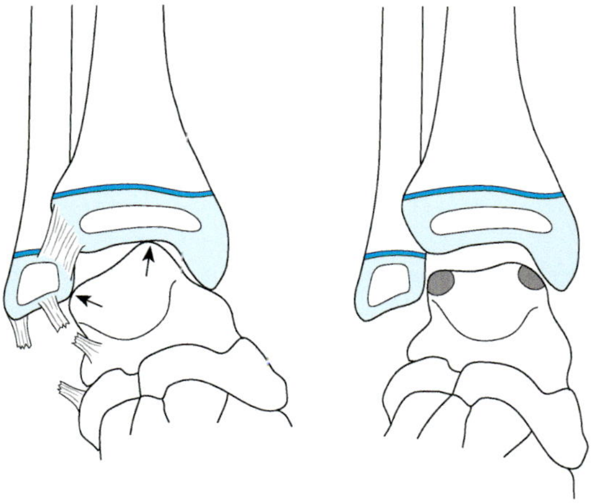

Fig. 15.39 Osteochondritis dissecans of the medial or lateral talus with mechanism of injury

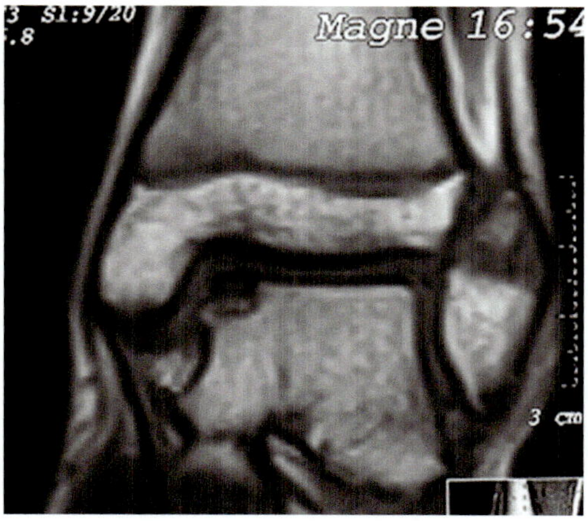

Fig. 15.40 MRI of osteochondritis dissecans of the medial talus shoulder

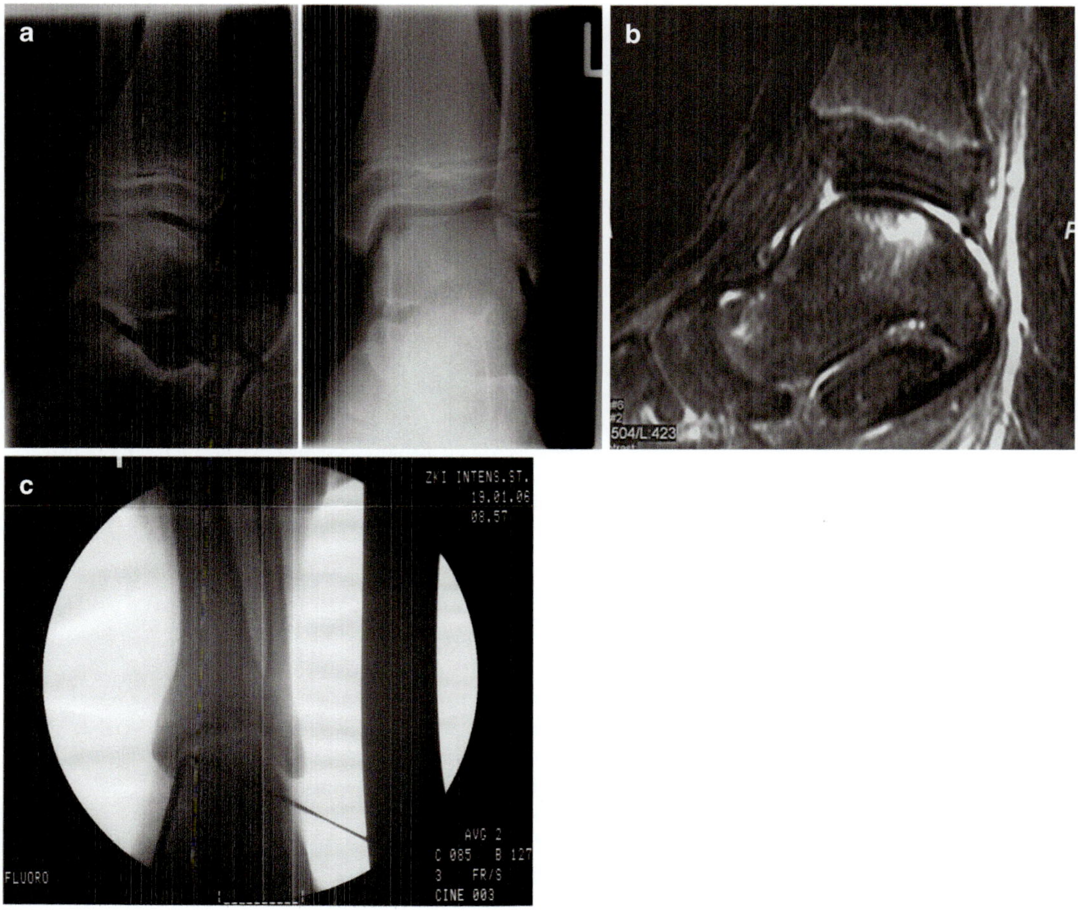

Fig. 15.41 Medial osteochondritis dissecans of the medial talus shoulder of a 13 year old boy. (**a**) X-rays, (**b**) MRI lateral view, (**c**) Intraoperative localization with fluoroscopy and drilling of the area

various approaches, but long-term data from prospective randomized studies are lacking. The importance of newer methods, such as growth factor application or cell transplants, remains to be seen in pediatric trauma. Overall, however, younger patients have a better prognosis than adults.

Technical considerations for the treatment of injuries to the distal tibia and ligament injuries of the ankle joint are given in Table 15.10.

Table 15.10 Shows the technical aspects to consider for the treatment of injuries or the distal tibia and the ankle joint

General material	Image intensifier
Positioning	Supine position, ankle tourniquet, draped above the knee (rotation control)
Approach - general	Medial malleolus (Fig. 15.42) Incision along the posterior border of the medial malleolus Lateral malleolus (Fig. 15.43) Incision along the posterior border of the lateral malleolus. Caution: Superficial peroneal nerve
Special clarification	Superficial peroneal nerve injury with lateral approach Osteochondritis dissecans: Loosening of the graft, iatrogenic cartilage damage
Hardware removal	K-wires: As needed under local anesthesia Screws: Under general anesthesia
Distal tibia fractures	
Material	Cannulated screws, self-tapping, reverse-threaded → titanium→ diameter: 3.5–4 mm
Approach	See general approaches Transition fractures: → usually lateral approach; in rare medial fractures, medial approach
Operative principle	Reduction 90° knee flexion and slight plantarflexion → muscle relaxation Reversal of mechanism of injury = reduction Compression screw fixation Closed reduction and fixation via stab incision with a cannulated cancellous screw/small fragment cancellous screw (3.5–4.5 mm), open reduction if needed (reduction obstacle, joint reconstruction) Salter III fracture: Epiphyseal screws parallel to the epiphyseal plate (Fig. 15.44), without crossing the growth plate; K-wires for tiny fragments if needed Salter IV fracture: Epiphyseal screws parallel to the growth plate, one screw is often sufficient, with a large metaphyseal fragment additional metaphyseal screws parallel to the plate Twoplane fracture: Epiphyseal screws, the growth plate may be crossed in a lateral fracture since it is largely closed (oblique course → better compression); no growth expected (Fig. 15.45) Triplane I/II fractures: First, metaphyseal fixation (anterior-posterior) followed by the epiphyseal fragment; the growth plate may be crossed in a lateral fracture (Fig. 15.46)
Lateral ligament rupture	
Approach	Curved skin incision over the lateral malleolus
Operative principle	Ligament reconstruction Divide the hyperextended ligaments 2 mm below the fibular tip Suture the overlapping stumps Modification: Lifting of a periosteal flap of the distal fibula, transosseous fixation of the ligament attachments and doubling with periosteal flap
Osteochondritis dissecans	
Approach	Arthroscopy only in cases of large defects and difficult localization Arthrotomy Anterolateral and anteromedial portals (Fig. 15.47) Open approach for large defects, medial malleolar osteotomy is problematic when growth is occurring because of the growth plate

Table 15.10 (continued)

Operative principle	Drilling/microfracturing
	Opening of the sclerosis (migrating mesenchymal stem cells → formation of fibrous cartilage)
	Retrograde drilling
	  Articular cartilage remains intact
	  Approach to the contralateral talar side
	Antegrade drilling (Pridie), microfracturing
	  Arthroscopically in plantar flexion; approaches: Anterior, posterior, transmalleolar
	  Drilling with K-wires (1.2 mm)
	Retrograde debridement and cancellous bone graft
	  Articular cartilage remains intact; filling with iliac crest cancellous bone or subchondral drilling if needed
	Antegrade debridement, cancellous bone graft and refixation
	  Arthrotomy
	  Removal of sclerotic zone on the articular side, filling with iliac crest cancellous bone graft and refixation of the fragment with fibrin glue and biodegradable pins
	Reconstructive methods
	Osteochondral transplantation: Transplantation of a cartilage-bone cylinder from the ipsilateral femoral condyle
	Autologous chondrocyte transplantation: Isolated case reports

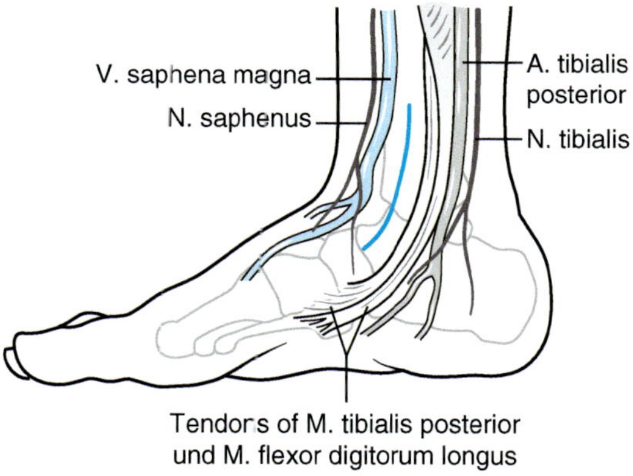

Fig. 15.42 Approach to the medial malleolus

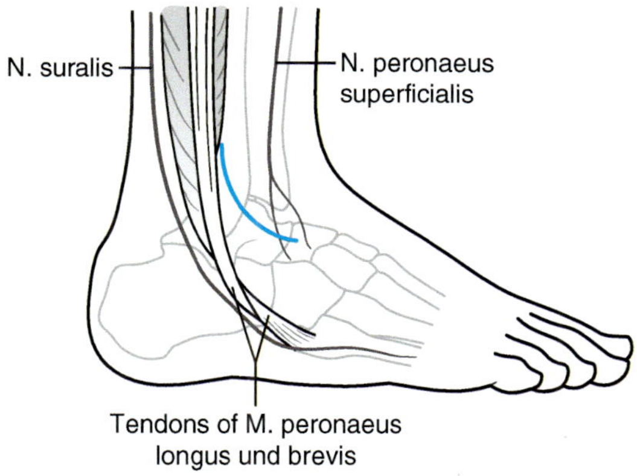

Fig. 15.43 Approach to the lateral malleolus

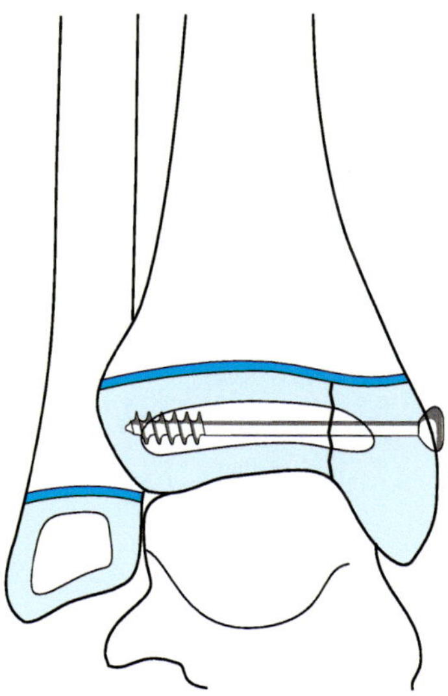

Fig. 15.44 Compression screw fixation for Salter III/IV fractures

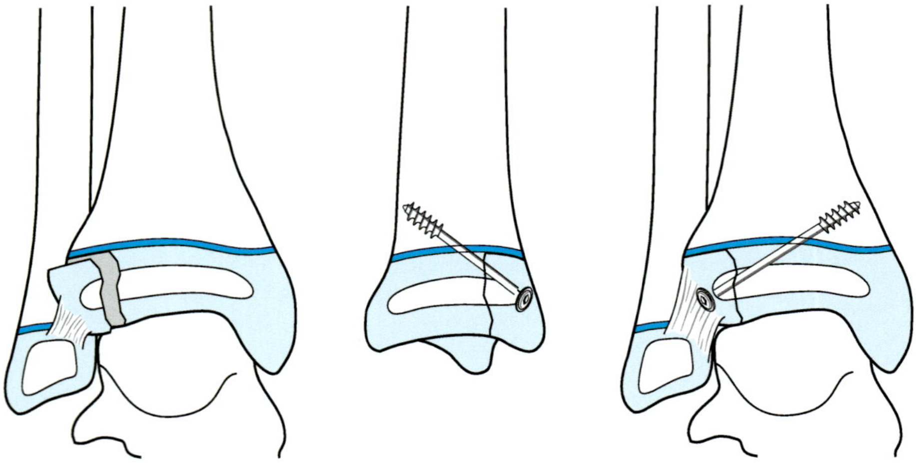

Fig. 15.45 Oblique-running fixation of a twoplane fracture. Compression of the anterolateral fragment

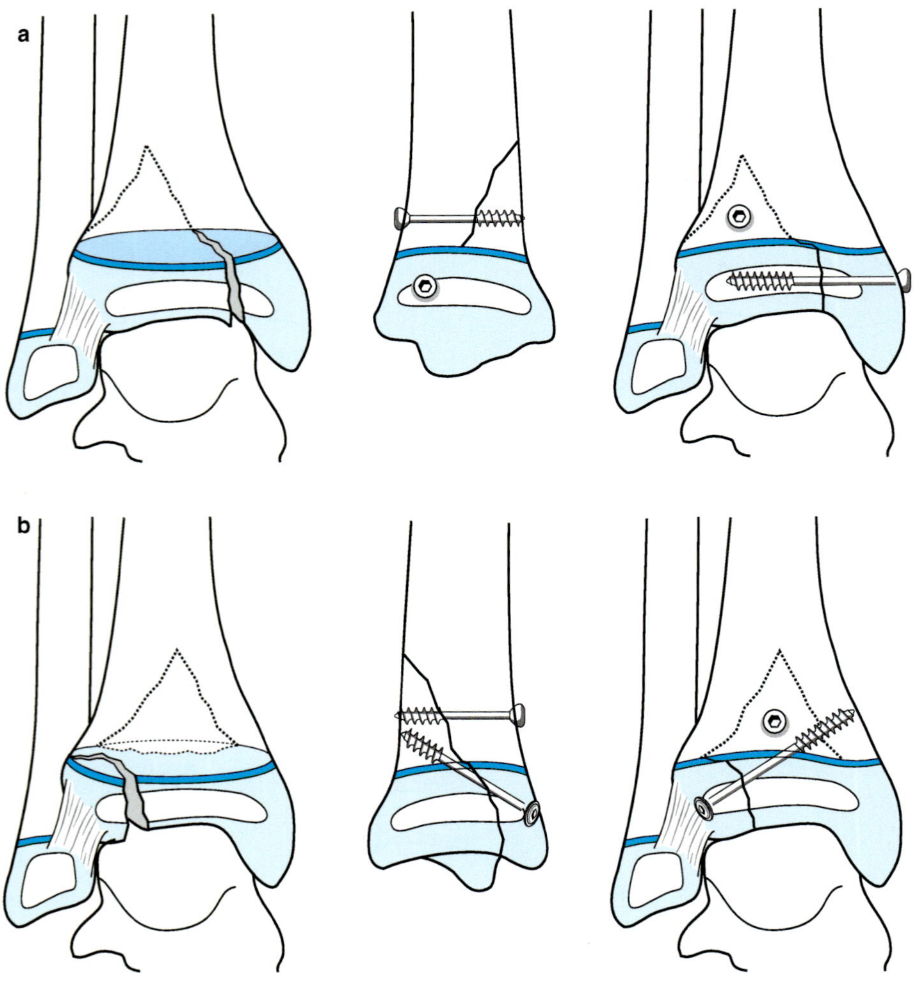

Fig. 15.46 Fixation of transition fractures. (**a**) Triplane I fracture. (**b**) Triplane II fracture

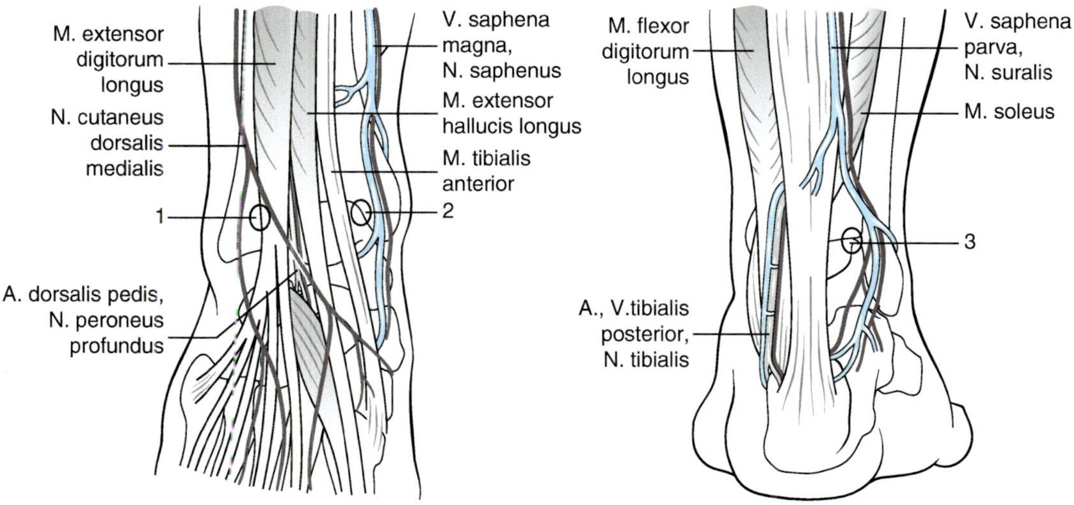

Fig. 15.47 Arthroscopic approaches to the ankle: (1) Anterolateral approach, (2) Anteromedial approach, (3) Posterolateral approach

Recommended Literature

Aitken AP (1936) The end results of the fractured distal tibial epiphysis. J Bone Joint Surg 18:685–691

Auner B, Marzi I (2013) Oberes Sprunggelenk. Trauma Und Berufskrankheit 15:217–223

Berndt AL, Harty M (1959) Transchondral fractures (osteochondrosis dissecans) of the talus. JBJS Am 41A:988–1020

Devries C, Meyer Z, Abzug JM, Baldwin KD, Milbrandt TA, Hosseinzadeh P (2019) Pediatric ankle fractures: when to operate and when to leave alone? Instr Course Lect 68:481–488

Hadad MJ, Sullivan BT, Sponseller PD (2018) Surgically relevant patterns in triplane fractures. J Bone Jt Surg 100:1039–1046

Lahm A, Erggelet C, Steinwachs M, Reichelt A (2000) Arthroscopic management of osteochondral lesions of the talus: results of drilling and usefulness of magnetic resonance imaging before and after treatment. Arthroscopy 16:299–304

Lurie B, Rysselberghe NV, Pennock AT, Upasani VV (2020) Functional outcomes of Tillaux and triplane fractures with 2 to 5 millimeters of intra-articular gap. J Bone Joint Surg 102:679–686

Marzi I (2016) Kindertraumatologie, 3rd edn. Springer, Berlin

Pallamar M, Eder T, Ganger R, Farr S (2021) Surgical treatment of atraumatic Osteochondrosis Dissecans of the immature talus – clinical results and prevalence of radiographic joint degeneration after a median follow-up of 72.5 months. Foot Ankle Surg. https://doi.org/10.1016/j.fas.2021.05.007

Rammelt S, Schneiders W, Fitze G, Zwipp H (2013) Foot and ankle fractures in children. Orthopade 42:45–54

Salter RB, Harris WR (1963) Injuries involving the epiphyseal plate. J Bone Joint Surg 45A:587–622

Schneidmüller D, Sander AL, Wertenbroek M, Wutzler S, Kraus R, Marzi I, Laurer HL (2014) Triplane fractures: do we need cross-sectional imaging? Eur J Trauma Emerg Surg 40:37–43

Schulz A, Jerosch J (2003) Therapiekonzepte bei osteochondralen Läsionen und der Osteochondrosis dissecans tali. Arthroskopie 16:51–56

Sjölin SU, Dons-Jensen H, Simonsen O (1991) Reinforced anatomical reconstruktion of the anterior talofibular ligament in chronic anterolateral instability using a periosteal flap. Foot Ankle 12:15–18

Ull C, Dudda M, Schildhauer TA, Seybold D, Geßmann J (2016) Osteochondrosis dissecans des Talus im Überblick. Trauma Und Berufskrankheit 18:48–55

Venkatadass K, Sangeet G, Prasad VD, Rajasekaran S (2021) Paediatric ankle fractures: guidelines to management. Indian J Orthop 55:35–46

Volmer E, Hauenstein C, Weber M-A (2020) Update: Übergangsfrakturen. Radiologe 60:1183–1194

von Laer L (2014) Growth behavior after epiphyseal plate injury. Unfallchirurg 117:1071–1084

Foot

16

16.1 Physiological Findings

Ossification Centers and Growth Plate Fusion

At birth, the only radiologically-evident ossification centers are those of the calcaneus and talus (Fig. 16.1).

- The last tarsal bone to become visible is the navicular bone, between three and five years of age.
- Between ages five and ten years, the calcaneal apophysis develops, often from several ossification centers.
- The phalanges and metatarsals each have a single epiphyseal plate.
- one basal growth plate: MT I, Phalanges I-V;
- one subcapital growth plate: MT II-V.

There are numerous accessory ossification centers in the foot (Fig. 16.2). Cleft sesamoid bones are common, but sesamoid fractures are rare in adolescents (Figs. 16.3 and 16.4).

Split epiphyseal plates can also appear during adolescence (Fig. 16.5).

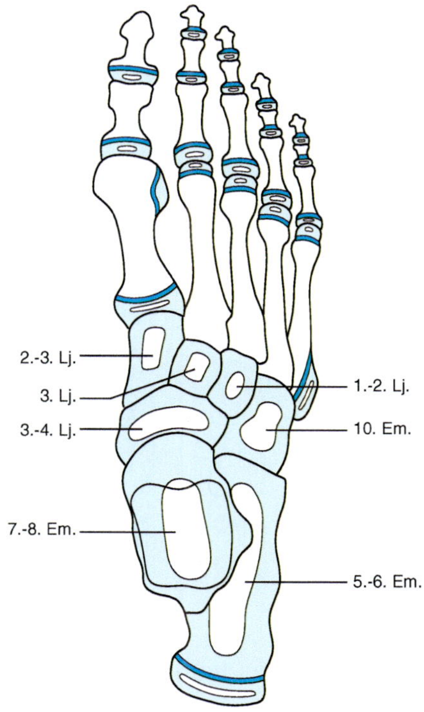

Fig. 16.1 Ossification centers and growth plate fusion. (*Lj*) life year; (*Em*) embryonal month

I. Marzi et al., *Pediatric Skeletal Trauma*, https://doi.org/10.1007/978-3-030-93685-3_16

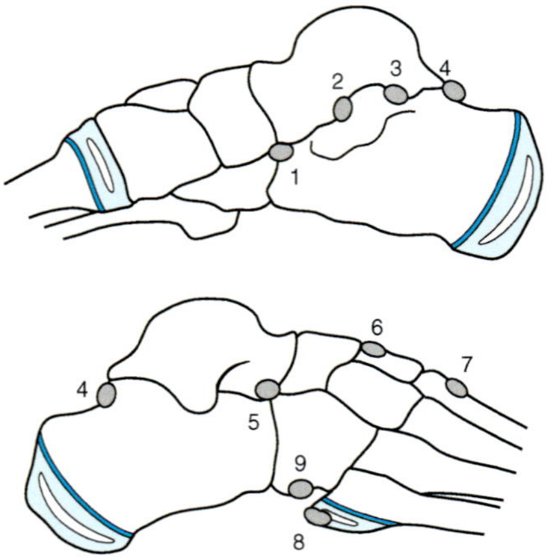

Fig. 16.2 Accessory ossification centers (1) Accessory navicular bone (10%), (2) Os sustentaculi (1.5%), (3) Talus secundarius, (4) Os trigonum (13%), (5) Calcaneus secundarius (.), (6) Os intercuneiforme (rare), (7) Os intermetatarseum (9%), (8) Os vesalianum, (9) Os subfibulare (10%)

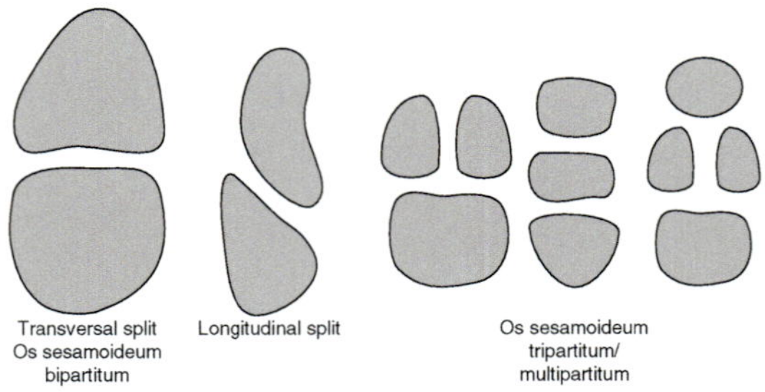

Fig. 16.4 Sesamoids—division variants

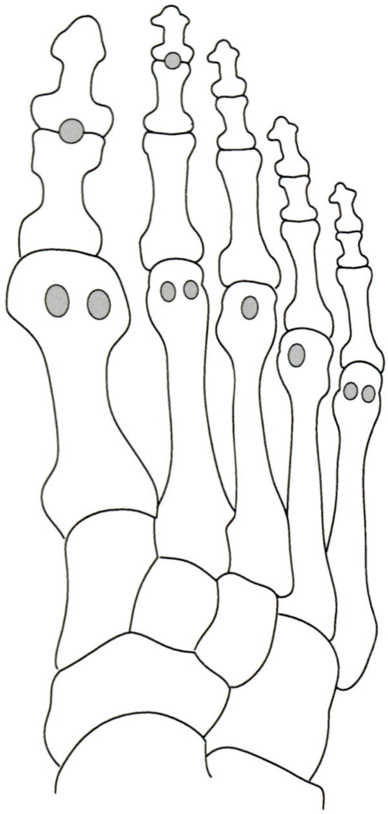

Fig. 16.3 Sesamoids—localization

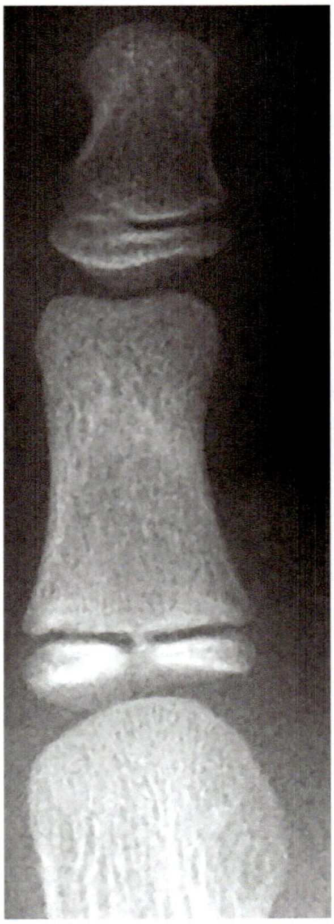

Fig. 16.5 Split epiphysis

16.2 Bony Foot Injuries

Incidence, Mechanism of Injury and Clinical Presentation

Bony foot injuries, primarily metatarsal and toe fractures, have an incidence of 13%. Tarsal injuries are uncommon and occur most often in the calcaneus, talus, and navicular bones. The child's foot changes throughout growth, with various axes, age-dependent growth plates and ossification centers, and overall increased ligament laxity. Radiological diagnosis of fracture can be challenging due to the many anatomical variations, particularly accessory bones. Accessory bones may mimic fractures on imaging, but they are mostly of no clinical significance (Fig. 16.2).

Compared to other body regions, the rate of longitudinal growth in the foot is particularly increased during the first few years of life. 50% of longitudinal growth has already occurred by one year in girls and one and a half years in boys; by age 12, it has reached 96% in girls and 88% in boys. This accelerated growth is an important factor when selecting treatment since proper reduction of displaced fractures must be prompt. Sufficient spontaneous correction can no longer be expected after 10–12 years of age because there is little residual growth. The majority of childhood foot injuries occur in the forefoot. These are usually uncomplicated except in direct crush injuries, and metatarsal fractures often heal well treated conservatively. In contrast, the treatment of tarsal fractures is technically demanding, without fixed recommendations in the literature.

Complex foot injuries such as rollover or crush injuries are rare, but they present an immense challenge. Soft tissue reconstructions are often necessary along with treatment for compartment syndromes and fractures/dislocations. The goal of treatment is to restore a functional, plantigrade foot. In the most severely injured children, the treatment approach is coordinated within a damage control framework based on the Zwipp five-point system. First considered are the number of involved structures, i.e., ankle joint, talus, calcaneus, midtarsal (Chopart) joint, tarsometatarsal (Lisfranc) joint (Fig. 16.6), and the degree of soft-tissue damage. One point is assigned per damage grade, with rollover trauma and subtotal amputation = 4 points. If the number of affected structures added to the point value of soft-tissue damage results in five or more points, the injury is considered a complex foot trauma. In adults, primary amputation is considered a valid option for extensive forefoot trauma in severely polytraumatized patients. More restraint is called for in children, however, because there is more healing potential. Thus, the best effort is made to follow a course of careful debridement with second-look operations and plastic reconstructions, with amputations only to the border zone, if at all.

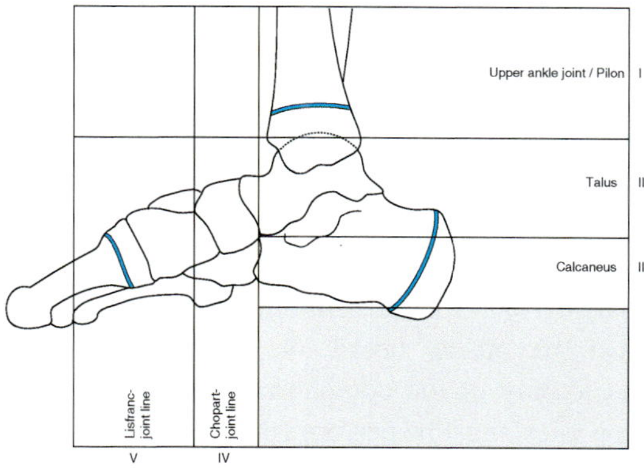

Fig. 16.6 Zwipp classification of anatomical injury regions of the foot

Treatment for complex injuries cannot be standardized; however, the following damage-control framework is used to guide the approach to severe soft-tissue injuries and open fractures:

- Thorough decontamination of wounds in the OR, if necessary, with jet lavage;
- Surgical wound debridement;
- Systemic antibiotic therapy (cephalosporins);
- Temporary coverage with artificial skin, vacuum system, and regular re-debridement, second-look procedures every two days;
- Minimally-invasive or percutaneous bony fixation to restore anatomical axes (hindfoot, midfoot, medial, and lateral columns) with K-wires (1.4–1.6 mm), cannulated screws (3.5 mm), or external fixators;
- if necessary, secondary tissue transfer (flaps, but also skin replacement; Integra).

Compartment syndromes can occur in both closed and open fractures and must not be overlooked in children. The foot has four compartments: medial, lateral, central, and interosseous. They are not easy to distinguish clinically. Clinical signs of compartment syndrome are swelling, severe pain, pain with passive toe movement, reduced pulse, reduced 2-point discrimination, and motor deficit. Pressure > 30 mmHg is also diagnostic, but direct measurement is practically impossible in children. The complex anatomy and small foot compartments make precise diagnosis and targeted compartment release difficult. Thus, decisions must be made based on clinical findings. Fasciotomy of the compartments, including the deep ones, must be performed at an early stage to avoid sequelae such as plantar contracture, pes cavus deformity, claw toes, restricted movement, sensory disorders, and chronic pain.

16.3 Talus Fracture

Incidence, Mechanism of Injury and Clinical Presentation

With an incidence of 0.008%, talar fractures are extremely rare. They typically result from severe force trauma. Most fractures are nondisplaced and can be treated conservatively in children. When there is displacement, the goal is anatomical reduction and fixation. Without it, there are poor long term results, with premature joint necrosis and osteoarthritis.

There are three zones of the talus typically affected by fracture. The talar neck is most common, and then the body and the lateral and posterior processes. In fractures of the talar neck (Table 16.1 and Fig. 16.7) and body, there is a risk of necrosis that increases with increasing age and ossification (incidence up to 25%). Necrosis usually becomes evident on radiographs only after 6–9 months. One indication is the missing Hawkins' sign, a subchondral hypodense zone in the talar dome area that appears after eight weeks. However, this applies only to children with sufficient ossification, over ten years of age. MRI can provide more timely information regarding circulation.

Indications and procedure of Talus fractures are indicated in Table 16.2.

Table 16.1 Hawkins classification of talar neck fractures (Fig. 16.7)

Type	Displacement	Treatment	Risk of necrosis
Type I	Mostly nondisplaced	Closed, as needed open reduction for joint step-off >12 years Short leg cast for 6 weeks non-weight-bearing (Fig. 16.8)	5–10%
Type II	Body displaced dorsally without dislocation from the malleolar fork; often associated with medial comminution (Fig. 16.9)	Anatomical reduction and screw fixation, In individual cases also K-wire fixation; Short leg cast for 6 weeks non-weight-bearing, emergency	40–50%
Type III	Body displacement from the malleolar fork	Emergency open reduction and screw fixation; Short leg cast for 6 weeks non-weight-bearing	80–100%
Type IV	Additional talar neck displacement from malleolar fork	Open reduction and screw fixation with additional K-wire transfixion of the talo-navicular and subtalar joints for 4 weeks; short leg cast for 6 weeks non-weight-bearing, emergency	80–100%

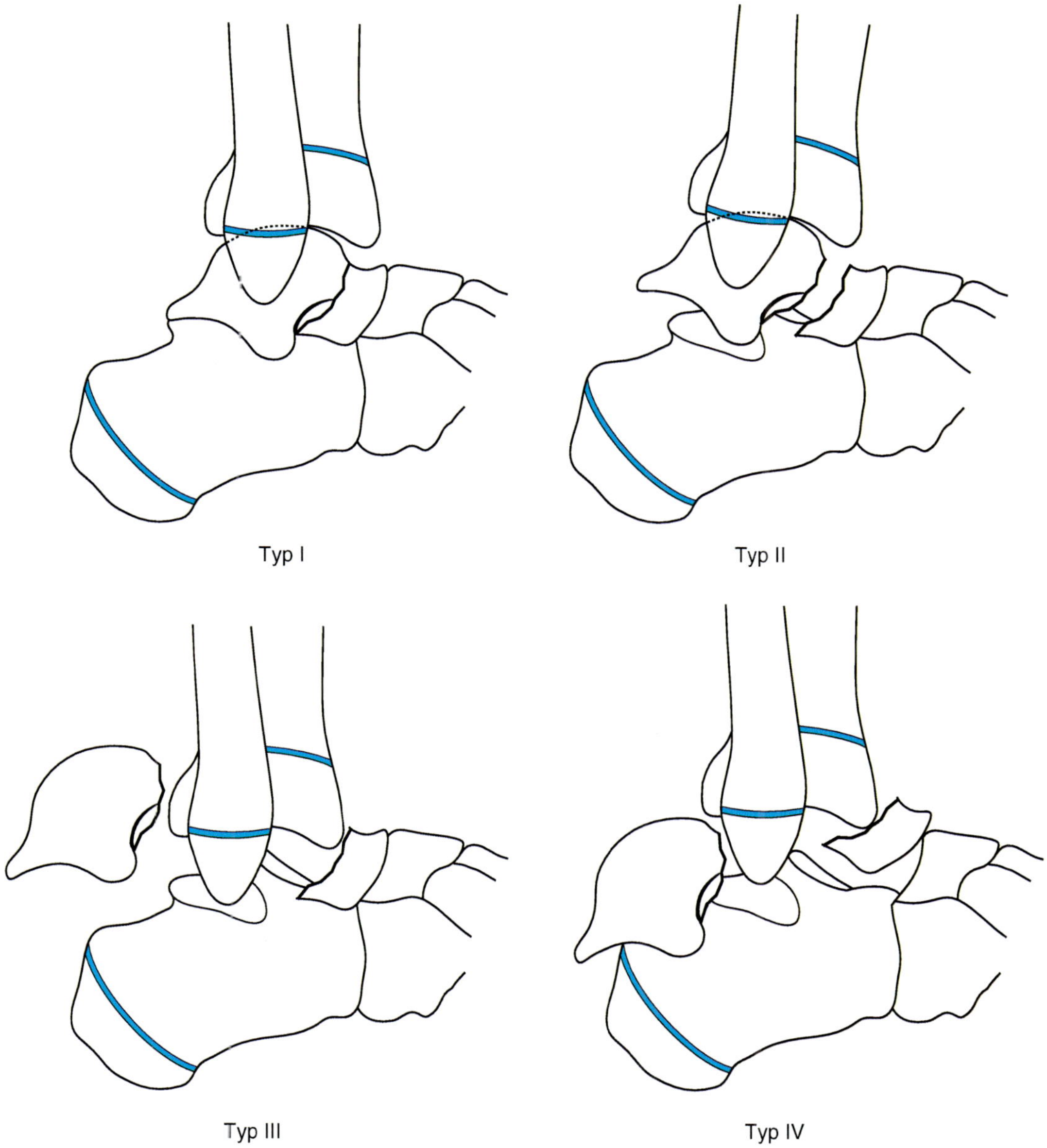

Fig. 16.7 Hawkins classification of talar neck fractures

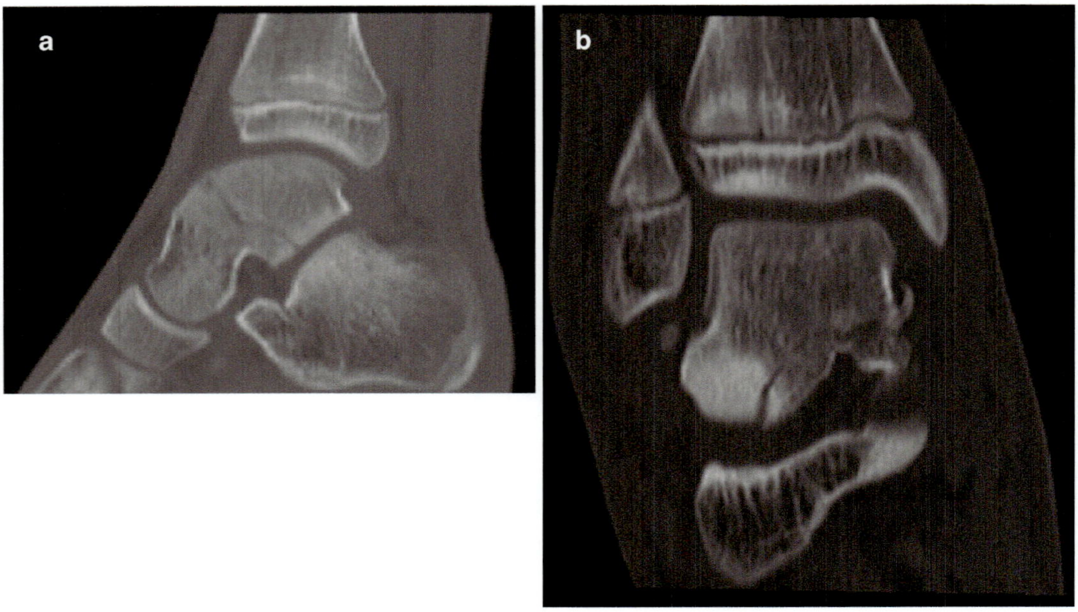

Fig. 16.8 Undisplaced talar fracture type Hawkins I of a 15 year old boy after fall from 4 m. Conservative treatment in a lower leg cast. (**a**) Longitudinal CT scan, (**b**) Coronar view of CT scan, showing the participation of the lower ankle joint

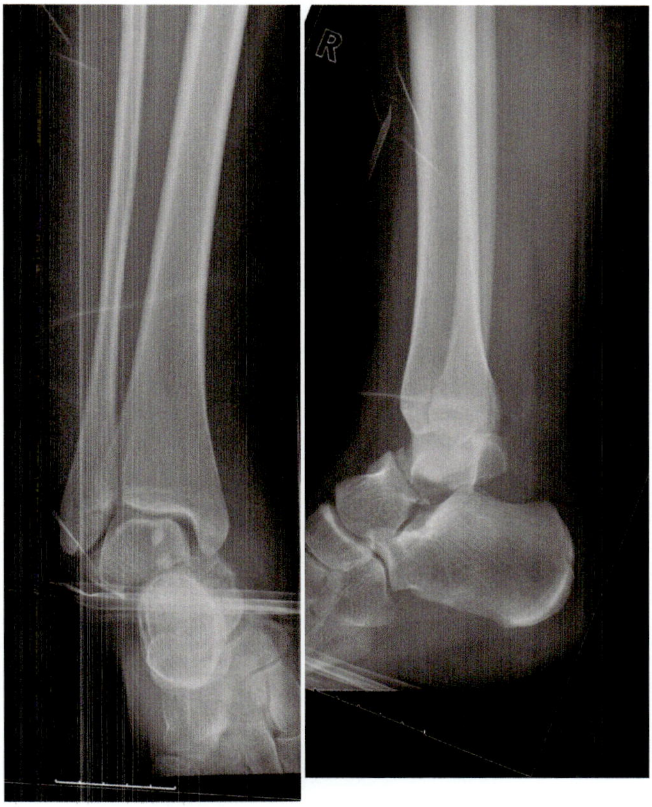

Fig. 16.9 Displaced talar fracture type Hawkins II

Table 16.2 Talus fractures

Special features	Rare Possible fractures: neck, body, processes Especially massive trauma (rollover trauma), often associated with complex foot trauma Luxation fractures (Fig. 16.10)
Diagnostic process	AP and lateral x-rays of the hindfoot MRI: Fracture course, circulation; visualization of non-ossified areas CT for older children if necessary, assessment of joint surfaces and fracture course
Treatment goals/limits of correction	Restoration of anatomy and joint surfaces, preservation of the foot axes
Primary treatment	Short leg plaster splint, medical analgesia as needed Open fracture, fracture-dislocation: Emergency surgery (risk of necrosis)
Conservative treatment	
Indication	Nondisplaced fractures, joint gap or step <2 mm
Approach	6–8 weeks short leg cast, non-weight bearing
Follow up	Weight-bearing as tolerated after cast removal Physical therapy is generally not necessary
Control X-rays	Consolidation check at 6–8 weeks (no cast)
Return to sports	Approximately 6 weeks after consolidation, with unlimited function
Operative treatment	
Indication	Joint displacement >2 mm; shortening, angulation; Hawkins type II-IV; open fractures
Approach	Closed reduction; screw fixation when possible, otherwise K-wire transfixion Open reduction is usually necessary; screw fixation Ankle dislocation: If necessary, supplemental transfixion with the ankle joint in individual cases with ligament reconstruction and drilling of the flake (Fig. 16.11)
Follow up	6 weeks of short leg cast (if necessary, in light flexion), non-weight-bearing 10 weeks non-weight-bearing if there is a risk of necrosis Weight-bearing as tolerated after cast removal
Control X-rays	Postoperative reduction control; consolidation check at six weeks (cast-free), MRI to rule out necrosis as needed for complaints
Hardware removal	At four weeks, transfixing K-wires At six months, screws
Return to sports	Approximately 6 weeks after consolidation, with unlimited function
Complications	Premature ankle joint osteoarthritis Talar necrosis Foot compartment syndrome in cases of rollover trauma and massive hematoma
Growth disturbance	–
Follow up	In cases of necrosis risk: MRI at 10 weeks (exclude necrosis) Checks every three weeks, until unlimited function and full weight-bearing achieved; At one year with unremarkable findings

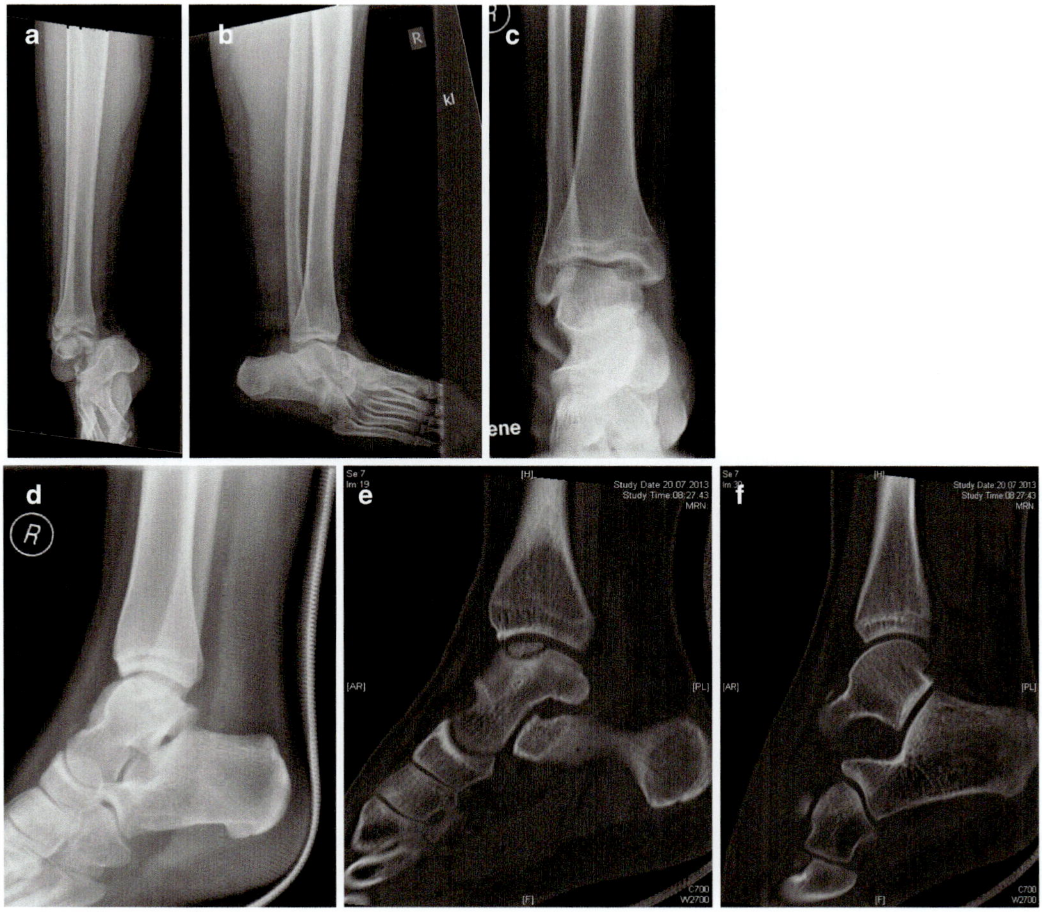

Fig. 16.10 Luxation fracture of the talus type Hawkins II with osteochondral lesion after Salto jump of a 16 year old boy. (**a**, **b**) Trauma images, (**c**, **d**) Reduction with a large medial osteochondral flake. (**e**, **f**) CT of the flake and after drilling

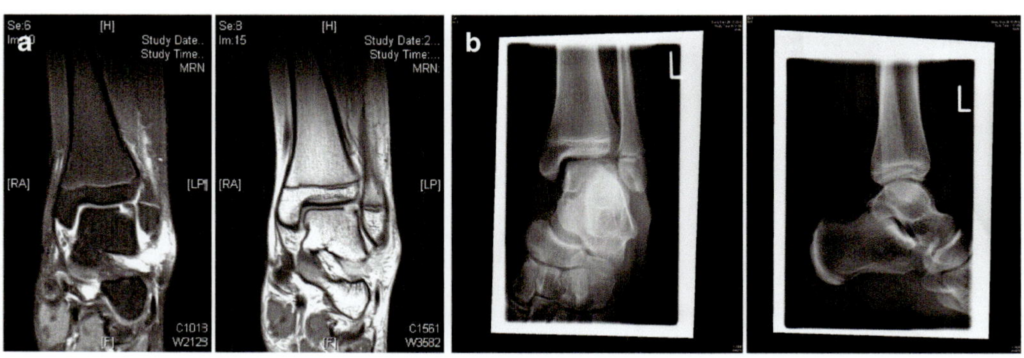

Fig. 16.11 Lateral osteochondral flake after severe distorsion trauma of a 12 year old girl. (**a**) MRI of the lateral flake of the talus, (**b**) x-ray view

16.4 Calcaneus Fracture

Incidence, Mechanism of Injury and Clinical Presentation

Calcaneus fractures are rare, with an incidence of 0.005% (Table 16.3).

The mechanism of injury is not always high-speed trauma or falls from height. In children up to three years, calcaneus fractures can also be caused by mild trauma. However, these fractures can be detected radiologically. Thus, in cases of negative x-ray findings and persistent complaints, it is recommended to repeat x-rays after two weeks in the cast to find evidence of fracture or callus formation.

One-third of calcaneus fractures are associated with additional injuries, and this should be noted particularly in cases of high-speed trauma. In children younger than seven years, fractures are predominantly extraarticular. These generally affect the calcaneal tuberosity. In adolescents, most calcaneus fractures are intraarticular and lead to a flattening of the tuber joint (Bohler) angle (<25–40°) (Fig. 16.12). There is insufficient long-term evidence available regarding displaced intraarticular calcaneus fractures that have been treated conservatively. Nondisplaced extraarticular fractures in young children are treated conservatively, and displaced intraarticular fractures of adolescents are anatomically reduced and stabilized as in adults.

Table 16.3 Calcaneus fractures (Fig. 16.15)

Special features	Etiology: <10 years simple fall; >10 years high-speed trauma Especially adolescents: intraarticular displaced fractures <8 years: extraarticular, mildly displaced fractures
Diagnostic process	AP and lateral x-rays of the hindfoot; calcaneus axial view With suspected fracture: MRI with reconstructions (Fig. 16.16) Alternatively, low dose CT + 3D reconstructions
Treatment goals/limits of correction	Restoration of congruent joint surfaces; preservation of foot axes and joint angles, stable healing
Primary treatment	Short leg plaster splint, medical analgesia as needed, anti-swelling measures
Conservative treatment	
Indication	No joint step-offs, acceptable tuber-joint (Böhler) angle Nondisplaced extraarticular fractures
Approach	4–6 weeks short leg splint, weight-bearing according to age
Follow up	Weight-bearing as tolerated
Control X-rays	Consolidation check at 6 weeks (no cast)
Return to sports	When complaint-free
Operative treatment	
Indication	Displaced intraarticular fractures Displaced extraarticular fractures Usually in intervals, after soft-tissue swelling has diminished Open fractures
Approach	Open reduction of axes, angles and joint surfaces, if necessary with cancellous graft or synthetic bone replacement (Figs. 16.17 and 16.18). Bony fixation in small children with K-wires, otherwise with flat profile plates. Fixed-angle adult calcaneus plates are usually too large; alternatives are small fixed-angle hand or foot plates. Indirect reduction and stabilization with external fixateur, soft tissue management in open fractures (Fig. 16.19).
Follow up	6 weeks non-weight-bearing in short leg cast After cast removal, weight-bearing as tolerated
Control X-rays	Postoperative reduction control; consolidation check at 6 weeks (no cast)
Hardware removal	One year post-surgery
Return to sports	Approximately 6–8 weeks after consolidation
Complications	Premature talotarsal osteoarthritis is most common;initial compartment syndrome (10%) with extensive displacement and trauma
Growth disturbance	Possible incongruity of the subtalar joint
Follow up	Every three weeks until unlimited function and full weight-bearing

Classification

There are several classifications for calcaneus fractures. Fractures are distinguished as extraarticular or intraarticular according to involvement of the central thalamic joint. The Essex-Lopresti Classification recognizes two main fracture entities: the joint depression type and the tongue type (Fig. 16.13). Only a few classifications refer to injuries in childhood; one example is the Wiley and Profit Classification (Fig. 16.14).

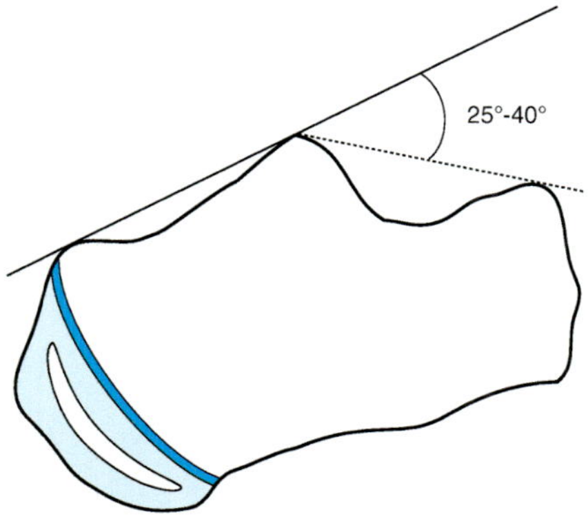

Fig. 16.12 Böhler angle (Tuber-joint angle)

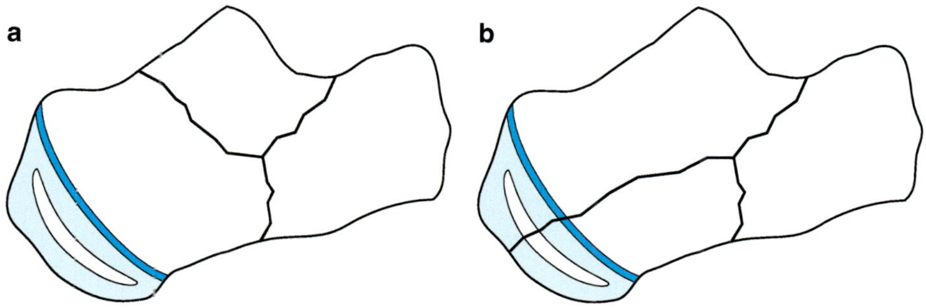

Fig. 16.13 Essex-lopresti classification of calcaneus fractures. (**a**) Joint depression type, (**b**) Tongue type

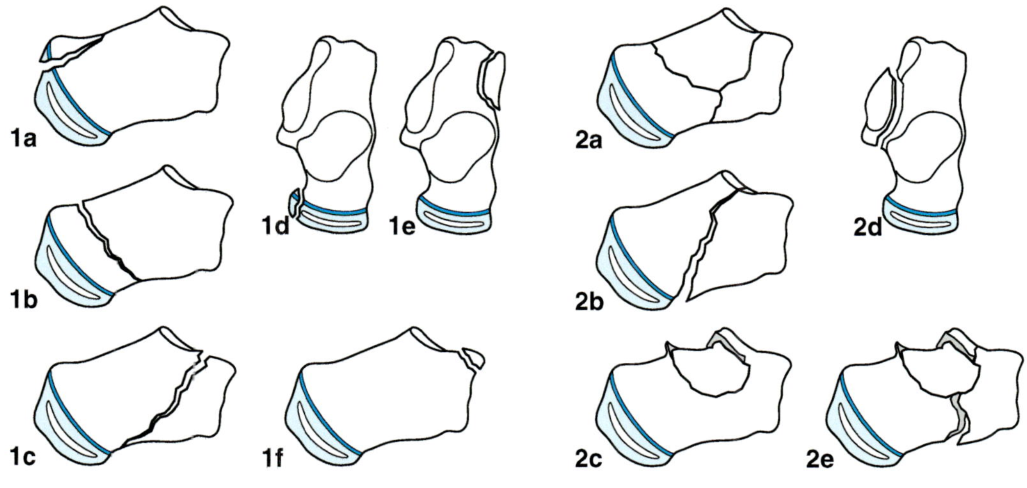

Fig. 16.14 Wiley and profit classification of calcaneus fractures (**1**) Extraarticular; (**a**) Tuberosity avulsion, (**b**) Vertical body fracture, (**c**) Horizontal body fracture, (**d**) Avulsion medial process, (**e, f**) Avulsion anterior process. (**2**) Intraarticular; (**a**) Nondisplaced, (**b**) Tongue type, (**c**) Displaced centrolateral fracture, (**d**) Sustentacular fracture, (**e**) Multi-fragment fracture

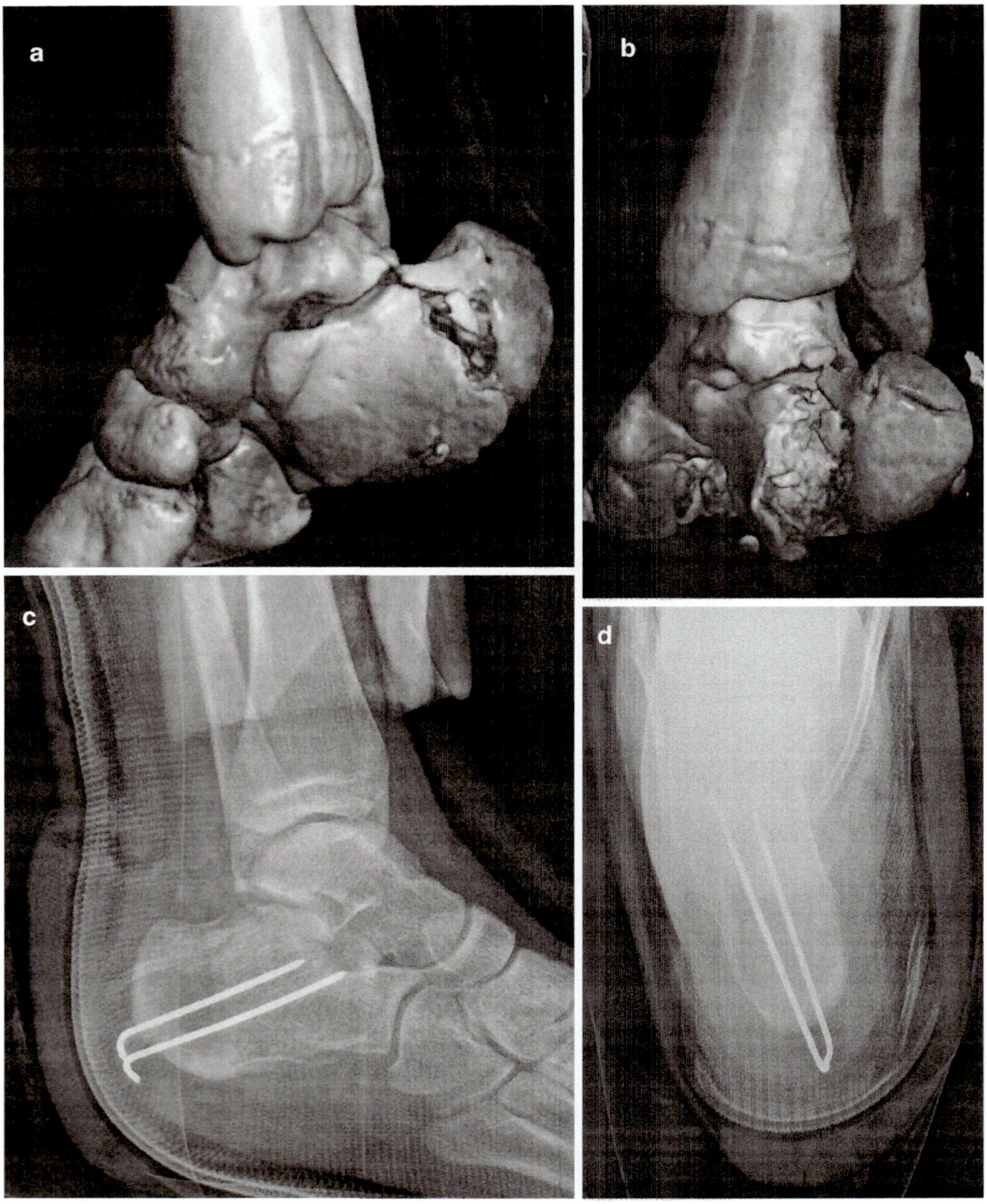

Fig. 16.15 Calcaneus fracture in a small child. (**a**, **b**) Trauma Image, (**c**, **d**) After Reduction and Stabilization with 2 K-wires and cast

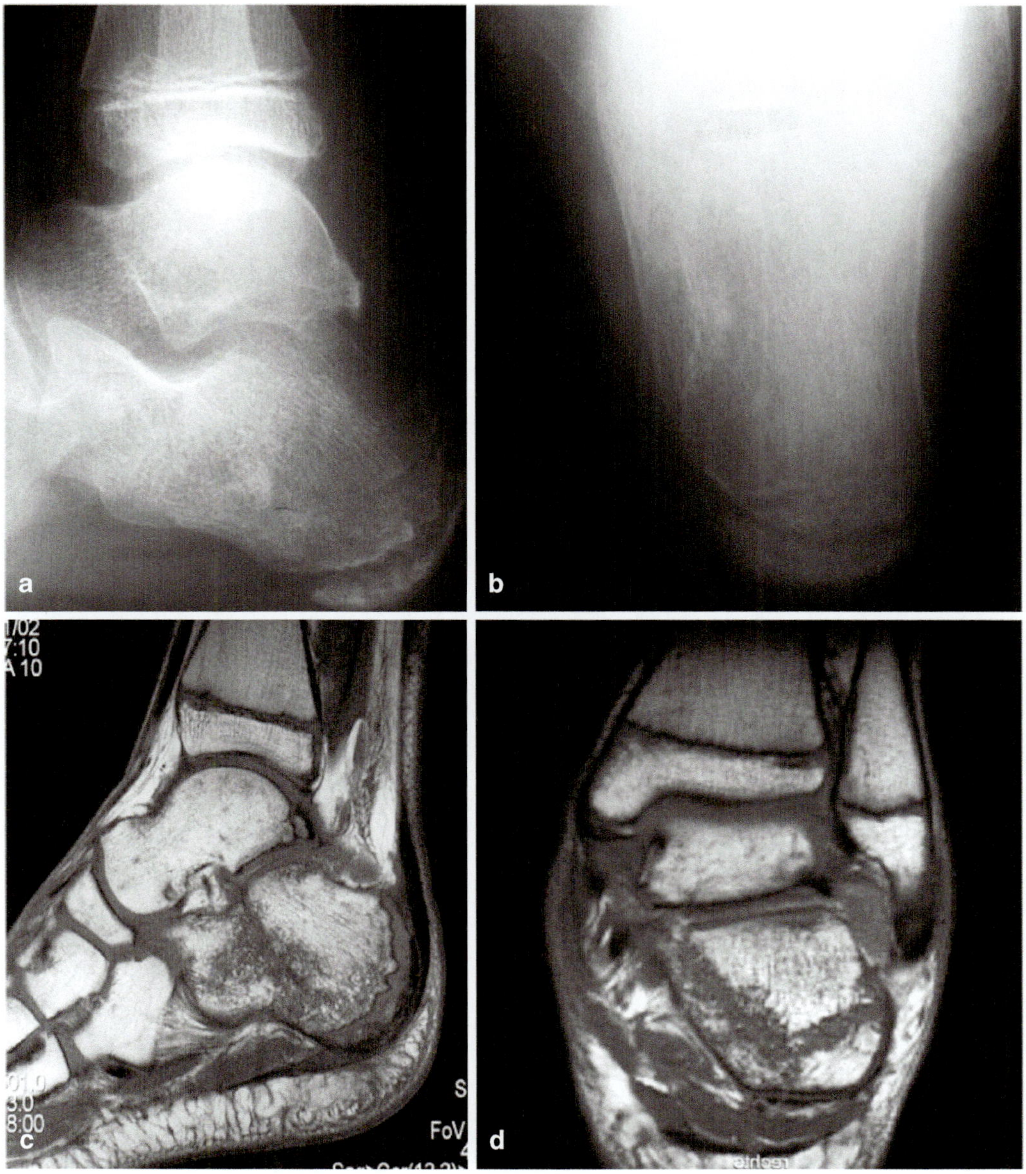

Fig. 16.16 Undisplaced intraarticular calcaneus fracture after soccer accident of a 10 year old boy. (**a**, **b**) Trauma images, (**c**, **d**) MRI images

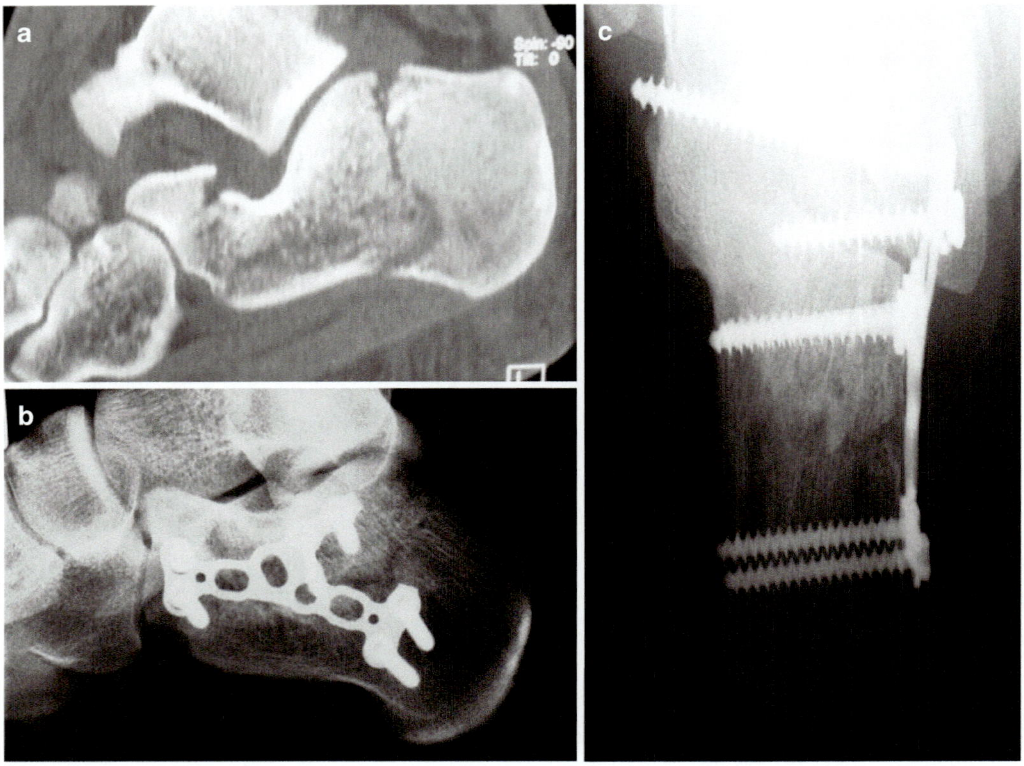

Fig. 16.17 Displaced intraarticular calcaneus fracture of an adolescent afrter jump from great height. (**a**) Trauma image, (**b**, **c**) Postoperative after open reduction and fixation with an anatomical calcaneus plate

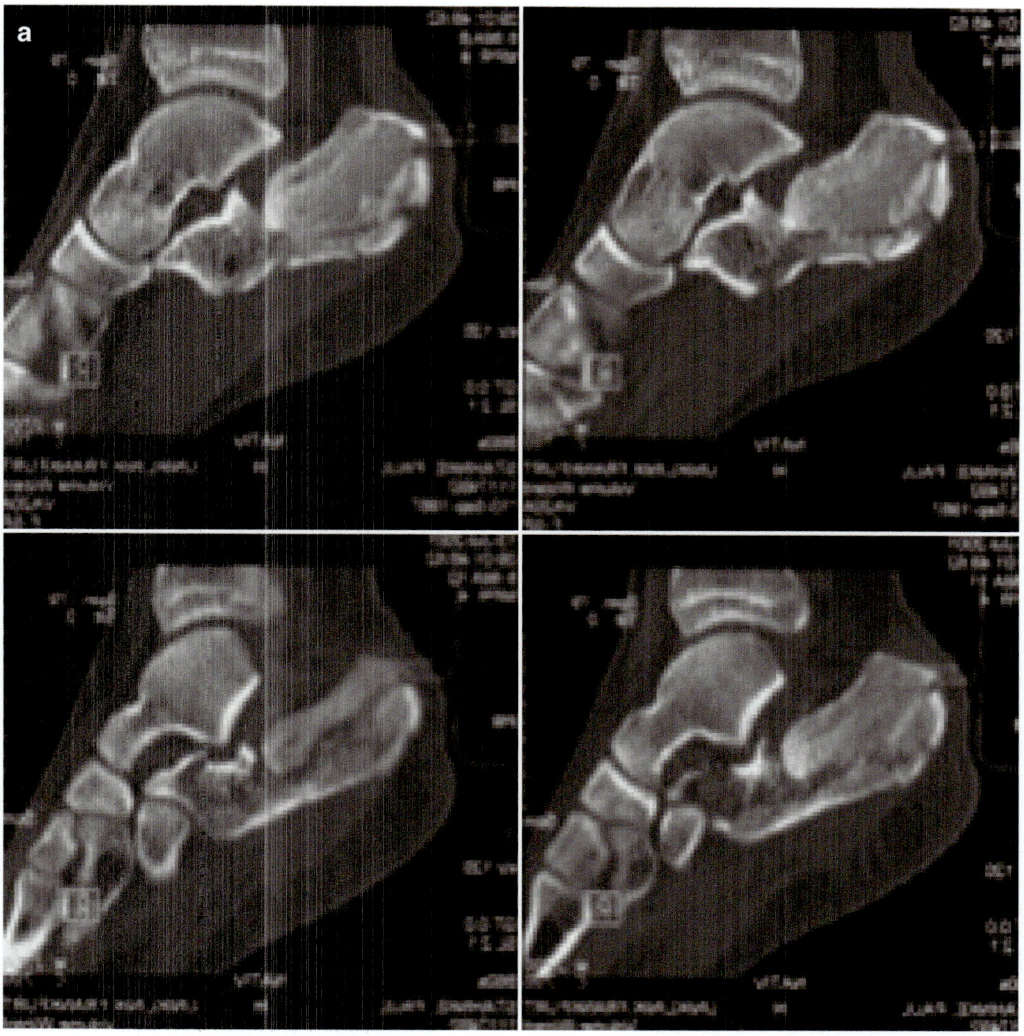

Fig. 16.18 Compound fracture of the calcaneus after fall from the third floor on both sides of a 13 year old boy. (**a**) CT Images of both sides with joint depression fractures, (**b**) Postoperative x-ray left side after open reduction and plate osteosynthesis, (**c**) Postoperative after open reduction and lateral angular stable plate osteosynthesis right side

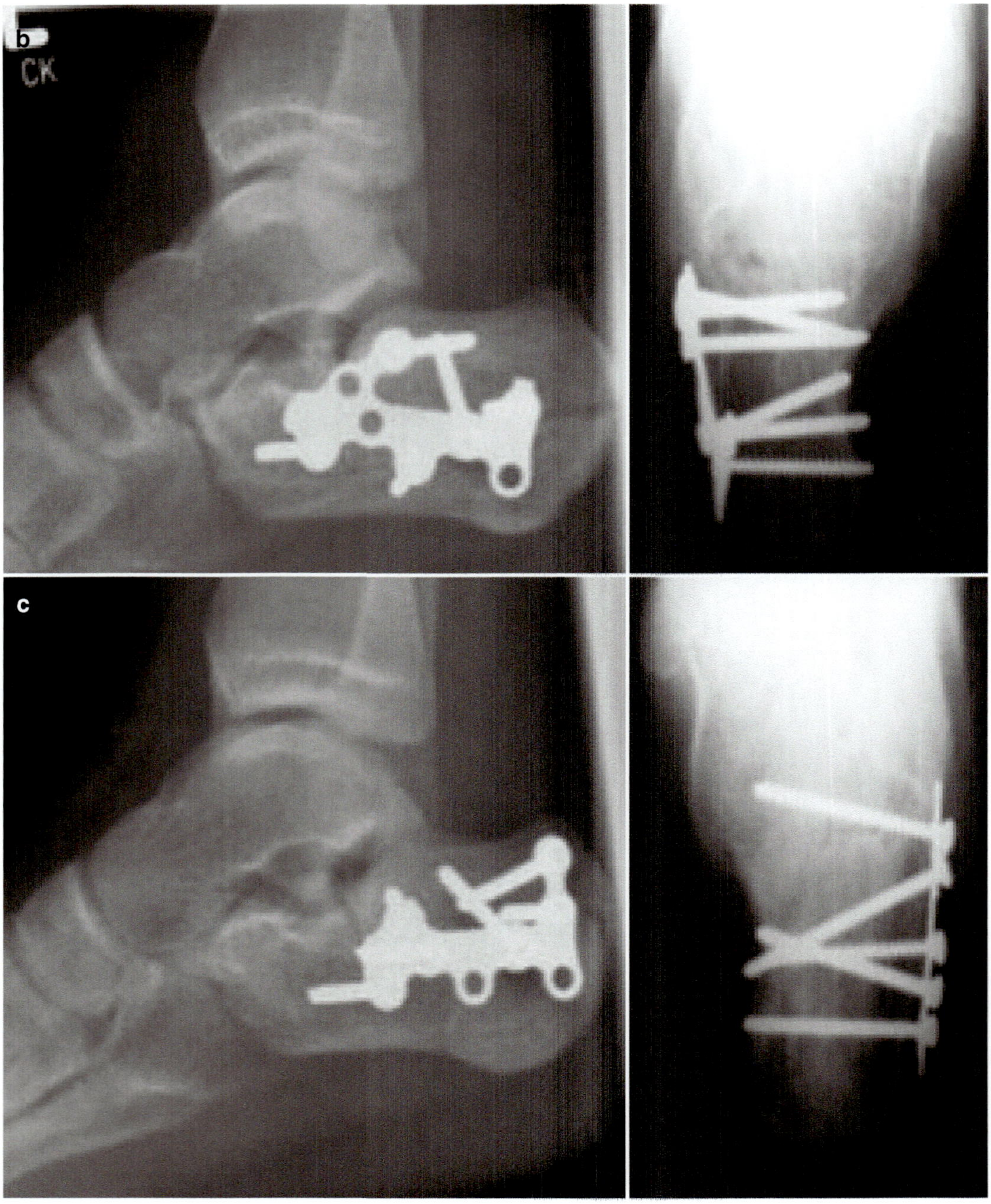

Fig. 16.18 (continued)

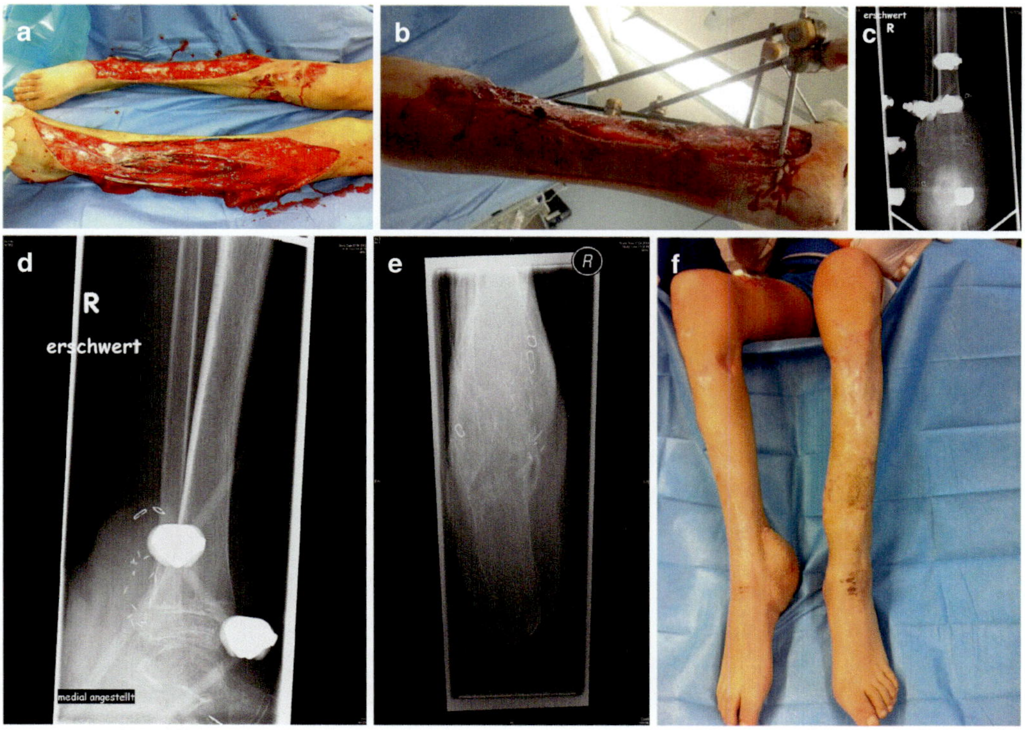

Fig. 16.19 11 year old boy after underground accident. Medial open calcaneus fracture und soft tissue defect of the right foot and both legs. (**a**) Trauma image after overroll trauma (**b**) Primary stabilization with transfixation in an external fixateur. (**c–e**) X-ray controls, (**f**) Healing after plastic reconstruction with a free flap and mesh graft

16.5 Tarsal Fracture: and Hindfoot Injuries

Incidence, Mechanism of Injury and Clinical Presentation

Tarsal Fractures These are very rare, but the goal is anatomical reduction due to the high risk of necrosis. If malalignment persists, premature osteoarthritis can be expected to cause considerable complaints, which are often only resolved eventually through arthrodesis.

Navicular Fractures These are rarely displaced but may be associated with dislocations in the transverse tarsal (Chopart) joint.

Cuboid Fractures These are typically compression fractures with shortening of the lateral foot column. The goal is anatomic reduction with length restoration.

Bony Foot Dislocations These injuries are rare in childhood. Most are interphalangeal dislocations that are easily reduced and stabilized with tape. Peri-talar and subtalar dislocations and subluxations occur most commonly in adolescents, often associated with talar fractures.

Lisfranc joint dislocations occur most often after hyperflexion or rollover trauma in older children. Lisfranc injuries are easily missed on primary imaging; thus, precise true lateral projections must be performed. Spontaneous reduction often occurs, leaving the clinical manifestations of pain and possible hematoma in the metatarsal area. The different forms of Lisfranc dislocations can occur also in children, although in individual cases, the extent of injury is only recognizable on MRI or low-dose CT. There are often associated fractures in the tarsal and metatarsal areas. A fractured second metatarsal can be an indicator of Lisfranc subluxation/dislocation. Treatment consists of reduction, generally closed, and temporary transfixion with K-wires for instability, followed by immobilization. The key point here is stabilization of the basal second metatarsal fracture. The goal is anatomical reduction. Without it, poor long-term results can be expected (Table 16.4).

Table 16.4 Tarsal fractures

Special features	Rare
Diagnostic process	AP and lateral x-rays of the hindfoot With suspected fracture: CT + 3D reconstructions Alternatively, MRI with reconstructions in toddlers
Treatment goals/limits of correction	Restoration of joint surfaces and foot axes
Primary treatment	Short leg plaster splint, medical analgesia as needed
Conservative treatment	
Indication	Usually conservative if there is no displacement
Approach	6 weeks short leg cast, non-weight bearing
Follow up	Weight-bearing as tolerated after cast removal Insoles as needed
Control X-rays	Consolidation check at 6 weeks (no cast)
Return to sports	Approximately 6 weeks after consolidation
Operative treatment	
Indication	Displaced fractures; dislocations of the Chopart joint (Fig. 16.20) or Lisfranc joints (Fig. 16.21)
Approach	Closed reduction and percutaneous K-wire transfixion Instability: Open reduction and screw or K-wire fixation In soft-tissue injuries: Temporary transfixion for 2–3 weeks Key fragment: Stabilization of the second metatarsal basal fracture

Table 16.4 (continued)

Follow up	6 weeks non-weight-bearing After cast removal, weight-bearing as tolerated Physical therapy is generally not necessary; insoles as needed
Control X-rays	Postoperative reduction control; consolidation check at 6 weeks (no cast)
Hardware removal	Transfixion wires at 4 weeks
Return to sports	Approximately 6 weeks after consolidation
Complications	Premature osteoarthritis Changes in foot dynamics Compartment syndrome
Growth disturbance	Little data available
Follow up	Weekly, until unlimited function and full weight-bearing

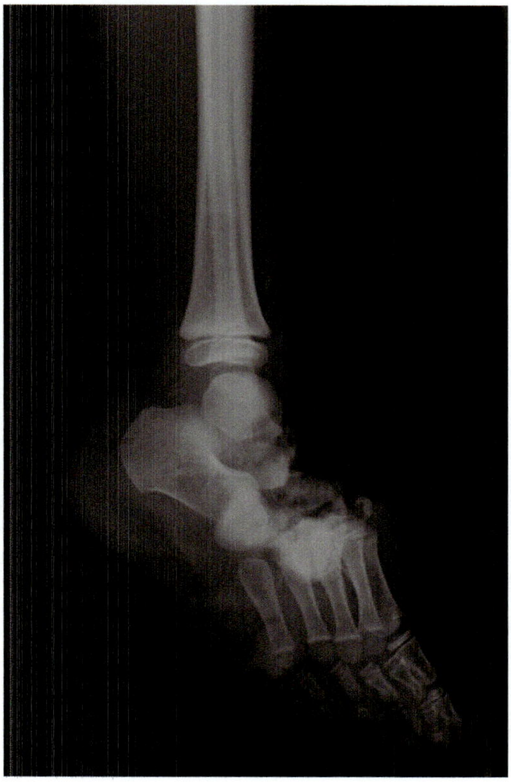

Fig. 16.20 Chopart luxation in a child

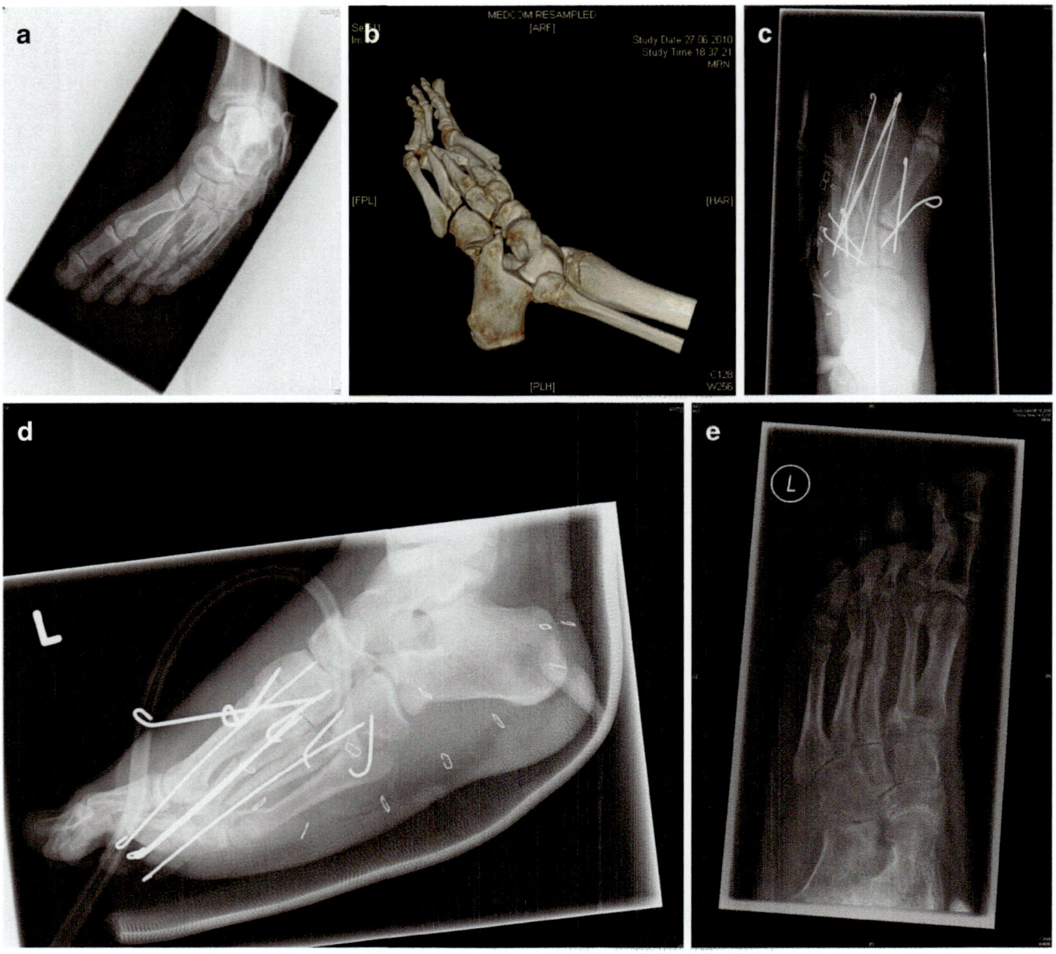

Fig. 16.21 Over-roll trauma with a stapler of a 15 year old boy. third degree open fractures of the hindfoot with subluxation of the Chopart and luxation fractures of the Lisfranc joints, calcaneus fracture and fractures of the Ossa cuneiforme laterale and intermedius as well as fractures of the metatarsal bones 2–4. (**a**) Xray of the foot, (**b**) CT 3D reconstruction, (**c**, **d**) Open reduction and stabilization with K-wires. (**e**) Healing after metal removal

16.6 Metarsal and Phalangeal Injuries

Metatarsal Fractures With an incidence of 4%, these account for up to 90% of all foot fractures in the literature. The majority of cases are subcapital fractures with slight displacement (Table 16.5). Conservative treatment is usually sufficient, even in small children when there is significant displacement. However, in the case of serial fractures, we recommend percutaneous axial K-wire transfixion because of instability. The first metatarsal is most commonly injured in children under ten years of age. In children over ten years, a fracture of the fifth metatarsal base is most prevalent. The typical mechanism of injury is supination trauma. Basal fractures of the fifth metatarsal run transversely. In contrast, apophyseal fractures run longitudinally and generally do not require further intervention (Figs. 16.22 and 16.23).

Toe and Phalangeal Fractures Along with metatarsal fractures, these are most common. The big toe is usually affected. These are typically basal epiphyseal separations and compression fractures. Shaft fractures can generally be treated conservatively through immobilization (with tape). On the other hand, intraarticular fractures and epiphyseal separations can lead to growth disturbances and premature osteoarthritis, and should be reduced when there is significant angulation, with K-wire fixation if necessary. Fractures of the phalanges can be observed after direct trauma (Table 16.6).

Fractures of the foot are usually treated conservative, or with closed reduction and with percutaneous K-wires. Instable fractures can be addressed by lag screws and plate osteoynthesis is rare, mostly on calcaneus fractures. Large soft tissue injuries or compartment syndromes might be addressed with an external fixateur (Table 16.7).

Table 16.5 Metatarsal fractures

Special features	Individual fractures through direct trauma Serial fractures from rollover trauma, wheel spoke injuries <10 years: mostly MT I; >10 years mostly MT V
Diagnostic process	AP, lateral and true lateral foot x-rays
Treatment goals/limits of correction	Length preservation; preservation of longitudinal and transverse arches No rotation deformity; no dorsal/plantar axis deformity
Primary treatment	Short leg plaster splint, medical analgesia as needed
Conservative treatment	
Indication	Usually conservative (Fig. 16.24) Mildly displaced shaft fractures Nondisplaced epiphyseal fractures
Approach	Approximately 4–5 weeks short leg cast, walking cast at 2–3 weeks Diaphyseal: 3–5 weeks; metaphyseal: 3 weeks
Follow up	Weight-bearing as tolerated after cast removal Insoles as needed
Control X-rays	Position control at one week; consolidation check at 4 weeks (no cast)
Return to sports	Approximately 4 weeks after consolidation
Operative treatment	
Indication	Displaced fractures
Approach	MT V base: Open reduction and tension-band fixation (Fig. 16.25) Closed reduction, or as needed open reduction and percutaneous K-wire transfixion (Figs. 16.26 and 16.27) If suitable, additional screws in adolescents Transfixation of the metacarpal bones and cast (Fig. 16.28).
Follow up	4 weeks non-weight-bearing; short leg cast/weight-bearing as tolerated after cast removal Physical therapy is generally not necessary; insoles as needed
Control X-rays	Postoperative reduction control; consolidation check at 4 weeks (no cast) MT V: Consolidation is radiologically evident only after a delay
Hardware removal	At 4 weeks (K-wire, tension-banding, screws)
Return to sports	Approximately 6 weeks after consolidation
Complications	Changes in foot dynamics/compartment syndrome/non-union (MT V)
Growth disturbance	Possible, but rare
Follow up	Every two weeks until unlimited function and full weight-bearing

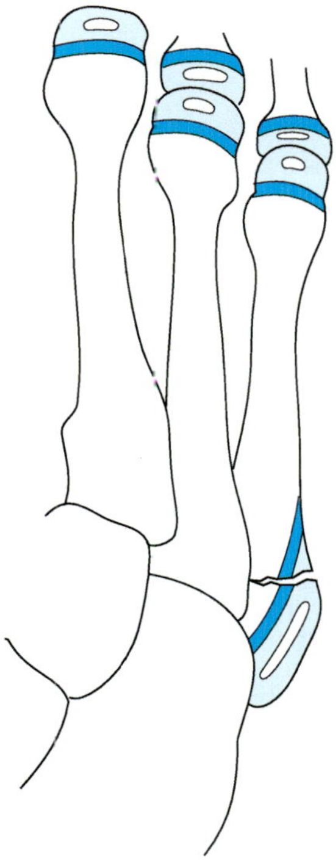

Fig. 16.22 MT V apophysis (longitudinal); differential diagnosis: basal fracture (transverse)

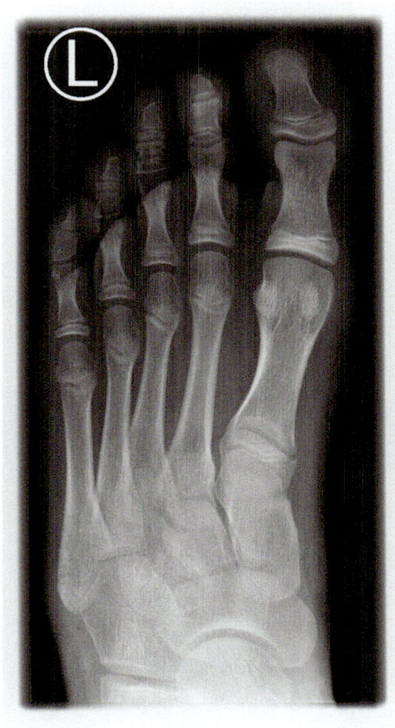

Fig. 16.24 Undisplaced fracture of the fifth metatarsal bone

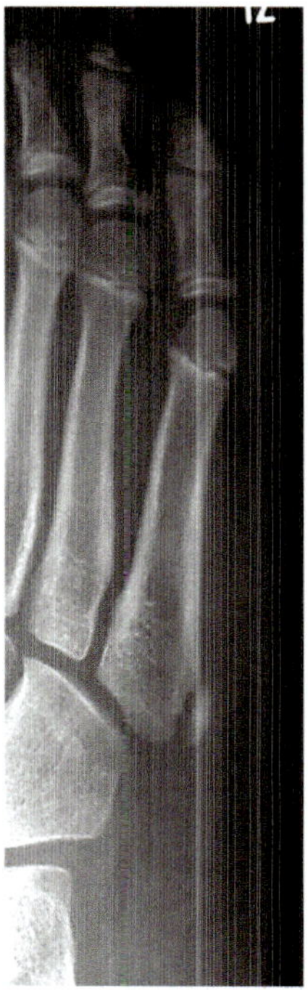

Fig. 16.23 Apophyseal fracture MT V (ten years of age)

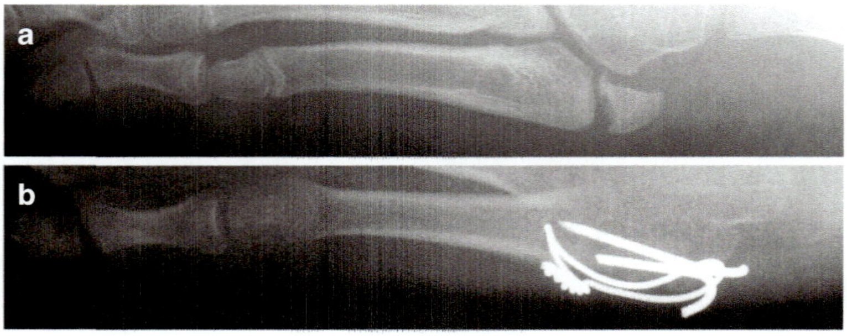

Fig. 16.25 Tension band fixation of a basal MT V fracture. (**a**) Trauma image, (**b**) Tension bend wiring

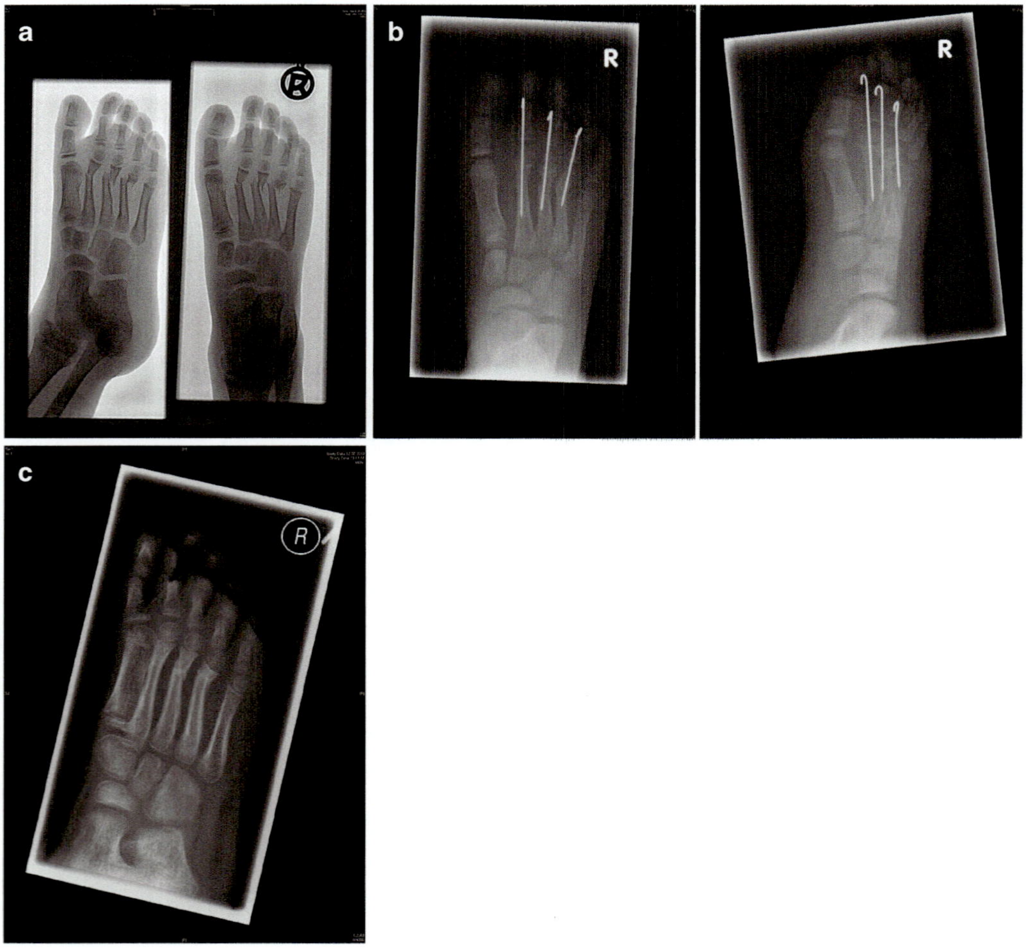

Fig. 16.26 Subkapital fractures of the second to fourth Metatarsal bones distally. (**a**) Trauma image, (**b**) Retrograde fixation with K-wires, (**c**) X-ray of consolidation after metal removal

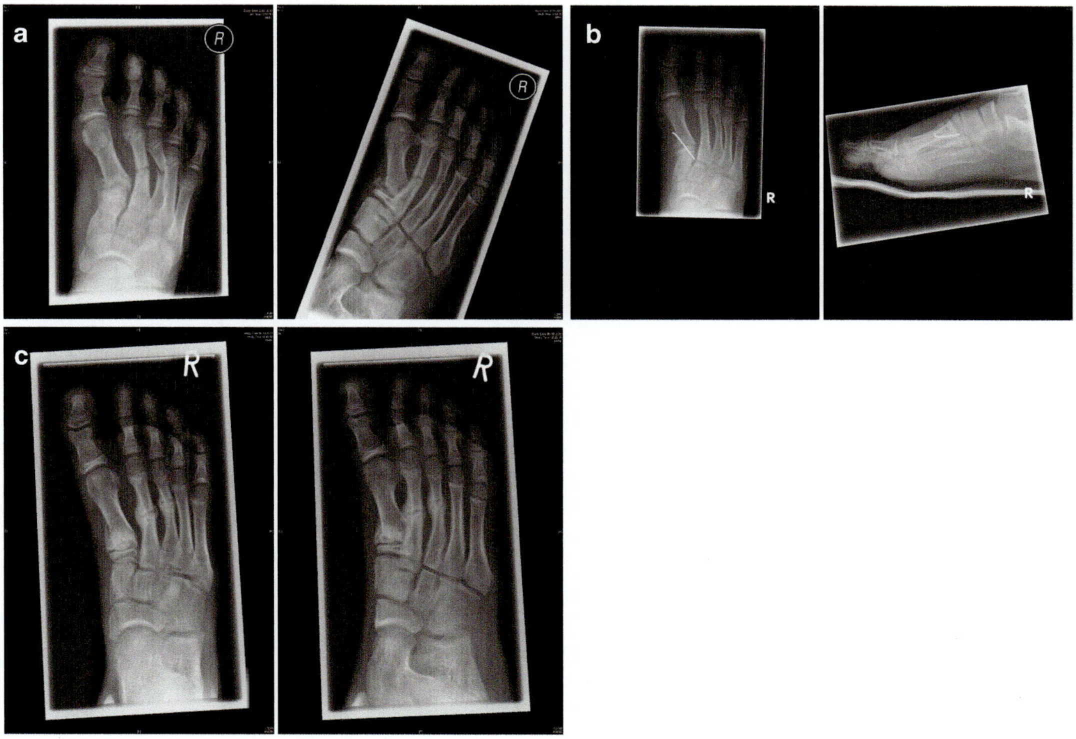

Fig. 16.27 Displaced fracture of the first metatarsalo bone (Salter-Harris II) and shaft fractures of the second and third metatarsal bone of a 12 year old boy after over-roll trauma by a car. (**a**) Trauma images, (**b**) Closed reduction and K-wire fixation, (**c**) X-ray of healing after metal removal

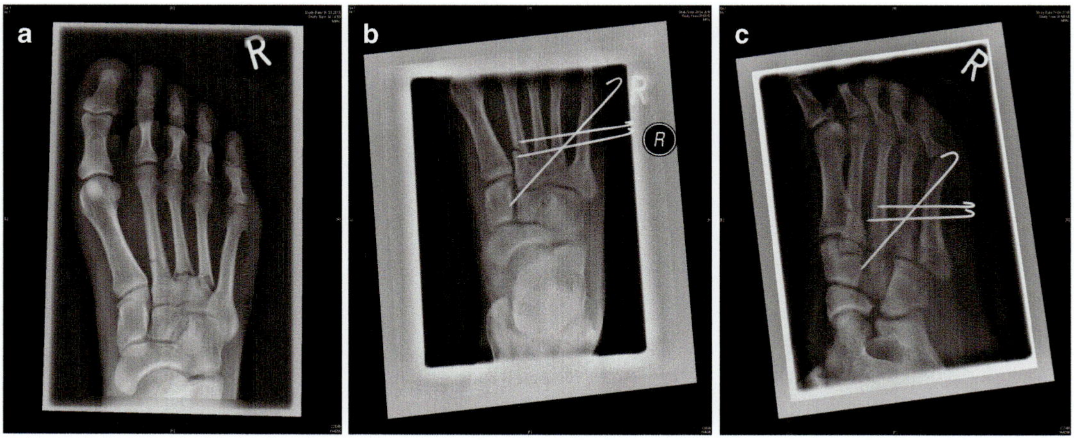

Fig. 16.28 Fractures near the basis of the second to fourth metatarsal bones after jump from 2 m in a 14 year old girl. (**a**) Trauma image, (**b**) Transfixation to the adjacent bones, (**c**) Consolidation of the fractures prior metal removal

Table 16.6 Phalanges fractures (Fig. 16.29)

Special features	Primarily direct trauma
Diagnostic process	AP and lateral x-rays of the forefoot and toes
Treatment goals/limits of correction	Length preservation Anatomical reduction
Primary treatment	Elastic bandage, as needed with short leg plaster splint, possibly medical analgesia
Conservative treatment	
Indication	Usually conservative (sometimes after closed reduction) (Fig. 16.30) Mildly displaced shaft fractures (Figs. 16.31 and 16.32). Nondisplaced epiphyseal fractures
Approach	Buddy toe bandaging or splinting; hard-soled shoe, If necessary, pain-related non-weight-bearing for 2 weeks If necessary, closed reduction with high block anesthesia
Follow up	After cast removal, weight-bearing as tolerated Physical therapy is generally not necessary
Control X-rays	Not necessary; clinical axis and functional checks
Return to sports	If pain-free, approximately 4 weeks after consolidation
Operative treatment	
Indication	Displaced fractures (>3 mm)
Approach	Closed reduction and percutaneous K-wire transfixion Basal and subcapital fractures: Crossed Shaft fractures: Intramedullary splinting
Follow up	3 weeks non-weight-bearing; plaster shoe if necessaryweight-bearing as tolerated after hardware removal
Control X-rays	Intraoperative or postoperative reduction control
Hardware removal	After 2–3 weeks transfixion wires
Return to sports	Approximately 4 weeks after consolidation
Complications	Changes in forefoot dynamics (hallux rigidus) Premature osteoarthritis
Growth disturbance	No reliable information
Follow up	Weekly, until unlimited function and full weight-bearing

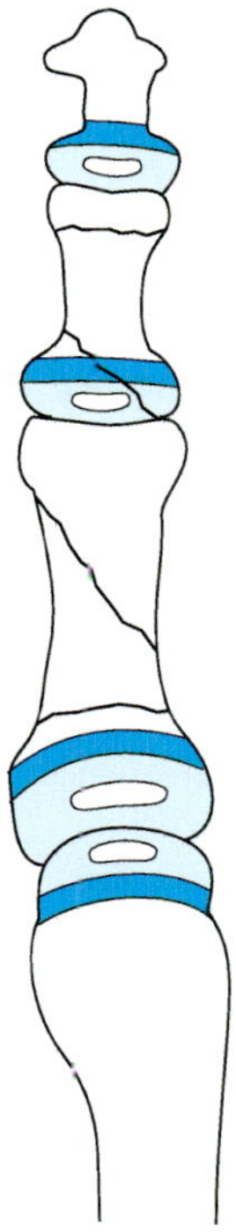

Fig. 16.29 Types of phalangeal fractures

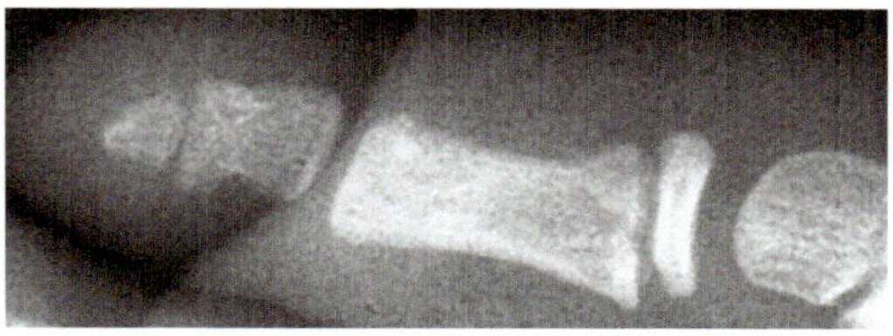

Fig. 16.30 Salter-Harris I fracture of the basis of the ground phalanx, conservative treatment

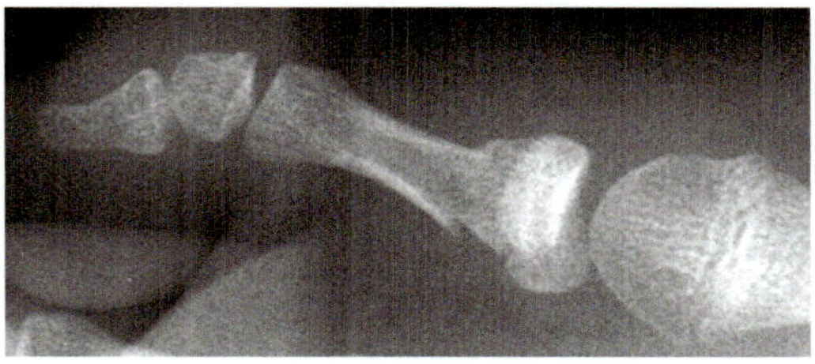

Fig. 16.31 Slightly displaced suprabasal fracture of the ground phalanx, conservative treatment

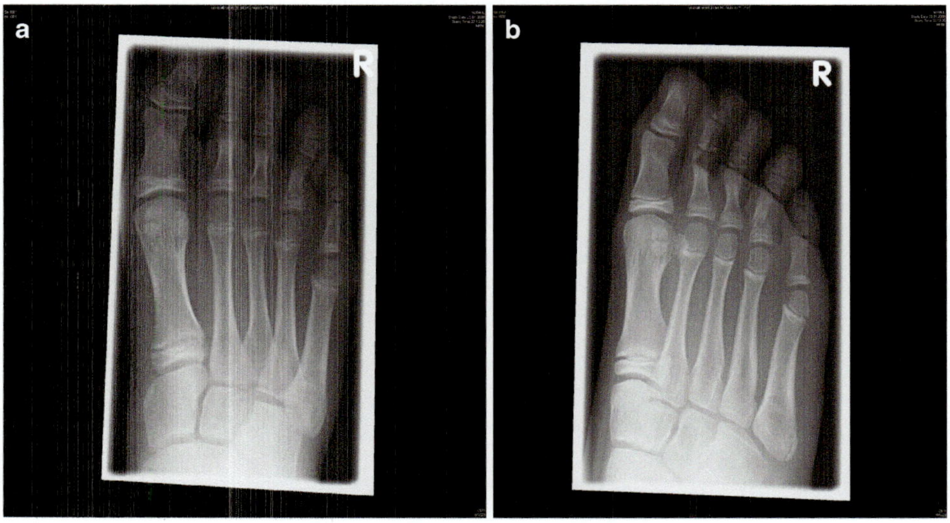

Fig. 16.32 Displaced fracture of the shaft of the fourth metatarsal bone. Conservative with a dressing, A.P. view and oblique view

Table 16.7 Technical aspects for the treatment of injuries to the foot

	General foot injuries
Positioning	Generally supine; tourniquet (optional) Draping to the knee joint; if necessary, with iliac crest
Approach	Hindfoot Caution regarding circulation: Approach as small as possible; preferably lateral(medial approach has greater risk of neurovascular injury) Medial approach: With direct screw fixation of the sustentaculum tali
Special clarification	Necrosis (especially tarsus) Premature osteoarthritis Compartment syndrome Tarsal fractures: Sensitive soft tissues → high risk of necrosis and infection Iliac crest cancellous bone graft only for very large defects (rare) An alternative is resorbable synthetic bone material Medial malleolar osteotomy only if unavoidable, if necessary for talar fracture
Hardware removal	Transfixion wires, percutaneous K-wires: 4 weeks post-surgery; outpatient Cannulated screws, flat anatomical plates: 6 months post-surgery
	Talus fracture
Material	Cannulated 3.5 mm screws, K-wires 1.6 mm
Approach	Lateral approach Medial approach only when inserting a screw into the sustentaculum tali (curved incision behind the medial malleolus; looping the neurovascular bundle)
Operative principle	Talus fracture Hawkins type I Closed reduction in plantar flexion, if needed via a stab incision Talus fracture Hawkins type II Bilateral approach Lag screws from medial and lateral via stab incision or central anterior longitudinal incision If necessary, anterior-posterior screw fixation via a posterolateral stab incision Talus fracture Hawkins type III Anteromedial approach (caution regarding vascular structures; deltoid ligament and protection of the soft-tissue connection between the talar neck and the navicular bone → risk of necrosis (Fig. 16.33) Insert screws parallel (otherwise blocking effect)
	Calcaneus fracture
Material	K-wires 1.6 mm Cannulated screws 3.5 mm Flat profile plate, if necessary fixed-angle (hand, foot set), titanium External fixator
Approach	Lateral approach (1 cm below the tip of the fibula; opening of the peroneal tendon sheath → lifting the peroneal tendons and the dorsal cutaneous nerve en bloc (Fig. 16.34)
Operative principle	K-wire fixation (Fig. 16.35) External fixator (Fig. 16.36) Reduction: If necessary, with a Steinmann nail inserted dorsolaterally and in the tibia for distraction
	Tarsal fractures
Material	K-wires 1.6–1.8 mm; mini screws (2.0–3.5 mm)
Approach	Dorsal, extensor side of the foot
Operative principle	Protection of the proximal and distal soft-tissue structures of the dorsal fragments Fixation with K-wires and 3.5 mm cannulated screws In cases of soft-tissue injuries: Talonavicular transfixion with 1.8 mm K-wires Cuboid fractures. Open reduction, lag screws as needed, cancellous bone graft as needed Transfixation with 2 K-wires (CC joint)
	Metatarsal fractures
Material	1.4–1.6 mm K-wires, mini-screws (2.0; 2.4) as needed
Approach	Dorsal, extensor side (Fig. 16.37)

Table 16.7 (continued)

	General foot injuries
Operative principle	Often closed reduction and percutaneous K-wire transfixion possible Open (impediment to reduction): Dorsal longitudinal incision K-wire fixation K-wire first threaded from the fracture into the distal fragment and pushed through the skin, then threaded retrograde into the proximal fragment (Fig. 16.38) Fixation with dorsal plate or crossed K-wires Serial fractures: Stabilization of the supporting pillars MT I and V Tension banding MT V basal fracture (Fig. 16.25) Lag screw Alternatively for basal MT V fracture at the start of growth plate fusion
	Toe fracture/dislocations
Material	Tape, brown plaster, K-wire 1.0 and 1.2 mm
Approach	Usually closed reduction
Treatment principle	Buddy taping for phalangeal fractures: Splint on the lateral toe in cases of primary varus angulation Splint on the medial toe in cases of primary valgus angulation Interdigital compress to avoid ulcers K-wire fixation Usually possible percutaneously (Fig. 16.39) Screws, rare 1.3 or 1.5 mm (Fig. 16.39)
	Lisfranc and Chopart dislocations
Approach	Closed reduction, if necessary open reduction with an approach over MT II and MT IV with K-wire transfixion of the Lisfranc joint Key area is the MT II and cuneiform bone II
	Compartment syndrome
Approach	Fasciotomy: Over two dorsal and one medial incisions Two parallel incisions over MT II and IV to the bone (leave sufficient skin bridge) One medial incision: Proximal MT I → dorsal heel Primary skin closure after approximately 6 days

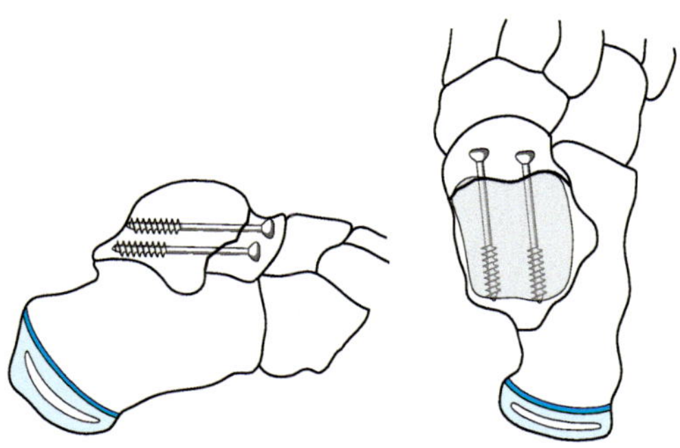

Fig. 16.33 Anteromedial screw fixation of the talus

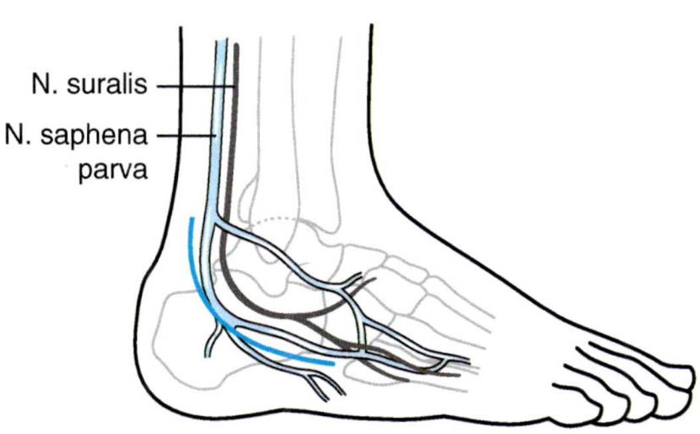

Fig. 16.34 Lateral approach to the hindfoot

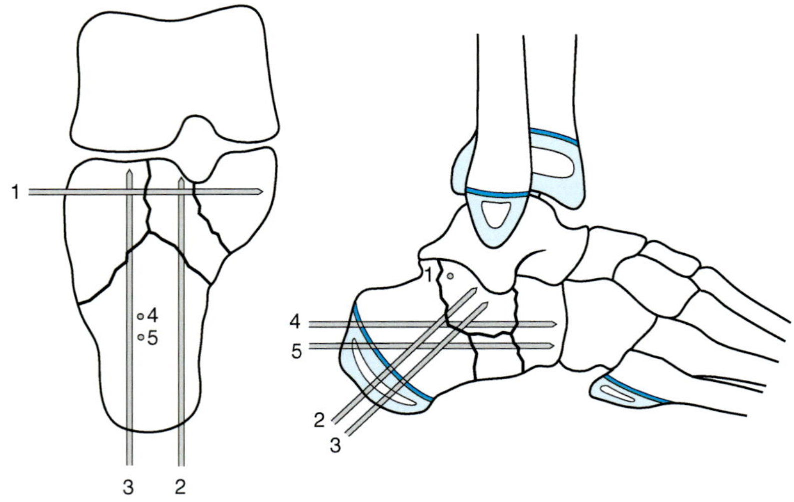

Fig. 16.35 K-wire fixation of the calcaneus

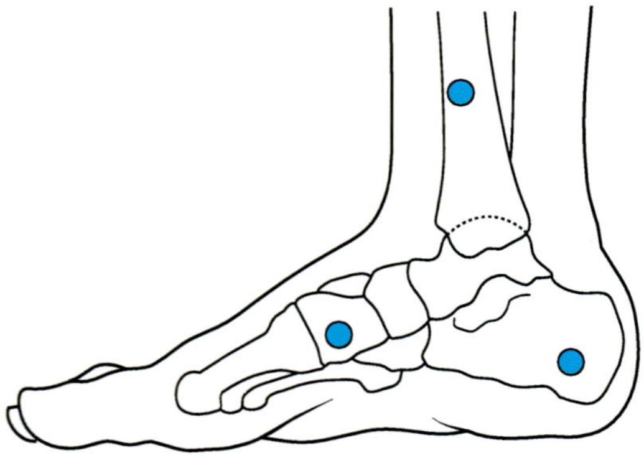

Fig. 16.36 Typical fixation points of an external fixator for calcaneus fracture

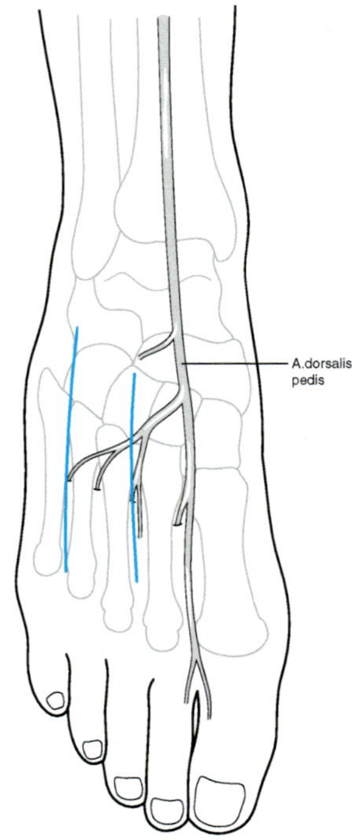

Fig. 16.37 Approach to the metatarsus

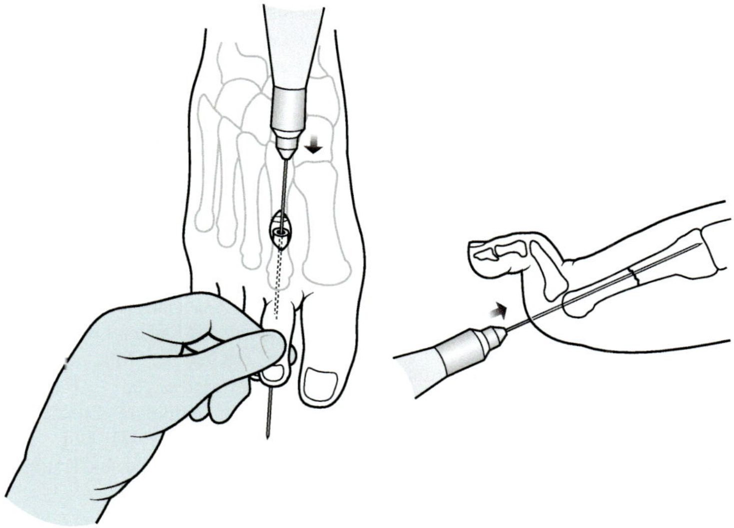

Fig. 16.38 Screws, K-wire fixation for a phalangeal fracture

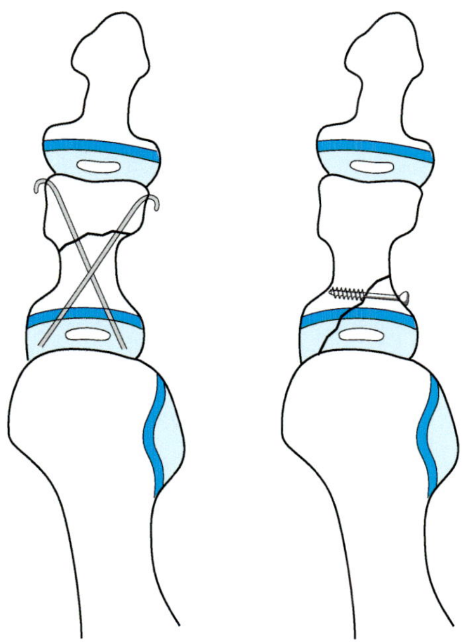

Fig. 16.39 Left side: K-wire fixation of a phalangeal shaft fracture, Right side: Screw fixation of a metaphyseal fracture

Recommended Literature

Ali-Asgar N, Alifyah N, Krishna V (2020) Paediatric calcaneal fractures: a guide to management based on a review of the literature. INJ 51:1432–1438

Babst R, Simmen BR, Regazzoni P (1989) Klinische Bedeutung und ein Behandlungskonzept der Lisfrancluxation und Luxationsfraktur. Helv Chir Acta 56:603–607

Crawford AH (1993) Fractures and dislocations of the foot and ankle. In: Green NE (ed) Skeletal trauma in children. Saunders, Philadelphia

Dudda M, Kruppa C, Geßmann J, Seybold D, Schildhauer TA (2013) Pediatric and adolescent intra-articular fractures of the calcaneus. Orthop Rev 5:82–85

Hawkins LG (1970) Fractures of the neck of the talus. JBJS Am 52:991–1002

Jaime RD, Charles TM (2019 Aug) The community orthopaedic surgeon taking trauma call: pediatric foot fracture pearls and pitfalls. J Orthop Trauma 33(Suppl 8):S27–S32

Prasad KSRK, Vali H, Hussain A (2013) Hawkins group I fracture of neck of talus and salter Harris type III tibial epiphyseal injury of medial malleolus. Foot (Edinb) 23:96–99

Rammelt S, Schneiders W, Fitze G, Zwipp H (2013) Foot and ankle fractures in children. Orthopade 42:45–54

Thermann H, Schratt HE, Hüfner T, Tscherne H (1998) Die Frakturen des kindlichen Fußes. Unfallchirurg 101:2–11

Tong L, Li M, Li F, Xu J, Hu T (2018) A minimally invasive (sinus tarsi) approach with percutaneous K-wires fixation for intra-articular calcaneal fractures in children. J Pediatric Orthop B 27:556–562

Veijola K, Laine H-J, Pajulo O (2013) Lisfranc injury in adolescents. Euro J Pediatr Surg: Official Journal of Austrian Association of Pediatric Surgery [et al] = Zeitschrift für Kinderchirurgie 23:297–303

Weber C, Klos K, Mückley T, Knobe M (2018) Rückfußverletzungen – Frakturen von Kalkaneus, Talus und peritalare Luxationen. Orthopädie und Unfallchirurgie 13:471–498

Zwipp H (2009) Foot injuries. Trauma und Berufskrankheit 11:249–260

Zwipp H, Rammelt S, Amlang M, Pompach M, Dürr C (2013) Operative treatment of central talar fractures. Oper Orthop Traumatol 25:554–568

Zwipp H, Rammelt S, Rammelt PDS (2014) Unfallchirurgie: Fuß. Springer, Berlin

Pelvis

17

17.1 Physiological Findings and Classifications

The pelvis of the child consists of multiple growth regions. Since the latter are equivalent to the epiphyses of the long bones, interpretation of secondary ossification in contrast to traumatic lesions might be difficult. Three primary growth centers namely the ileum, ischium, and pubis configurate the hip joint creating the Y-shaped triradiate cartilage (Fig. 17.1). Secondary growth centers are apophyses of the iliac crest, the anterior superior and inferior iliac spines as well as the ischial tuberosity (Fig. 17.2). The joint between the ischium and the pubis closes around the third year of life, and the triradiate cartilage between 12 and 14 in girls and between 14 and 16 years in boys. Traumatic injury to the triradiate cartilage especially in younger children may cause secondary deformity of the acetabulum up to complete hypoplasia of the hemipelvis.

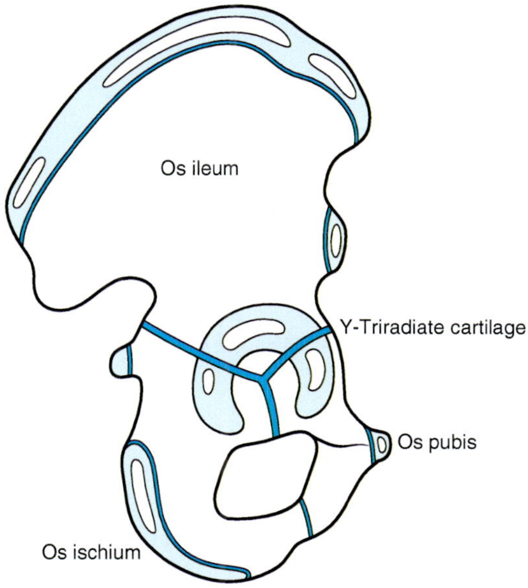

Fig. 17.1 Triradiate cartilage and primary growth centers

Epiphyseal-like growth areas are present at the ischiopubic and symphysis pubic bone. Widening of the symphysis region may substantially vary during growth. Thereby in children under 10 years of age, interpretation of width should be taken with caution. In older children adequate trauma and pain in the symphyseal region must be adequately diagnosed and substantial injury or instability excluded.

I. Marzi et al., *Pediatric Skeletal Trauma*, https://doi.org/10.1007/978-3-030-93685-3_17

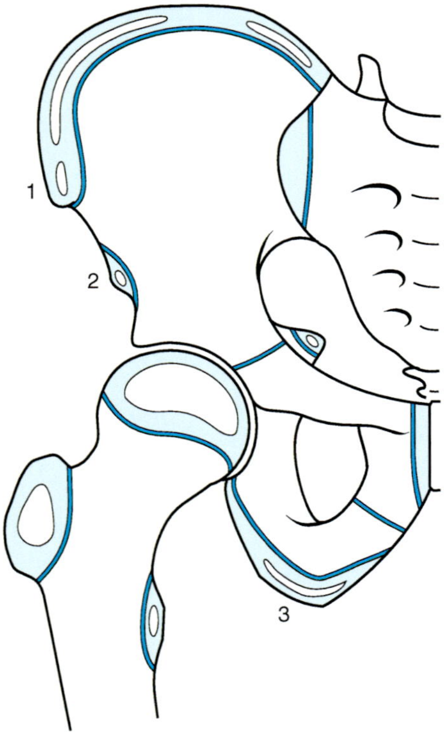

Fig. 17.2 Apophyses (secondary growth centers): (1) Anterior superior iliac spine, (2) Anterior inferior iliac spine, (3) Ischial tuberosity

The apophyseal ischial tuberosity may present quite irregular until adolescence and interpretation of radiological findings could be difficult, as well as the anterosuperior and anteroinferior apophysis of the iliac crest, which both appear between 13 and 15 years and fuse between 20–25 and 16–18 years may cause diagnostic problems, respectively. Apophyseal avulsion fractures are typically seen only in adolescents.

The thick periosteal coverage on the pediatric pelvic bones results in a very fast callus formation and might in some cases prevent bony displacement. Moreover, the combination of strong ligaments and multiple cartilaginous growth centers produce a high pelvic elasticity which reasonably absorbs and neutralizes external forces without producing classical fractures. In fact, substantial traumatic deformation with anatomical restoration of both the large cartilaginous areas and chondro-osseous interfaces might occur and distinguishes the pediatric pelvis from the osseous and ligamentous traumatic lesions of the adult. As a consequence of these anatomical features, injuries to the cartilaginous areas can be missed on radiological examinations. Unlike in adults, the elasticity of the hemi-pelvis joints enables isolated ring fracture formation, even in cases of considerable deformity resulting in a higher risk for accompanying organ injuries in especially of the bladder, urethra, rectum or even gynecologic organs.

Age-Dependent X-Ray Findings (Figs. 17.3, 17.4, and 17.5)

- Width of symphysis and sacroiliac joint varies considerably during growth
- Three primary growth centers are already evident in infants

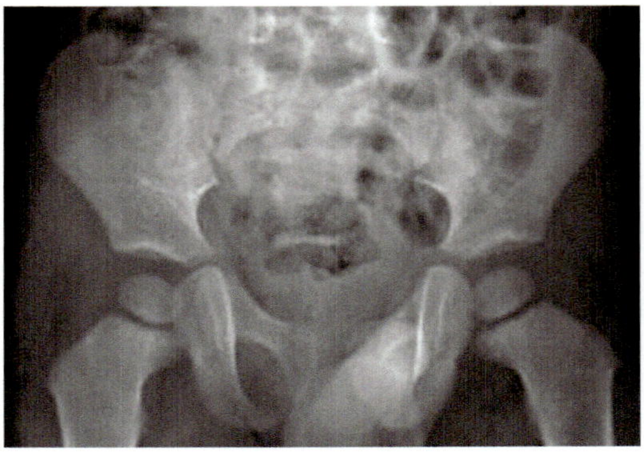

Fig. 17.3 Pelvic X-ray: 2-year-old boy. The primary growth centers and the triradiate cartilage are clearly visible

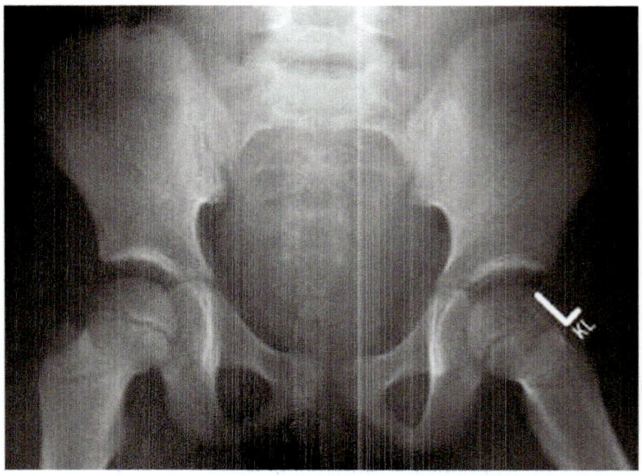

Fig. 17.4 Pelvic X-ray: 6-year-old boy. The gaps between the ischium and the pubis are closed

- The gap between the ischium and pubis closes between ages four and seven
- The triradiate cartilage is detectable until ages 12–16
- The apophyseal centers (secondary growth centers) appear between 12 and 17 years and fuse completely with the ilium between 20 and 25 year

Classification

Pelvic fractures in children, either of the pelvic ring or the acetabular region, are rare. However, the incidence might rise up to 4% Fractures of the growing pelvis may be classified by different aspects, e.g. anatomy, type of injury, instability, prognosis etc. Although, gross pelvic instability seems to be rare in children, clear decision making concerning the stability is necessary, since persistent instability causes deformity. Due to the crucial importance for walking and weight bearing anatomic "bony" restoration especially of the triradiate cartilage is of prognostic importance. So far, there is no clear definition of a specific age differentiating between a pediatric or an adult pelvic injury pattern. However, classification systems as used as in adults might adequately be used with increasing age and maturity of the bony regions during adolescence.

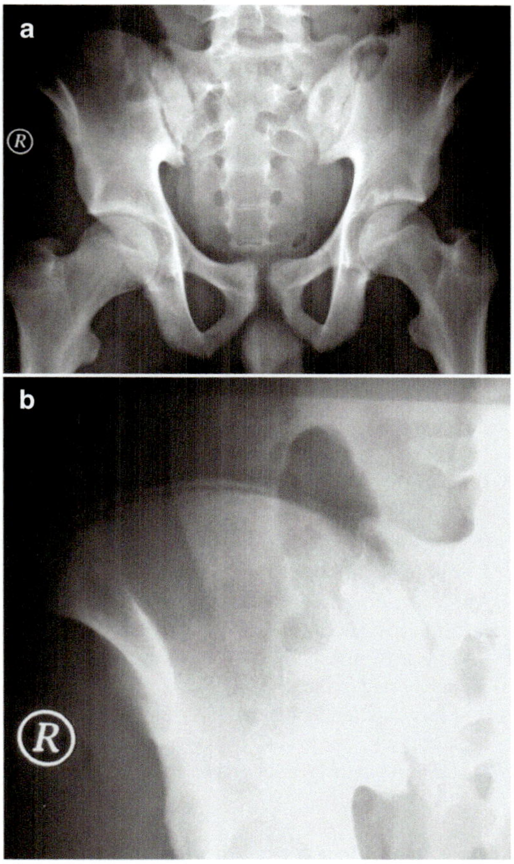

Fig. 17.5 (**a**, **b**) Pelvic X-ray: 16 year-old boy. The triradiate cartilage is closed, the apophyses are already recognizable

In this chapter we follow the common the AO Classification (see below), although there are several other classification systems which try to cope with the specific injury patterns in children. Nevertheless, a precise classification might be

Table 17.1 Classification of pelvic fractures according to Key and Cornwell

1. Fracture without interruption of the pelvic ring
(a) Avulsion Fracture
(I) Anterior Superior Iliac Spine (ASIS)
(II) Anterior Inferior Iliac Spine (AIIS)
(III) Ischial Tuberosity
(b) Fracture of the Ischium or Pubic bone
(c) Iliac Wing Fractures
(d) Sacrum or Coccyx Fractures
2. Simple Pelvic Ring Disruption
(a) Fracture of two ipsilateral rami
(b) Pubic symphysis rupture or fracture near the symphysis
(c) Sacroiliac joint (SIJ) rupture or fracture near the SIJ
3. Double Ring Fracture
(a) Bilateral Ischium and Pubis fractures
(b) Fracture of the anterior and posterior pelvic ring
(c) Multiple Fractures
4. Acetabular Fractures
(a) Hip dislocation with small acetabular rim fracture
(b) Linear fracture combined with non-displaced pelvic ring fracture
(c) Linear fracture combined with hip joint instability
(d) Central hip dislocation fracture

Table 17.2 von Laer classification of pelvic injuries

Lesions without serious consequences	Lesions with possible serious consequences
Apophyseal Avulsions Iliac Wing Fractures Isolated Ileum Fractures Isolated Pubic Fractures Isolated Sacroiliac Joint loosening	Pubic Symphysis Ruptures Malgaigne Fractures Acetabular Fractures

Table 17.3 Classification of pelvic fractures according to Torode and Zeig

– Type 1. Avulsion Fractures
– Type 2. Iliac Wing Fractures
– Type 3. Simple pelvic ring fractures with symphysis diastasis and without rupture of the posterior SIJ
– Type 4. All fractures producing a free bony fragment

Table 17.4 Classification of complications in children after pelvic fractures

– Grade 1. None
– Grade 2. Potentially impaired growth with secondary remodeling
– Grade 3. Potentially delayed fracture healing
– Grade 4. Nonunion, malunion, damage to the triradiate cartilage, SIJ fusion and leg length variation

difficult in children for pelvic ring and acetabular fractures.

Key and Cornwell specified the following fracture-oriented classification (Table 17.1).

Von Laer classified fractures as those without consequences and those expected to heal with grave consequences (Table 17.2).

Various other classifications have been introduced to account specifically for pediatric injuries like Torode and Zeig who have developed the following system based on the Watts classification (Table 17.3).

In addition, the same authors also suggested a classification of complications (Table 17.4).

We present the pediatric pelvic lesions in the following order: (1) Avulsion injuries, (2) Pelvic rim and pelvic ring fractures, (3) Acetabular fractures

17.2 Avulsion Injuries (Apophyseal Avulsion Fractures)

Incidence, Mechanism of Injury and Clinical Picture

Avulsion injuries are rare. They account for 4–13.4% of all pediatric pelvis fractures. Some authors have found avulsion of the anterior inferior iliac spine (AIIS) to be most common, and others of the anterior superior iliac spine (ASIS).

Avulsion fractures occur mainly in young athletes aged 12–16 years. Overloading the muscles attached to the apophyses during sport activities leads to avulsion of the growth center from the pelvis. According to the AO classification, these pelvic injuries could be classified as AO type A1 lesions since the ventral and dorsal pelvic rings are intact.

Avulsion of the Anterior Superior Iliac Spine (ASIS)

Cause. Overload from traction of the sartorius muscle with extended hip and flexed knee. Occurs mainly in athletes.

Symptoms. Local swelling and pain after athletic loading.

Avulsion of the Anterior Inferior Iliac Spine (AIIS)

Cause. Traction of the rectus femoris muscle with hyperextension of the hip and flexion of the knee, predominantly while playing football (soccer) (Fig. 17.6).

Symptoms. Localized pain and swelling after football play.

Avulsion of the Ischial Tuberosity

Cause. Overload of the hamstring muscles through abduction of the leg with the flexed hip and extended knee, predominantly while performing gymnastic exercises (Fig. 17.7).

Symptoms. Pain when sitting, local tenderness on digital rectal examination. Bony consolidation might produce excessive callus formation ("tumor").

Table 17.5 gives an overview of the common avulsion injuries of the pelvis.

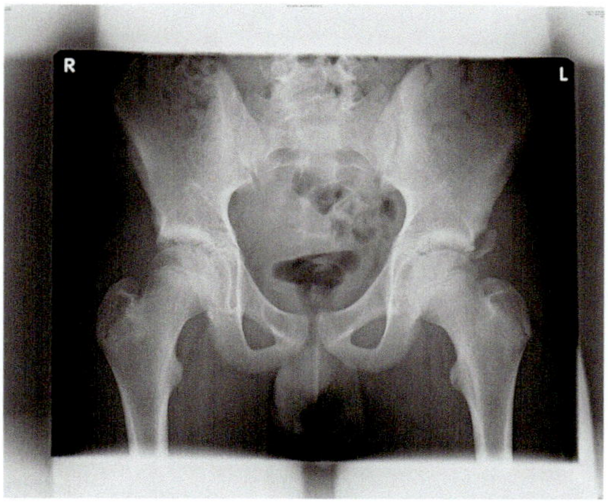

Fig. 17.6 Avulsion fracture of the Anterior Inferior Iliac Spine (AIIS) on the left side in a 14 year old boy

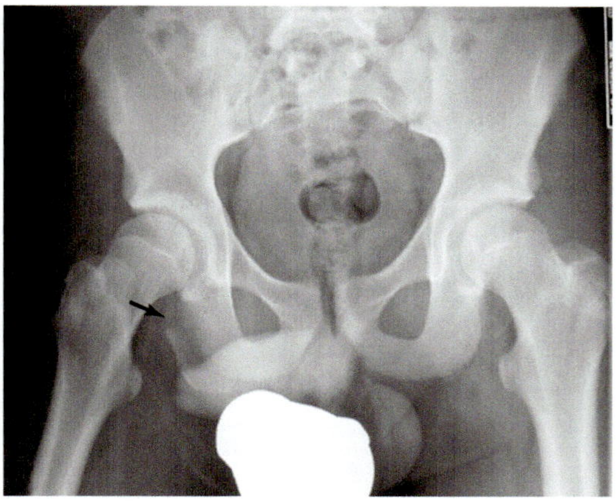

Fig. 17.7 Avulsion fracture of the ischial tuberosity on the right side

Table 17.5 Avulsion injuries (Fig. 17.8)

Particularities	Often first evidence by callus formation and sometimes misinterpreted as bony tumor, especially at the ischium
Diagnostic Assessment	Pelvic X-Ray, if necessary Ultrasound or MRI (Fig. 17.9)
Goals of Therapy/Limits of Correction	Lack of pain, ability to participate in sport activities, displacement less than 2–3 cm depending also on pain and disability (Fig. 17.10)
Primary Treatment	Pain therapy, bed rest, thromboprophylaxis depending on age, when possible functional treatment
Conservative therapy	
Indication	Standard
Procedure	Pain-adapted immobilization with flexed hip joint (extended for avulsion of the ischial tuberosity), followed by early functional therapy with partial load-bearing using underarm crutches for 2–4 weeks
Follow Up	Rapid load building
Radiographic Control	Only with persisting symptoms
Sports Participation	After 6–12 weeks
Operative therapy	
Indication	Rarely, only when grossly displaced fractures or large avulsion fragments, painful malunion or persisting functional impairment, large painful hematoma
Procedure	Reduction, single-screw fixation or tension banding; for non-unions, resection of the avulsed fragments
Follow Up	Short-term immobilization, gradual loading at 2–4 weeks
Radiographic Control	Only with persisting symptoms
Hardware Removal	Optional after 12 weeks
Sports Participation	After 12 weeks
Complications	Bony overgrowth, malunion, fixation failure
Growth Disturbances	No serious consequences should be expected
Follow-Up	Clinical wrap-up examination one year post-trauma, particularly in cases of excessive callus formation

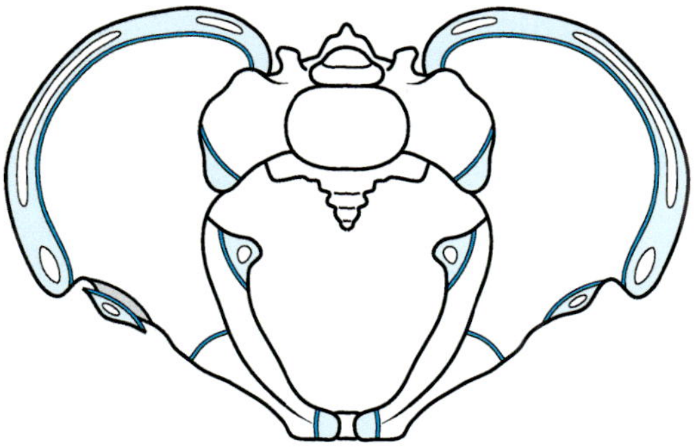

Fig. 17.8 Avulsion injuries of the pelvis

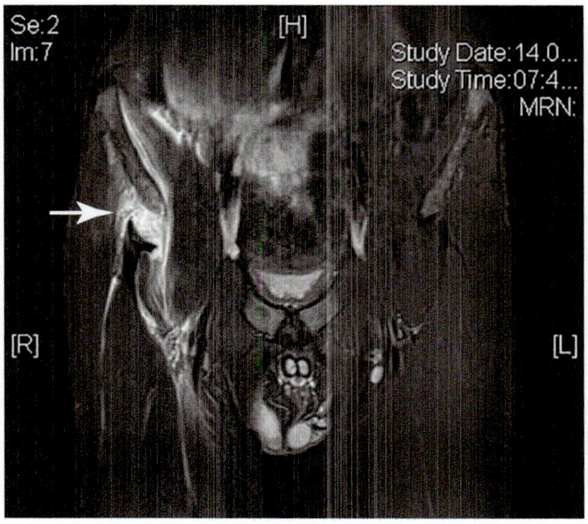

Fig. 17.9 Avulsion fracture of the tendon of the M rectus femoris from the AIIS in MRI of a 16 year old boy

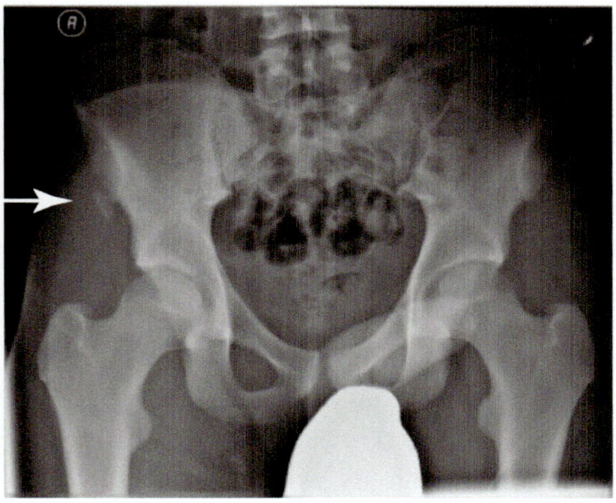

Fig. 17.10 Avulsion fracture of the Anterior Inferior Iliac Spine (AIIS) on the right side of a 15 year old boy

17.3 Pelvic Rim and Pelvic Ring Fractures

Incidence, Mechanism of Injury and Clinical Picture

Pelvic fractures in children result from considerable forces and associated injuries must always be expected and searched for. The most common causes are traffic accidents or falls from a height. A large proportion of these children succumb multiple injuries, and about 25% have additional traumatic brain injury depending on the study design. Pelvic fractures and lesions should be presumed in every child with multiple injuries and ruled out in any case.

Anterior pelvic ring fractures are caused by direct impact. Because of the elasticity and restoring forces, a considerable amount of energy must be assumed for the injury even in lightly displaced fractures, and thus, concomitant injuries, particularly of the genitourinary tract and the rectum, must be excluded. Subcutaneous degloving injuries may be initially largely unapparent due to the skin elasticity. Clinically, local swelling and pain are evident, especially when pressure is applied to the symphysis.

The simple pelvic ring fracture is an uncommon injury in children. Injuries of the pelvic ring are rare (2.7%) and only 10 % of the injuries are unstable. A prospective pelvic trauma registry analyzing 9684 patients found 1433 pelvic fractures in children. There is an increase with age comprising 6.6% up to an age of 5 years, 10.5% between 6 and 10 years and 15.3 between 11 and 14 years. In AO type C lesions hospital mortality rose up to 19.9%. Other studies showed that about half of the pelvic ring lesions are AO A-type fractures. The majority of pediatric fractures of the Ischium and Pubis (>90%) are stable and requires no surgical intervention.

Whereas in adults a variety of pelvic lesions may be classified as a single trauma mostly without further complications, the abovementioned mechanisms in the pediatric population need full attention to avoid complications. In any case, stable hemodynamics, stability of other vital functions and the assessment for organ and soft-tissue damage are of first priority. Fracture care has second-line priority.

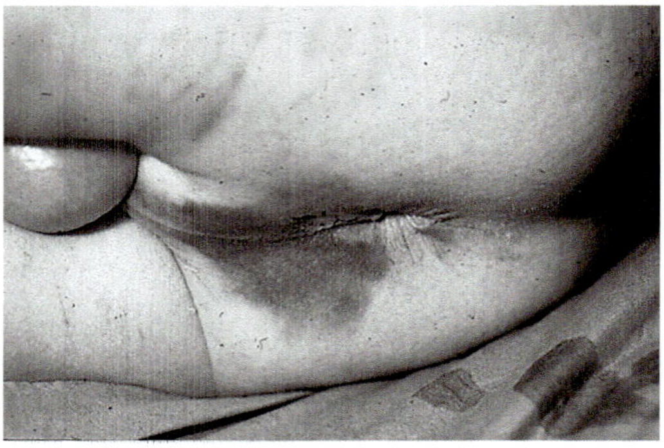

Fig. 17.11 Perianal hematoma with rectal lesion

Inspection of the pelvic region for open wounds and hematoma follows the examination for stability. A digital rectal examination is mandatory in anesthetized patients. Perianal hematoma formation is pathognomonic for rectal lesions (Fig. 17.11). Further clinical signs of pelvic fracture are: localized pain on pressure, formation of large superficial inguinal and scrotal hematoma (Destot sign), reduced distance between the greater trochanter and the pubic symphysis compared to the contralateral side in lateral compression fractures (Roux sign), and palpable fracture ends or hematoma formation on rectal examination (Earle sign). Bilateral pubic fractures are often associated with injuries to the genitourinary tract. A retrograde urethrogram is mandatory in these cases.

In general, a pelvic X-ray is indicated and still gold standard with a suspicious pelvic lesion. However, due the above-mentioned elasticity of the pediatric pelvis, hidden bony lesions and moreover lesions of the dorsal and acetabular elements cannot not be ruled out safely. A low-dose computerized scan is more and more frequently used also as a routine diagnostic tool and should be applied with any suspicion of a more complex contribution of the dorsal ring.

In case of multiple trauma the algorithm used in primary care and diagnosis for this group of patients has to be followed.

Classification

Basically, classifications differentiate stable and unstable fracture forms or fractures that heal without consequences versus those that heal with deformity.

Pediatric pelvic injuries are mainly classified using the adult systems, not least in order to achieve comparability. Around the age of 14 (closure of the triradiate cartilage), the fracture forms correspond to those of adults and are classified and treated according to adult surgical principles.

Nowadays, the frequent use of low dose computerized scans in both primary survey of pelvic injuries and severely injured children lead to a higher detection of lesions of the dorsal pelvic ring. As a consequence, a more precise classification of specific fracture patters also in children is possible.

The most commonly used classification, the AO (Arbeitsgemeinschaft für Osteosyntesefragen) Classification, is based on the Pennal and Tile Classification and categorizes stable A-type, partially (rotational) unstable B-type, and (vertically) unstable C-type injuries (Fig. 17.12).

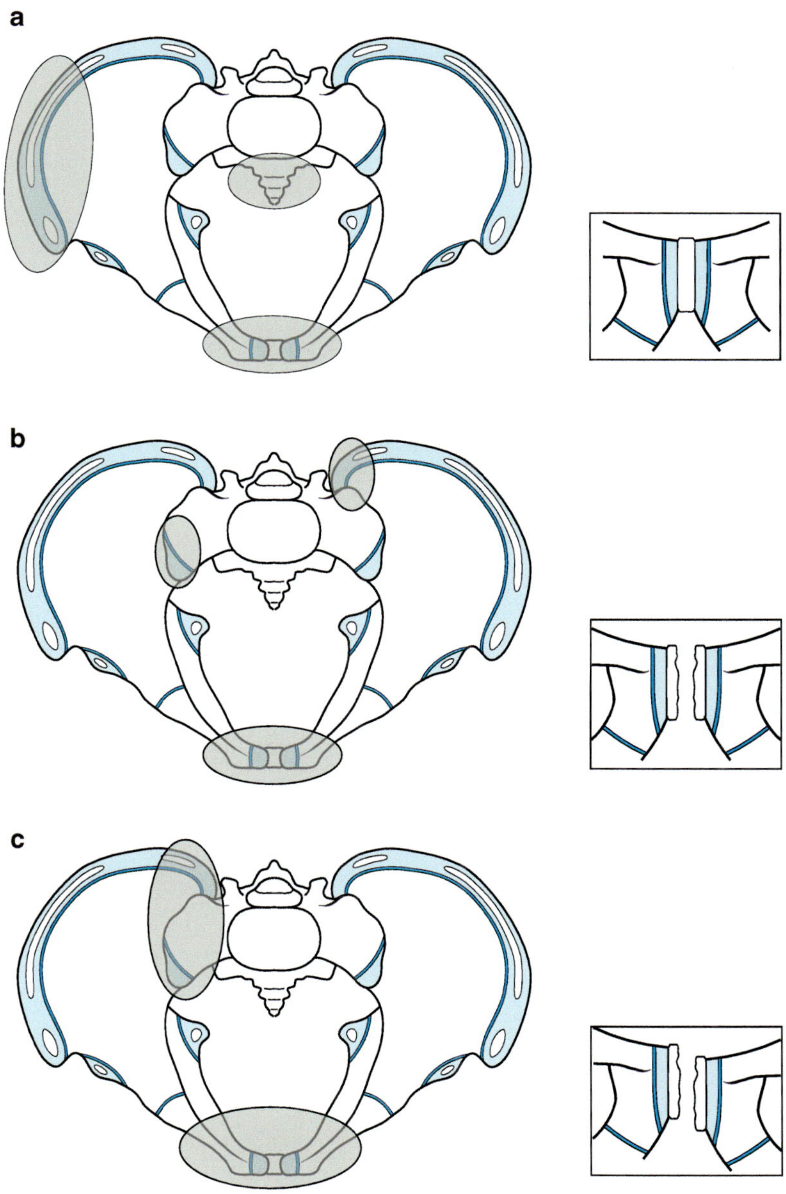

Fig. 17.12 Pennal and Tile classification of pelvic ring fractures. (**a**) type A, (**b**) type B, (**c**) type C

A-type pelvic fractures

The characteristics, diagnostic and treatment options for A-type pelvic fractures are shown in Table 17.6 pelvic rim, Table 17.7 anterior pelvic rim and Table 17.8 for symphysis ruptures.

Table 17.6 Pelvic rim fracture type A1 (Fig. 17.13)

Particularities	Dorsal and ventral pelvic ring stable, fractures of anterior iliac spine and pelvic crest, ischial tuberosity, mostly direct impact, combination with pelvic ring injuries possible
Diagnostic Assessment	Pelvic X-Ray or low dose CT (Fig. 17.14)
Goals of Therapy/Limits of Correction	No pain, sports participation, lack of cosmetic deformity
Primary Treatment	Pain therapy, bedrest, thromboprophylaxis
Conservative therapy	
Indication	Normal case
Procedure	Pain-adapted immobilization, then early functional therapy with crutch-assisted partial weight bearing 2–4 weeks
Follow Up	Rapid load building (Fig. 17.15)
Radiographic Control	Only with persisting symptoms
Sports Participation	After 6–12 weeks
Operative therapy	
Indication	Rare, for grossly displaced fractures
Procedure	Open reduction, single-screw fixation or K-wire fixation
Follow Up	Short-term immobilization, gradual loading at 4–6 weeks
Radiographic Control	Post-operative
Hardware Removal	Optional after 12 weeks
Sports Participation	After 12 weeks
Complications	Malunion, fixation failure, displacement from muscle tension, cosmetic deformity
Growth Disturbances	No serious consequences should be expected
Follow-Up	Clinical wrap-up examination one year post-trauma, particularly in cases of excessive callus formation
Classification	AO: A1

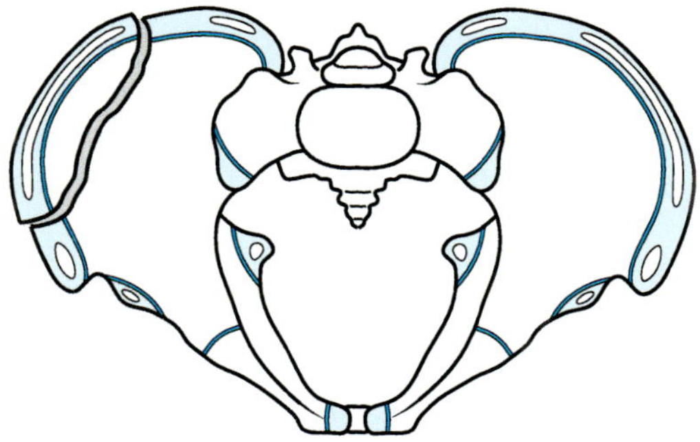

Fig. 17.13 Pelvic rim fracture, type A1

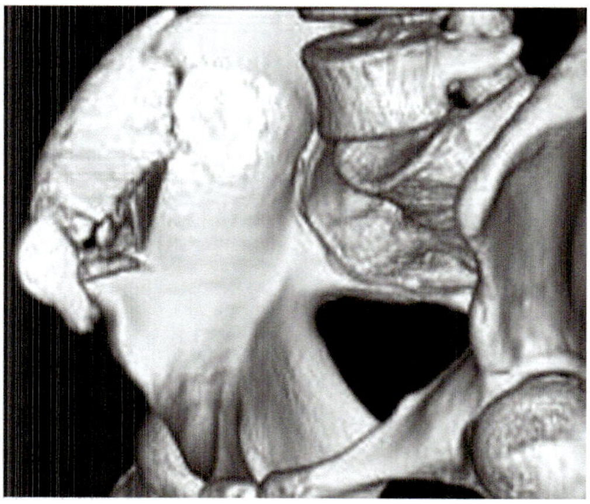

Fig. 17.14 Pelvic rim fracture of the iliac crest with moderate dislocation and contact. Conservative treatment

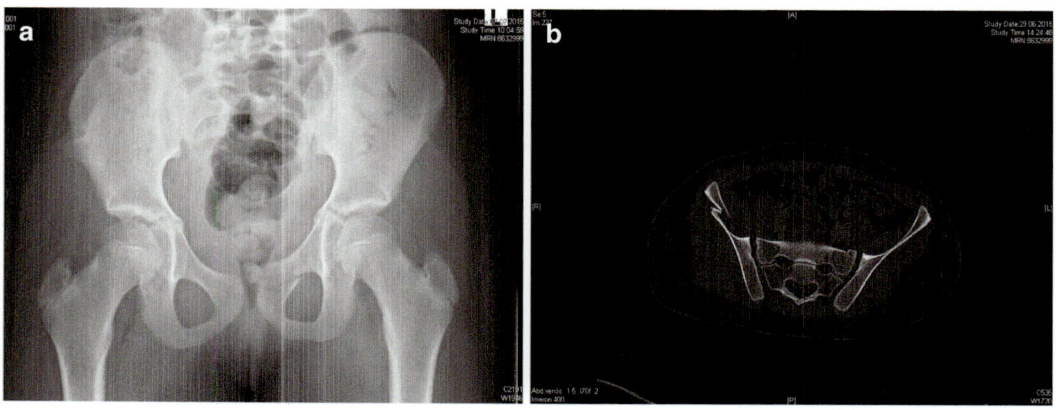

Fig. 17.15 Fracture of the ileum on the right side of a 11 year old girl after collision with a car on a roller; in addition liver laceration and lung contusion. (**a**) X-ray; (**b**) CT scan. Conservative treatment

Table 17.7 Anterior pelvic ring fracture type A2 (Fig. 17.16) (dorsal pelvic ring intact, fractures of ilium, single or bilateral transpubic fracture)

Particularities	Due to elasticity of the bony pelvis and especially the hemi-pelvis, "single-ring" injuries are possible in children despite considerable deformity.
Diagnostic Assessment	Clinical examination (concomitant injuries!); abdominal ultrasound, pelvic X-ray, CT, MRI
Goals of Therapy/Limits of Correction	Exclusion of concomitant injuries, ability to mobilize early
Primary Treatment	Bedrest, pain therapy, thromboprophylaxis
Conservative therapy	
Indication	Generally for closed fractures and moderate displacement (no open book situation) (Figs. 17.17 and 17.18)
Procedure	Pain-adapted immobilization (Fig. 17.19)
Follow Up	Early functional partial loading at 2–4 weeks, full load bearing at 6–8 weeks
Radiographic Control	Only with persisting symptoms
Sports Participation	After 12 weeks
Operative therapy	
Indication	Rare, with fracture displacement inflicting the bladder, with organ injury, or open fractures
Procedure	Reduction, possible periosteal suture, organ care
Follow Up	Short-term immobilization, gradual loading at 2–4 weeks
Radiographic Control	Only with persisting symptoms
Hardware Removal	Not necessary
Sports Participation	After 12 weeks
Complications	Secondary uterine or bladder injury; re-displacement
Growth Disturbances	No serious consequences should be expected
Follow-Up	Clinical wrap-up examination one year post-trauma

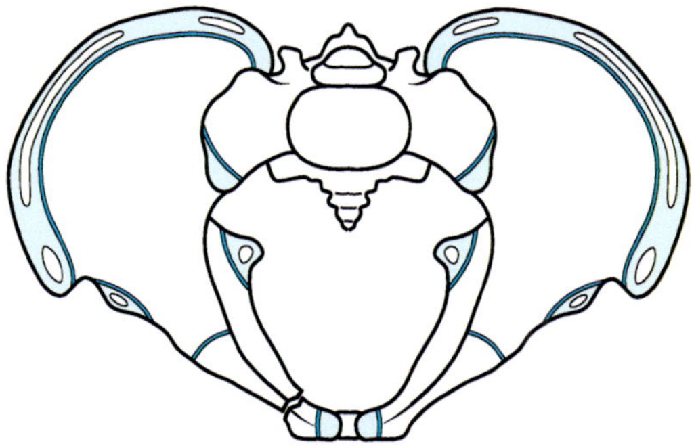

Fig. 17.16 Anterior pelvic ring fracture type A2

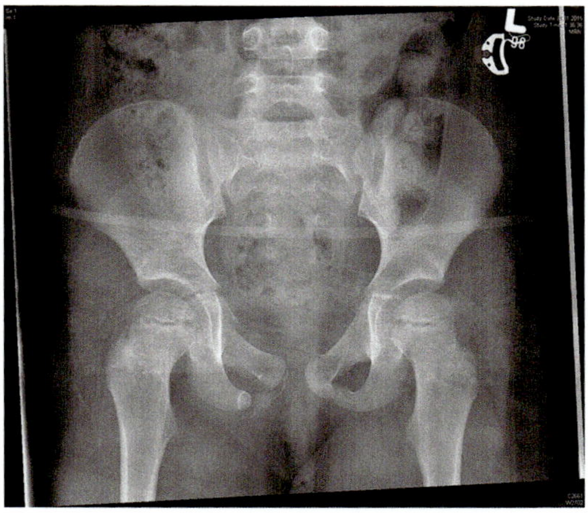

Fig. 17.17 Anterior pelvic ring fracture with bony and periosteal tears in a 4 year old girl; type A2

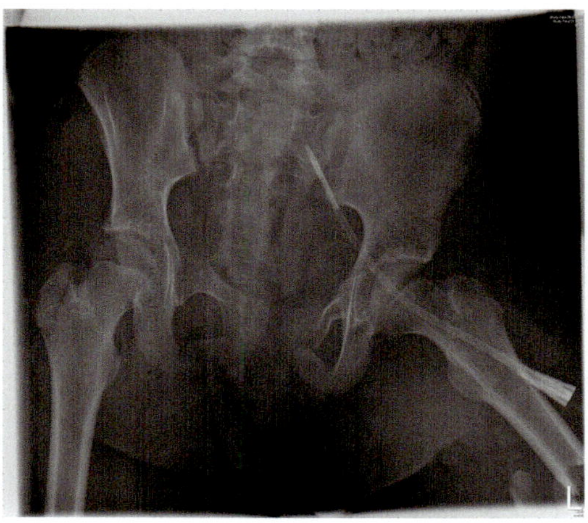

Fig. 17.18 Displaced bilateral anterior pelvic ring fracture in a 13 year old girl, type A2

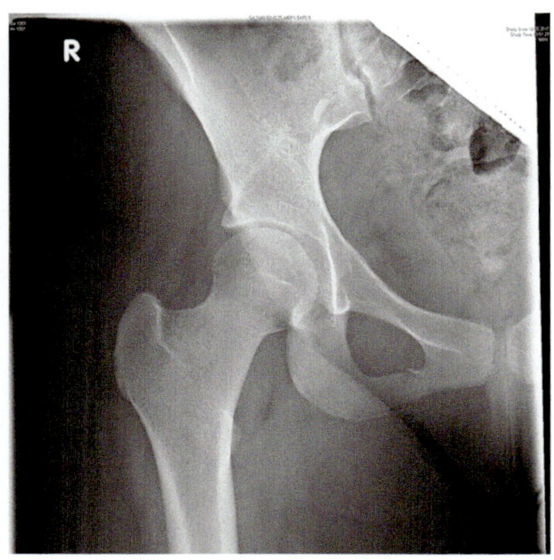

Fig. 17.19 Undisplaced fracture of the os ischiii right side in a 13 year old girl

Table 17.8 Isolated symphysis rupture (Fig. 17.20)

Particularities	Mostly bony rupture due to ligament laxity; symphysis gap is age-dependent enlarged, AO A type lesion if dorsal structures are intact, B type with dorsal structures associated
Diagnostic Assessment	Clinical examinations (concomitant injuries!); abdominal ultrasound, pelvic X-ray, CT, MRI (Fig. 17.21)
Goals of Therapy/Limits of Correction	Exclusion of concomitant injuries, displacement <1 cm (age-dependent)
Primary Treatment	Bedrest, pain therapy, thromboprophylaxis
Conservative therapy	
Indication	In general, for closed fractures, displacement <1 cm
Procedure	Pain-adapted immobilization, with displaced ruptures in a crossed sling
Follow Up	Partial load bearing at 3–4 weeks, full load bearing at 6–8 weeks
Radiographic Control	Within the first 5 days to control adequate reduction, longer only if symptoms persist
Sports Participation	After 12 weeks
Operative therapy	
Indication	Rare, with ruptures displaced more than 2 cm, with organ injuries or open fractures
Procedure	Closed or open reduction, possible periosteal suture with tension banding or plate fixation if necessary while organ injuries are treated
Follow Up	Bedrest, gradual loading at 3–4 weeks
Radiographic Control	Post-operatively, then only with persisting symptoms
Hardware Removal	At 3–6 months
Sports Participation	After approximately 12 weeks
Complications	Metal loosening; urethral, bladder, or uterine lesions
Growth Disturbances	Potential serious complications such as pubic symphysis ossification
Follow-Up	Clinical and radiological control after 3 months, clinical wrap-up examination one year post-trauma

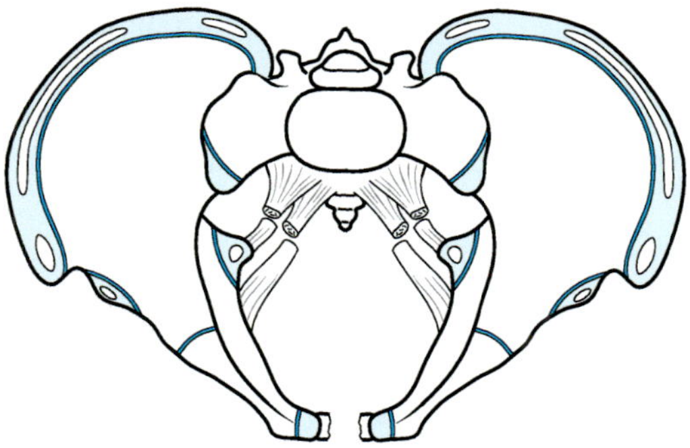

Fig. 17.20 Isolated rupture of the symphysis

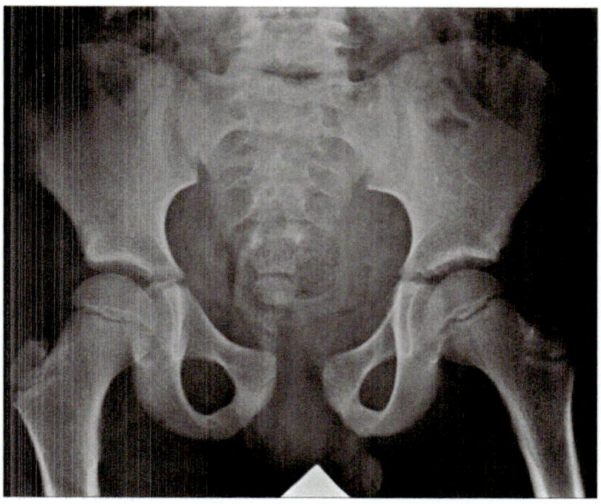

Fig. 17.21 Wide rupture of the symphysis in a child

B-type pelvic fractures

AO B type lesions are defined as lesions of the anterior and dorsal pelvic ring with incomplete dorsal instability. In general, stabilization and closure of the ventral lesion will cause stability and healing. Table 17.9 shows the B1 fracture and Table 17.10 the B2 fractures

Table 17.9 Pelvic ring fracture type B1 (Fig. 17.22)

Particularities	Incomplete unilateral lesion of dorsal pelvic ring, outer rotation commonly associated with genitourinary injuries (especially bilateral anterior fractures) or rectal injuries, large blood loss possible (Fig. 17.23)
Diagnostic Assessment	Pelvic X-Ray, inlet/outlet views, CT
Goals of Therapy/Limits of Correction	Closure of the pelvic ring, reduction of pelvic volume
Primary Treatment	Depending on concomitant injuries, mechanical decrease of pelvic volume e.g. with cloth belting, circulatory stabilization
Conservative therapy	
Indication	Minimally displaced or nondisplaced fractures without concomitant injuries, children under 6
Procedure	Bedrest for 3–4 weeks in crossed sling
Follow Up	Partial load bearing of the affected side for a further 2–4 weeks
Radiographic Control	Reduction check within the first 5 days; prior to load bearing
Sports Participation	After 12 weeks
Operative therapy	
Indication	Displaced fractures with circulatory instability, with accompanying organ injuries during treatment of those injuries
Procedure	Preferably with external fixator, possibly with tension banding or plate fixation of the symphysis (Fig. 17.24)
Follow Up	Bedrest for about 4 weeks then partial load bearing for another 4 weeks
Radiographic Control	Post-operative and after fixator removal
Hardware Removal	Fixator removal usually at 4 weeks, symphysis-bridging implants at about 3–6 months
Sports Participation	After 12 weeks
Complications	Infection; injuries to the urethra, bladder, or uterus
Growth Disturbances	Serious complications such as ossification of the sacroiliac joint or pubic symphysis are possible
Follow-Up	Clinical and radiological controls at 4 and 12 weeks and at approximately one year
Classification	AO: B1

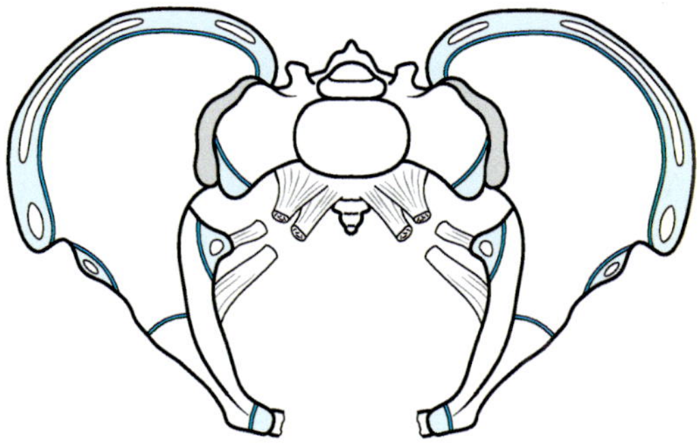

Fig. 17.22 Pelvic ring fracture type B1 (open book fracture B1)

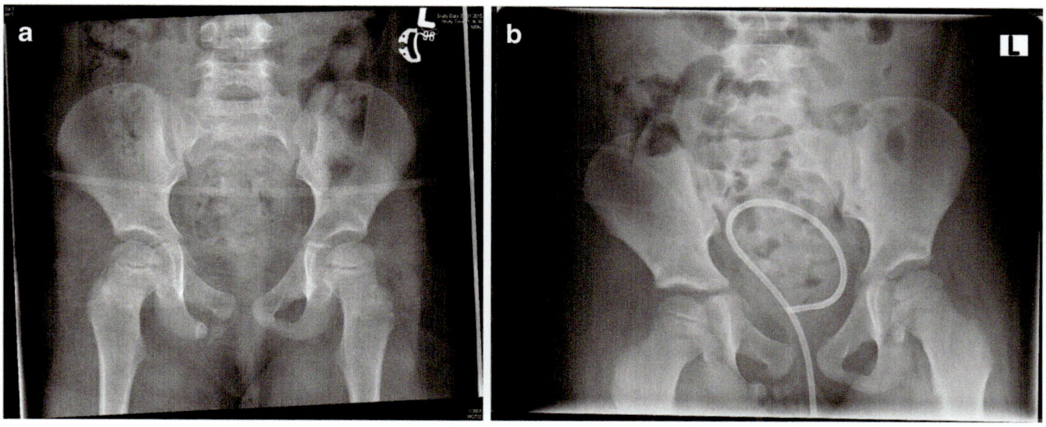

Fig. 17.23 Open book injury with fracture close to the symphysis on the right side and injury to the urethra in a 4 year old girl; type B1. (**a**) Trauma image, (**b**) 14 days with ongoing consolidation and urinary catheter. Standing already possible

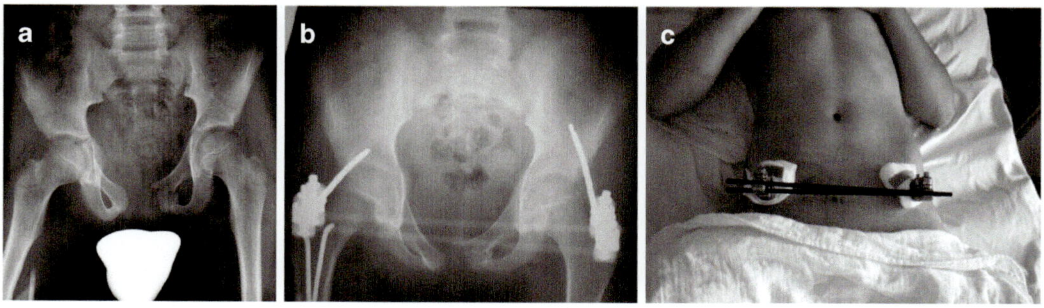

Fig. 17.24 Open-book injury and femoral shaft fracture, boy, 12 years old, moped accident; type B1. (**a**–**c**) Treatment of pelvic injury using external fixator and the femur fracture with intramedullary elastic titanium nail

Table 17.10 Pelvic ring fracture type B2 (lateral compression) (Fig. 17.25)

Particularities	Incomplete unilateral lesion of dorsal pelvic ring, inner rotation, relatively frequent on the left (in countries driving on the right side), mostly stable
Diagnostic Assessment	Pelvic X-Ray, inlet/outlet views, CT
Goals of Therapy/Limits of Correction	Preservation of pelvic symmetry, gross displacement more than twice the shaft width should be eliminated
Primary Treatment	Pain therapy, bedrest, thromboprophylaxis
Conservative therapy	
Indication	Mildly displaced or non-displaced fractures without concomitant injuries (Fig. 17.26)
Procedure	Bedrest for 2–3 weeks
Follow Up	Partial load bearing of the affected side for a further 2–4 weeks
Radiographic Control	Prior to gradual loading
Sports Participation	After 12 weeks
Operative therapy	
Indication	Significantly displaced fractures, possibly with concomitant organ injuries during intervention for organ injuries
Procedure	Preferably closed reduction, possibly with external fixator or plate fixation of the pubic symphysis (Fig. 17.27)
Follow Up	Short-term bedrest for 1–2 weeks then pain-adapted partial to full load-bearing within the next 2–4 weeks
Radiographic Control	Post-operative and prior to full load-bearing
Hardware Removal	Symphysis-bridging implants should be removed at about 3–6 months
Sports Participation	After 12 weeks
Complications	Injuries to the genitourinary tract, re-displacement
Growth Disturbances	Serious consequences such as sacroiliac joint or pubic symphysis closure are possible
Follow-Up	Clinical and radiological controls at 4 and 12 weeks and at approximately one year
Classification	AO: B2

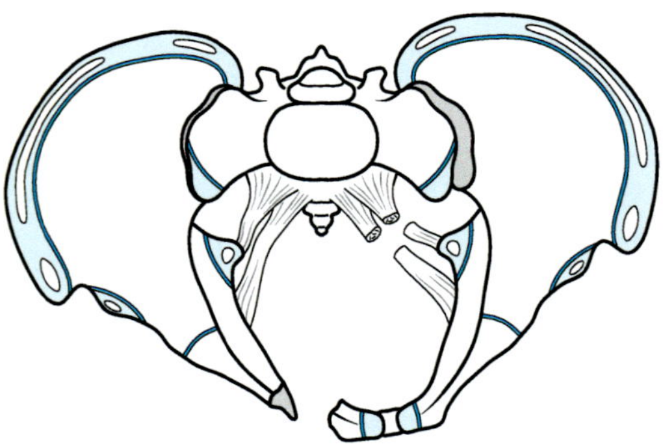

Fig. 17.25 Ten pelvic ring fracture type B2 (lateral compression)

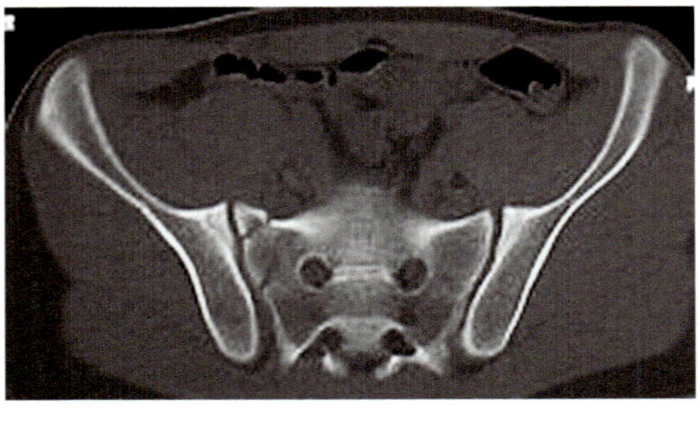

Fig. 17.26 Lateral compression fracture right side with participation of the sacrum and the ileo-sacral joint. Conservative treatment

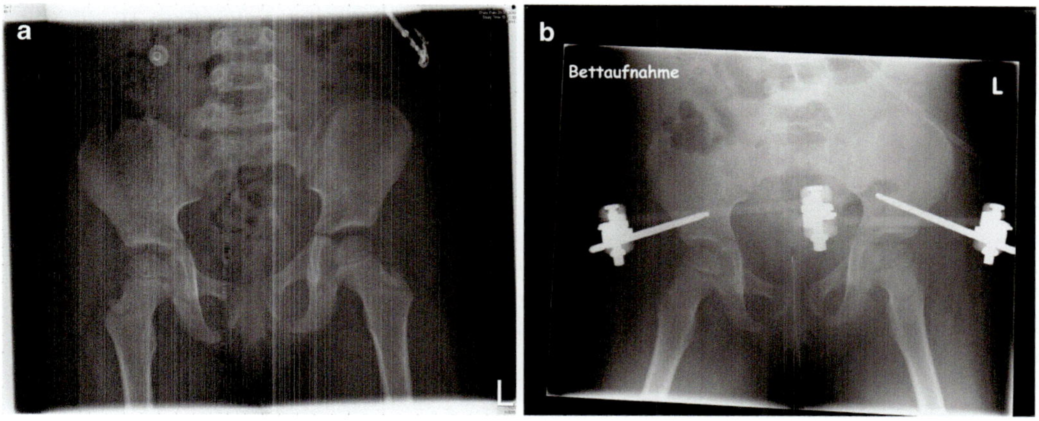

Fig. 17.27 Fracture of the dorsal ileum left side of a 4 year old boy. (**a**) Trauma image, (**b**) Stabilization and reduction with external fixation

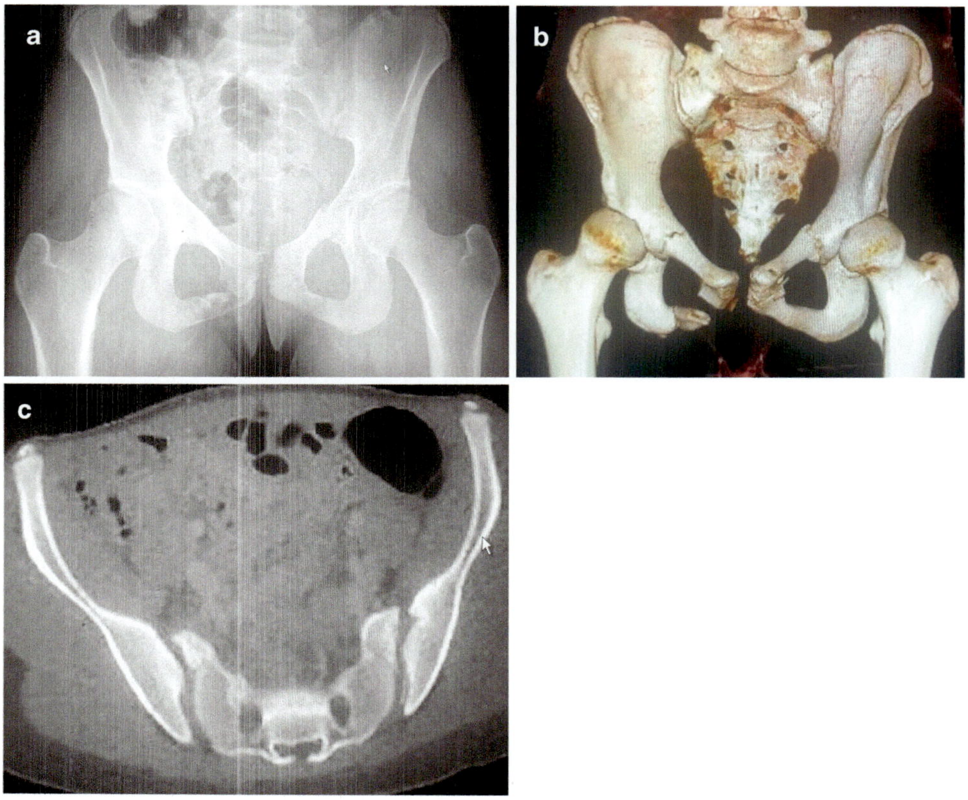

Fig. 17.28 16 years old girl after fall from horse with pelvic lesion type B2. (**a**) Trauma image. Multiple fractures of the ventral pelvic ring. (**b**, **c**) CT scan shows stable bilateral ventral sacral fractures. Conservative treatment, 4 month later painless healing without deformation

C-type pelvic fractures

Complex pelvic ring fractures are rare, but are often associated with a polytraumatized children and other organ or skeletal injuries. Table 17.11 gives all relevant information on these Type C – injuries.

Table 17.11 Pelvic ring fracture type C (Fig. 17.29)

Particularities	Complete uni- or bilateral disruption of the dorsal pelvic ring (Fig. 17.30), vertical instability; in 25% of cases concomitant traumatic brain injury; often local concomitant injuries; circulatory instability more likely from concomitant injuries
Diagnostic Assessment	Pelvic X-Ray, (Polytrauma) CT
Goals of Therapy/Limits of Correction	Most emergency stabilization in cases of hemodynamic instability or to enable positioning stability in intensive care; instability of the sacroiliac joint should be eliminated
Primary Treatment	External compression e.g. with pelvic sling, trauma bay management, external fixator or pelvic C-clamp
Conservative therapy	
Indication	Mildly or non-displaced fractures, age less than 6 years, poor general condition
Procedure	Bedrest for 4–6 weeks, extension treatment, unloading of the affected side
Follow Up	Partial load-bearing at 4–6 weeks, full loading at 6–8 weeks
Radiographic Control	Within the first 5 days as position check, prior to gradual loading and prior to full load-bearing
Sports Participation	After about 12 weeks
Operative therapy	
Indication	Displaced fractures (Fig. 17.31) concomitant organ lesions requiring intervention, circulatory instability, necessary positioning therapy, displacement with conservative therapy
Procedure	Supra-acetabular external fixator, possibly with additional single-screw fixation of the posterior pelvic ring, tension banding or plate fixation of the pubic symphysis (Fig. 17.32)
Follow Up	No full loading until removal of the external fixator
Radiographic Control	Direct post-operative radiographic control, further controls after external fixator removal, CT is optional
Hardware Removal	Removal of the external fixator is generally possible after 4 weeks, removal of the sacroiliac joint-crossing or pubic symphysis bridging implants at 3–6 months
Sports Participation	After 3–6 months
Complications	Pin infections, screw malposition, secondary neurological disorders, delayed or non-union, periarticular calcification, especially with concomitant traumatic brain injury
Growth Disturbances	Serious complications though growth plate injury or fusion of the SI joint/pubic symphysis are possible
Follow-Up	Clinical and radiological controls at 4 and 12 weeks, then in 6-month intervals until two years post-trauma
Classification	AO: C

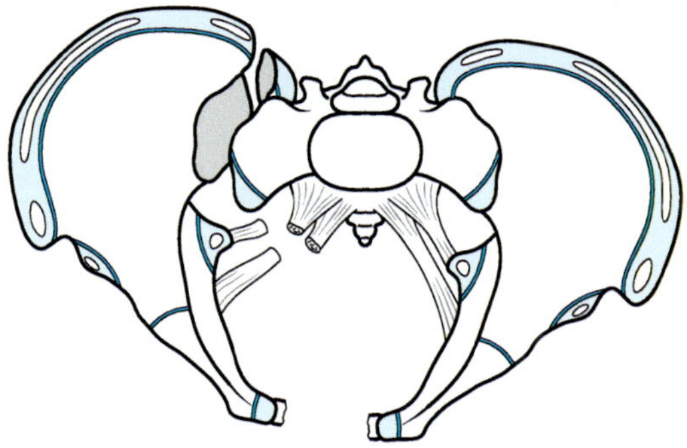

Fig. 17.29 Pelvic ring fractures type C

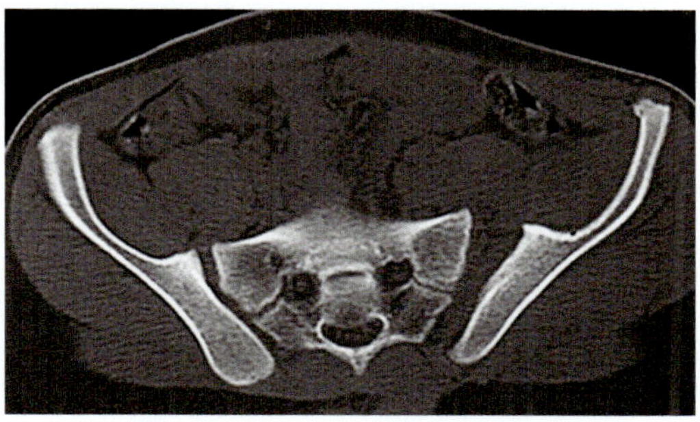

Fig. 17.30 C-type injury of the pelvis with complete dislocation of the ileo-sacral joint

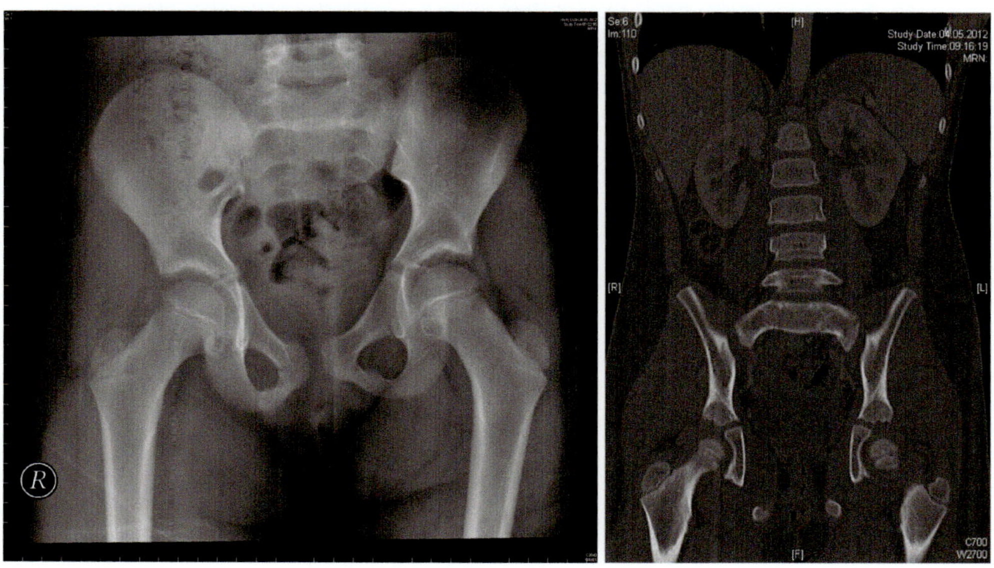

Fig. 17.31 Diagonal C type injury of the pelvis with anterior pelvic ring fracture right side and displaced sacrum-ileosacral joint injury left side

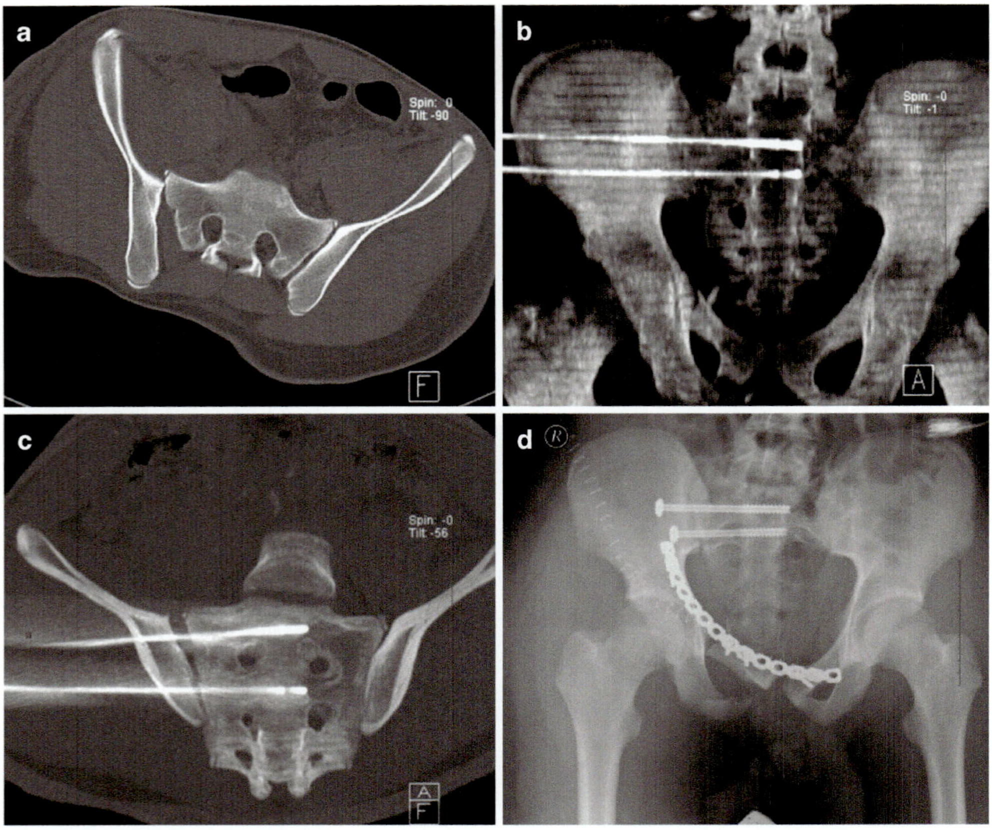

Fig. 17.32 Two complex pelvic trauma in an adolescent, boy, 14 years old, fall from bridge. (**a**–**d**) CT-guided percutaneous screw fixation of the transforaminal sacral fracture and open plate fixation of the anterior pelvic ring

17.4 Acetabular Fractures

Incidence, Mechanism of Injury and Clinical Picture

Acetabular fractures are extremely rare. They account for 0.8–15% of all pediatric pelvic fractures.

The pediatric acetabular fracture is caused by direct impact (lateral force) or (femoral) compression. Force via the femoral shaft (compression) usually occurs with hip dislocation. About every 7th hip dislocation in children is accompanied by bony injury to the hip joint. Hematoma often forms over the greater trochanter. Lateral force can lead to pure joint injuries such as epiphyseal separation or compression, but also to accompanying bony injuries corresponding to Salter-Harris I. Growth plate injuries are often not visible on native X-ray. Mildly displaced fractures are difficult to detect.

Classification

Prior to closure of the triradiate cartilage, the Salter-Harris Classification is used. With this, estimates regarding prognosis are also possible (Fig. 17.33).

However, acetabular fractures are generally classified according to Letournel and Judet. This classification is used to understand the biomechanics and is necessary for operative planning.

Table 17.12 gives the relevant information about acetabular fractures.

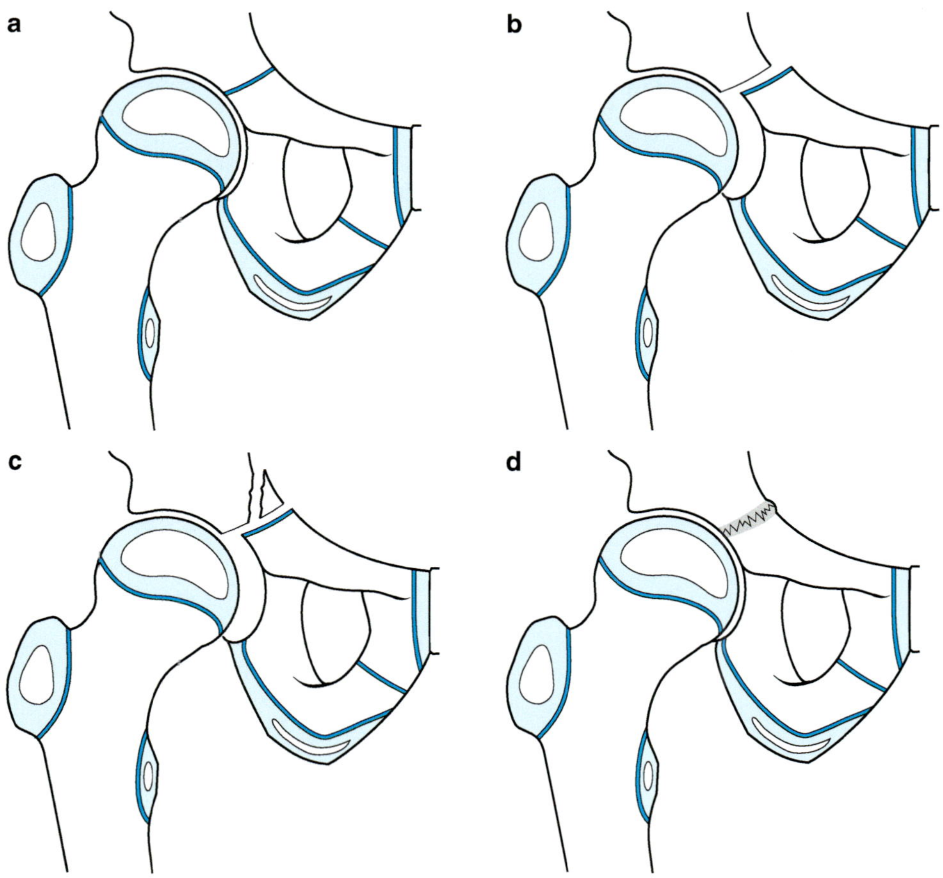

Fig. 17.33 Salter/Harris classification for pediatric acetabular fractures (according to Scuderi et al.). (**a**) Normal growth plate, (**b**) Salter-Harris I fracture, (**c**) Salter-Harris II Fracture, (**d**) Salter-Harris V fracture

Table 17.12 Acetabular fractures (Fig. 17.33)

Particularities	Rare, can result in growth disturbances
Diagnostic Assessment	Pelvic X-Ray, Judet and Obturator views, CT, possibly MRI to exclude injury to the growth plates (triradiate cartilage)
Goals of Therapy/Limits of Correction	Closest possible anatomical reconstruction of the joint surface, displacement <1 mm
Primary Treatment	Bedrest, possible extension therapy
Conservative therapy	
Indication	Non-displaced fractures, concomitant injuries
Procedure	Non-load-bearing of the affected leg for 4–6 weeks, optional initial extension of the leg
Follow Up	Gradual loading after 6–8 weeks; joint mobilization, possible physical therapy
Radiographic Control	Pelvic X-Ray, possible MRI
Sports Participation	About 12 weeks post-trauma
Operative therapy	
Indication	All fractures with >2 mm displacement
Procedure	Open or closed reduction, single-screw fixation or plate osteosynthesis via established approaches (Stoppa approach, Kocher-Langenbeck approach, Letournel approach or trochanter flip osteotomy) as appropriate (Figs. 17.34, 17.35, 17.36, 17.37 and 17.38)
Follow Up	Non-load-bearing of the affected leg for 4–6 weeks
Radiographic Control	Post-operative CT, further controls during healing only for complaints
Hardware Removal	Removal of joint-spanning implants as soon as possible
Sports Participation	After about 12 weeks
Complications	Growth disturbances, delayed or non-union, hip dislocation as a result of growth disorders around the acetabulum, hemi-pelvic hypoplasia, leg shortening, post-traumatic arthritis, ankylosis
Growth Disturbances	Serious complications, especially with compression of the triradiate cartilage (Salter-Harris V) are possible, can lead to hemi-pelvic aplasia or to acetabular dysplasia with consequent hip dislocation
Follow-Up	Clinical and radiological: at 2 and 6 weeks, then in 6-month intervals until 2 years post-trauma to detect and treat growth disorders early

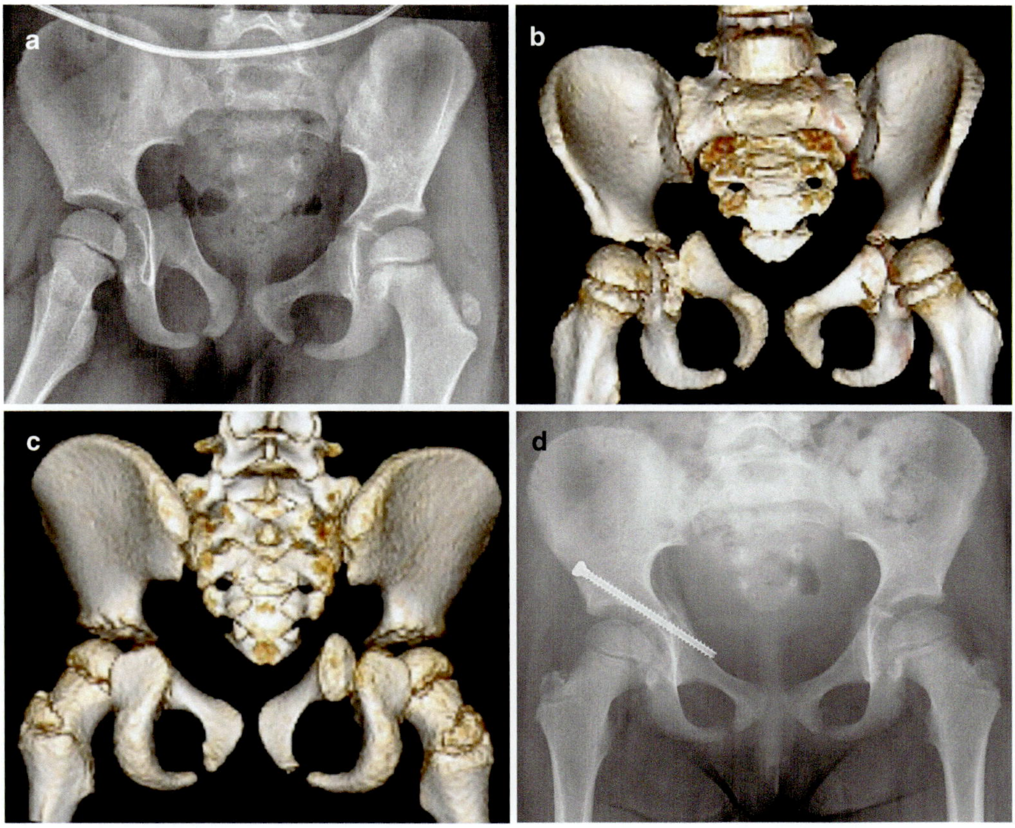

Fig. 17.34 4 years old girl rolled over by a truck. (**a**) Triradiate actebular injury Salter-Harris II with dislocated superior pubic ramus of the right side, undisplaced on the left side. No further lesions of inner organs. (**b**, **c**) Ventral and dorsal CT reconstruction, (**d**) Bony consolidation 6 weeks after open reduction and screw fixation. Immobilisation in wheel chair for 6 weeks postoperatively then implant removal. Follow up after 4 years shows no complications (Courtesy of Drs. Frühwirt, Flossmann, Universitätsklinikum St.Pölten, Austria)

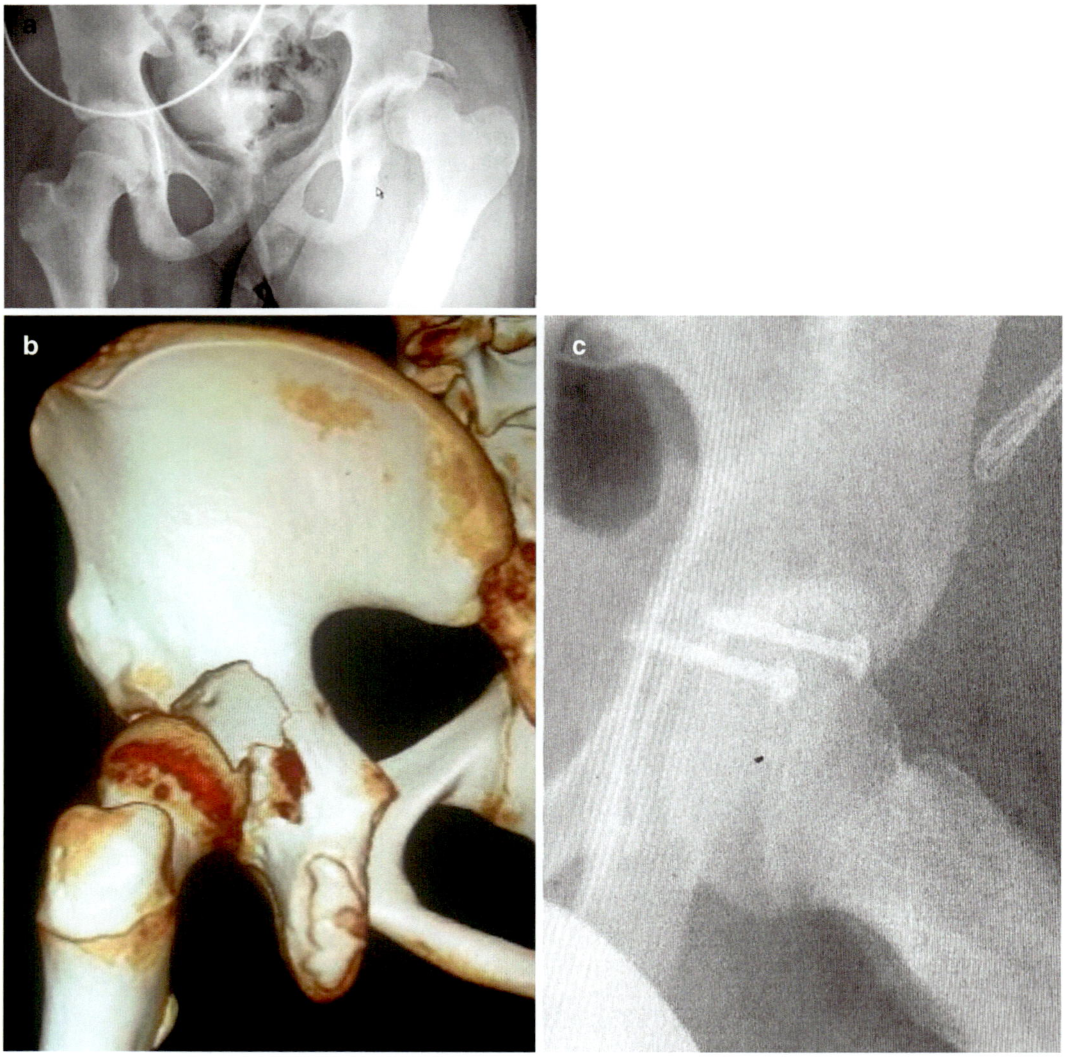

Fig. 17.35 13 years old girl falling when running. (**a**) dorsal hip luxation with dislocated fracture of the dorsal acetabular rim. (**b**) reduction in general anasthesia, (**c**) elective dorsal cannulated 4.0 mm screw osteosynthesis. Implant removal after 6 months

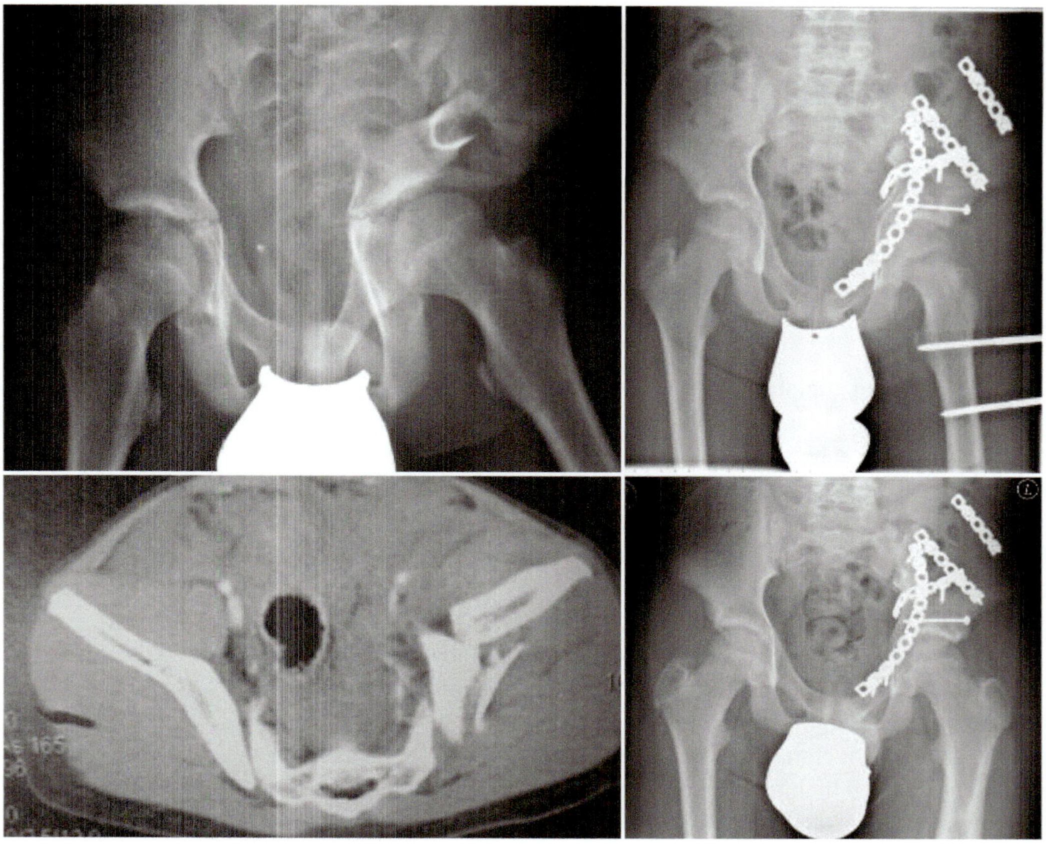

Fig. 17.36 Plate osteosynthesis of a pelvic ring fracture with large impression of the left acetabulum of 12 year old boy (sozius motobike), see also femur fracture lift side

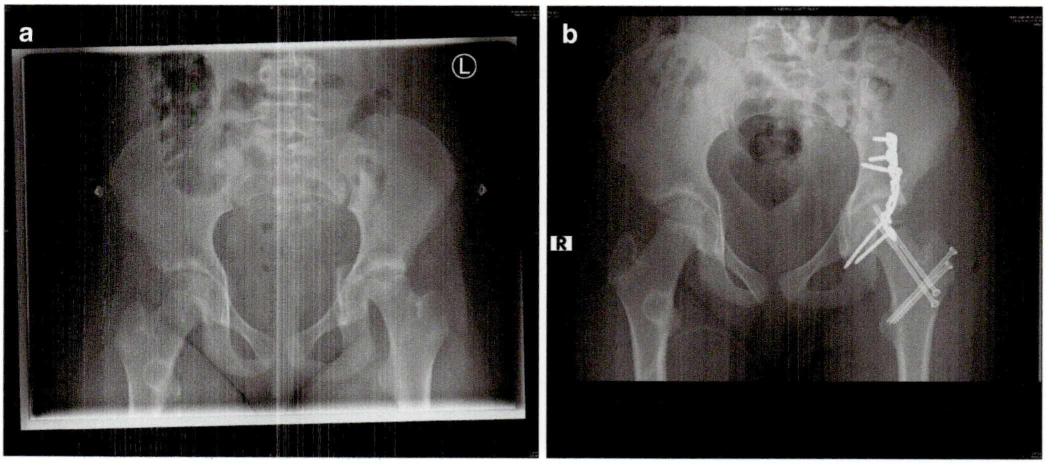

Fig. 17.37 Eleven year old girl with heavy accident to a beton wall. Luxation fracture of the femoral head and the dorsal acetabulum. (**a**) Trauma image. (**b**) After immediate trochanter flip osteotomy, fixation of the femoral head and stabilization of the dorsal acetabulum

17.5 Complex Injuries

Incidence, Mechanism of Injury and Clinical Picture

According to Bond, the incidence of concomitant intra-abdominal or genitourinary injuries with isolated pubic fractures is 6%, much higher at 33% with ileum and pelvic ring fractures, and even higher at 80% with severe, unstable pelvic fractures.

The etiologies of complex injuries to the pediatric pelvis are high-speed or roll-over trauma and falls from a great height. Thus, they are generally found in children with acute, vital, polytrauma injuries. The clinical picture often obscures the severity of injury. Soft-tissue degloving injuries can remain initially unobserved due to high skin elasticity.

Genitourinary and intra-abdominal injuries can also occur even with simple fracture presentations. Especially unstable pelvic fractures (Malgaigne fractures) and bilateral pubic rami fractures show high incidence of concomitant intra-abdominal and genitourinary lesions Concomitant injuries should be definitively excluded in all children with pelvic fractures. Perianal hematoma is pathognomonic for rectal lesions, and a rectal examination can sometimes reveal palpable puncturing fracture fragments. Children compensate much longer than adults even with considerable volume loss, but then decompensate rapidly. Pelvic bleeding is rarely the cause of death in children with pelvic injuries; intra-abdominal bleeding is much more often to blame. Thus, treatment of potentially life-threatening concomitant injuries has absolute priority over fracture care. Here generally, a multidisciplinary approach under direction of a pediatric surgeon or traumatologist is necessary. However, in severe bleeding a contrast enhanced CT can demonstrate an arterial blood blush which would allow an angioembolisation. This might be prior or after an indicated stabilization of the pelvis (Fig. 17.38).

Classification

Most classifications focus on bony injuries. Quinby and Rang differentiate pediatric fractures into three categories:

1. Uncomplicated Fractures
2. Fractures with abdominal organ injuries requiring surgical exploration
3. Fractures with associated massive bleeding

Table 17.13 gives the particularities of complex pelvic injuries.

Table 17.14 gives some technical aspects for the treatment of the pelvis.

Table 17.13 Complex injuries

Particularities	Relatively common in pediatric pelvic fractures; degloving injuries especially can easily escape primary diagnostic assessment
Diagnostic Assessment	Pelvic X-Ray, CT, possible MRI, soft-tissue ultrasound, rectal examination, retrograde urethrocystography (not when blood is present at the meatus), angiography (Figs. 17.38 and 17.39)
Goals of Therapy/Limits of Correction	Hemostasis, elimination of gross displacement and restoration of pelvic symmetry, prevention of secondary damage such as abscess formation from contamination or skin/organ perforation from bony fragments
Primary Treatment	According to shock treatment protocol; cardiovascular stabilization; external pelvic stabilization
Conservative therapy	
Indication	Small surface-area degloving, solid organs injuries that can be conservatively managed, controllable bleeding, mildly displaced fractures
Procedure	Clinical and ultrasound controls, generally intensive care monitoring
Follow Up	Dependent on fracture type
Radiographic Control	Corresponds to fracture type
Sports Participation	About 12 weeks post-trauma
Operative therapy	
Indication	Hollow organ injuries, bladder injuries (see above), large surface-area degloving, solid organ injuries that cannot be treated conservatively, open fractures, presence of neurological disturbances from displaced fracture fragments
Procedure	Organ care through a midline laparotomy; Pfannenstiel incision and primary repair of bladder rupture; primary or secondary reconstruction for urethral injury; ileostomy for intestinal injury with stool contamination; pelvic stabilization with external fixator and local K-wires or small-fragment screw fixation if needed; debridement and drainage in degloving injuries; interventional angiography of bleeding if needed
Follow Up	Generous indication for staged lavage in cases of contamination; soft-tissue reconstruction, urethral reconstruction; mobilization dependent on fracture type
Radiographic Control	Dependent on fracture type
Hardware Removal	Removal of external fixator at 4 weeks, screw removal at 3–6 months
Sports Participation	–
Complications	Infection, abscess formation, urethral strictures
Growth Disturbances	Serious complications can be expected from concomitant injuries
Follow-Up	Corresponding to fracture type and concomitant injuries

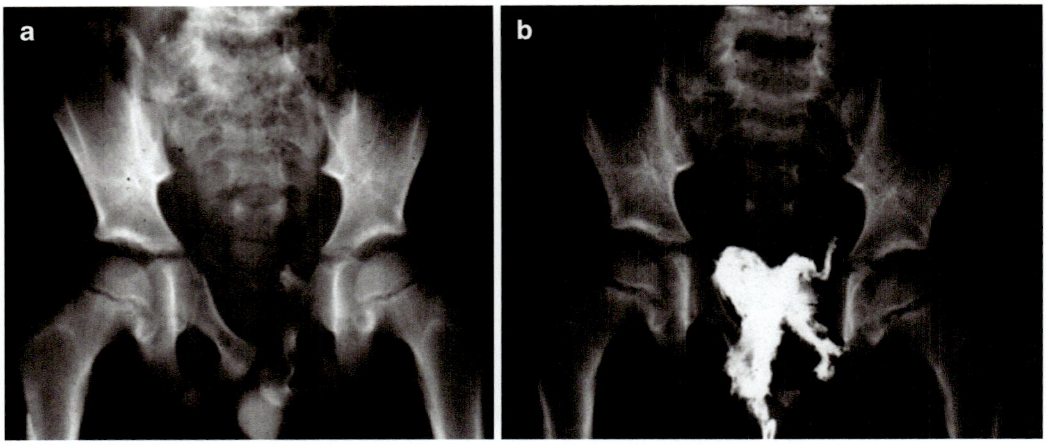

Fig. 17.38 Complex injury of the pelvis with bladder rupture; retrograde filling of the bladder

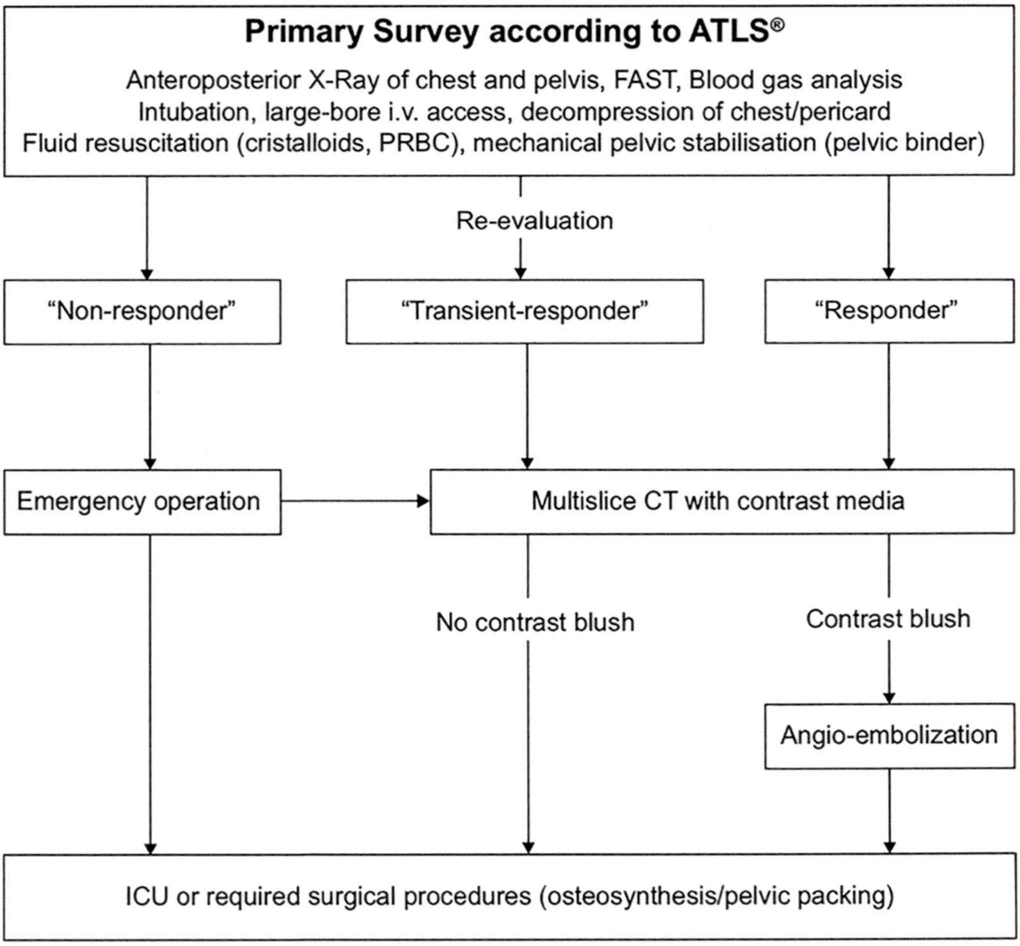

Fig. 17.39 Diagnostic algorithm for severe pelvic injures. ATLS Advanced Trauma Life Support, BGA Blood gas analysis, DCO (Damage Control Orthopedics) FAST Focused Assessment with Sonography for Trauma, ICU Intensive Care Unit. (Adapted to Marzi and Lustenberger 2014)

Table 17.14 Technical aspects pelvis

Hardware	External Fixator Cannulated screws → titanium, diameter 3.5–4 mm K-wires → titanium, diameter 1.4–2 mm Small-Fragment Plates
Positioning	Supine for external fixator, Stoppa approach, Letournel approach and covered SIJ screw placement (Fig. 17.40) Lateral positioning for Kocher-Langenbeck approach Prone position for open SIJ screw placement, Kocher-Langenbeck approach
Approach	Pubic symphysis: Pfannenstiel incision, possibly median in cases of laparotomy, incision median to the symphysis or bow-shaped transverse in the lower abdomen about 2 finger-widths superior to the symphysis Anterior acetabular column: Modified Stoppa approach seems to be more appropriate than ilioinguinal approach according to current developments Stoppa Incision above the Symphysis and preparation to the side. Take care of the Corona Mortis and adapted plates for children For the Ilioinguinal (Letournel) approach, incision from iliac crest over the ASIS to 2 finger widths superior to the symphysis, take care around the femoral vessels and nerve. SIJ anterior: 1. window of the ilioinguinal approach, incision as above Posterior column/posterior cup edge: Kocher-Langenbeck approach, bow-shaped incision from the posterior rim of the greater trochanter towards superior-posterior External Fixator: preferably supra-acetabular, possibly iliac wing, stab incision about 3 finger widths superior to the trochanter tip or on the iliac crest about one finger width posterior to the ASIS
Special Information	Sciatic nerve lesion during Kocher-Langenbeck approach Femoral nerve/vessels lesions during ilioinguinal approach Lateral femoral cutaneous nerve lesion during fixator application and Ilioinguinal approach Bladder injury during symphysis access Bleeding of the corona mortis and the femoral vein for Stoppa approach Root injury during SI joint screw fixation Growth disturbances with acetabular fractures
Operative Principles	*External fixator* Closure of the anterior pelvic ring with lateral compression Application of Schanz screws supra-acetabular or on the iliac crest through stab incisions under image intensification *Plate fixation* Open reduction of the pubic symphysis or acetabulum with small-fragment plates *Tension screw fixation* Closed reduction and fixation through a stab incision with cannulated cancellous tension screws or fully-threaded cortical screws, in case no tension is desired (S1 nerve root); introduction with image intensification; inlet/outlet and lateral views for the SI joint, Judet-obturator views for the acetabulum, CT-guided screw fixation of sacral factures through minimally-invasive stab incisions is possible *K-wire fixation* Closed or possible open reduction of acetabular or pelvic rim fractures and stabilization preferably with percutaneously introduced K-wires
Hardware Removal	All percutaneously introduced implants can be removed as an outpatient procedure
Other features	Pediatric pelvic injuries are rare, and thus, the indicated procedures should be performed by a surgeon experienced in pelvic surgery for adults

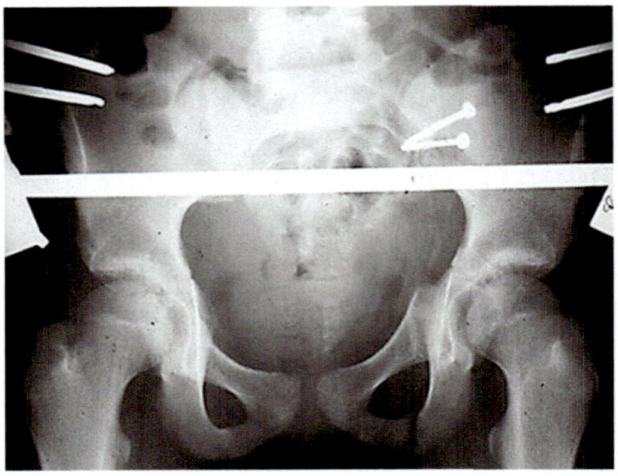

Fig. 17.40 Stabilization of a complex pelvic instability with an external fixateur in combination with a screw osteosynthesis of the left ileo-sacral joint

Recommend Literature

Blasier RD, McAtee J, White R, Mitchell DT (2000) Disruption of the pelvic ring in pediatric patients. Clin Orthop 376:87–95

Canale ST, King RE (2003) Pelvic and hip fractures. In: Rockwood CA, Wilkins KE, King RE (eds) Fractures in children. JP Lippincott, Philadelphia

Gaensslen A, Heidari N (2013) Weinberg AM Fracture of the pelvis in children: a review of the literature. Eur J Orthop Surg Traumatol 23:847–861

Gaensslen A, Pohlemann T (1998a) Kindliche Acetabulumfrakturen. In: Tscherne H, Pohlemann T (eds) Tscherne Unfallchirurgie. Becken und Acetabulum. Springer, Heidelberg, pp 442–445

Gaensslen A, Pohlemann T (1998b) Kindliche Beckenringfrakturen. In: Tscherne H, Pohlemann T (eds) Tscherne Unfallchirurgie. Becken und Acetabulum. Springer, Heidelberg, pp 205–211

Gänsslen A (2019) Verletzungen des Beckenrings bei Kindern. JATROS Orthopäd Traumatol Rheumatol 2:228–230

Heeg M, de Ridder VA, Tornetta P, de Lange S, Klasen H (2000) Acetabular fractures in children and adolescents. Clin Orthop 376:80–86

Leonard M, Ibrahim M, Mckenna P, Boran S, McCormack D (2011) Paediatric pelvic ring fractures and associated injuries. Injury. 42(10):1027–1030

Letournel E (1980) Acetabulum fractures: classification and management. Clin Orthop 151:81–106

Lustenberger T, Wutzler S, Störmann P, Laurer HL, Marzi I (2015a) The role of angio-embolization in the acute treatment concept of severe pelvic ring injuries. Injury 46(Suppl 4):S33–S38. Elsevier Ltd

Lustenberger T, Wutzler S, Störmann P, Marzi I (2015b) The role of pelvic packing for hemodynamically unstable pelvic ring injuries. Clinical medicine insights: trauma and intensive medicine, vol 6. Sage, London. https://doi.org/10.4137/CMTIM.S12257

Lustenberger T, Störmann P, Eichler K, Nau C, Janko M, Marzi I (2020) Secondary angio-embolization after emergent pelvic stabilization and pelvic packing is a safe option for patients with persistent hemorrhage from unstable pelvic ring injuries. Front Surg 7:601140

Marzi I, Lustenberger T (2014) Management of bleeding pelvic fractures. Scand J Surg 103(2):104–111

Nowack K, Schlickewei W (2013) Injuries of the pelvis and apophysis in childhood and adolescence. Unfallchirurg 116(12):1069–1075

Ogden JA (2000) Pelvis. In: Skeletal injury of the child. Springer, New York, pp 790–830

Oransky M, Arduini M, Tortora M, Zoppi AR (2010) Surgical treatment of unstable pelvic fracture in children: Long term results. Injury 41(11):1140–1144

Salter RB, Harris WR (1963) Injuries involving the epiphyseal plate. J Bone Joint Surg 45A:587–622

Schneidmüller D, Wutzler S, Kelm A, Wyen H, Walcher F, Marzi I (2011) Beckenverletzungen im Kindes- und Jugendalter: Eine retrospektive Analyse eines überregionalen Traumazentrums über 5 Jahre. Unfallchirurg 114(6):510–516

Slongo TF (2013) Acetabulum injuries in infancy and childhood. Unfallchirurg 116(12):1076–1084

Smith W, Shurnas P, Morgan S, Agudelo J, Luszko G, Knox E, Georgopoulus G (2005) Clinical outcomes of unstable pelvic fractures in skeletally immature patients. J Bone Joint Surg 87-A(1):2423–2431

Swiontkowski MF (2003) Fracture and dislocations about the hips and pelvis. In: Green NE, Swiontkowski F (eds) Skeletal trauma in children. Saunders, Philadelphia

Tile M (1995) Fractures of the pelvis and acetabulum. Williams & Wilkins, Baltimore, pp 210–218

Torode I, Zieg D (1985) Pelvic fractures in children. J Pediatr Orthop 5:76–84

Vitale MG, Kessler MW, Choe JC, Hwang MW, Tolo VT, Skaggs DL (2005) Pelvic fractures in children: an exploration of practice patterns and patient outcomes. J Pediatr Orthop 25(5):581

Watts HG (1976) Fractures of the pelvis in children. Orthop Clin North Am 7:615–624. New York

Wirth PDT (2016) Avulsionsverletzungen der Hüftregion des Jugendlichen. Der Orthopäde 45(3):213–218. Springer, Berlin

Zwingmann J, Lefering R, Maier D, Hohloch L, Eberbach H, Neumann M, Strohm P, Südkamp N, Hammer T (2018) Pelvic fractures in severely injured children: results from the TraumaRegister DGU. Medicine 97:e11955. https://doi.org/10.1097/MD.0000000000011955

Spine

18

18.1 Physiology, Anatomy and Development of the Spine

Data regarding range of movements, size ratios, and "physiological" findings of the pediatric spine are subject to high variation according to the investigator, mode of examination, and age.

Joints. In younger children, the cranium articulates horizontally with the atlas (C1). The atlantooccipital joint (condyloid joint) exerts tight control, predominantly allowing flexion/extension with less rotation and lateral inclination. The more horizontal and level articular facets are held together by weak musculature and lax ligamentous structures. Due to the large head-to-body relationship in children any force generates high loads. The dens of the axis (C2) and anterior arch of C1 are connected with the cruciform ligament of C1, composed of the transverse ligament of C1 and longitudinal bands (from the anterior edge of the foramen magnum to the posterior C2 body). The alar ligaments are secondary stabilizers, first connecting the sides of the dens to the foramen magnum and medially to the occipital condyle, and second drawing the pars toward the anterior arch of the Atlas. Since the pediatric ligament structures of the atlanto-axial joint (combined swivel joint) allow approximately 20–60° rotation, ligament ruptures and injuries to the facet joints with subluxation are possible. 60% of axial c-spine rotation arises between C0 and C2 (of this, 50% between C1 and C2), and the remaining 40% in the lower c-spine. With growth, joint surface inclination of C1/C2 increases from 55 to 70° and of C2–C4 from 30 to 60–70°, resulting in higher bony stability. While the ligaments, joints, and discs can withstand severe strain and displacement up to 5 cm with no apparent damage, the spinal cord has minimal tolerance of only a few millimeters, which explains common neurological disorders.

Bony Development. The atlas has three primary ossification centers (OFC): one in the center of each arch and a third in the anterior body, which is formed in 20% of children at birth or only ossifies within the first year. The third OFC can also be formed from two centers or completely absent, so that the two arches close anteriorly without a body or leaving a gap. The posterior bony arch normally closes before the third year, but can remain open and, along with other variations and synchondroses, should not be misinterpreted as posttraumatic. With 7 years, the two anterior arches join with the body in the neurocentral synchondrosis. The C1 ring reaches adult size around the 4th or 5th year of life (spinal canal diameter approximately 22 mm), although it can be absent altogether or not ossify. Third rule: approximately one third of the canal is occupied by the dens, one third by the spinal cord, and one third by free space.

The axis has four OFCs (two in the arches, one in the body, one in the dens). Ossification of the dens begins prenatally with two oblong primary centers that unite at birth. However, a vertical line

I. Marzi et al., *Pediatric Skeletal Trauma*, https://doi.org/10.1007/978-3-030-93685-3_18

can persist until the 7th month. All centers are present at birth and fuse between 3 and 6 years of age. The dens is separated from the C2 body by a growth cartilage zone (the dentocentral synchondrosis) that grows in the superior-inferior vectors and disappears between ages 5 and 7 years It is inferior to the plane of the articular facets and the dens-body transition, and can remain a small radiolucent structure for years. It can easily be confused with a fracture because pediatric dens fractures also arise in this region. This synchondrosis appears as an H on transoral radiograph views (Fig. 18.1). Because circulation of the dens occurs via connective tissue at the tip and through vessels of the synchondrosis medial to the joint facets, perfusion is not disrupted in fractures (good prognosis). Coalescence of the two primary ossification centers of the dens leads to a V-shaped cartilage area, between or over which there is a secondary apical OFC of the dens tip. This does not appear before the sixth or seventh year and fuses around twelve. Lack of ossification results in a persistent ossiculum terminale of Bergmann. The fusion boundaries can remain for a long time. Fusion may be incomplete and thus complicate differentiation from fracture. There is a standard variant of about 4% with the dens angulating posteriorly. The ring apophysis at the base of C2 can remain open until age 25.

Below the C3 body, all vertebral bodies ossify in the same manner. An OFC forms in the vertebral body and two others in the neural tubes (vertebral arches). Ossification of the body occurs in a semi-sphere, first in the superior-inferior directions, then laterally and posteriorly. From 2 years of age, growth develops primarily towards anterior and in the width. The anterior neurocentral synchondrosis separates these three between ages three and six and doesn't ossify until after age 5 or 6 years. Closure of the spinal canal is variable and depends on the level. The cervical spine closes between ages 6 and 7 years, thoracic between 7 and 9 years, and lumbar between 9 and 10 years. It can be confused with a spina bifida.

In the cervical and thoracic vertebrae, five other secondary OFCs appear during adolescence on the tips of the spinous (fusion at 25 years) and transverse processes (fusion in puberty) as well as on the borders of the superior and inferior endplates (apophysis or apophyseal ring; Fig. 18.2). The spine does not have classic bony epiphyses as found in the long bones, so the cartilaginous vertebral endplates are not recognizable as growth plates at a young age and directly border the disc. At age 6 or 7 years, the thin, ring-shaped cartilage layer of the ring apophysis forms a varied fine interlocking with the OFC of the body. As slow-growing ossification centers, the ring apophyses are barely involved in height increases of the vertebrae, but act as anchors for the annulus fibrosis and the insertion of the lumbar diaphragm. The epiphyseal synchondrosis of the endplates does not fuse until the age of 25 years. The lumbar vertebrae grow greatly in height, especially during adolescence, through epiphyseal growth zones. There are two additional OFCs for the mammillary processes. Injuries to the secondary OFCs can only be demonstrated radiographically to a limited extent. Approximately 20% of the population retains an open posterior synchondrosis (spina bifida) at L5. Trauma can result in injury to the cartilage-bone transformation, with sclerotic bony areas within the vertebra.

The spinal canal diameter measures approximately 18 mm at C7. Earlier closure of the spinal canal, e.g. after trauma, can lead to spinal canal stenosis. Maturation of the c-spine occurs more quickly than the extremities and other parts of the

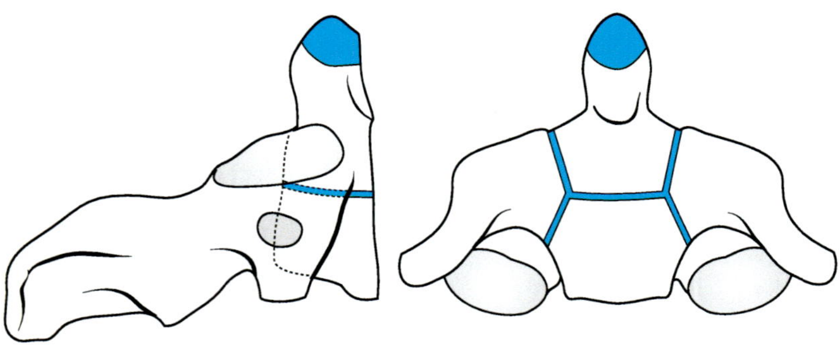

Fig. 18.1 Synchondrosis and ossification centers of the second cervical vertebra

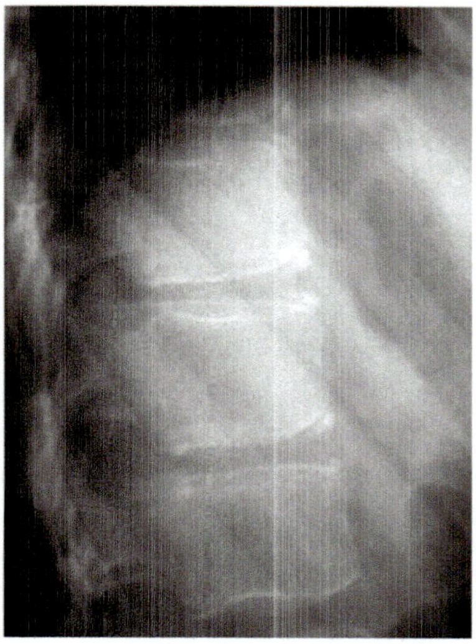

Fig. 18.2 Growth zone of the spine, ring apophysis (13 years)

skeleton. Ossification is complete between 8 and 10 years so that little height increase is seen after age ten.

In summary, from age 8 to 10 on, the spine matures with stable ligaments and joints, steeper articular facets, and rectangular vertebral bodies, approaching adult spine anatomy. Thus, from this age on, injuries and healing processes are similar to those of adults.

18.2 Injuries to the Spine: General

Incidence

Injuries of the spine are rare in children and affect only some 1.5% of pediatric trauma, of whom 5% are under age 16 years. However, incidence statistics are only estimates because often additional diagnostic studies are not performed or they are difficult to interpret. Age plays an essential role in the type, localization, and appearance of the injury. Birth trauma is most common under 2 years of age, with other age peaks in 3–4-year-olds (traffic accidents, falls, child abuse) and adolescents (sports, traffic). The thoracolumbar spine is most commonly injured. The younger the child, the more likely a c-spine injury. Severe c-spine injuries are often not survived.

Neurological Complications

Spine injuries in children have a good prognosis overall since posttraumatic wedge vertebrae will compensate. For injuries of the growth plates or posttraumatic paralysis, however, growth disturbances and deformities are possible. A high percentage of unstable injuries lead to neurological disorders, in certain populations as high as 14–57% and 19–25% for complete transverse spinal cord syndromes. Significant c-spine injuries have the highest risk with neurological complications in 22–30%. It is sometimes very difficult to judge stability of an injury because of the elastic and weak ligament anatomy as well as the limited ability to evaluate chondro-osseous injuries. Immobilization is recommended and is obligated for the injured regions (rigid collar, bedrest) until the questionable lesion is safely excluded. Up to 30% (5–67%) of severe injuries show non-specific neurological symptoms (SCIWORA = Spinal Cord Injury Without Radiographic Abnormalities).

Diagnostic Assessment

Growth-related characteristics of the spine place high demands on imaging assessments (Fig. 18.3). In addition to technical quality of CT and MRI especially, the experience of the radiologist and the surgeon plays an important role. Depending on the age of the child and level of consciousness, taking a good history and identifying the affected spinal region can also be problematic. The extent of X-ray examination should nevertheless be determined according to the level of consciousness and ability to perform clinical assessment. An overall complete diagnostic series (c-spine, t-spine, and l-spine in two planes) should be reconsidered in isolated trauma.

Appropriate c-spine immobilization with a rigid pediatric collar (Stiff neck) should be applied, usually at the scene, once life-threatening injuries (airway, breathing, circulation) have been excluded, if not before. Special positioning with thoracic support or head recess (spine board) is used to avoid hyperflexion of the c-spine due to the proportionally large head.

Mobilization over the body axis is possible with head and torso stabilization once severe trunk and extremity injuries have been excluded. Inspection (soft tissues, abrasions, bruises, posterior bleeding), assessment of mobility or painful limitations, palpation (tenderness, interspinous gap), and repeated neurological examination are performed.

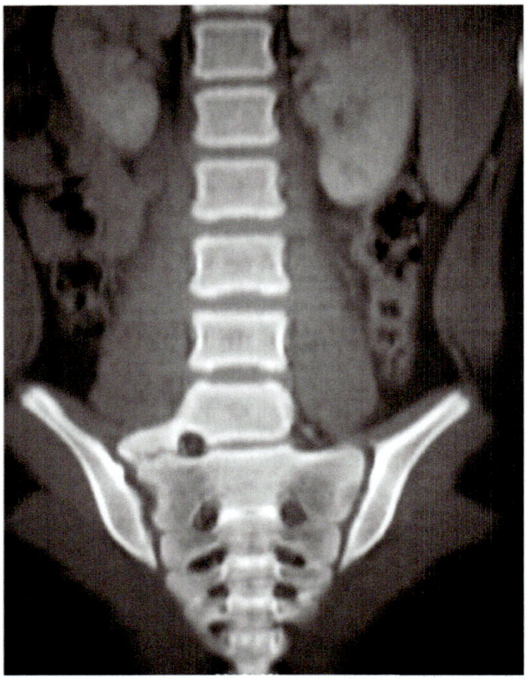

Fig. 18.3 Lumbosacral transition vertebra (12 years)

Standard Assessment of Spine Injuries. Spine anatomy changes constantly during growth. Ossification of the c-spine is normally completed between ages 8 and 10 years. Injury to the c-spine must always be excluded when the following clinical findings are present: unconsciousness or GCS < 13, disorientation, local complaints, neurological deficits, corresponding history (traffic accident, seat belt marks, lack of seat belt, severe head or face trauma, falls). The c-spine in particular offers a diagnostic challenge, because the primary and secondary OFCs as well as the adjacent synchondroses are difficult to differentiate from pathological changes.

The evaluation of c-spine radiographs should follow the following key points:

A.P. views of the c-spine (and transoral dens view; Fig. 18.4a, c):

- Position of the lateral mass
- Dens fracture
- Interpedicular distance
- Pseudosubluxation C2/C3 (normal: ≤4 mm) (Fig. 18.5); Pseudosubluxation C3/C4 (normal: ≤3 mm)

Lateral views of the c-spine with T1 (Fig. 18.4b):

- A.P. vertebral body alignment, spinolaminar and spinous process lines

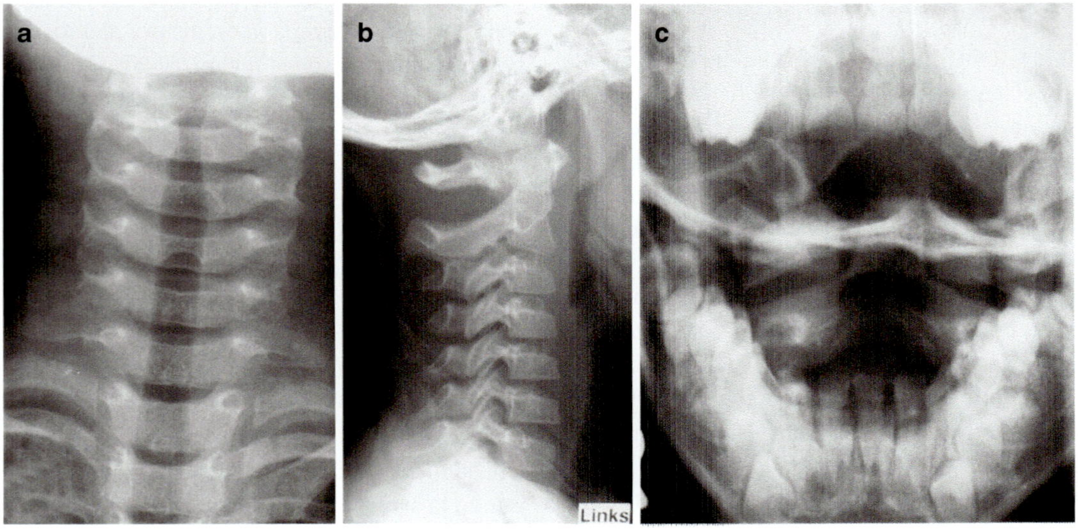

Fig. 18.4 Conventional c-spine X-rays of a 4-year-old girl. (**a**) A.P. view, (**b**) Lateral, (**c**) Transoral

- Atlas-Dens Interval (≤4 mm)
- Distance C1 joint to occiput (≤5 mm)
- Retropharyngeal (≤8 mm for C2) and retrotracheal space (≤14 mm for C6 under 15 years)
- Spinal canal diameter (spinolaminar line to posterior edge distance at C1 ≥14 mm)

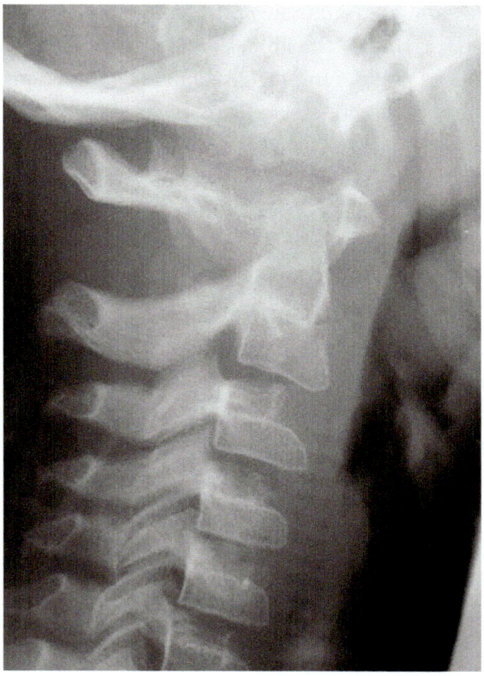

Fig. 18.5 Pseudosubluxation C2/C3 (4 years)

Table 18.1 shows the variations of the X-ray findings.

According to Woodring and Lee, high-quality conventional X-rays of the c-spine show most fractures of the body, dens, and spinous processes as well as dislocations. Dietrich et al. found that lateral c-spine X-rays were sufficient at detecting injuries in 98% of cases. The trans-oral X-ray, which is also recommended, is technically difficult with the limited cooperation of a child, but may be helpful in the absence of CT. When there is urgent suspicion of injury, MRI or CT are necessary due to the difficult assessment of the upper c-spine joints and the axis dens on X-ray.

When there is suspected instability, functional views in flexion/extension should be performed by experienced physicians (Caution: iatrogenic injury!) on conscious patients, or in exceptional cases (severe pain) also under anesthesia with direct fluoroscopic control.

Suggestions of ligamentous injury (according to Blauth):

- Severe trauma mechanism
- Posterior tenderness to palpation, pain on traction or compression, spasm, limited movement
- Distinct monosegmental step formation of the posterior vertebral line with distorted lateral alignment
- Incongruent joint facets, 50% subluxation of the intervertebral joints

Table 18.1 Differential diagnosis of growth-dependent physiological-anatomical X-ray normal findings and questionable instability

X-ray findings	Variations
Dens-basion (anterior lip of the foramen magnum) distance approximately 5 mm	Smaller children to 10 mm (McGregor or Chamberlain line; Wholey et al.)
Increased distance between the dens and anterior Atlas arch in flexion (pseudosubluxation)	3+ mm in 20%, to 4 mm in flexion normal, when injury is suspected, the atlantodental interval >5 mm is pathological
C1 overriding the dens tip in extension	In approximately 20% of lateral X-rays up to 8 years; enlarged space due to cartilage zones of Atlas and dens tip
Pseudosubluxation of C2/C3	Lateral, particularly between C2 and C3, less in C3/C4 (approximately 20–40% of all children until age 8), in flexion, lateral step of 4 mm acceptable (Cattell and Filtzer). Cause: lax ligaments, horizontal joints, under-developed uncinate process. The spinolaminar line can show an interval of 1.5 mm to C1, but must correct in extension
Segmental kyphosis of the mid cervical spine	Is physiological for ages 2–7 years, for 14% of children under 16 years, but must correct in extension
Lack of cervical lordosis	Muscle spasms (approximately 14% under 8 years)

- Lack of correction in extension (Caution: often spontaneous reduction after hyperextension trauma)
- Swelling of the pre-vertebral fat
- Spinous process fractures (apophyseal avulsions)
- Late signs: small avulsed bone of the ossified vertebra, late ossification of the posterior ligaments, compensatory lordosis beneath the lesion
- Widening of the interspinous distance on AP views by about 1.5 times (Naidich rule)
- Widening of the posterior intervertebral disc space
- Kyphosis with narrowing of the intervertebral disc space
- Wedging of two or more vertebrae per fracture, kyphosis and widened distance of the spinous processes
- Swischuk's line (of the posterior vertebral arch C1–C3) is not a reliable diagnostic tool

CT of the c-spine should always be done in cases of severe traumatic brain injury (intubation, bleeding, etc.). In cases of polytrauma, severe mechanism of injury, and children who cannot be evaluated (intubation, loss of consciousness), primary assessment follows the polytrauma protocol, i.e. trauma CT series (head and neck, thoraco-abdominal with contrast) without conventional X-rays. The spine is only cleared from spine-protective positioning when a c-spine injury is definitively excluded. This is often difficult if there are additional sources of pain, traumatic brain injury prevents adequate assessment, and analgesia or anesthesia have been administered.

MRI is always indicated in cases of suspected spine or spinal cord injury (e.g. SCIWORA) when there are no pathological findings on conventional X-rays or CT. Because of the ligamentous and cartilaginous elasticity, severe spinal cord injury is possible without morphological changes. Widening of the intervertebral space should be noted particularly in cases of injury to the growth plates. MRI should also be carried out here when there is doubt, because it often offers evidence of the underlying injury.

Injuries to other sections of the spinal cord are targeted through history, complaints, and physical examination. Difficulties with conventional techniques regarding the evaluation of the upper and mid-thoracic spine are similar to those in adults. Injuries to the thoracic and lumbar spine should be assessed as in adults.

Differential Diagnosis of Growth-Related Findings

Tables 18.2 and 18.3 give an overview and clues for the differential diagnosis of growth-related as well as systemic spinal and post-traumatic changes.

Table 18.2 Growth-related physiological-anatomically normal X-ray findings and questionable fractures

X-ray findings	False interpretation/differential diagnosis
Atlas "Pseudospread"	Fracture
Open Synchondrosis of the Atlas	Fracture
Angulation of the dens tip	Dens fracture
Persistent dentocentral synchondrosis	Dens fracture (Cause: Epiphyseal line at the base is physiological until age 6/7 years. This can persist until 11 years, but it is more sclerotic and inferior to the dens base).
Synchondrosis of the Axis arch	Traumatic spondylolisthesis
Incomplete ossification of the ring apophysis	Avulsion fracture
Indentations of the anterior/posterior vertebral body wall	Fracture (Cause: anterior vascular canal up to 1 year)
Soft borders of the epiphyseal zones	Compression fracture
"Mach effect"	Artificial lines on the borders of various X-ray densities (e.g. dens base)
Soft tissue shadows c-spine	Prevertebral variable, retropharyngeal space >7 mm and retrotracheal space >14 mm abnormal (Wholey)
Wedge-shaped Vertebrae	Compression fracture (exception: → wedge shape is normal in upper c-spine and children up to 8 years)

Table 18.3 Differential diagnosis congenital anomalies and other spine changes (incidence unclear, often incidental findings)

Changes	Differential diagnosis
Os odontoideum (congenital hypoplastic tip or base of the dens)	Dens fracture
Agenesis or hypoplasia of the dens	Dens fracture
Down syndrome (dens hypoplasia)	Atlanto-occipital instability; weak ligaments reduce the Atlas-Dens distance, narrowed spinal canal, risk of myelopathy
Klippel-Feil Syndrome	Congenital fusion of two or more vertebrae with increased risk of fracture due to the lever arm
Osteogenesis imperfecta	Absent separation of C1 from the occiput with narrowing of the foramen magnum and neurological deficits; wedge-shaped and split vertebrae, also in combination
Thoracolumbar block vertebra, split vertebra	Fractures
Bifid structures without sclerosis	Non-ossified synchondroses, fracture, spina bifida, facility-dependent (see above)
Persistent lumbar separation	Fracture
Lumbarization and sacralization	Fracture
Spondylolisthesis	Fracture, segmental instability
Pathological fracture (acute neck pain)	Physiological wedge vertebra, eosinophilic granuloma, leukemia, bone cysts and necrosis, Scheuermann's disease, spondylitis, metabolic disorders, juvenile rheumatoid arthritis, renal osteodystrophy
Spinal cord tumors	Fractures

Classification

Classification of injuries from C3 to C7 is carried out with the AO classification in older children, and with the Salter-Harris classification in younger children.

All types of injury observed in adults are also seen in children over 8–10 years of age and adolescents. Thus, classical AO (Magerl et al.) differentiation according to compression, flexion-distraction and rotational injuries can be used (Fig. 18.6a–c).

In children under 8 years, there are cartilaginous injuries (fractures of the cartilaginous vertebral endplates and growth plates). In detail (according to Blauth):

1. Rupture of the lower cartilaginous vertebral endplate (Salter-Harris I lesion) (Fig. 18.7a) of the lower c-spine and upper t-spine; secondary deformity is possible due to the potential for growth in height.
2. Destruction of the anterior inferior vertebral edge (Aitken 2, Salter-Harris III fracture) (Fig. 18.7b); predominantly in adolescents, good prognosis.

Fractures of the ring-shaped vertebral edge (apophyseal ring) have been reported in older children and adolescents. These are a fractured growth plate, which can reduce spontaneously and remain hidden on conventional X-rays. Apophyseal separations, generally in male adolescents, occur in the upper lumbar and occasionally in the thoraco-cervical spine, but then inferiorly. The cause is generally violent monotrauma or chronic overloading during sports. Typically there is lumbar pain with or without neurological symptoms (symptoms of disc herniation are possible). According to Takada and Epstein, there is a

1. Anterior displacement (avulsion fractures of the anterior longitudinal ligament and the annulus fibrosis)
2. Posterior displacement, more common (Fig. 18.8):
   (a) Type 1: simple separation of the entire posterior edge (11–13 years)
   (b) Type 2: border edge with cancellous parts of the vertebra (13–18 years)
   (c) Type 3: lateral border edge with parts of the vertebra (older than 14 years)
   (d) Type 4: fracture of the entire posterior wall between the endplates, possible narrowing of the spinal canal, decompression necessary with neurological findings; potential for secondary deformity

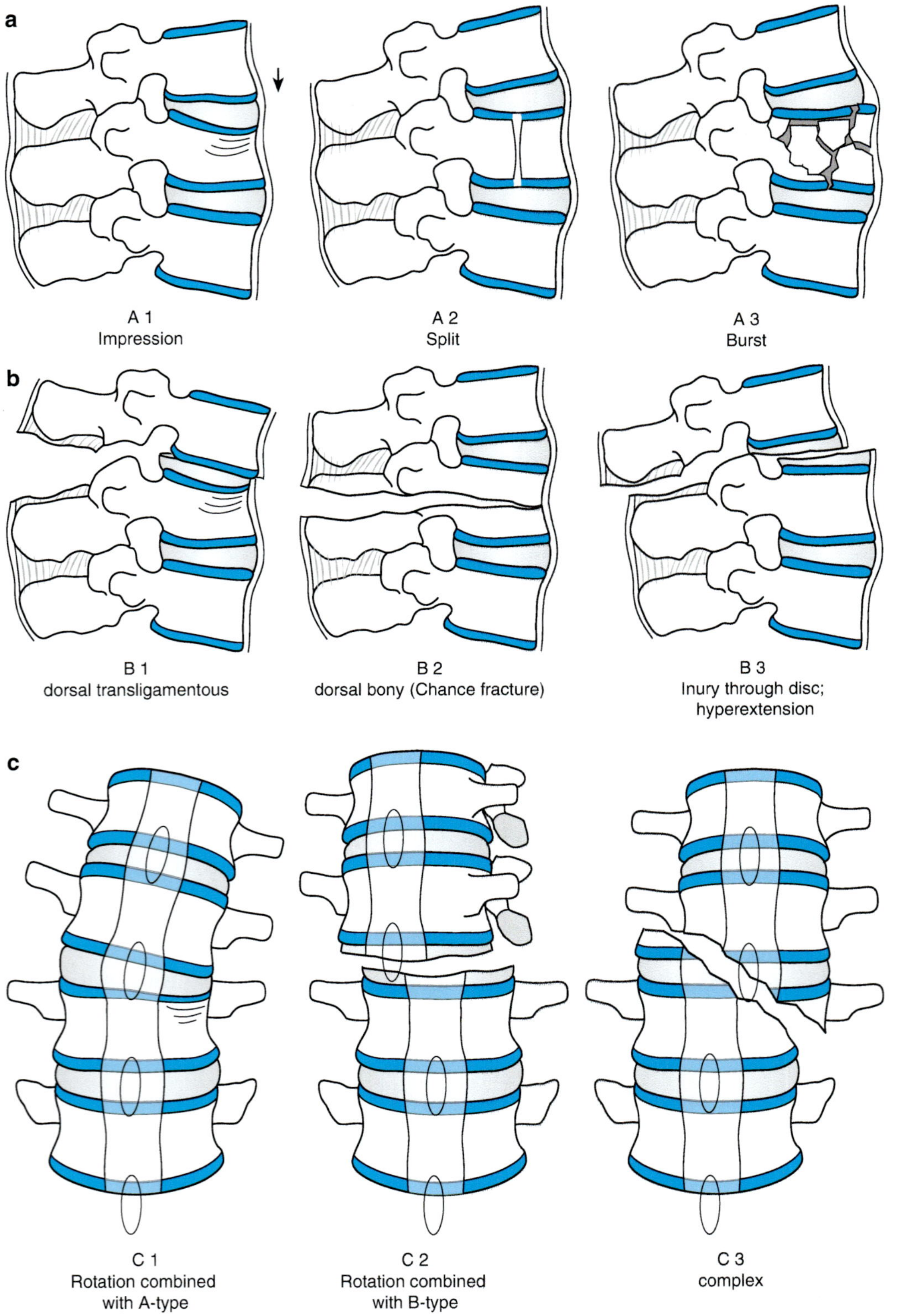

Fig. 18.6 AO classification of spine injuries. (**a**) Compression fractures, (**b**) Flexion-distraction fractures, (**c**) Rotation and translation fractures

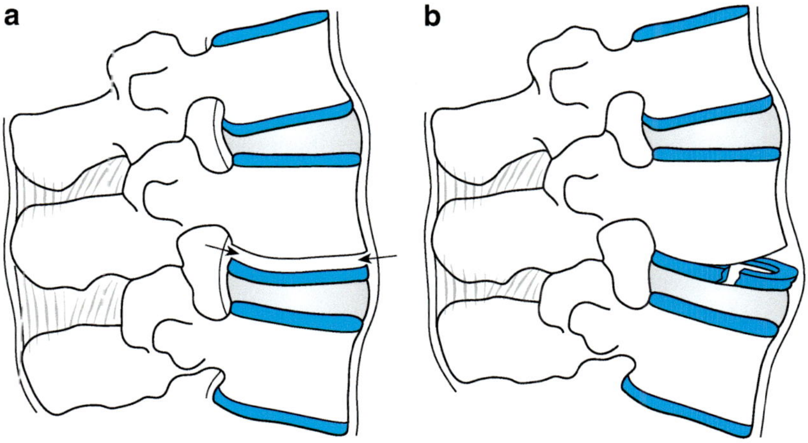

Fig. 18.7 (**a**) Disruption of the lower cartilaginous vertebral endplate (Salter-Harris I lesion), (**b**) Avulsion of the lower anterior vertebral edge (Aitken 2, Salter-Harris III injury)

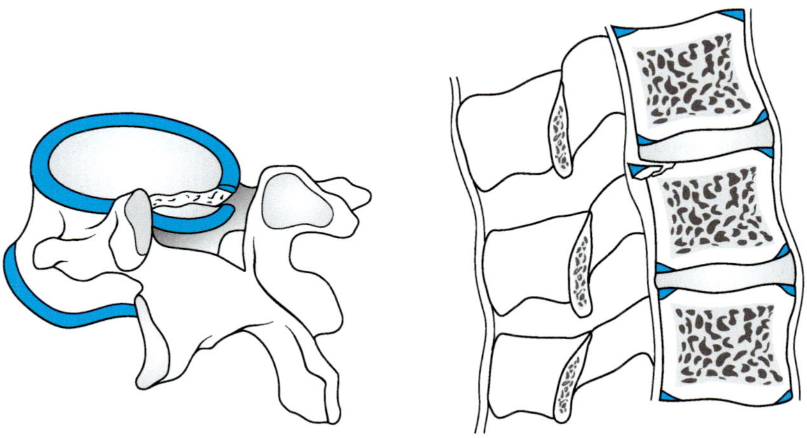

Fig. 18.8 Apophyseal fracture with posterior displacement

In the thoracic and lumbar spine, disruptions of the synchondroses between the bipolar neurocentral cartilage and the growth centers of the arch are possible in the form of spondylolysis.

Treatment

The goal of treatment is a stable, healed spine, since missed instability can lead to progressive deformity or neurological deficits. Follow-up investigations are necessary for (unstable) injuries for which development of posttraumatic deformity can be expected. It should be noted that posttraumatic deformities will undergo varying levels of compensation, for example, the pediatric c-spine matures earlier than the rest of the spine. The potential for good regeneration (remodeling) allows a better prognosis for many fractures, so that predominantly conservative therapy can be used. For example, conservative therapy in a corset is recommended for thoracic fractures as well as functional treatment for stable compression fractures. Unstable bony deformities can only be stabilized to a limited extent with braces or bed rest as these measures cannot completely prevent displacement.

The indications for operative stabilization are the criteria for instability. Alignment lines, with consideration of growth-related variants, are crucial in the c-spine. Most fractures here are stable, but the specific pattern of injury is of high importance. In the thoracic and lumbar spine, initial kyphosis over 20% is an indication for surgery. Here in older children, the criteria of the Denis Classification (mechanical, ligament, bony-ligament according to Denis and Frank) and the Magerl concept (compression, flexion-distraction, rotation) can be used.

In older children and adolescents, thoracic and lumbar injury fusions are performed according to the principles of adult care. Operative stabilization in small children is particularly difficult because of the anatomy and difficulties in implant selection. However, pronounced instability should be treated with internal stabilization or alternatively with traction. Ligamentous injuries are rare, and most endplate fractures achieve bony healing. Laminectomy in children produces significant growth-related deformities and is therefore contraindicated provided there is no evidence of mechanical spinal canal stenosis with correlated neurological complications. The extent of the spinal canal injury is assessed by the bony or discal compression of the spinal cord. Because of the good healing potential in children, unstable injuries that are purely ligamentous can also be treated conservatively or with a posterior spondylodesis.

Unstable bony lesions are difficult to be sufficiently supported externally. Fractures with neurological damage and incomplete neurological syndromes with spinal canal narrowing require operative stabilization, especially in cases of progressive neurological deficit with confirmed spinal cord damage.

18.3 Injuries to the Cervical Spine

Incidence, Mechanism of Injury and Clinical Picture

Cervical spine injuries are relatively uncommon (approximately 2% of all spine injuries). However, they are the most common spine lesions for children under 10 years. Under 8 years, the increased head-to-body ratio yields primary loading of the upper c-spine. Approximately 70% of all pediatric c-spine lesions affect C1 and C2 with a high mortality risk in complex injuries. In approximately 50% of cases there is additional injury to the skull.

Injuries from child abuse ("shaken baby syndrome") are caused by torsion of the heavy head against the upper c-spine. Under 2 years of age, birth trauma is the most common. In head-first births, high spinal cord injuries can occur through rotation, and lower cervical and upper thoracic lesions (SCIWORA) from traction during forceps-assisted births.

Classification

The respective classification is listed under the specific injuries.

Particulars

It is often necessary to make the differential diagnosis from pseudosubluxation (see segment C2/C3). Anterior rotational displacement of C1 over C2 (see AAD) is also a consideration.

Grisel's Syndrome: The lymphatic drainage of the c-spine region occurs through the retropharyngeal and deep cervical lymph nodes that also drain the nasopharynx. Cervical pseudosubluxation can also occur in cases of pharyngitis and lymphadenopathy. Subluxation with torticollis can be caused by inflammation, an atlantoaxial subluxation by local hyperemia and edema after pharyngitis, otitis, tonsillar abscess, osteomyelitis, or tumors. Tuberculosis must also be excluded when the traumatic etiology is not clear.

Diagnosis

In cases of skull injury, additional c-spine injury must always be excluded. Radiographs of the cervical spine are carried out in two planes, possibly with oblique views. Correct positioning of the head during X-ray and complete imaging of the c-spine must be ensured. Additional assessments are MRI and CT. Interpretation of radiographic findings of the upper c-spine can be difficult (see age-related X-ray findings). Caution: spontaneous reduction of fractured growth zones.

Rare pathological fractures and battered child syndrome must be considered.

Occipital Fracture

Incidence, Mechanism of Injury and Clinical Picture

Occipital fractures are very rare. The cause for this injury is severe axial compression (Table 18.4).

Classification

In adolescents, the Anderson-Montesano classification for adults is also used.

Table 18.4 Occipital fracture

Particulars	Very rare (case study in children), severe trauma, axial compression
Diagnostic Assessment	Method of choice: CT
Therapy goal/Limits of correction	Prevention of growth distortion, diagnosis and therapy for possible concomitant injuries
Primary treatment	Immobilization with hard collar (Stiffneck)
Conservative therapy	
Indications	Method of Choice
Procedure	Philadelphia collar depending on extent, concomitant injuries (instability), and complaints
Follow Up	Symptomatic
X-ray Controls	Only CT is meaningful (Fig. 18.9)
Return to sports	Earliest at 16 weeks
Operative treatment	
Indications	Instability in cases of concomitant ligament injuries (see AOD)
Procedure	Halo fixateur for 4–6 weeks
Follow Up	Pin control and cleaning
X-ray Controls	CT or MRI at 6 weeks
Return to sports	Earliest at 16 weeks
Complications	Subdural hematoma, growth disturbances
Growth Disturbances	Possible because of chondro-osseous growth regions
Follow Up	Optional regarding potential growth disturbances

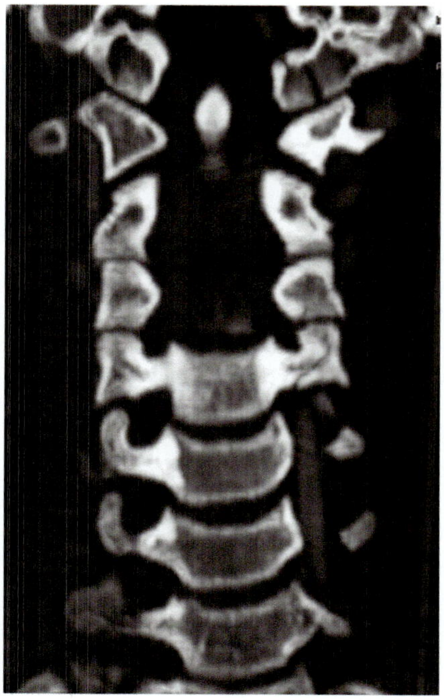

Fig. 18.9 Fracture of the occipital condyle without displacement—conservative treatment

Occipitoatlantal Dislocation

Incidence, Mechanism of Injury and Clinical Picture

Occipitoatlantal dislocations are very rare and often primarily fatal. In cases of survival for often only a few hours, the mortality is ≥50%. Occipitoatlantal dislocation occurs twice as often in children as in adults. It often occurs in traffic accidents where the patient has been driven into.

The mechanism of injury is a strong acceleration of the head with horizontal joint line and incongruent joint surfaces. The result is usually polytrauma with traumatic brain injury (Table 18.5).

The neurological findings are diffuse, and with deficits and injuries of the lower cranial nerves, the brainstem, the proximal spinal cord, and the first three spinal nerves, the results can be cardiac arrhythmias, asymmetrical paralysis, apnea and respiratory failure.

Table 18.5 Occipitoatlantal dislocations

Particulars	Very rare; often fatal
Diagnostic Assessment	Massive soft-tissue swelling in the head and neck region, clinical suspicion (ambulance), neurological findings Radiology: lateral X-rays of the c-spine with often significant dislocation (caution: spontaneous reduction); distinct retropharyngeal/retro-tracheal swelling; normal basion to dens interval 4–5 mm; borderline values are problematic because of variable magnification factors, eventually functional X-rays in flexion-extension 3D-CT: with sagittal and coronal reconstruction MRI: ligament ruptures, bleeding (angio-MRI: a. vertebralis lesion) Harris sign: reliable, independent of variations and position. Cranial extension of the posterior vertebral line of C2 may be located not less than 6mm and not more than 12mm from the basion (midpoint of the anterior rim of the foramen magnum), applicable in adults and children. The center of the dens tip should be perpendicular beneath the basion; from 13 years on the distance should not be >12 mm
Therapy goal/Limits of correction	Stability, smaller children can survive
Primary treatment	Rapid detection at the scene of the trauma; c-spine immobilization to prevent secondary damage; cautious intubation with complications
Conservative therapy	
Indications	Method of Choice
Procedure	Rapid closed reduction (without extension), immobilization in halo (also combined with plaster vests) when neurologically asymptomatic (Fig. 18.11)
Follow Up	In cases of minimal instability, Halo fixator or Minerva cast for 2 months (8–10 weeks), consider postoperative corrections, new functional views after treatment
X-ray Controls	Close X-ray controls
Return to sports	Depends on stability and overall course
Operative treatment	
Indications	Older children and adolescents; with persistent instability and neurological deficits also in younger children since failure of conservative therapy is possible
Procedure	Occiput-C1/C2 fusion, as short as possible! Technique: posterior midline approach, wire cerclage and bone graft
Follow Up	additional temporary protection with a stiff soft collar
X-ray Controls	Regular
Hardware removal	If needed once consolidated and stable
Return to sports	Depends on the course
Complications	Increasing number of survivors, sometimes with unexpectedly positive clinical course but with possible neurological (>80%, approximately 40% tetraplegic) and vascular complications; Caution: excess distraction; halo complications
Growth Disturbances	Possible, if spondylodesis
Follow Up	Course-dependent

Classification

Occipitoatlantal dislocations are classified according to the direction of dislocation (Fig. 18.10).

- Type 1: Anterior head dislocation; most common
  1a: sagittal head dislocation
  1b: head dislocation combined with axial instability
- Type 2: posterior head dislocation, very rare
- Type 3: axial dislocation with global instability, also complete separation; incomplete sub-luxate forms possible

Atlas Fracture

Incidence, Mechanism of Injury and Clinical Picture

C1 fractures are rare in children. The cause is often birth trauma (can be confused with congenital defects), usually an indirect trauma caused by axial force over the head on the lateral mass. Fractures of the lateral mass and ruptures of the transverse ligament are possible. Clinically there is a feeling of instability and pronounced pain posteriorly over the proximal c-spine. Spinal cord injuries are rare (Table 18.6).

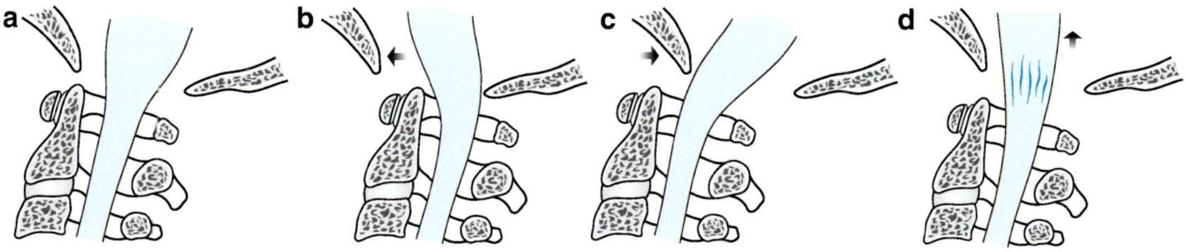

Fig. 18.10 Atlanto-occipital dislocation. (**a**) Normal situation, (**b**) Dislocation of the head to the ventral side, (**c**) Dislocation of the head to the dorsal side, (**d**) Axial extension of the myelon due to distraction of the head

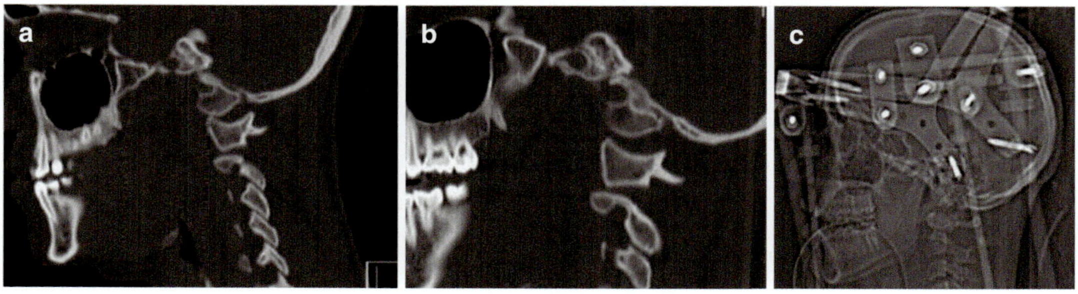

Fig. 18.11 20 Year girl with dislocation of the occipital condyle to the ventral side after traffic accident. (**a**) Trauma image CT, (**b**) Reduction in anesthesia, (**c**) Stabilization with HALO fixateur. Good healing without problems

Table 18.6 Atlas fracture

Particulars	Microfractures in the ossification centers, in smaller children mostly through the neurocentral synchondrosis (fusion at 7 years), often undetectable on X-ray
Diagnostic Assessment	Conventional X-rays are problematic, transoral views when possible Method of choice: CT, accurate fracture morphology (Fig. 18.12) Caution: C1 grows faster than the C2, and can project laterally between the 3rd month and 4th year of age with the lateral masses (called "pseudospread" by Suss et al.); synchondroses of C1 can be confused with fracture
Therapy goal/Limits of correction	Stable healing
Primary treatment	Immobilization
Conservative therapy	
Indications	Method of Choice
Procedure	Smaller children: Philadelphia collar (or Minerva cast) for 6–8 weeks, then well-fitting soft brace; halo fixator for older children and adolescents (Fig. 18.13)
Follow Up	May be a long immobilization (up to 6 months) until complete consolidation
X-ray Controls	CT controls regarding consolidation
Return to sports	With consolidation and lack of complaints
Operative treatment	
Indications	Very rare, only with persistent complaints of instability and non-union
Procedure	Depends on individual situation and age
Follow Up	Specific to the procedure, individual
X-ray Controls	Specific to the procedure, individual
Hardware removal	Specific to the procedure, individual
Return to sports	Specific to the procedure, individual
Complications	Rare
Growth Disturbances	Possible, but rare
Follow Up	After treatment is completed, only when complaints are present

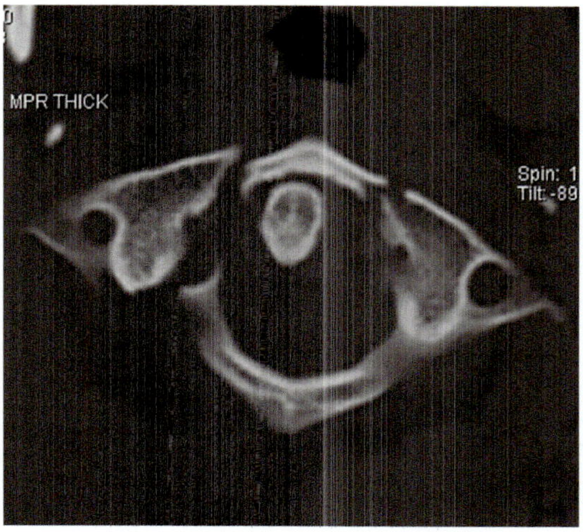

Fig. 18.12 Fracture of the Atlas in a child. Jefferson fracture right side (from Nau et al. Thieme Verlag)

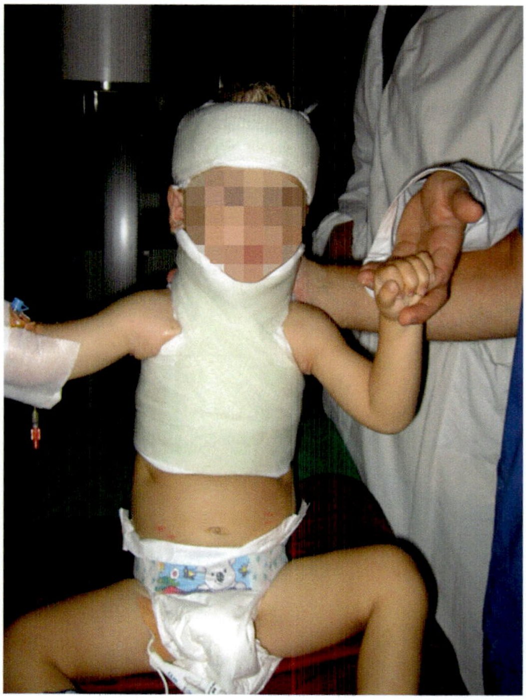

Fig. 18.13 Minerva cast in a small child

Atlantoaxial Dislocation (AAD)

Incidence, Mechanism of Injury and Clinical Picture

Atlantoaxial dislocations are relatively common lesions in the C1/C2 region. They occur as translational or rotational instability of C1 on C2 with traumatic and atraumatic history. There are fluid transitions (Table 18.7).

Ligamentous translational AAD. The clinical picture is of neck pain and often secondary neurological deficits. Traumatic translational anterior AAD is caused by (isolated) rupture of the transverse ligament with anterior shift of C1 on C2. This is distinct from non-traumatic translational anterior AAD that is caused by increased ligament laxity with spinal canal stenosis in Down syndrome, inflammatory processes (Grisel syndrome) and rheumatoid arthritis.

Rotatory AAD. This is associated with painful torticollis, stiff neck, occipital neuralgia and cervical muscle spasm. The clinical picture shows symmetrical shoulders, head not inclined laterally, with hardened sternocleidomastoid muscles on the side to which the head is turned. Traumatic rotatory AAD is often accompanied by fractures of the superior body, capsular ligament tears with tilted dislocation of a joint, and rotation of C1 over C2. Bilateral locking of the articular processes is possible, and in ligament ruptures also an anterior shift of C1. There is pronounced pain on motion despite unremarkable still X-ray images (Fig. 18.14).

Non-traumatic rotatory AAD (also called atlanto-axial rotatory subluxation = AARS or atlanto-axial rotatory fixation) is distinguished by the fact that it occurs predominantly in girls with diffuse etiology. Causes include inflammation-related decalcification and ligament laxity (ruptures) in juvenile rheumatoid arthritis, infections

Table 18.7 Atlantoaxial dislocation (AAD)

Particulars	Common; traumatic and atraumatic forms
Diagnostic Assessment	Difficult. Anterior shift of C1 over C2 through the horizontal facet joint is common and normal in small children. Cave: superior "pseudosubluxation" of C1 and C2 in 20% of children <8 years. With lax transverse ligaments of C2, the physiological limit for anterior shift of C1 is 3 mm, or 5 mm when flexed. In extension, posterior shift of C1 arch and overriding the tip of the dens is possible (Fig. 18.15) Clinically there is muscle spasm, pain, limited extension; the history is crucial Radiology: X-rays of the c-spine in two planes, lateral X-rays of the upper c-spine: sagittal C1-Dens distance (anterior dens cortex to the posterior C1 cortex) ≥4 mm means suspected rupture of transverse ligament, with distance of 10–12 mm all ligaments ruptured Transoral radiographs: in rotatory AAD, asymmetrical atlanto-axial joint and dens, varied size of the lateral masses. C2 spinous process out of the midline CT: retro-odontoid distance enlarged, sagittal and rotatory deformity MRI: Ruptured transverse ligament, visualization of nerve and bony lesions Differential diagnosis: (a) hypermobility of C1/C2 in syrinx, spinal tumors, pseudospread, Down's syndrome, (b) dens hypoplasia: in approximately 15% shift >5 mm, approximately 10–15% are neurologically symptomatic, incidence unclear, (c) upper respiratory tract infections, (d) agenesis of the dens, (e) Os odontoideum, (f) dens shortening due to missing terminal ossification center
Therapy goal/Limits of correction	Stability
Primary treatment	With traumatic etiology, external halo fixator
Conservative therapy	
Indications	Atlantoaxial deformity is usually temporary and reversible, disco-ligamentous instability is problematic to treat conservatively
Procedure	Traumatic translational AAD: immobilization in halo ring or Minerva vest for 6–12 weeks possible (see below) Acute rotatory AAD is generally reducible; halo ring. Technique: traction and rotation, manipulation and normal positioning. In cases of intact transverse ligament, healing is possible with immobilization in a Philadelphia collar
Follow Up	Complaint-dependent
X-ray Controls	Regular, depends on initial CT
Return to sports	Case-dependent
Operative treatment	
Indications	Traumatic translational AAD: C1–C2 fusion, since no healing is expected with conservative management Rotatory AAD: dorsal fusion when the transverse ligament is ruptured. In situ C1–C2 fusion for non-reducible deformities. C1–C2 fusion when there is posttraumatic instability after 2–3 months of halo treatment and shift >5 mm persists on functional views
Procedure	Posterior C1–C2 spondylodesis: cerclage, bone graft; screws
Follow Up	Procedure-dependent
X-ray Controls	Procedure-dependent
Hardware removal	Halo after 2–3 months
Return to sports	Questionable
Complications	Survivors of traumatic AAC: neurological complications, persistent instability after conservative treatment, neurological complications from traction, non-correctible deformity with the need for fusion (in deformed position), hypermobility of adjacent segments after fusion
Growth Disturbances	Possible
Follow Up	Long-term

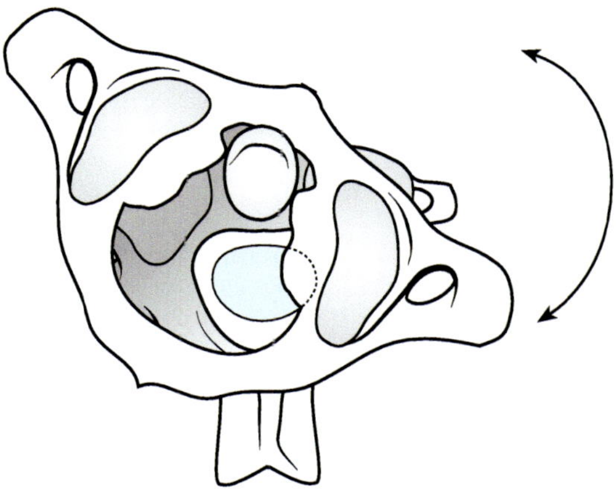

Fig. 18.14 Rotation instability with enormous narrowing of the spinal canal

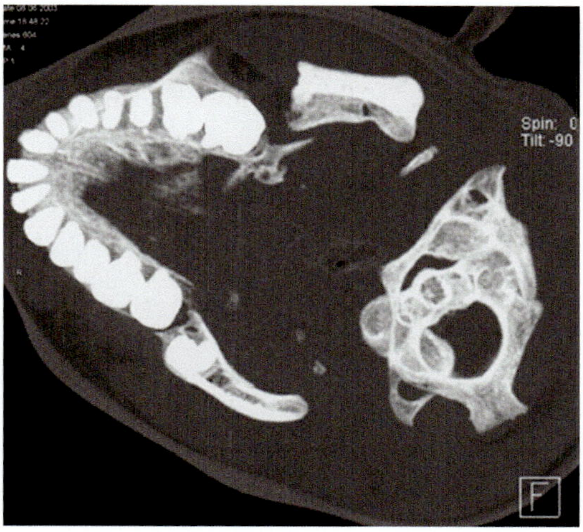

Fig. 18.15 CT projection of a rotation injury C1–C2

of the upper respiratory tract (Grisel's syndrome), ENT procedures, mild trauma, as well as muscle contraction and spasms. Signs of this are torticollis (pain, limitation of movement), approximately 20° lateral inclination of the head, 20° of rotation to the opposite side with slight flexion.

Classification

The Fielding and Hawkins Classification of rotatory AAD is based on 17 patients (two trauma) and accounts for only "fixed" deformities.

- Type I: most common; rotatory displacement without anterior movement of C1, intact transverse ligament, normal C1-Dens distance; fulcrum in the dens.
- Type II: second most common, rotatory displacement with 3–5 mm shift of C1, possible transverse ligament insufficiency; fulcrum in the lateral mass.
- Type III and IV non-traumatic.
- Type III: rotatory displacement on C1> 5 mm; insufficiency of the transverse ligament and other stabilizers; both lateral masses anterior.
- Type IV: posterior rotatory displacement of C1 with absent dens.

Axis and Dens Fractures

Incidence, Mechanism of Injury and Clinical Picture

Axis and dens fractures are rare in children under 7 years, even rarer in children under 3 years. However, it is one of the most common cervical spine injuries (Table 18.8).

The cause is usually massive trauma with flexion (traffic accidents, falls from a height, falls on the head). History is important, it is possible even in mild trauma with negative X-rays. Clinically, there is a heterogeneous picture ranging from mild pain and neck stiffness to severe pain at the occipital base, worsened with head movement.

A diagnostic clue is that the patient holds head to prevent extension.

Patients feel instability, as if the head would fall down. Also acute torticollis can be observed. The injured person prefers lying or standing position.

Fracture localization is in the body, beneath the level of the facet joint. The subdental synchondrosis is vulnerable until 10 years of age, and fractures occur along the basal cartilage plate (growth zone).

Table 18.8 Axis and dens fractures

Particulars	Confusion with synchondroses (Fig. 18.16)
Diagnostic Assessment	C-spine X-rays in two planes, trans-oral views: usually confirm diagnosis, occasional wide displacement on lateral image. Anterior translation and angulation of the dens in kyphosis. Spontaneous reduction is possible with correct positioning. Retropharyngeal soft-tissue swelling is a diagnostic clue Flexion/extension views: dens moves with C1 Differential diagnosis: (a) open dentocentral synchondrosis, (b) Os odontoideum (trauma history!), (c) H-form synchondrosis of the horizontal synchondrosis along the base and two vertical synchondroses along the transition from body to arch, which merge between ages 3 and 6 years. They may be visible until age ten When in doubt, CT: Injuries of the C2 synchondroses are only visible on CT
Therapy goal/Limits of correction	Anatomic healing
Primary treatment	Immobilization
Conservative therapy	
Indications	Conservative treatment until age 8 years
Procedure	With mild displacement: light traction in stable brace (Fig. 18.17) With further displacement: reduction under traction and retention in Minerva cast or halo (6–12 weeks), prognosis good with good reduction, immobilization sometimes up to 4 months Rare fractures of the C2 body or the vertebral arch also heal conservatively
Follow Up	Complaint-dependent
X-ray Controls	Regular, possibly CT, MRI
Return to sports	Case-dependent, after 3–4 months when asymptomatic for approximately 3–4 months
Operative treatment	
Indications	Rare; in older children with unstable Anderson Type II (adult classification) fractures; in smaller children with persistent movement of the dens like a pseudarthrosis (see Os odontoideum); high-grade instability, fractures displaced at least the width of the dens
Procedure	Posterior C1–C2 fusion, in older children also direct screw fixation
Follow Up	Stable orthosis for 4 weeks
X-ray Controls	At 2 and 6 weeks
Hardware removal	Not applicable
Return to sports	At 3–4 months
Complications	Myelopathy with longer unrecognized instability and dens displacement, temporary kyphosis after C1–C2 fusion
Growth Disturbances	In cases of epiphyseal damage, earlier closure of the dens growth plates, although without major consequences; in children over 7 years complications as in adults, particularly regarding delayed healing, that applies for Anderson Type II fractures and posterior displacements that often mandate fusion. Os odontoideum can often be interpreted as non-union after missed dens fracture in smaller children
Follow Up	Delayed occipitoatlantal instability is possible; thus follow-up is required until growth ceases

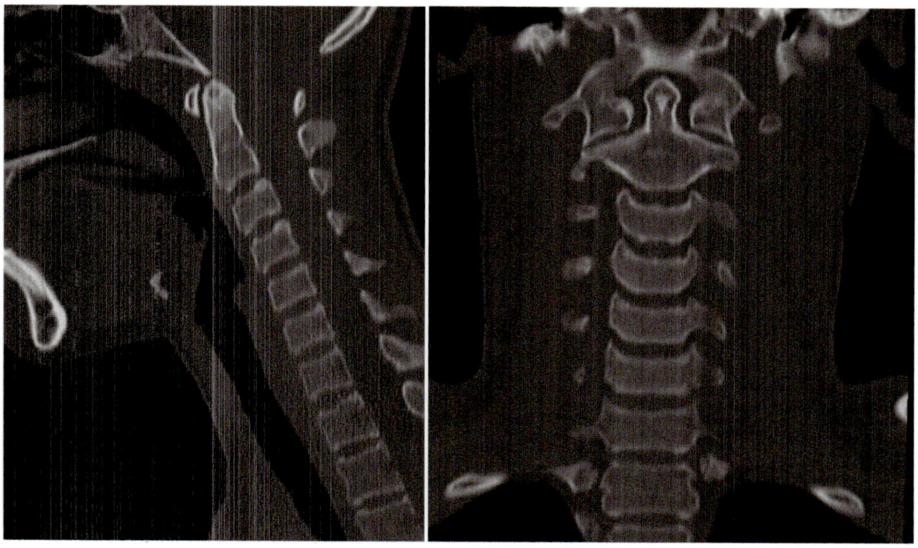

Fig. 18.16 Synchondrosis of the dens axis of a 12 year old girl in CT scan

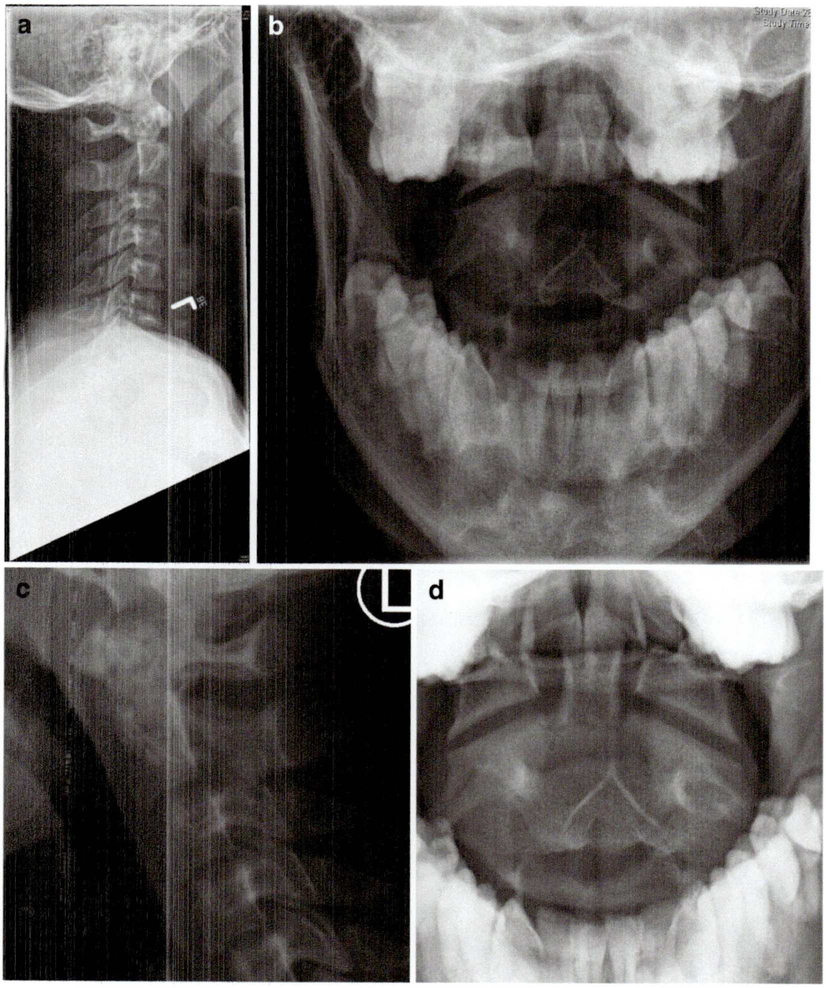

Fig. 18.17 14 Year old boy after mountain bike stand with fracture of the dens axis, type Anderson II, undisplaced and conservative treatment in stiff-neck. (**a**, **b**) AP and LATERAL VIEW, (**c**, **d**) magnification, AP and oblique view

Os Odontoideum

Mechanism of Injury and Clinical Picture

Real congenital Os odontoideum. This is a deformed dens that has not fused with the base, also a hypertrophied remnant with dens hypoplasia and lacking distal ossification center (Table 18.9).

Post-traumatic Os odontoideum. It occurs after unrecognized trauma with non-union and fibrous replacement as a result of an untreated fracture in the cartilaginous growth zone of the dens, the "dens stump" of the Axis body with sagittal translational instability (AAD).

Table 18.9 Os odontoideum

Particulars	Congenital and posttraumatic origin theory
Diagnostic Assessment	Functional X-ray images in flexion/extension, in exceptional cases also flexion/extension CT or MRI: extent of instability, exclude spinal cord compression. In symptomatic patients, the os odontoideum moves anteriorly with C1 up to a centimeter CT: big gap between the odontoid tip and the base
Therapy goal/Limits of correction	Stability
Primary treatment	–
Conservative Therapy	Method of Choice
Indications	Congenital: no treatment
Procedure	Post-traumatic: 6 weeks orthosis
Follow Up	Not applicable
X-ray Controls	Post-traumatic: 6 weeks, 3 months, 1 year
Return to sports	Complaint-dependent
Operative treatment	
Indications	In cases of pathological mobility, persistent instability or evidence of acute/potential spinal cord damage with or without neurological symptoms. Difficult indications in asymptomatic patients. Potential instability/risk in case of trauma!
Procedure	Posterior C1–C2 fusion, very rare
Follow Up	6 weeks stable orthosis
X-ray Controls	At 6 weeks
Hardware removal	Implant-dependent
Return to sports	At 4–6 months
Complications	See Growth Disturbances
Growth Disturbances	Are possible because of fusion
Follow Up	At 6 and 12 months

Injuries to the C2/C3 Segment and Pseudosubluxation

Incidence, Mechanism of Injury and Clinical Picture

In contrast to pseudosubluxation, discoligamentous instability occurs rarely, and when it does, in children over 10 years. In consideration of the posterior vertebral borders, pseudosubluxation of C2/C3 occurs distinctly in some 10% of children and moderately in 15%. 40% of children under 8 years show this anterior shift (Table 18.10).

C2/C3 subluxation/dislocation is possible as a consequence of trauma, often associated with injuries to the head, face or chest and localized pain without evidence of fracture. Until age 7–8 years, the C2/C3 segment is the flexion/extension fulcrum. Traumatic facet dislocations without fracture are possible, often isolated injuries, as are apophyseal fractures. A C2 pedicle fracture (Hangman's fracture) is the result of flexion or extension trauma.

Table 18.10 Injuries to the C2/C3 segment pseudosubluxation

Particulars	True instability is rare; pseudosubluxation is common
Diagnostic Assessment	Pseudosubluxation: C2/C3 is the main segment of motion under 8 years, on lateral views of this segment in flexion, 2–4 mm shift is normal (Figs. 18.18 and 18.19). Diagnostic challenge in case of local symptoms. Cause: inclination of the joint surfaces changes from 55° to 70° in C1/C2 and 30° to 60–70° in C2–C4. Pseudosubluxation is not easily quantifiable due to absent landmarks. The spinolaminar Swischuk's line between the arch borders of C1–C3 should remain within 1.5 mm at C2. It's possible to confuse it with primary spondylolysis or synchondroses of the posterior arch. Pseudosubluxation resolves in extension. MRI is the method of choice to exclude discoligamentous injury/instability
Therapy goal/Limits of correction	Exclude traumatic instability
Primary treatment	Immobilization after trauma and exclude instability
Conservative therapy	
Indications	Method of Choice
Procedure	For fractures, closed reduction and halo for approximately 8 weeks; for subluxation/dislocation in children under 8 years, closed reduction and halo immobilization
Follow Up	Halo care
X-ray Controls	At 4 and 12 weeks
Return to sports	Complaint-dependent
Operative treatment	
Indications	Persistent posterior instability when there is discoligamentous instability (C2/C3 subluxation) or non-union
Procedure	Posterior fusion (C1–C3); however, after careful verification of posterior instability. Vertebral body involvement can result in bony healing. With posttraumatic subluxation and dislocation in children over 8 years, posterior fusion
Follow Up	Rigid orthosis for 4–6 weeks
X-ray Controls	At 4 and 12 weeks
Hardware removal	Implant-dependent
Return to sports	Complaint-dependent
Complications	In cases of fusion
Growth Disturbances	Possible
Follow Up	Until growth conclusion in cases of fusion

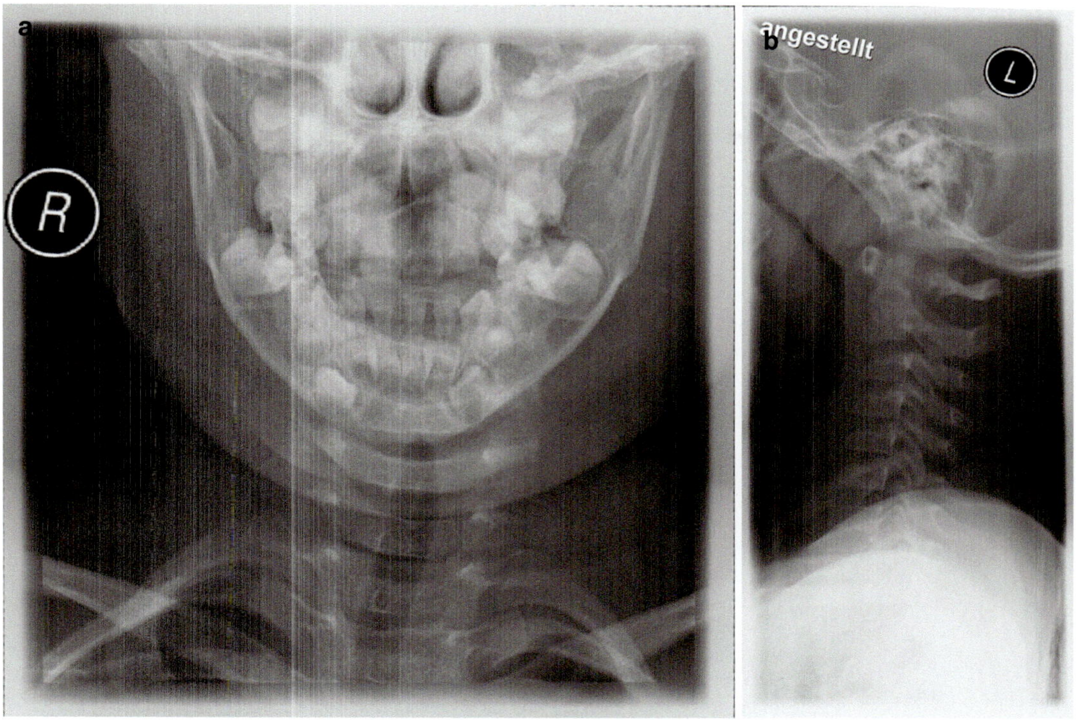

Fig. 18.18 Child with subluxation with slight pseudoluxation C2/C3. (**a**, **b**) AP and lateral view

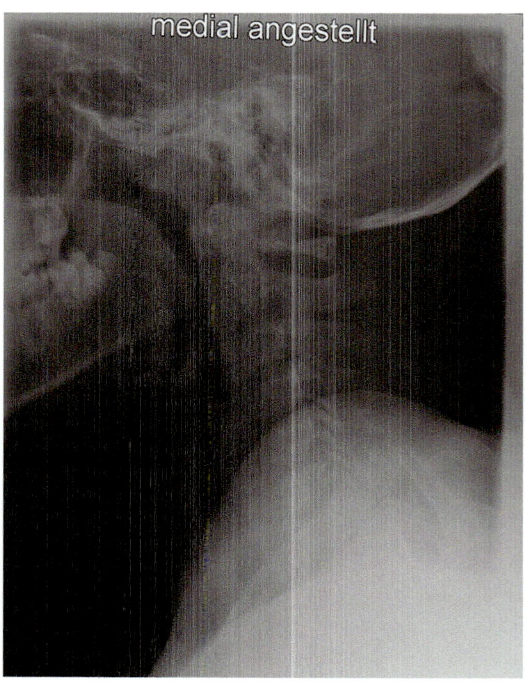

Fig. 18.19 Pseudoluxation C2/C3 in a child

Classification

The Effendi Classification can be used for injuries of the C2 segment in adolescents.

Injuries to C3–C7

Incidence, Mechanism of Injury and Clinical Picture

Injuries in the C3–C7 area are rare in children under 10 years; the average age of patients is 13 years.

It is often a compression fracture.

A flexion/extension mechanism can lead to discoligamentous injury, hyperflexion to ruptures of the secondary OFC in the tips of the spinous processes. Ruptures of the lower epiphyseal endplates can be caused by hyperextension-distraction traumas, e.g. in car accidents, jumps into shallow water, or child abuse. Predisposing congenital factors are generally associated with posterior instability (Table 18.11).

Table 18.12 gives some technical aspects for the treatment of cervical spine injuries.

Table 18.11 Injuries to C3–C7

Particulars	Salter-Harris I Injuries = Epiphyseal separation (usually in younger children); Salter-Harris III (Aitken 2) injuries occur as anterior rupture of the growth plate and epiphyses (in adolescents) Fractures of the apophyseal ring have to be excluded
Diagnostic Assessment	C-spine views in two planes (including T1). Under 8 years, X-ray functional views in flexion/extension to assess segment mobility in cases of pseudosubluxation (better visualized with longitudinal distraction). MRI when there are radiographic signs of instability T3 and T4 can have a variety of shapes (wedge, rounding, etc.). Caution: injuries to the growth plates and painful fractures of the secondary ossification centers (often only visible radiographically beginning between 10 and 12 years, soft-tissue swelling). Spontaneous reduction is possible. Displaced ring apophyseal injuries can be confused with secondary ossification centers
Therapy goal/Limits of correction	Avoiding post-traumatic kyphosis
Primary treatment	Immobilization in stable orthosis (Philadelphia collar)
Conservative therapy	
Indications	Compression fractures usually heal conservatively in orthoses. Spontaneous correction after compression fractures C3–C7 is limited compared to the thoracic/lumbar spine because of more rapid maturation (Fig. 18.20). No mandatory treatment recommendations to tolerate fracture displacement, kyphosis or necessary positional corrections. Course is important. Closed reduction and retention of compression fractures is only possible to a limited extent, corrected position is often lost. Serial compression fractures are generally treated conservatively and corrected as needed after healing. Ligamentous injuries can heal with immobilization; however, there is a risk of kyphotic deformity and complications as in adults. In cases of persistent instability and increasing kyphosis, posterior stabilization is needed. In adolescents, anterior bridging spondylodesis (as possible with disc conservation)
Procedure	Children under 8 years with rare extended compression or serial fractures: 6 weeks halo and 6 weeks in rigid orthosis. Salter-Harris III injuries will heal within weeks because of the osteogenic potential of the anterior longitudinal ligament. In cases of discoligamentous injuries, halo for 8–12 weeks is possible (see below)
Follow Up	Consistent immobilization will lead to healing of the injured ligamentous and chondro-osseous structures
X-ray Controls	6 weeks, 3 months, 1 year
Return to sports	Course-dependent
Operative treatment	
Indications	Ligamentous instability rarely heals but in children there are exemptions (Fig. 18.21). Indications for operative stabilization depend on age, grade of displacement/instability and extent of bony destruction with potential instability and expected secondary deformity (Fig. 18.22) Posterior fusion with radiographic evidence of instability after 3+ months of conservative treatment. Because mostly flexion injuries and mechanisms, anterior approach is contraindicated. Impaired growth of the anterior ossification center and posterior instability make spontaneous fusion improbable in adolescents. Early surgical stabilization is needed for unstable fractures and spinal cord injury
Procedure	Posterior wire fusion of the spinous processes and autologous bone graft. Anterior fusion is contraindicated in small children because of endplate destruction; however, bridging plate fixation with hardware removal is possible in older children (see Figure above) Laminectomy only in exceptional cases with progressive neurological symptoms and verified spinal compression since significant damage to posterior stabilizing elements (swan neck deformity) can be expected. Facet joints can be stabilized with cerclage and bone graft Resection of painful non-unions of the spinous processes. Minimize surgical exposure due to risk of spontaneous adjacent segment fusion

Table 18.11 (continued)

Follow Up	Course-dependent
X-ray Controls	Control of fusion and kyphotic deformity. Cave: Halo pin penetration (severe pain) and local osteolysis
Hardware removal	After 1 year following anterior bridging procedure
Return to sports	Symptom-free
Complications	Halo care: pin infections or penetration. Salter-Harris I injuries are often not survived. Halo treatment is difficult with smaller children (see below)
Growth Disturbances	Premature growth plate closure, narrowing of the disc space, ossification of the longitudinal ligament in type III injuries
Follow Up	At 6 weeks, 3 months and 12 months

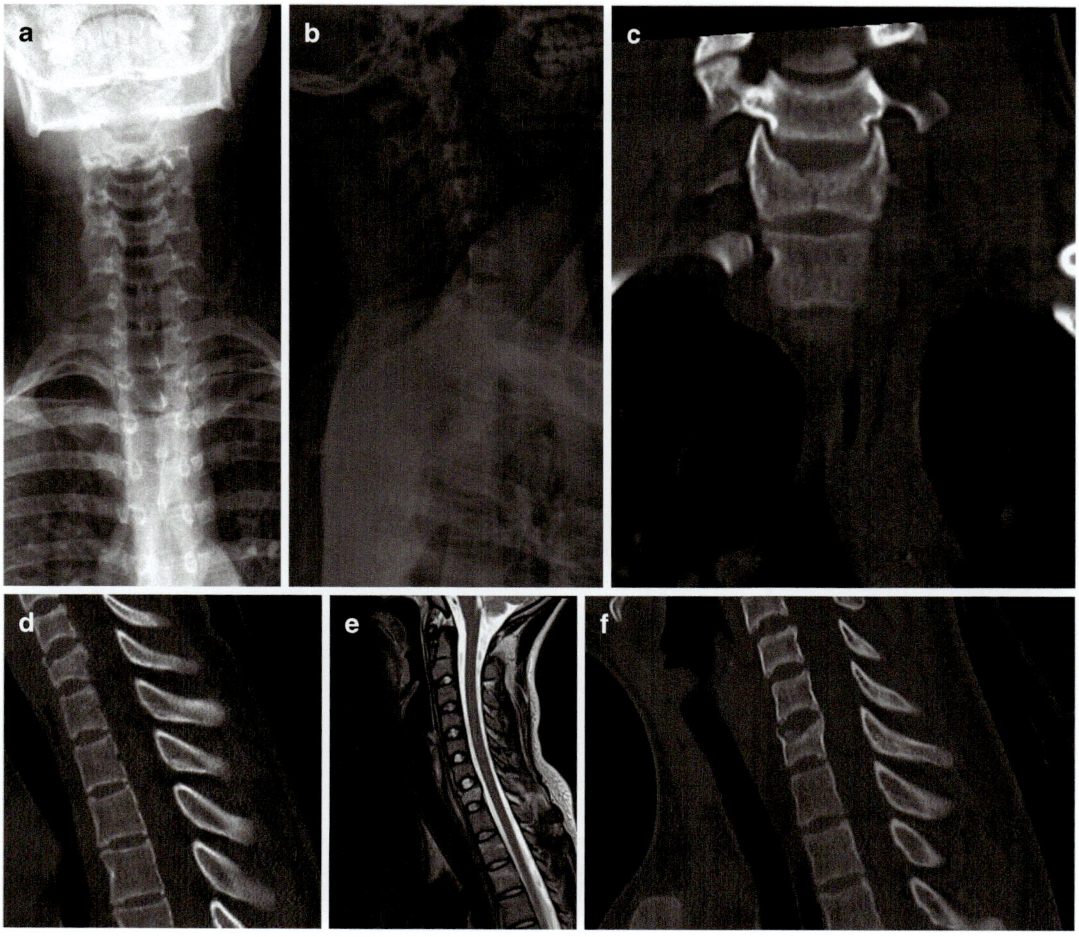

Fig. 18.20 Compression fracture of the seventh cervical spine after jump into water. (**a**, **b**) X-ray, (**c**, **d**) CT scan, (**e**) MRI, (**f**) Healing in CT after conservative therapy

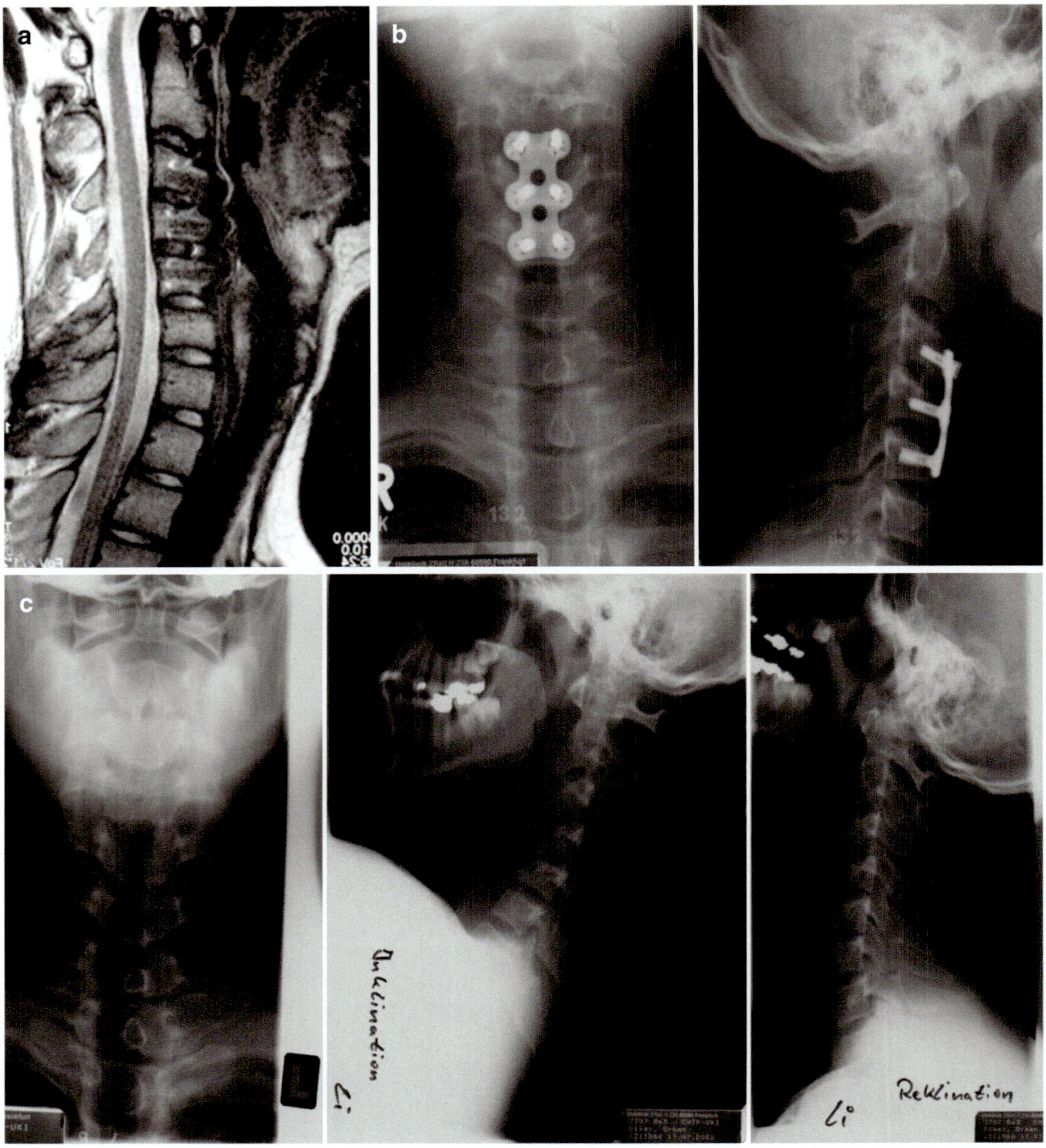

Fig. 18.21 Discoligamentous B-type injury of a 15 year old boy after jump into low water. (**a**) MRI with disc and ligamentous injuries C3/C4 and C4/C5. (**b**) Operative transfixation of the C3 to C5 without taking out the discs with angular stable plate. (**c**) Good function with stability after taking out the plate 1 year later and healed injuries

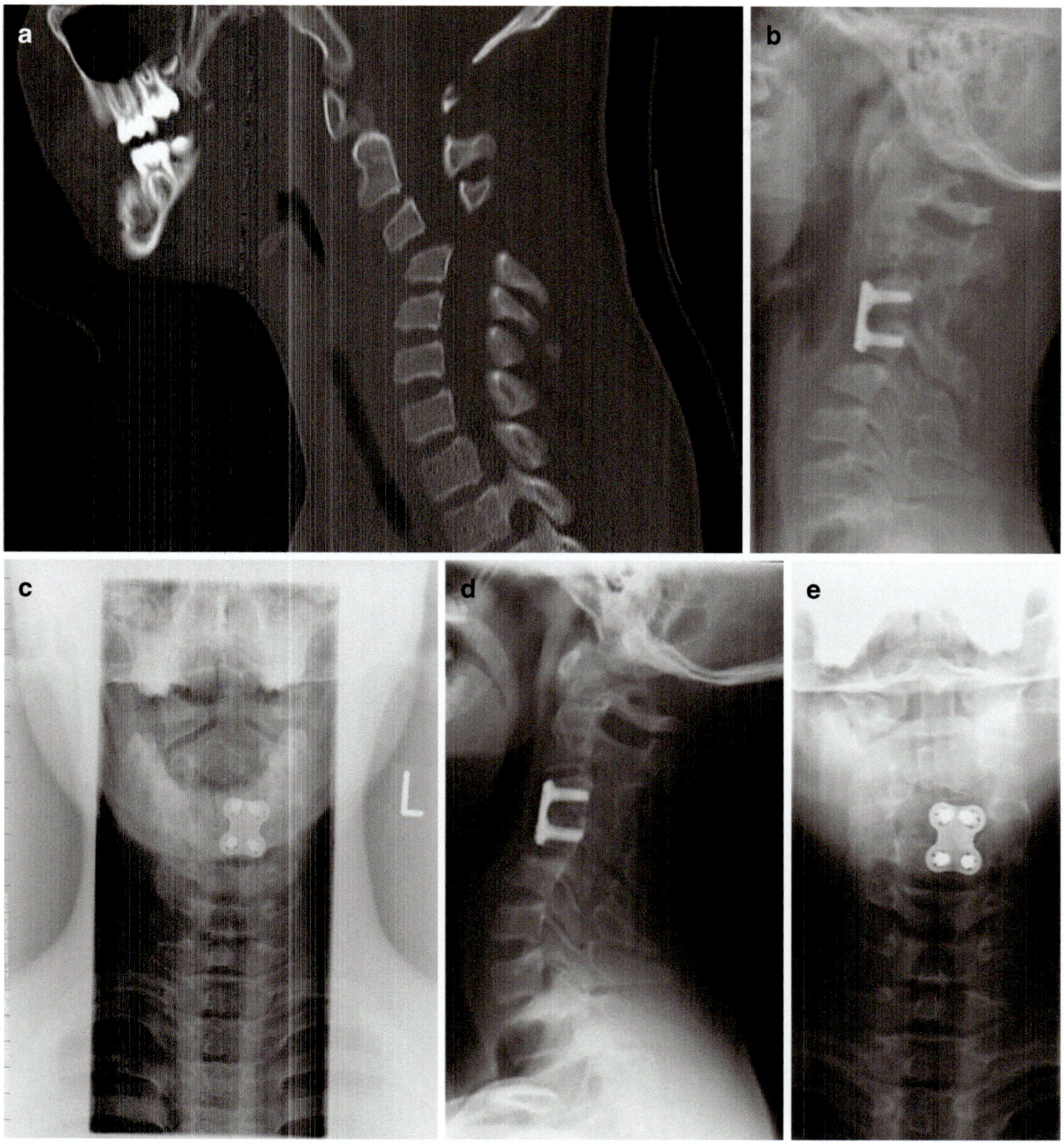

Fig. 18.22 12 Year cld boy with a swing in the back of the cervical spine. (**a**) Trauma image with severe instability C3/C4 without neurology. (**b**, **c**) Postoperative after ventral fusion with iliac crest and angular stable plate. (**d**, **e**) Image after 2 years. No complaints 15 years later now and normal activity and function

Table 18.12 Technical aspects cervical spine

Material	Halo fixator Carbon ring Sterile torque screws Halo vest (various sizes)
Positioning	Prone with overhanging forehead, head must be held Intermittent X-ray fluoroscopy is necessary to check positioning of the c-spine
Approach	HALO fixation: pin placement anterolateral and posterolateral If necessary, determination of thickest bone area with CT Use of as many pins as possible, which must be tightly controlled Caution regarding over-distraction and frequent pin infections Other complications: dural penetration and injury to the supraorbital nerve, not with open sutures Special considerations of the use of halo fixator in children (Fig. 18.23) Anticipation of bone thickness with CT in children under 6 years Ring beneath the widest skull diameter, approximately 1 cm above the ears At least 6 pins with low torque (2–5 ft/lb) Avoid the thin regions temporally and frontal sinus Anterior safety zone: 1 cm above the orbital rim, lateral 2/3 of the orbit Place anterior pins with eyes closed so lid closure isn't jeopardized Simultaneous tightening of opposing pins to avoid slipping of the ring Pins can be re-tightened once there is resistance Remove loose pins and replace with new ones
Special Explanation	Effort of treatment Pin infection Perforation of the cortex
Operative principle	In children endotracheal anesthesia Halo fixator secured in thick areas of the external table of the skull Assembly of the halo ring Longitudinal stability with slight distraction and support of the halo vest
Hardware removal	At 8–12 weeks

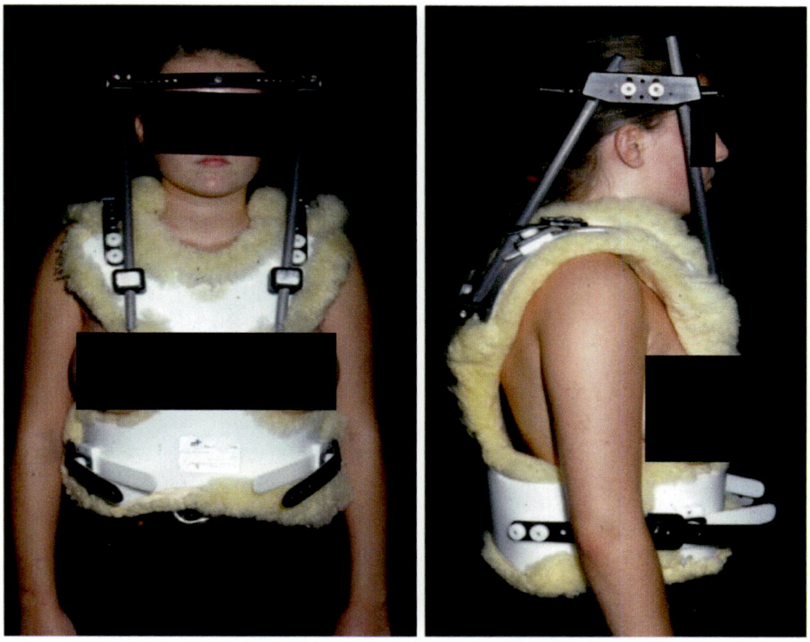

Fig. 18.23 Halo fixateur of a girl

18.4 Injuries to the Thoracic Spine

Incidence, Mechanism of Injury and Clinical Picture

Injuries to the thoracic spine are more common than those of the lumbar spine; in younger children they occur in the mid-thoracic and in adolescents in the thoracolumbar regions.

The cause of injury is often a motor vehicle accident, but also falls while playing or during sports can be responsible. However, child abuse must also be considered (approximately 2–3% of thoracolumbar compression fractures).

The elastic thorax and the ribcage are protective, so that often fractures are stable hyperflexion injuries (<20°) of the mid-thoracic spine without posterior spine involvement (A fractures). The superior endplate is affected twice as often as the inferior. Stable discs induce advanced serial compression fractures of the softer vertebral body, and in older children, burst fractures are commonly seen. The disc-epiphyseal complex, posterior wall, and posterior structures remain intact. Wedge fractures are caused by cancellous bone compression and anterior wall fractures in the thoracolumbar transition. Instability can be observed in cases of injury to the ligamentous and/or posterior chondro-osseous structures (including articular processes). In the thoracolumbar transition, facet displacement can occur without evidence of fracture or spinal cord injury because of ligament. Neurological deficits, transverse spinal cord syndrome (artery of Adamkiewicz) and thoracic spinal cord damage is often seen without evidence of fracture (SCIWORA). With lesions of the thoracolumbar transition, often there are only symptoms of root injury.

Classification

In adolescents, the AO three column classification is used (compression, flexion-distraction, rotation) (Fig. 18.6). Endplate disruptions can occur, but rarely. Impact fractures of the endplates and wedge impact fractures AO Type (A1.1; A1.2) occur (Table 18.13).

Table 18.13 Injuries to the thoracic spine

Particulars	Narrow bony spinal canal; high risk of spinal cord compression
Diagnostic Assessment	Skin abrasions over the back. Neurology. X-rays of the t-spine in two planes (centered). Fractures usually occur in the middle t-spine, often discreet or spontaneously reduced. Mediastinal extension? MRI to assess spinal compression, rare disc damage, in cases of posterior ligament stability. Accompanying findings: often additional occult fractures of the superior endplate series 3D CT reconstruction: preoperatively, in severe bony lesions and suspected apophyseal fractures Differential diagnosis: pathological fractures (eosinophilic granuloma, cysts, leukemia)
Therapy goal/Limits of correction	Stability. High potential for correction. Under 10 years of age, sagittal deformities with height decrease to half can restore completely. Minimal correction capacity of lateral compression with risk of scoliosis and worse prognosis of combined fronto-sagittal deformities
Primary treatment	Immobilization, analgesia
Conservative therapy	
Indications	Method of Choice—in particular single or multiple bone bruise in MRI and moderate compression fractures (Fig. 18.24)
Procedure	Short-term bedrest (stable hyperflexion compression fractures), orthosis in exceptional cases. Pain-dependent mobilization after bedrest. According to Hasler/Jeanneret: wedge vertebrae under 10° undergo early functional treatment with physiotherapy, 3 months no sporting activities (Fig. 18.25). When there is a Risser sign ≤2, 1 year support corset for the anterior wedge vertebrae with more than 10° (pressure relief in the growth zone, stimulation of anterior vertebral growth). Conservative healing of purely osseous Chance fractures and stable facet dislocation without neurological deficits and immobilization can be done in a reclining corset, Conservative treatment with longer immobilization is theoretically possible, but there is risk of secondary deformity (Fig. 18.26)
Follow Up	Rest for 3 months
X-ray Controls	At 6 months and 1 year
Return to sports	At 6 months, depending on complaints and kyphosis development

Table 18.11 (continued)

Operative treatment	
Indications	Instability in older children and adolescents since healing of unstable fractures is difficult to guarantee with orthosis. Posterior fusion in: (a) facet dislocation with neurological damage, (b) unstable flexion/extension (T1 and T2), (c) Chance fractures and rotation injuries (type C). Rare involvement of the endplates and growth zones (type A3). With kyphosis of 20° and more, progression of deformity can be expected. In children over 10 years and adolescents, the spine should be anatomically reconstructed
Procedure	Short-range posterior fusion with cerclage, no fixed-angle implants; decompression indicated only with progressive neurological deficits and partial nerve root and spinal cord lesions
Follow Up	Stable fixation, rest for 8–12 weeks
X-ray Controls	Procedure-dependent
Hardware removal	After consolidation
Return to sports	Consolidation-dependent
Complications	Unstable flexion/distraction and rotation injuries often have concomitant intraabdominal injuries (small bowel, etc.)
Growth Disturbances	Often a balanced scoliosis (<10°) forms around the fractured region, usually only slightly progressive. Under 12 years in the absence of neurological symptoms, persistent kyphotic deformity is rare, because the spinal growth zones are balanced. Segmental kyphosis is rare >10°, however, frontal deformities barely compensate, there is often post-traumatic scoliosis that rarely exceeds 20°. Also in the frequent series compression fractures and wedge impact fractures, posttraumatic deformities are not generally expected. Endplate fractures do not correct themselves, growth disturbance is a consequence. Injuries to the endplates and intervertebral discs usually lead to spontaneous segment fusion. However, persistent instability can lead to progressive deformity, especially when there is accompanying neurological damage
Follow Up	Regular over the course of further growth

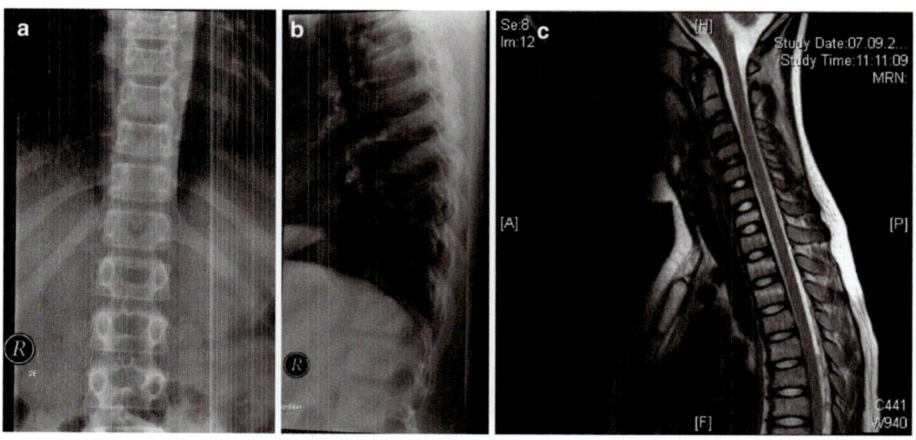

Fig. 18.24 'Bone bruise' of the seventh cervical body to the tenth thoracal body of a 11 year old boy after bicycle fall. (**a**, **b**) X-ray with almost invisible fractures, (**c**) MRI with bone bruise without impression of vertebral bodies. Functional treatment

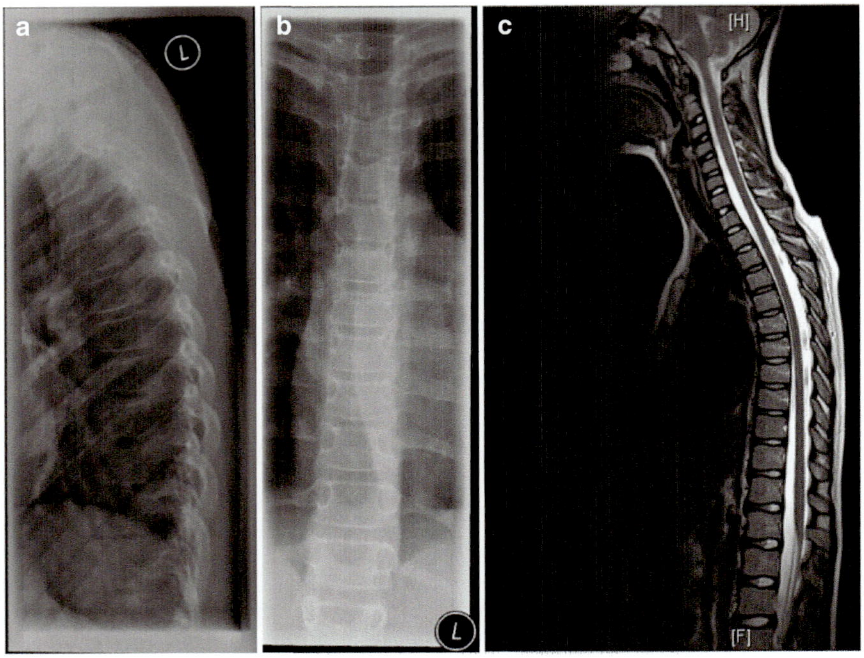

Fig. 18.25 Thoracic serial fractures with end plate impression and bone bruise vertebral bodies 6–9, (**a**, **b**) X-ray of the thoracic spine. Fractures are barely visible. (**c**) MRI with bone bruise and vertebral body upper end-plate impressions. Functional therapy

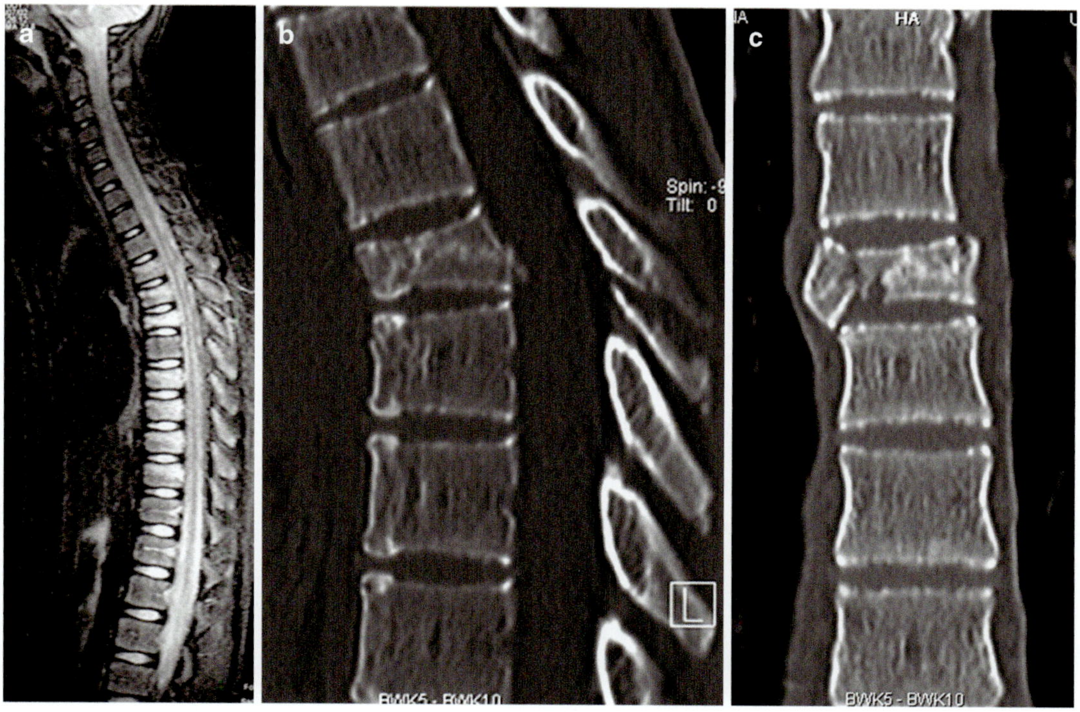

Fig. 18.26 Vertebral body compression fracture without impairment of the spinal canal and dorsal structures. (**a**) MRI, (**b**, **c**) CT scan. Conservative treatment still possible in the thoracic upper spine

18.5 Injuries to the Lumbar Spine

Incidence, Mechanism of Injury and Clinical Picture

Injuries to the lumbar spine in children are rarely severe injuries (Table 18.14). The mechanism of injury is compression with/without flexion; distraction and shear/rotation injuries (e.g., from the seat belt in a motor vehicle accident) are also possible. Compression fractures can also occur as apophyseal injuries in adolescents. Burst fractures are observed with mostly intact posterior elements. The disc is pressed into the vertebral body. Special case: lumbar apophyseal injuries occur in sports such as gymnastics and weightlifting. Intervertebral discs/ring apophyses as well as metaphyseal fragments can be pressed posteriorly into the spinal canal.

Classification

There are four types of apophyseal fractures in adolescents.

Table 18.14 Injuries to the lumbar spine

Particulars	Discoligamentous instability must be excluded
Diagnostic Assessment	X-rays of the lumbar spine in two planes (centered) 3D CT reconstruction: preoperative planning, differentiation of bony injuries, especially of apophyseal fractures. Apophyseal fractures in adolescents usually affect the posterior lumbar endplates. Parts of the disc with or without bony components are displaced posteriorly into the spinal canal, often between L5 and S1. There is often acute pain on effort and sport activities. Can be overlooked on conventional X-ray. CT method of choice to detect fragment size and extent of canal narrowing MRI with spinal compression and to exclude rare disc injuries. Special form: unstable Chance fracture equivalents (flexion-distraction type) as horizontal shear fracture with anterior displacement/compression and posterior distraction (region T12–L3). Classic Chance fracture is a pure bony lesion Blunt abdominal trauma from seat belt (lap belt syndrome), often ileus/intraabdominal injuries (Fig. 18.27)
Therapy goal/Limits of correction	Prevent neurogenic damage and static misalignment
Primary treatment	Positional treatment, progressive kyphosis
Conservative therapy	
Indications	Fractures with intact posterior elements. Before puberty also spinal canal stenosis through impinging parts of the disc and progressive axial deviation. Conservative treatment possible with sufficient vertebral height and impaction of the fractured vertebra (Figs. 18.28 and 18.29)
Procedure	Stability is generally reached at 12 weeks. Flexion/extension views are evidence of stability. In prepubertal children, the orthosis may be worn until growth ceases (girls 14 years, boys 16 years) Whether external support prevents the development of deformity is questionable, however
Follow Up	Functional
X-ray Controls	In the interval to exclude progressive deformity or instability
Return to sports	Case and complaint-dependent
Operative treatment	
Indications	Chance fractures with predominantly bony lesions can be treated with closed reduction and corset immobilization; however, most recommend posterior tension banding and internal fixator. The goal is restoration of lordosis. Ligamentous injuries are treated with open reduction and posterior fusion. In smaller children, the spinous processes can be connected (e.g. PDS suture), with follow up in a corset. For adolescents, posterior internal fixator (Fig. 18.30) Vertebral endplate fractures (and also trans-osseous instability Chance type) are decompressed with symptomatic disc protrusions and fragments to prevent spinal stenosis depending on age. Lumbar apophyseal damage with tissue displaced into the spinal canal must be surgically removed when neurological symptoms are present

Table 18.14 (continued)

Procedure	Posterior tension banding, cerclage, internal fixator (Figs. 18.31, 18.32, and 18.33) and in destructed vertebral bodies additional minimal-invasive anterior decompression and titanium replacement of vertebrate (Fig. 18.34)
Follow Up	Case-dependent
X-ray Controls	Case-dependent
Hardware removal	After healing
Return to sports	After healing
Complications	Progressive deformation with conservative treatment and instability
Growth Disturbances	Possible with growth plate injuries
Follow Up	At 6 months and 1 year

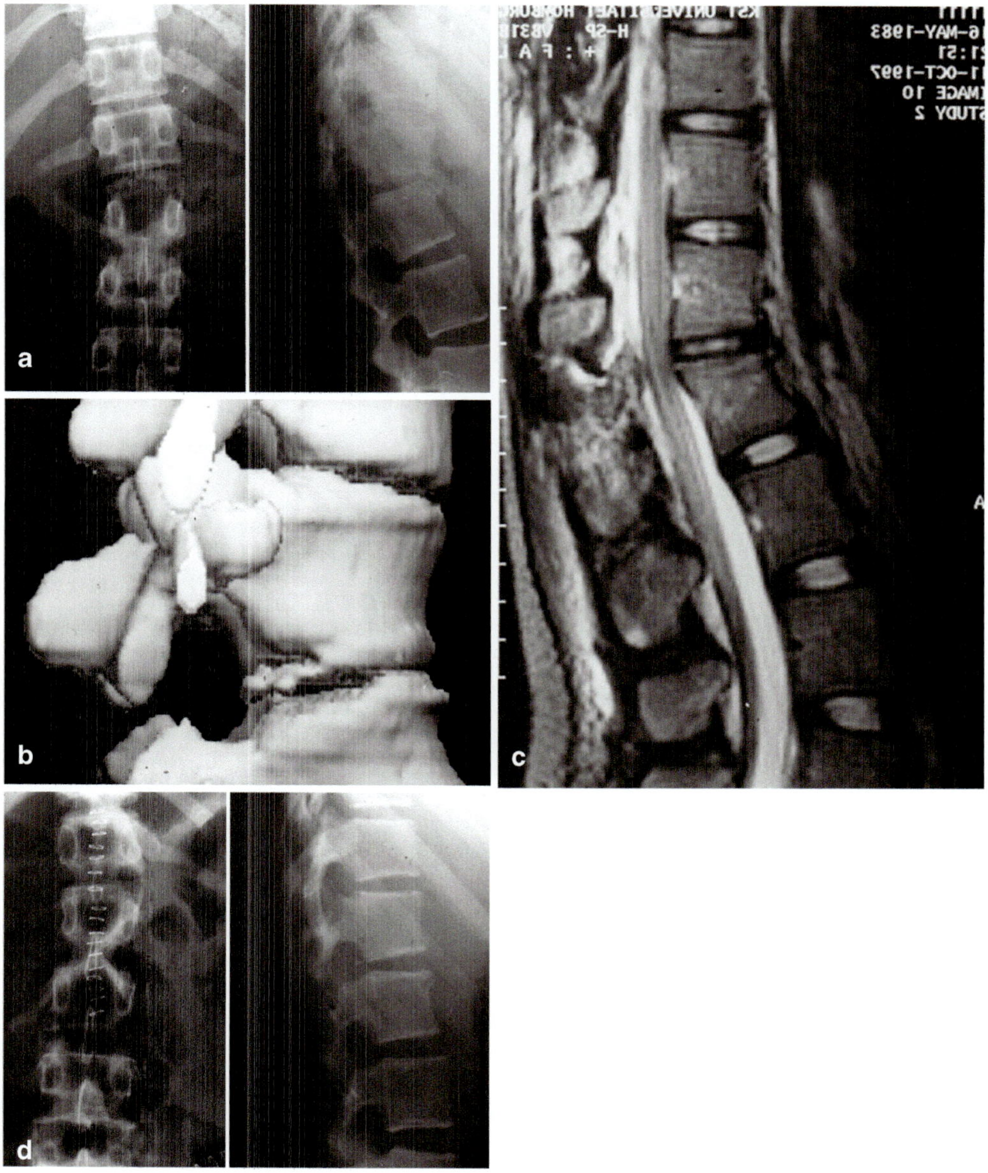

Fig. 18.27 Type B Injury of a 14 y old girl after car accident with a simple belt in the middle seat. (**a**) Trauma Image, (**b**) CT, (**c**) MRI, (**d**) Dorsal reduction and tension bend fixation with PDS-band

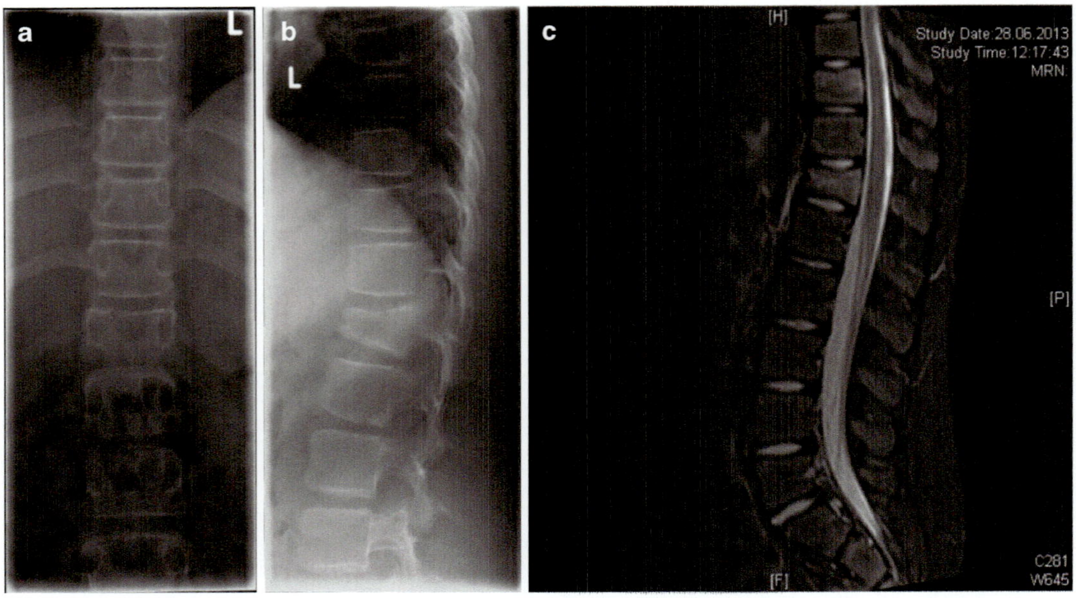

Fig. 18.28 Stable vertebral body compression fracture of the 12 thoracic vertebrate with functional treatment. (**a**, **b**) X-rays, (**c**) MRI with bone bruise also of the tenth vertebrate and stabile fracture situation

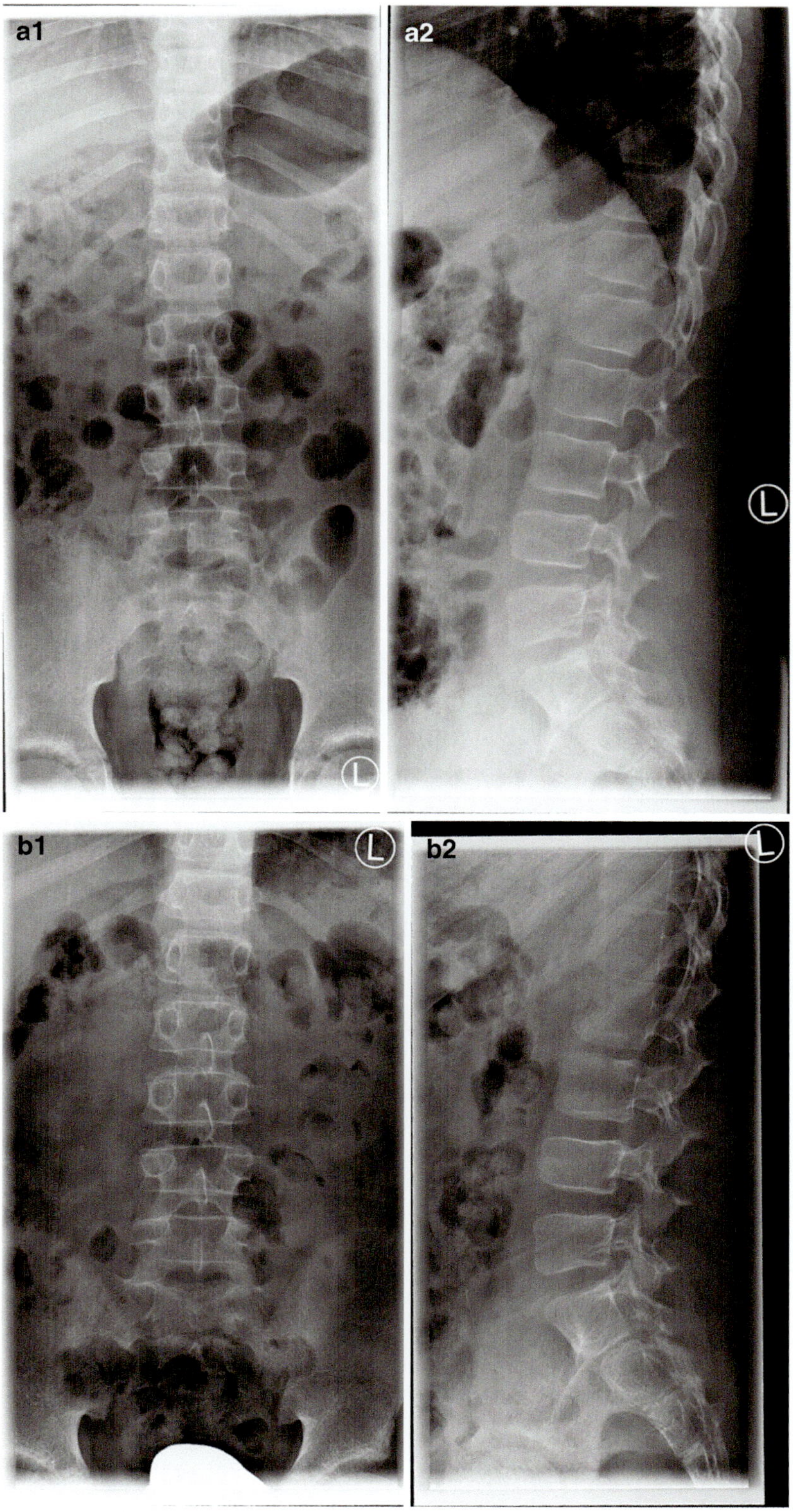

Fig. 18.29 13 Year old boy with stable compression fracture of the fourth lumbal vertebrate, (**a1**, **a2**) Trauma Imgae, (**b1**, **b2**) conservative treatment and healing

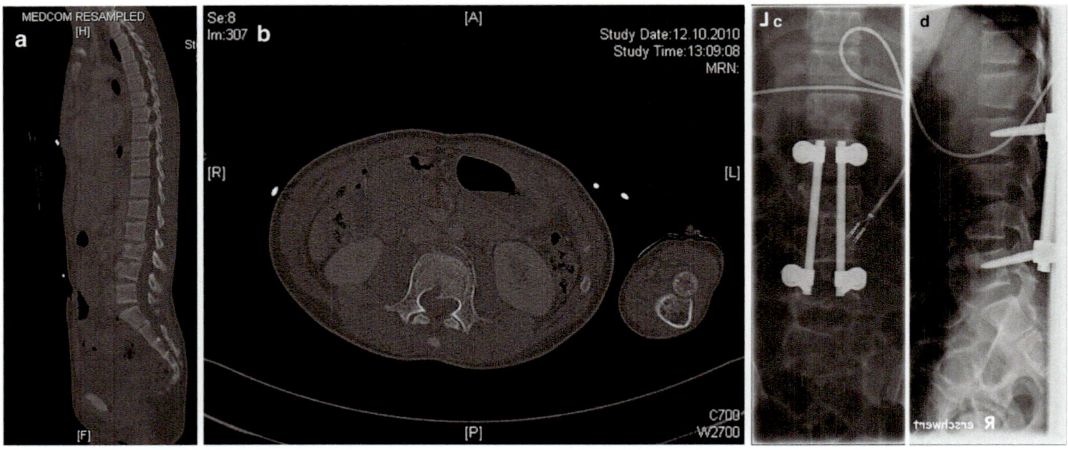

Fig. 18.30 L1 burst fracture with incomplete transverse spinal cord syndrome, girl, 14 years, suicide attempt, jump from third floor. (**a**, **b**) Trauma images, considerable spinal canal narrowing (**c**, **d**) Bisegmental posterior-anterior spondylodesis including thoracoscopic spinal canal decompression

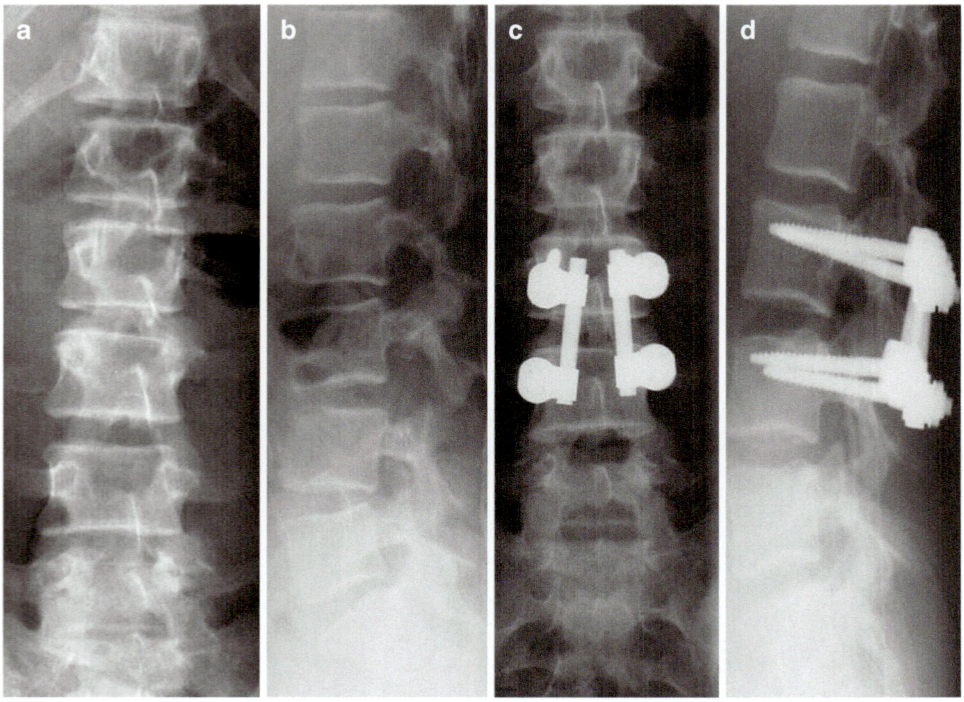

Fig. 18.31 Flexion-distraction injury of the L3/L4 lumbal spine of a 14 year old boy after traffic accident with pelvic-binder. (**a**, **b**) Trauma images. (**c**, **d**) Dorsal monosegmental reduction and stabilization

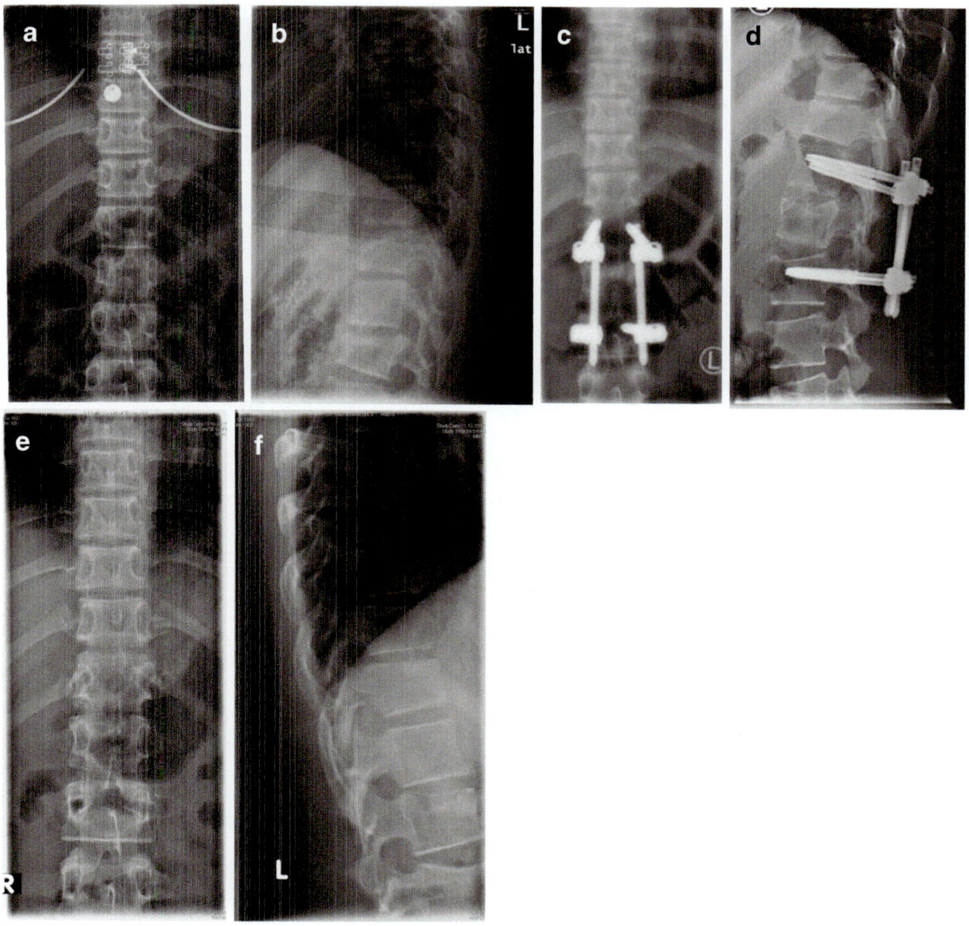

Fig. 18.32 Burst fracture of the L1 vertebrate of a 13 year old girl after suicide jump. (**a**, **b**) Trauma image, (**c**, **d**) X-ray after 4 weeks, (**e**, **f**) X-ray after metal removal

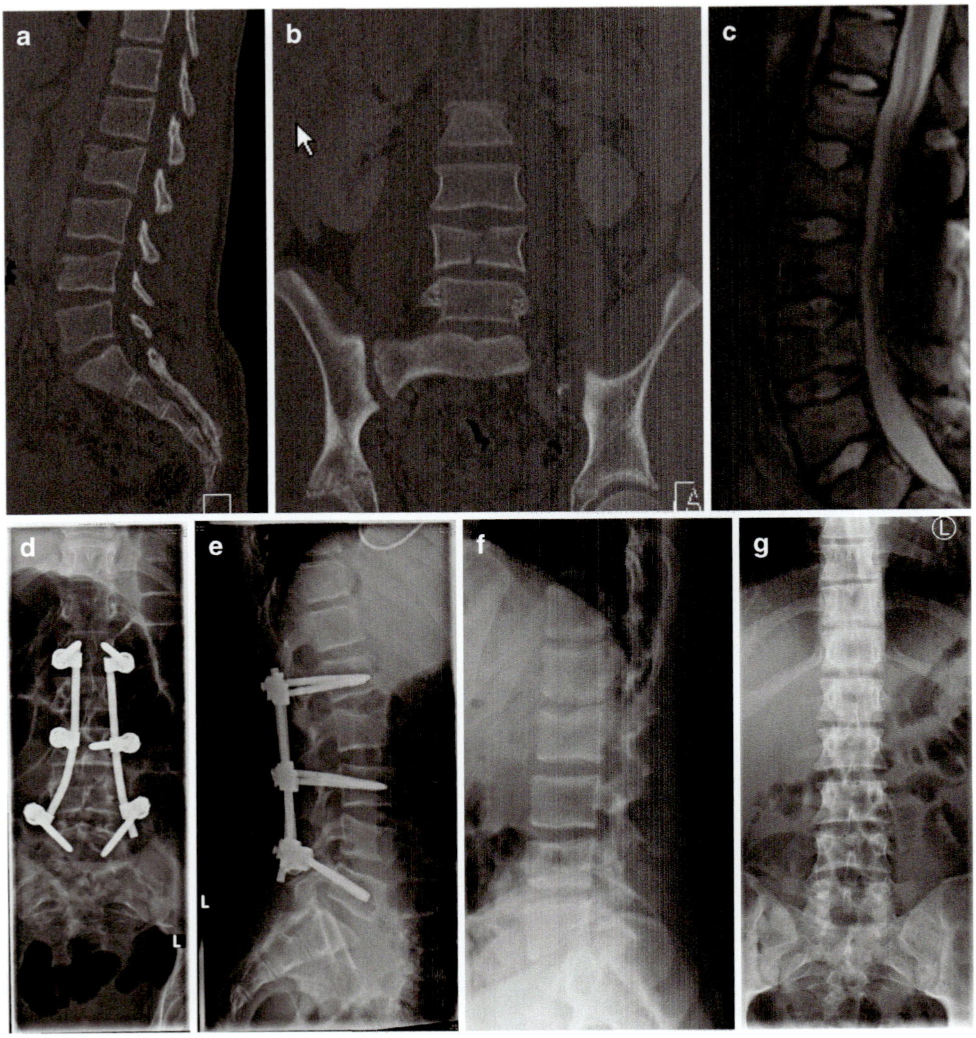

Fig. 18.33 Burst fracture of the L2 and L4 spine after fall from 10 m high of a 13 year old boy; in additional bilateral calcaneal fractures. (**a–c**) Trauma images with gap and compression fractures, (**d**, **e**) After dorsal stabilization from L1 over L3 to L5. (**f**, **g**) X-ray 3 years after metal removal

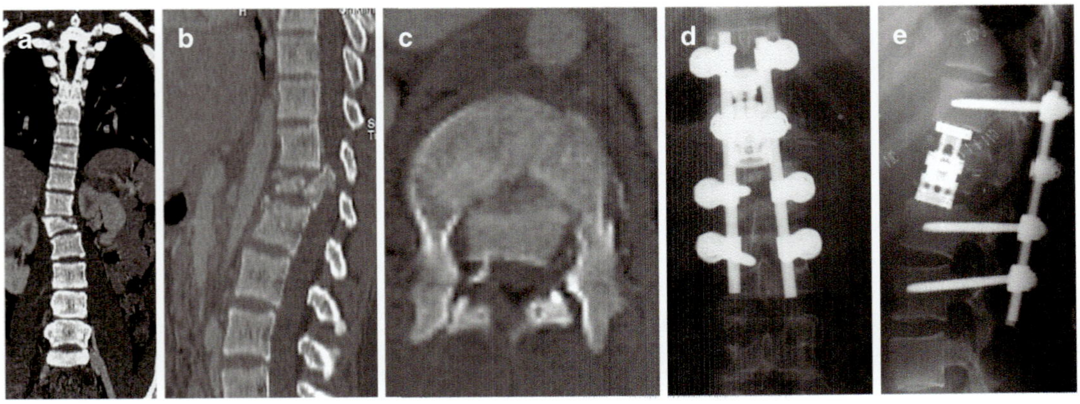

Fig. 18.34 Burst fracture of the first lumbal vertebrate of a 14 year old girl after suicide jump from second floor with incomplete neurological deficit. (**a–c**) Trauma CCDT with impressive narrowing of the spinal canal. (**d**, **e**) X-ray after posterior reduction and decompression immediately after trauma and secondary anterior fusion with titanium cage

18.6 Spinal Cord Injuries

Incidence, Mechanism of Injury and Clinical Picture

Up to 30% (5–67%) of spine injuries in children give a clinical picture of "SCIWORA." High resolution MRI can determine the cause in many cases (Fig. 18.35). In younger children (<8 years), the c-spine and mid-t-spine (cervicothoracic transition) are often affected (70% of significant spinal cord injuries occur at the C3/C4 level), but the potential for recovery is very good. In the case of birth trauma (head distraction), the picture is a flaccid child without a progressive lesion. In adolescents, injuries to the thoracolumbar transition dominate, because the thoracic spinal cord is vulnerable with the narrow spinal canal and complicated perfusion. In adolescents there are often also thoracolumbar fractures, with incomplete neurological deficits (Fig. 18.34). Because the spine is much more elastic than the spinal cord, longitudinal distraction, hyperextension, flexion and spinal ischemia play important pathogenetic roles. Open injuries are rare, and the prognosis is generally dependent on the mechanism of injury (Fig. 18.36).

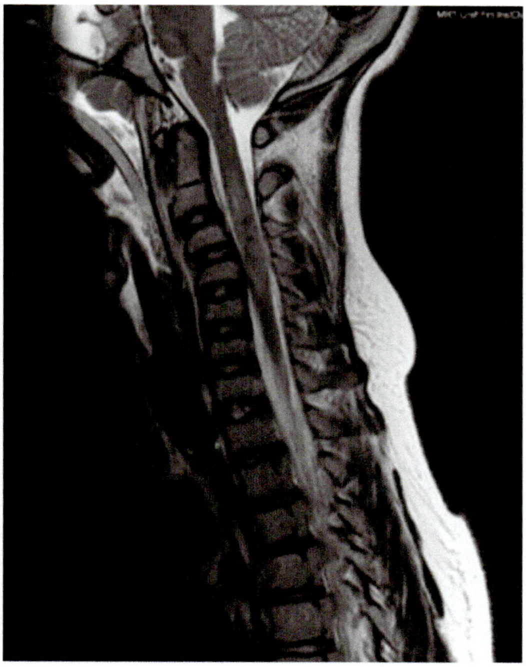

Fig. 18.35 Primary transverse spinal cord symptoms with multisegmental instability of the c-spine

Diagnostic Assessment

MRI is the method of choice. It shows ruptures of the anterior and posterior longitudinal ligaments, disc herniation, spinal cord transections, bleeding, and edema as well as bone edema (bone bruise) in spontaneously reduced endplate fractures. The goal is to exclude unstable injuries (fractures, ligament instability). In many cases, however, the MRI shows no cause (SCIWORA) and the neurological symptoms increase in hours to days.

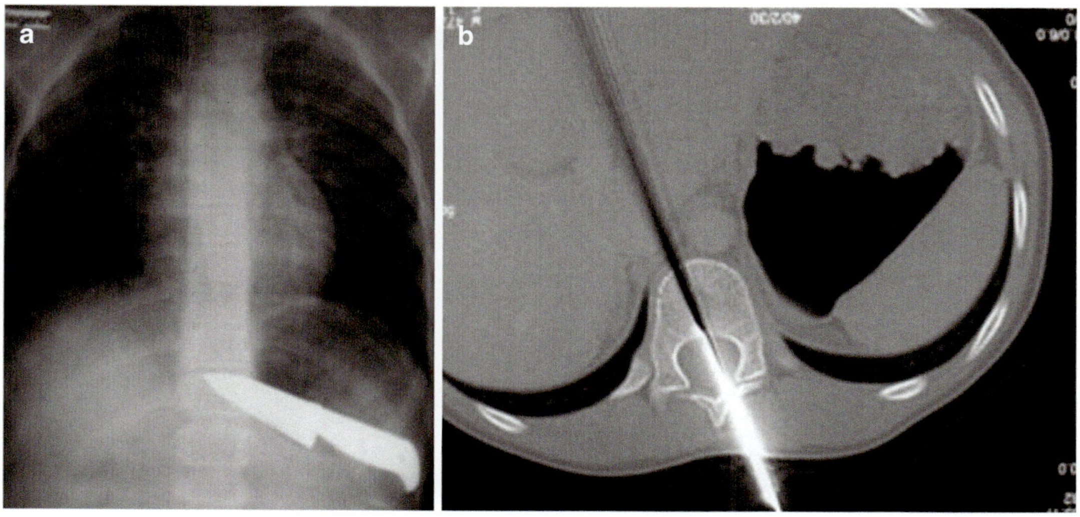

Fig. 18.36 (**a**, **b**) Open spinal cord trauma without significant neurological consequences

Treatment and Prognosis

Operative decompression is critical because of significant consequences with further growth and kyphotic deformity. However, the indication must be considered with persistent spinal bony or disc compression. In any case, the joint facets and capsules should be preserved and not injured if possible. Conservative immobilization is a stiff soft collar or thoracolumbar brace. In pronounced forms, rest and movement restriction is prescribed for 3 months, especially considering that renewed trauma can lead to exacerbation and worsening of symptoms. There should always be controls to determine and prevent any worsening. The administration of methylprednisolone has not been scientifically evaluated in children under 13 years of age. Late consequences can be expected especially when the injuries occurred in children under 10 years; thus, deformity, increasing neurological deficits and syrinx can result.

Prognosis correlates with the primary severity of neurological deficits. Around 90% of children with incomplete SCIWORA improve. Thoracic spinal cord damage has the worst prognosis.

Recommended Literature

Auner B, Marzi I (2014) Polytrauma des Kindes. Chirurg [Internet] 85(5):451–461. Quiz 462–3. Available from: http://link.springer.com/10.1007/s00104-013-2680-z

Copley PC, Tilliridou V, Kirby A, Jones J, Kandasamy J (2019) Management of cervical spine trauma in children. Eur J Trauma Emerg Surg 45(5):777–789. Springer

Dauleac C, Beuriat P-A, Di Rocco F, Szathmari A, Mottolese C (2019) Surgical management of pediatric spine trauma: 12 years of experience. World Neurosurg 126:e1494–e1502. Elsevier

Hasler C, Jeanneret B (2002) Wirbelsäulenverletzungen im Wachstumsalter. Orthopäde 31:65–71

Herman MJ, Brown KO, Sponseller PD, Phillips JH, Petrucelli PM, Parikh DJ et al (2019) Pediatric cervical spine clearance: a consensus statement and algorithm from the pediatric cervical spine clearance working group. J Bone Joint Surg 101(1):e1. LWW

Gonschorek O (2015) Spinal injuries in children and adolescents. Trauma und Berufskrankheit 17(S1):235–240

Jarvers JS, Spiegl U, Höh von der N, Josten C (2016) Verletzungen der kindlichen thorakolumbalen Wirbelsäule. Der Orthopäde

Kraus R, Stahl JP, Heiss C, Horas U, Dongowski N, Schnettler R (2011) Fractures of the thoracic and lumbar spine in children and adolescents. Unfallchirurg 116(5):435–441

Magerl F et al (1994) A comprehensive classification of thoracic and lumbar injuries. Eur Spine J 3:184–201

Nau C, Rose S, Laurer HL, Marzi I (2010) Wirbelsäulenverletzungen im Kindesalter. Orthopädie und Unfallchirurgie up2date 5(01):23–38

Phillips N, Rasmussen K, McGuire S, Abel K-A, Acworth J, Askin G et al (2021) Projected paediatric cervical spine imaging rates with application of NEXUS, Canadian C-Spine and PECARN clinical decision rules in a prospective Australian cohort. Emerg Med J 38(5):330–337. BMJ Publishing Group Ltd and the British Association for Accident & Emergency Medicine

Powers B, Miller MD, Kramer RS, Martinez S, Gehweiler JA Jr (1979) Traumatic anterior atlanto-occipital dislocation. Neurosurgery 4:12–17

Srinivasan V, Jea A (2017) Pediatric thoracolumbar spine trauma. Neurosurg Clin 28(1):103–114. Elsevier

Tscherne H, Blauth M (1998) Unfallchirurgie: Wirbelsäule. Springer, Berlin

Voth M, Nau C, Marzi I (2013) Thoracic and lumbar spinal injuries in children and adolescents. Unfallchirurg 116(12):1062–1068

Weiß T, Disch AC, Kreinest M, Jarvers J-S, Herren C, Jung MK et al (2020) Diagnostics and treatment of thoracic and lumbar spine trauma in pediatric patients: Recommendations from the Pediatric Spinal Trauma Group. Unfallchirurg 123(4):269–279

Part III

Secondary Reconstructions

Secondary Reconstruction of the Elbow

19

19.1 Mechanism of Injury

The elbow joint is involved in more than 10% of injuries in children and adolescents. Depending on the specialization of the admitting department/hospital (e.g., hand surgery inclusive) or participation in a trauma network as Level I hospital (polytrauma patient care—including children), the numbers vary regarding frequency and location of bony injuries. Our data estimates that of approximately 2000 injured children visiting our Emergency Department each year, around 25% have relevant injuries. The proportion of fractures in these relevant injuries is over 80%, with elbow involvement in approximately 13%. Thus, for our patient population, it is one of the most common fracture sites.

The proportion of longitudinal growth in the distal versus proximal humerus is relatively small (20%). Thus, there is little spontaneous correction of fractures. In general, this limited potential is gone by the age of seven. The complex joint situation with three coordinated articulations must also align precisely to enable good mobility in all directions. Today, elbow deformities result mostly from inadequate primary diagnosis and treatment. Either the significance of injury is underestimated, or optimal treatment is unsuccessful. Table 19.1 lists relevant elbow injuries. The most important are supracondylar humerus fracture, lateral condyle fracture, and Monteggia lesion with radial head dislocation. These fractures are called "Kadi" lesions by von Laer because they often have legal consequences if not adequately treated. Increased awareness has led to a range of advanced training courses in recent years. With changes to worker's compensation insurance in 2011, advanced pediatric trauma training became mandatory for worker's compensation specialists every five years in Germany.

Table 19.1 Relevant pediatric elbow injuries

• Supracondylar humerus fracture	6.5%
• Lateral condyle fracture	1.8%
• Elbow dislocation and medial epicondyle	1.3%
• Radial head fracture	1.3%
• Monteggia injury	1.3%
• Olecranon injuries	0.5%

19.2 Deformities of the Distal Humerus

Table 19.2 lists the familiar deformities of the distal humerus and their etiologies. The most common is the supracondylar humerus fracture. These results are generally good revealed by a multicenter review study of the German Trauma Society. However, in more severe injuries (grades III and IV), there is number of patients approaching 20% poor results (Table 19.3). The advanced training and associated content, which have become widespread, have unquestionably

I. Marzi et al., *Pediatric Skeletal Trauma*, https://doi.org/10.1007/978-3-030-93685-3_19

Table 19.2 Posttraumatic deformities of the distal humerus

Deformity	Etiology
Cubitus varus	Mostly after supracondylar fractures Ulnar epiphyseal closure Lateral stimulation—condylar fracture
Cubitus valgus	Lateral nonunion—condylar fracture Medial stimulation—condylar fracture
Nonunion	Lateral condyle fracture Medial epicondylar fracture
Fishtail deformity	Central epiphyseal closure—condylar fracture/Y-fracture

Table 19.3 Score for the classification of treatment result after supracondylar humerus fractures

Points	Radiological results	Clinical results
0 = ideal	No axial deviation AP, lateral good	No functional deficits, axes symmetrical
1 = good	To 5° varus/valgus, anteverted, retroverted defects to 10°	Up to 10° extension/flexion deficits, axial deviation to 5°
2 = tolerable	5–10° Varus/valgus	10–20 extension/flexion deficits Valgus and Varus 5°–10°
3 = poor	**10° Varus- valgus Or more deviations**	**20° difference In one plane, or more**

Additional radiological and clinical points (Min 0—Max 6)

increased the number of adequate reductions and stabilization. Thus, a relevant varus deformity occurs in a maximum of 3% of cases. Historically, rates have been as high as 60% based on conservative treatment. Valgus deformities are usually secondary to lesions of the lateral condyle and occasionally lead to nonunion.

Treatment

Underlying Principles

If reduction and fixation of the joint surface at the distal humerus is inadequate, typical results are multi-dimensional mal-alignment with varus deformity, internal rotation, and anteversion deformity (Fig. 19.1). Functional limitations, cosmetic concerns, and occasional nerve irritation are indications for corrective surgery. A valgus deformity is less obvious, and corrective interventions are rare, mainly because appearance and function are less impaired. Problems that occasionally indicate corrective procedures are medial ligament instability due to overload with associated ulnar nerve irritation. If nonunion develops after lateral condyle fracture, operative treatment is usually necessary to eliminate radial column instability, which is generally associated with this entity (Fig. 19.2).

Operative Therapy

Preoperative Preparation

The first preparation step is to analyze the deformity precisely, measuring deviation, range of motion, joint function, and stability. The common deformity seen after supracondylar humerus fractures leads to flexion deficits in anteversion and extension deficits in retroversion of the distal humerus.

If there is evidence of nerve irritation, this should be verified with neurophysiological measurements. With extreme valgus deformity, ulnar nerve irritation should be evaluated as this can be an indication for surgery. Further treatment and alternatives must be discussed in detail with the child and parents. If there is an indication for surgery, then the individual steps should be discussed—if necessary, with potential deviations/additional measures. In cases of complex procedures such as a fixator, the child must receive informations and careful explanation of the situation according to the age. Various planning programs are useful for this. Optimized calibration can be used to determine dimensions such as the osteotomy to the joint line, wedge size, extent of shift/translation needed according to the desired axis correction (Fig. 19.3). Such planning, also as a sketch, can help prepare for potential problems and variants even before surgery.

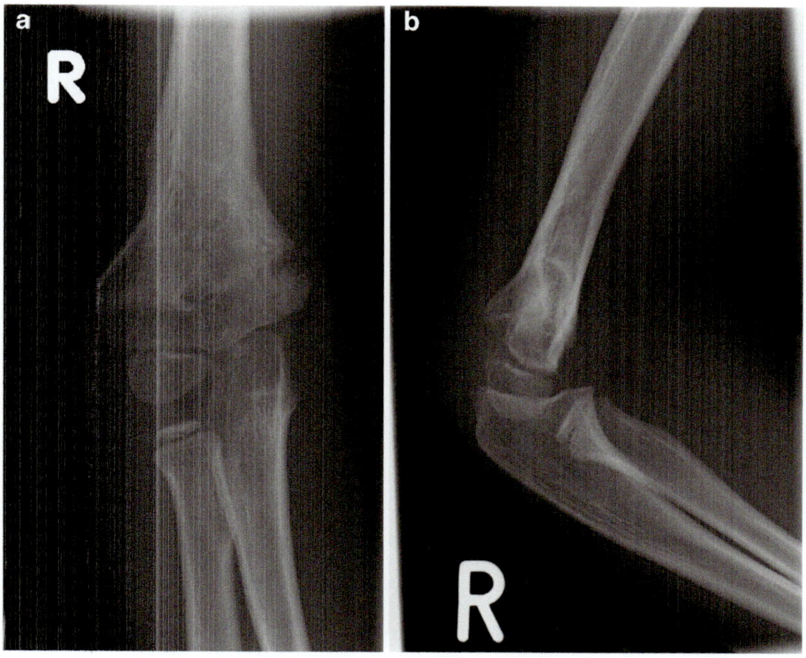

Fig. 19.1 Xray image of an incorrectly-healed supracondylar humerus fracture with Cubitus varus. (**a**) A.P. view (**b**) larteral view

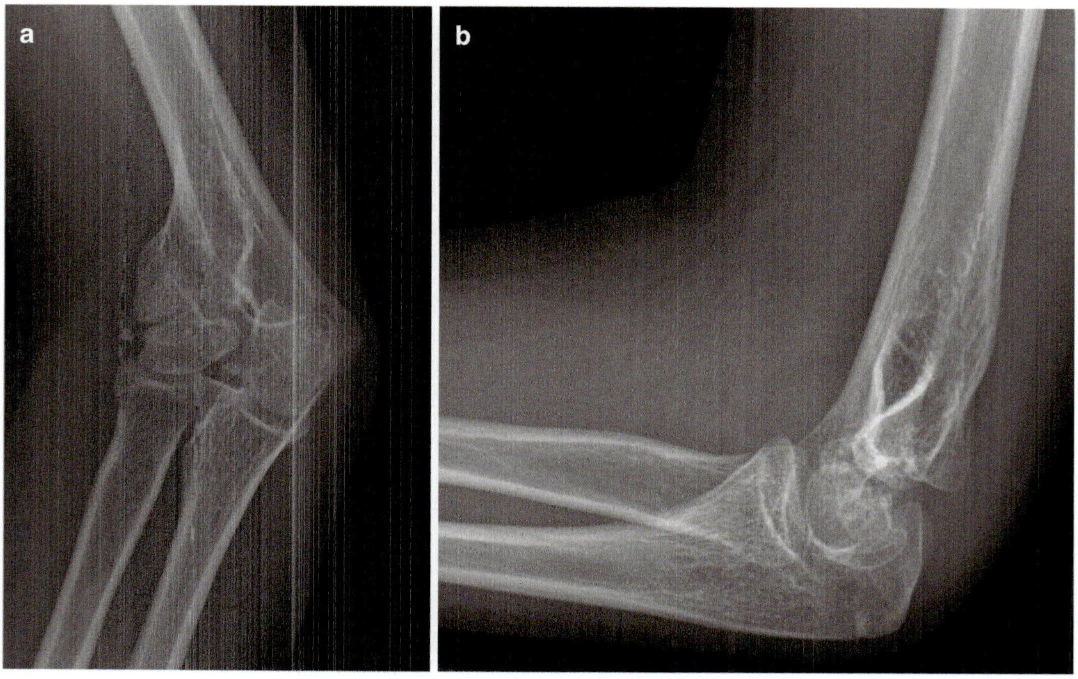

Fig. 19.2 Xray image of the distal humerus. Nonunion of the lateral condyle with valgus deformity. (**a**) A.P. view (**b**) larteral view

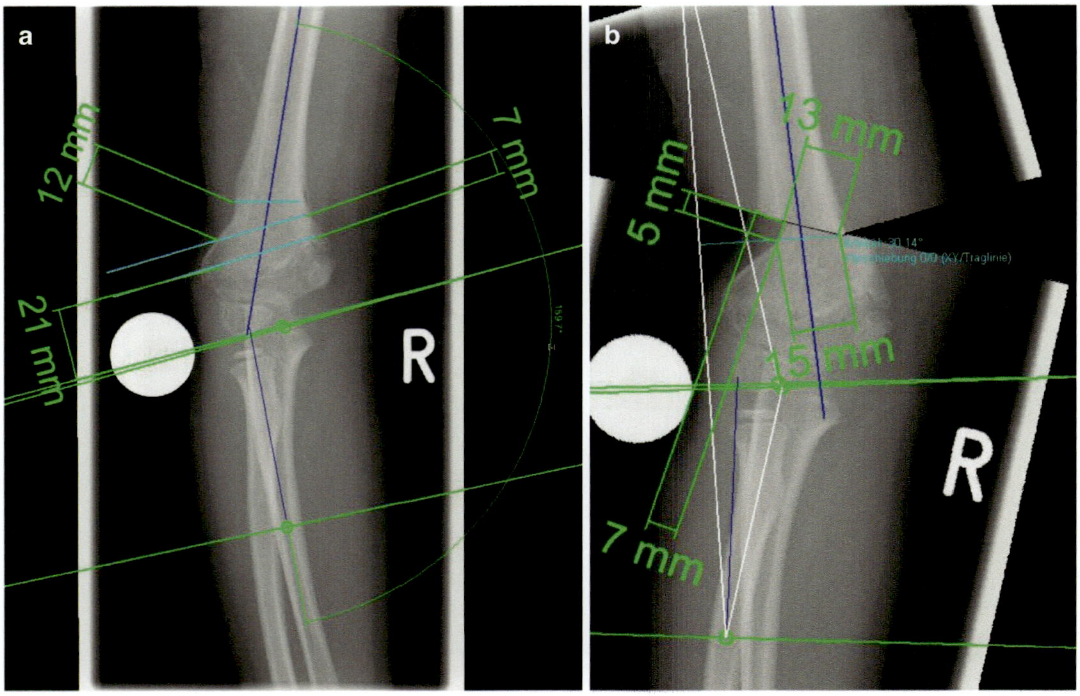

Fig. 19.3 Xray and digital planning before performing the corrective osteotomy. (**a**) measurements, (**b**) correction plan

Operative Methods

Nonunion is generally associated with lesions of the lateral condyle and should have screw fixation to regain stability. Autologous cancellous bone graft can be used according to the defect or the extent of distalization needed to compensate for the valgus deformity (Fig. 19.4). In some cases, screw fixation alone is enough after debridement.

The surgical technique for correcting valgus or varus deformities depends on the child's age. A distinction must be made between fixation and corrective osteotomy techniques. In adolescents and towards the end of growth, fixation can be performed as in adults, with fixed double-plates (Fig. 19.5) or special Y-plates. For younger children, K-wire fixation or external fixators are used, depending on the corrective technique.

In terms of osteotomy techniques, the lateral "closed wedge" or French osteotomy is probably the easiest technically and is usually performed today using a fixator together with K-wire stabilization. Dome osteotomy (similar to a pendular osteotomy of the tibial plateau) is widely used in younger children. The literature reports a slightly higher complication rate with this technique. An additional modification is the step-cut osteotomy. In this case, rotation and medialization are made possible by removing a triangular wedge of the distal humerus. This can reduce the unsightly lateral bony prominence and improve stability through fragment balancing. Because of the bony prominence and visible scarring, some authors prefer correction via a medial approach. This can also be an open-wedge osteotomy (Fig. 19.6). Stabilization is usually performed with an external fixator and can also be carried out using callus distraction.

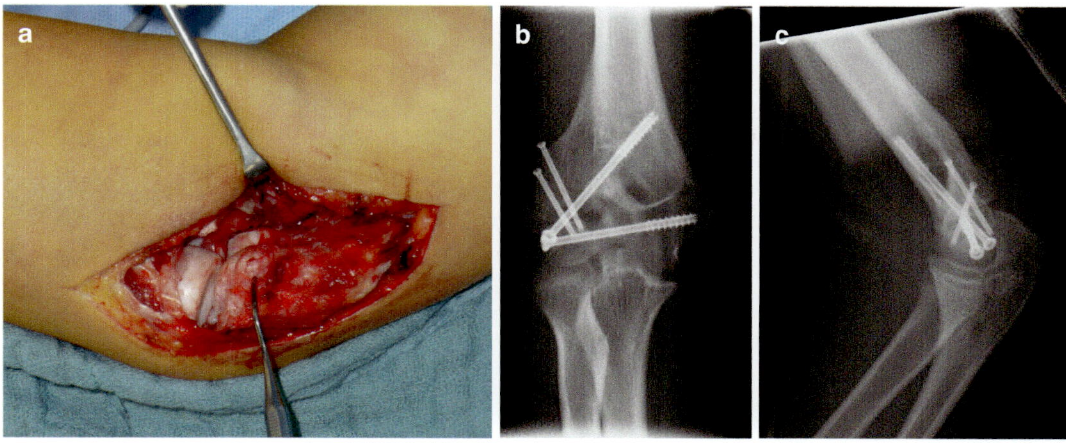

Fig. 19.4 Reconstruction of nonunion of the lateral condyle with bone graft and screw osteosynthesis. (**a**) intraoperative finding, (**b**) A.P. view, (**c**) lateral view

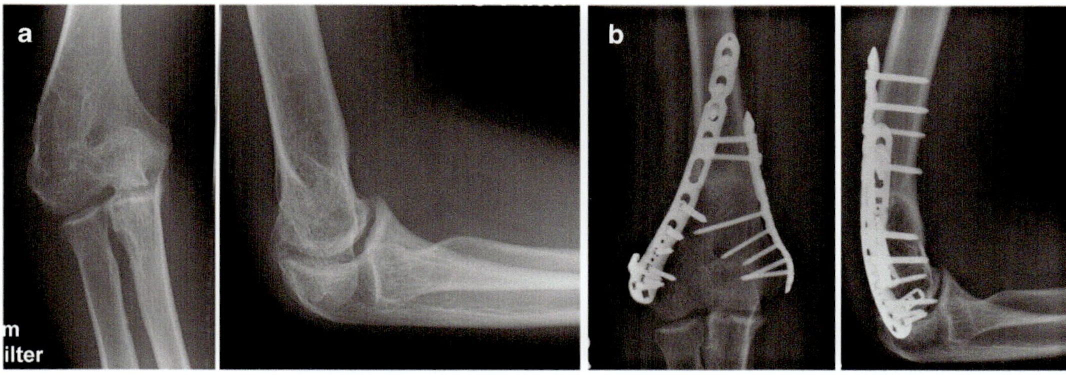

Fig. 19.5 Varus deformity after distal humerus fracture, (**a**) Preoperative radiograph, (**b**) Postoperative xray after correction, and stabilization with double-plate fixation

Our preferred method corresponds to that of Linhart and Kraus and is performed using an external fixator and three-dimensional supracondylar derotation osteotomy. Implantation of the fixator pins is carried out according to preoperative planning (see Fig. 19.3). The distal pins, introduced first, lie proximal to the growth plate, and the proximal pins are introduced through an open exposure of the humerus to ensure preservation of the radial nerve. After a test assembly, the osteotomy is performed. During planning, care should be taken to place the osteotomy as close as possible to the CORA (Center of Rotation and Angulation). In cases of deviation, the resulting translation must be considered. This is especially true when the distal pins need to be placed more proximally for open growth plates. Then the osteotomy and free adjustment of the distal joint block are performed according to the malalignment (Fig. 19.7a–c). External fixators are generally well-tolerated by children. The elbow can be moved as much as possible according to appropriate care instructions (Fig. 19.8 and Table 19.4).

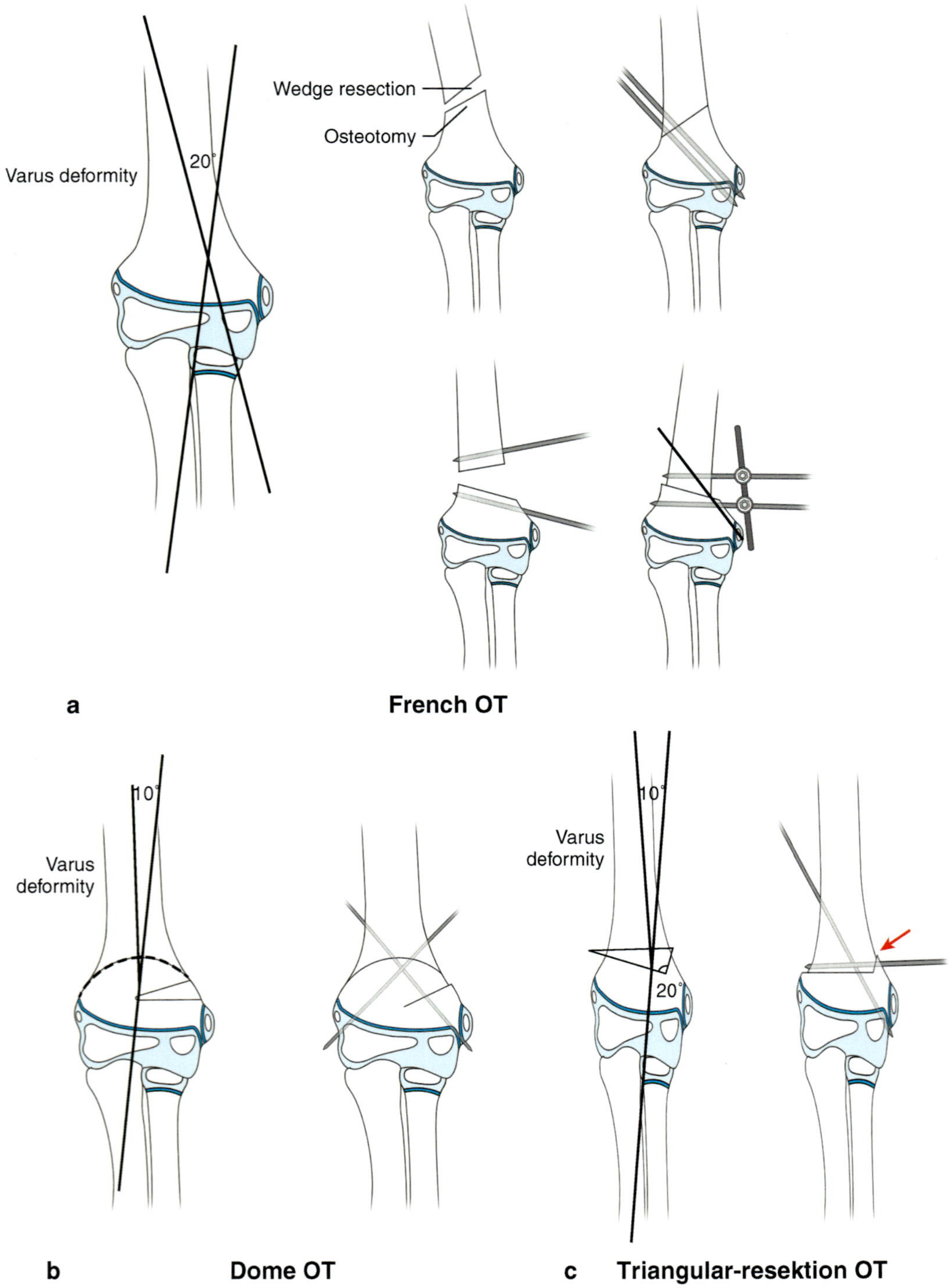

Fig. 19.6 Various possibilities for corrective osteotomies after post-trauma deformities due to supracondylar fractures. These examples illustrate the correction using a simple French osteotomy with examples for stabilization (**a**), dome osteotomy (**b**) and triangular resection osteotomy (**c**), in this case sometimes a small additional triangle needs to be resected radially to adjust medialization and fitting of the osteotomy (marked with arrow). (*OT*) osteotomy

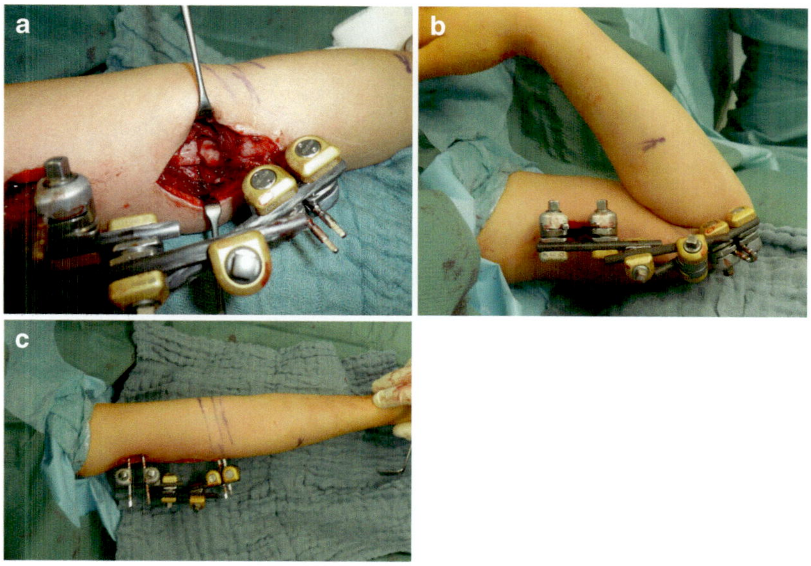

Fig. 19.7 Intraoperative image of the correction of a varus deformity after supracondylar humerus fracture. (**a**) View of the osteotomy, (**b**) Functional control with flexion, and (**c**) Extension

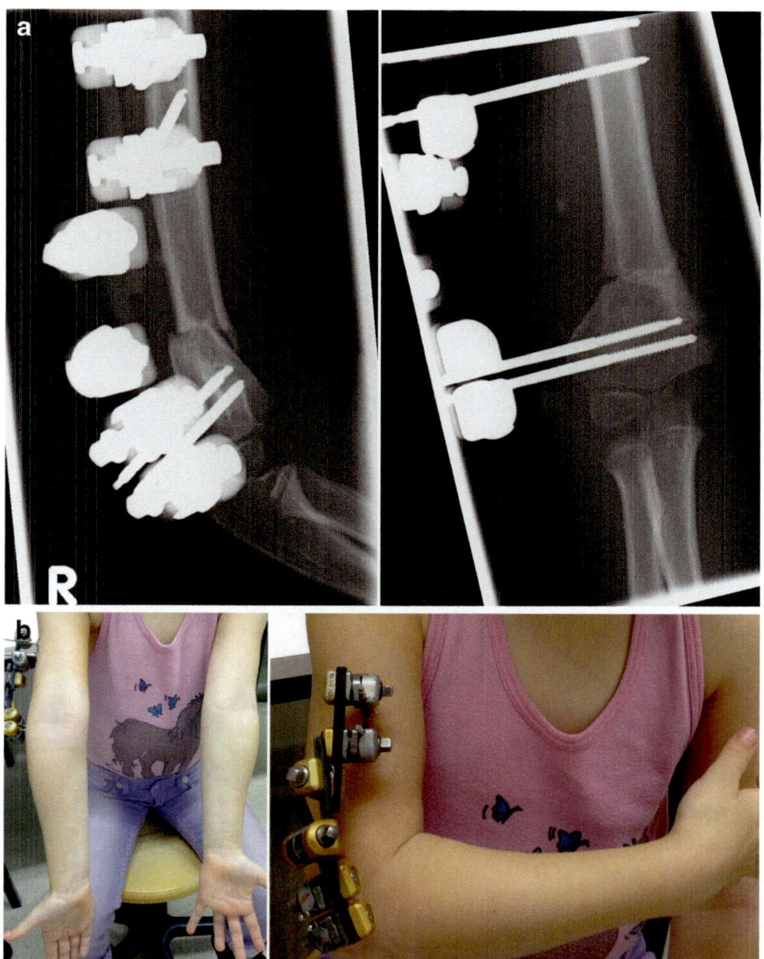

Fig. 19.8 Postoperative images after correction of Cubitus varus, (**a**) Postoperative radiographic image, (**b**) Clinical function

Table 19.4 Key points for care in cases of external fixation

Topics	Estimated time
Early wound care, compressin, padding, bandage	2–3 weeks
Pin care with local antiseptic solutions	Permanent
Tape dressing of the wound and pin area	After 2–3 weeks
Control of tightness, screws, pins, bars	Permanent weekly
Showering	After 2–3 weeks. Allowed
Distraction osteogenesis around 1–2 mm a day	Start at day 6–8
Clinical direction and X-ray controls during osteogenesis	Weekly
Patient and family education	Permanent

19.3 Deformities of the Proximal Forearm

In the proximal forearm, it is essential to discuss radial head deformities, e.g., those occurring after radial neck fractures, and ulnar deformities, e.g. after olecranon fracture. Particular attention should be paid to radial head dislocation after a Monteggia lesion. This lesion appears in various forms and can be classified according to Bado as in adults or according to Letts et al., who created an adaptation for pediatric injury patterns. Here, "ulnar bowing" is also included. In such cases radial head dislocations are particularly difficult to identify due to the lack of an obvious fracture (Fig. 19.9).

Chronic dislocation can lead to severe joint changes, and primary recognition is critical. Thus, the following three rules apply:

1. **Rule:** For every ulnar shaft fracture (including "bowing" fractures), elbow x-rays should be performed in two planes. Conversely, forearm x-rays should be carried out when there is radial head dislocation.
2. **Rule:** On every elbow image and in each plane, the radial head must be centered on the capitellum.
3. **Rule:** If congenital dislocation is suspected (lack of sufficient trauma), a comparison to the other side should be done (forearm, wrist).

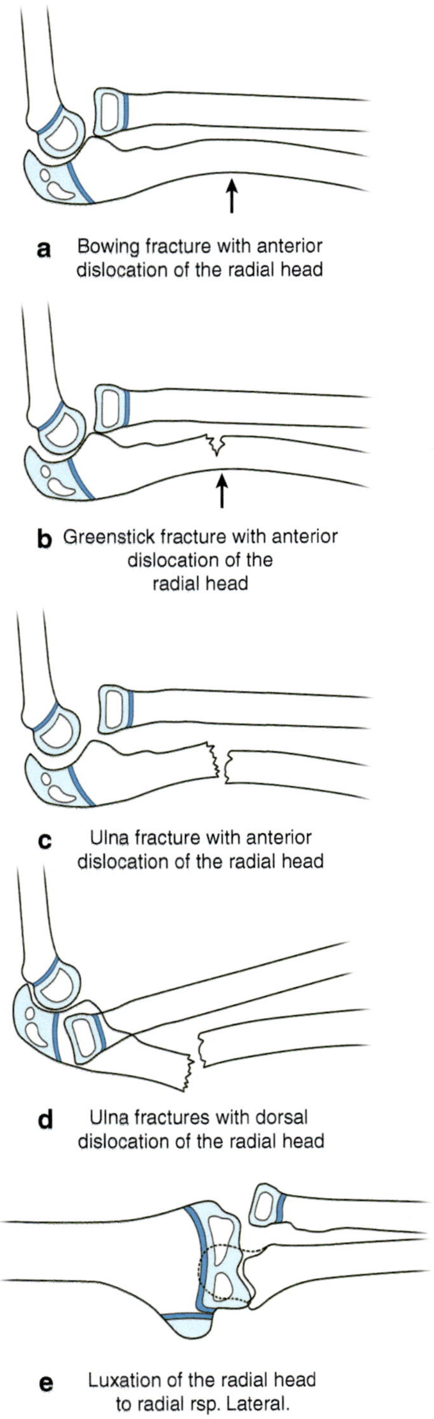

Fig. 19.9 Classification of pediatric Monteggia lesions. Modification of the Bado classification according to Letts et al. The 5 types are indicated (**a**–**e**)

An acute dislocation is relatively easy to treat surgically, whereas chronic dislocation with malunion requires a sophisticated approach, both for diagnosis and correction. Nerve lesions have also been reported in up to 10% of cases of soft tissue irritation caused by radial head dislocation.

Treatment

Underlying Principles

The date of injury and time point of dislocation is very helpful to plan a treatment of chronic radial head dislocation or Monteggia lesions, because secondary deformities can occur over time, which make an optimal reconstruction difficult or impossible. In cases of acute dislocation, the crucial joint structures remain intact. In an older, posttraumatic chronic dislocation, considerable deformities may be present regardless of whether it is purely congenital or developmental. The typical features of congenital dislocation are listed in Table 19.4. If there are chronic changes, assessment for the deformities listed in Table 19.5 must be carried out because they might prevent successful correction (Figs. 19.10 and 19.11). Principally, indications for correction include:

1. Instability
2. Irritation of the ulnar nerve
3. Restricted movement/Elbow joint impairment
4. Progression of deformity
5. Pain
6. Cosmetic impairment

Table 19.5 Features of congenital dislocation

Anatomical area	Features
Capitellum	Hypoplasia
Ulna	Shortened, anterior arch for anterior, posterior arch for posterior dislocation
Radius	Dome-shaped in anterior, elongated/narrow in posterior dislocations.
Radial head	Dislocation vector 43% posterior, 47% anterior, 10% radial dislocation
Contralateral elbow	Often bilateral
Other area, e.g., hand	Combination with other anomalies/syndromes

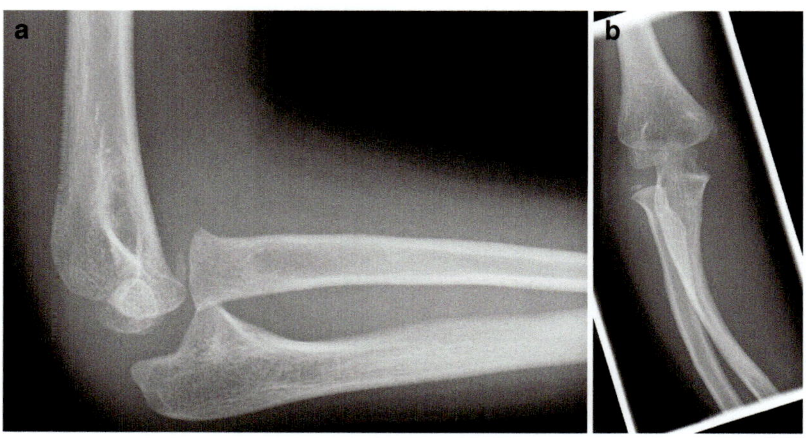

Fig. 19.10 Chronic posttraumatic deformity of the proximal ulna with radial convex deformity and radial head dislocation from the humeroradial joint. (**a**) latral view, (**b**) A.P. view

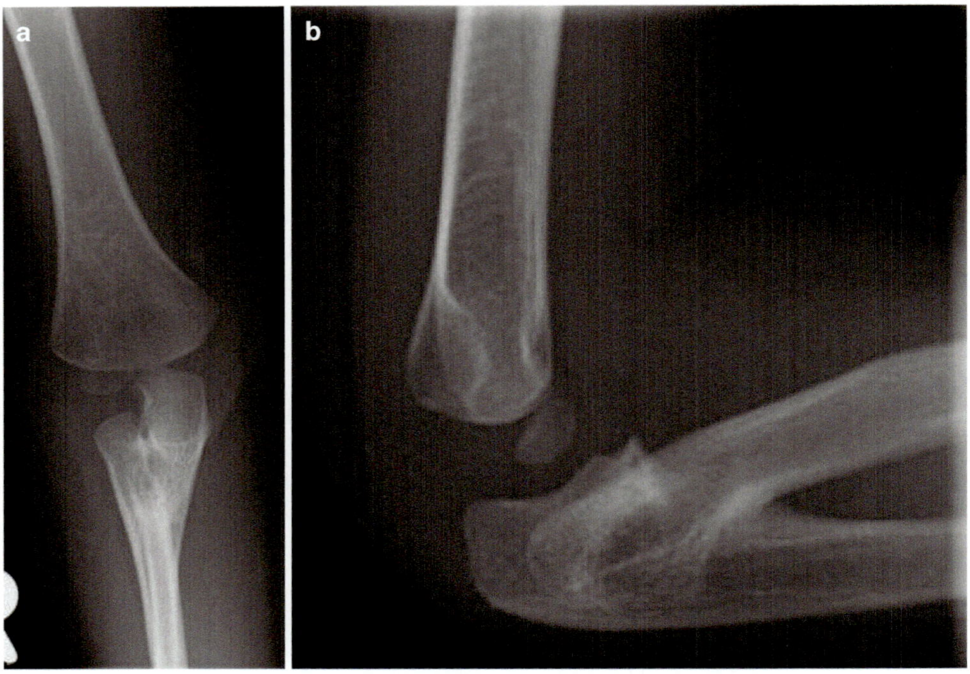

Fig. 19.11 Congenital deformity of the proximal radius with synostosis formation. (**a**) A.P. view (**b**) larteral view

Operative Therapy

Preoperative Preparation

According to the presenting circumstances, steps for correction must be discussed with the child and parents as precisely as possible. Initial function must be recorded, and the chances of eliminating existing functional impairments must be evaluated. If necessary, it must be discussed that only partial success can be achieved. When correcting a Monteggia lesion, the primary goal is to improve flexion since the typical form of acute injury involves anterior dislocation that limits elbow flexion (see Fig. 19.9).

Operative Methods

If the diagnosis is made promptly—within the first 6–12 weeks—correction is usually relatively strait forward because of mild deformity. The situation can often be remedied using an angled osteotomy with open reduction of the radial head, checking all axes of motion. Good function can be expected after treatment (Fig. 19.12a–g).

In chronic radial head dislocation, proximalization of the radial head must be considered along with anterior dislocation and the deformities listed in Table 19.5. This makes direct reduction almost impossible, since it would require extreme angulation that shortens the ulna relative to the radius. Forcing the reduction too much can lead to excessive pressure in the humeroradial joint, causing deformity or worse, osteonecrosis. Redislocation is also more likely.

Distalization of the radial head is necessary before these problems can be overcome and the joint aligned. This is accomplished through ulnar osteotomy and lengthening with callus distraction. To avoid disruption at the wrist or relative ulnar advancement, the radius could be fixed distally and move together with the distal ulnar fragment during the lengthening process. The distance from the proximal radial head to the capitellum should reach approximately 1.5 cm. After a resting phase of about three weeks, angulation and open reduction are performed as described above. In most cases you can see a spontaneous repositioning of the radial head. Changing the procedure to plate fixation can increase comfort and avoid long external fixator application times (Fig. 19.13a–f). Elbow exercises without loading should be performed throughout the treatment phase.

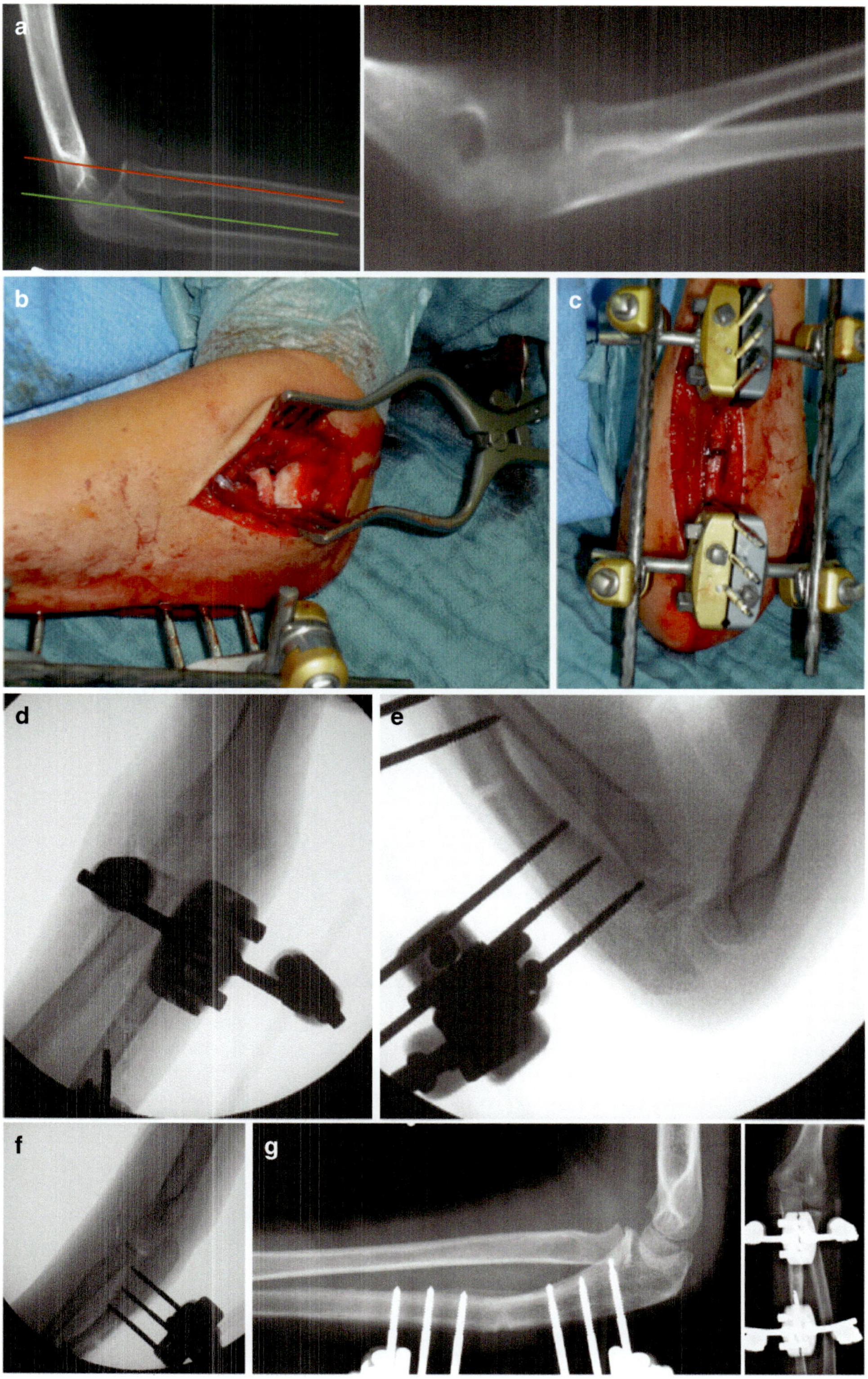

Fig. 19.12 Correction of a Monteggia lesion with radial head dislocation without significant deformity or proximalization of the radial head: (**a**) Preoperative radiograph, the red line marks the dimensions of the anterior dislocation, the green lines are the expected position, (**b**) Open adjustment of the radial head (**c**) Clinical images of angulation, (**d–f**) Intraoperative xray controls in various planes, (**g**) Recovery image

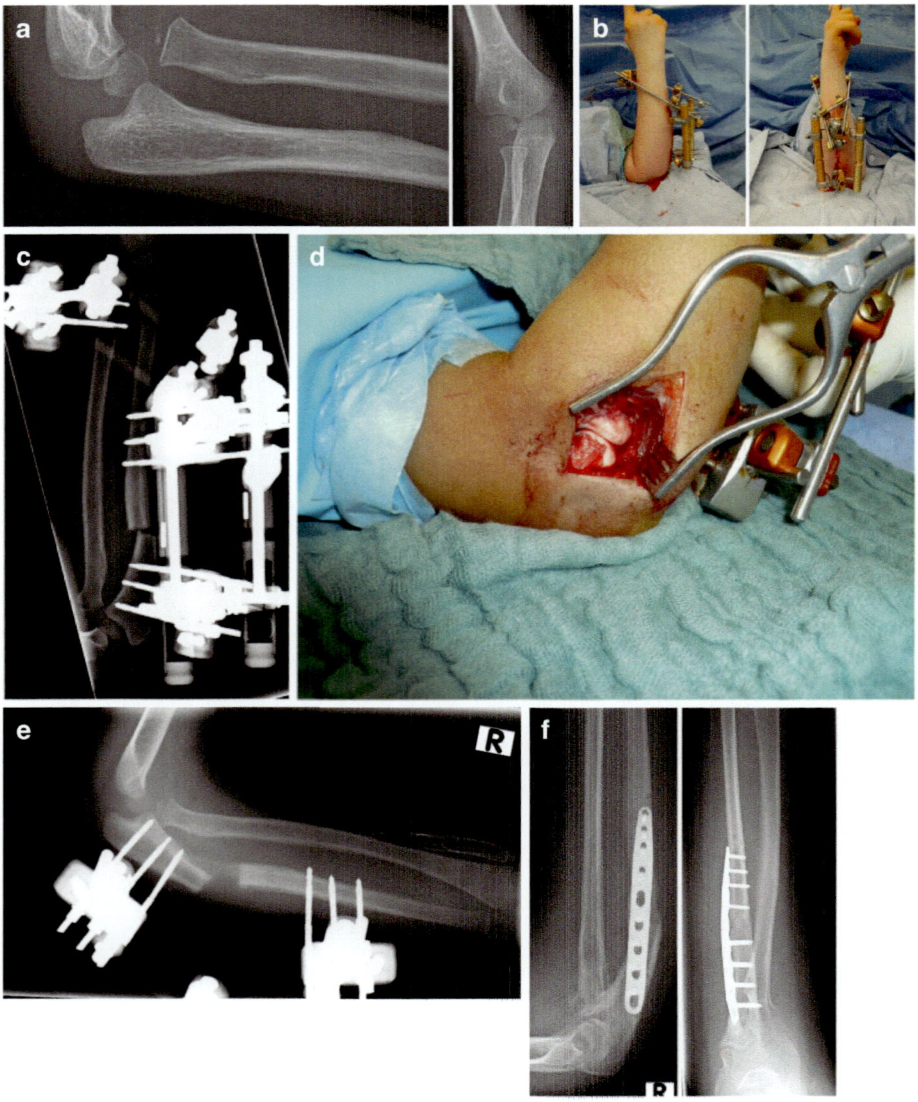

Fig. 19.13 Correction of a chronic Monteggia lesion with radial head dislocation and marked proximalization: (**a**) Preoperative xray, (**b**) Intraoperative appearance correcting possible fixator assembly for correction (Hoffmann II Compact System from Stryker), (**c**) Xray control of the callus distraction, (**d**) Open reduction and fixator remodeling, (**e**) Xray control with increasing consolidation of the distraction callus, (**f**) Example of a procedure change with stabilization of the ulna or the distraction callus with plate fixation (e.g., ulnar osteotomy plate from Synthes)

19.4 Complications

For corrective interventions on the elbow, there are acute complications that can occur during or immediately after surgery. All three nerves in the elbow region are at risk of injury. As with primary treatment, ulnar and radial nerve injuries are most common because of exposure and manipulation. Radial nerve involvement is challenging during the ongoing therapeutic course because of the associated drop hand. Individual cases with perfusion complications and compartment syndromes have also been reported. Specific problems are associated with age and method of fixation. For example, an external fixator can yield pin infections and insufficient consolidation that can lead to refracture or renewed deformity. This applies particularly to primary Monteggia lesions where forearm callus distraction is necessary and also critical, deformity-related adjustments must be made that can lead to redislocation and treatment failure. Pre-existing changes to the radial head and reduction manipulations, with associated risks of soft-tissue calcification and ossification, can lead to synostosis development, resulting in forearm rotation deficits (Table 19.6). Sometimes an additional osteotomy can help to improve the diaphysis-neck angle allowing alignment in relation to the capitulum at any point of rotation, flexion and/or extension (Fig. 19.14). The effects on the wrist and, as needed, the secondary correction (leveling of a relative ulnar advancement) should be emphasized: In most cases this final alignment is carried out after complete consolidation of the needed corrections at the elbow level as well as after stabilization of the soft tissue, since there is a significant force for relaxation, e.g. due to the changes also in the interosseous membrane between ulna and radial bone. We consider a good time about 1 year after elbow alignment (Fig. 19.15). Nonunion after correction of the distal humerus or even re-nonunion after lateral condyle revision must be mentioned. Despite a good healing process and cosmetic results, decreased range of motion remains the most common complication and can be up to five times more frequent than the problems mentioned above.

Table 19.6 List of consequential changes after chronic Monteggia lesions

Anatomical area	Secondary deformities
Radial head	Convex radial head
Proximal radius	Axial deviation, e.g., radial neck
Proximal ulna	Deformities with radial convexity, expansion of the proximal ulna over the capitellum
Deformity PRUJ (proximal radioulnar joint)	Neojoint, synostosis

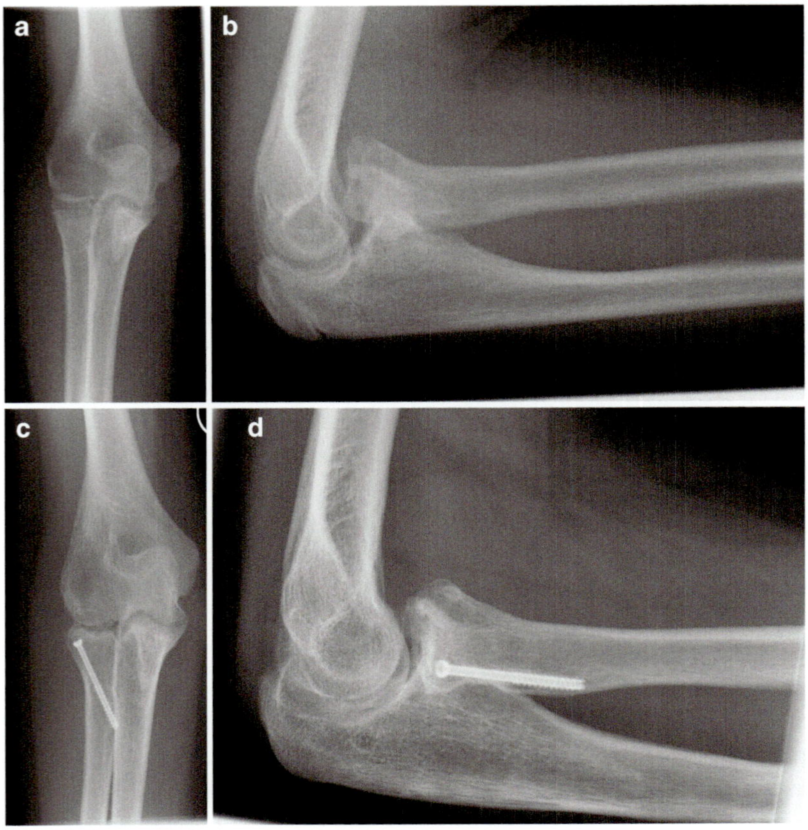

Fig. 19.14 Luxation of the proximal radial head with significant secondary deformity of the proximal radius and diaphysis-neck—angle (**a**) A.P. view (**b**) Lateral view. Postoperative appearance after bone lengthening and secondary realignment of the radial head together with a corrective osteotomy at the proximal radial neck (**c**) A.P. view (**d**) Lateral view

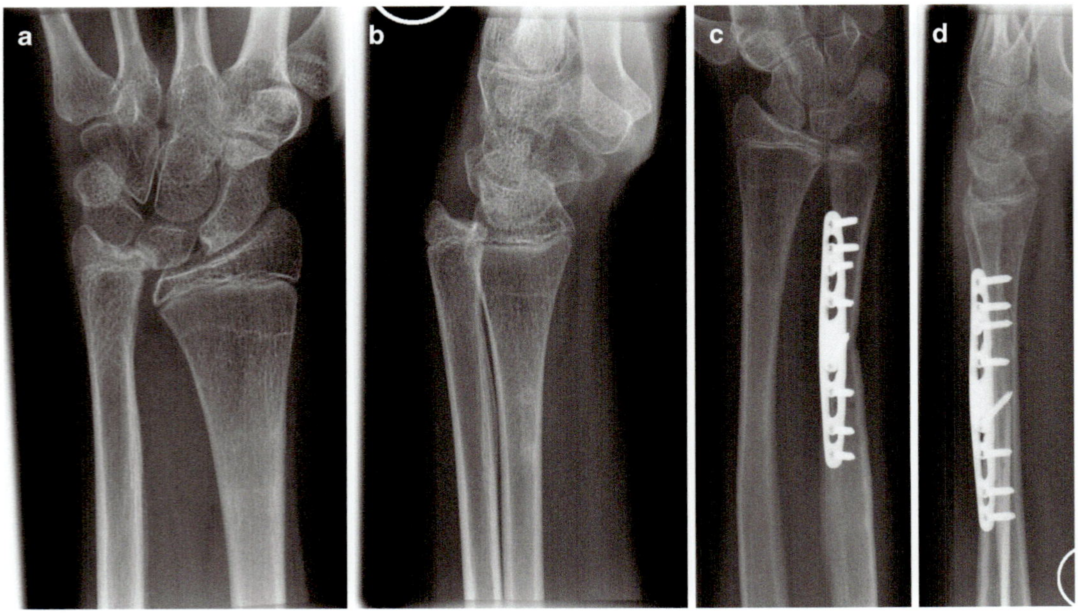

Fig. 19.15 Dislocation of the distal radio-ulnar-joint after correction of a monteggia lesion, dorsal luxation and relative ulna advancement are obvious, (**a**) A.P. view (**b**) Lateral view. Postoperative appearance after corrective osteotomy of the ulna with shortening, (**c**) A.P. view (**d**) Lateral view

19.5 Practical Conclusions

Operative therapy of posttraumatic elbow deformities is a unique challenge due to the complex articular anatomy with three joints and two degrees of freedom as well as growth plates. The best solution is adequate treatment of the acute injury. If facing posttraumatic deformity in this region, there is a sophisticated process to identify indications for corrective procedures. This includes evaluating realistic goals, especially when there are functional deficits, and considering the adjustments necessary for various structures and joints affected by the deformity. For cases with cosmetic concerns, the rate of complications (sometimes quite high in the literature) must be considered and the decision for surgery carefully considered. Particularly with chronic radial head dislocation after Monteggia lesions, congenital and developmental deformities must be differentiated and preferably followed through with conservative therapy. This always calls up a detailed discussion with the child and parents as well as explanations of treatment, including various deviations and potential problems with further treatment options.

Recommended Literature

Bado JL (1967 Jan) The Monteggia lesion. Clin Orthop Relat Res 50:71–86

Bellemore MC, Barrett IR, Middleton RW, Scougall JS, Whiteway DW (1984 Aug) Supracondylar osteotomy of the humerus for correction of cubitus varus. J Bone Joint Surg Br 66(4):566–572

Best TN (1994) Management of old Unreduced Monteggia Fracture Dislocations of the elbow in children. J Pediatr Orthop 14(2):193

Degreef I, De Smet L (2004 Jul) Missed radial head dislocations in children associated with ulnar deformation: treatment by open reduction and ulnar osteotomy. J Orthop Trauma 18(6):375–378

Frank J, Sander AL, Voth M, Marzi I (2017a Jan 10) Long-term clinical and radiographic outcomes after open reduction for missed monteggia fracture-dislocations in children. Trauma und Berufskrankheit [Internet]. 2nd ed. 40(6):1394. Available from: http://jbjs.org/article.aspx?doi=10.2106/JBJS.H.00644

Frank J, Sander AL, Voth M, Marzi I (2017b Aug 1) Sekundäre Rekonstruktionen am Ellenbogengelenk im Kindesalter. Trauma und Berufskrankheit. 2nd ed. Springer Medizin 19(2):126–134

French PR (1959 Sep 26) Varus deformity of the elbow following supracondylar fractures of the humerus in children. Lancet 2(7100):439–441

Hasler CC (2001 Feb) Supracondylar fractures of the Humerus in children. Eur J Trauma 27(1):1–15

Hasler CC, Laer von L, Hell AK (2005 Jan 1) Open reduction, ulnar osteotomy and external fixation for chronic anterior dislocation of the head of the radius. Bone Joint J 87-B(1):88–94

Horst M, Altermatt S, Weber DM, Weil R, Ramseier LE (2010 Dec 3) Pitfalls of lateral external fixation for supracondylar humeral fractures in children. Euro J trauma Emerg Surg 37(4):405–410. Springer-Verlag

Horstmann HM, Blyakher AA, Quartararo LG, Cavalier R (2000 May) Treatment of cubitus varus with osteotomy and Ilizarov external fixation. Am J Orthop 29(5):389–391

Hui JHP, Torode IP, Chatterjee A (2004 Sep) Medial approach for corrective osteotomy of cubitus varus: a cosmetic incision. J Pediatr Orthop 24(5):477–481

Josten C, Freitag S (2008 Dec 8) Monteggia and Monteggia-like-lesions: classification, indication, and techniques in operative treatment. Eur J Trauma Emerg Surg 35(3):296–304

Karatosun V, Alekberov C, Alici E, Ardiç CO, Aksu G (2000 Sep) Treatment of cubitus varus using the Ilizarov technique of distraction osteogenesis. J Bone Joint Surg Br 82(7):1030–1033

Kemnitz S, De Schrijver F, De Smet L (2000 Oct) Radial head dislocation with plastic deformation of the ulna in children. A rare and frequently missed condition. Acta Orthop Belg 66(4):359–362

Kim HT, Lee JS, Yoo CI (2005 Apr) Management of cubitus varus and valgus. J Bone Joint Surg Am 87(4):771–780

Koch PP, Exner GU (2003 Mar) Supracondylar medial open wedge osteotomy with external fixation for cubitus varus deformity. J Pediatr Orthop B 12(2):116–122

Korner J, Hansen M, Weinberg A, Hessmann M, Rommens PM (2004 Dec) Monteggia fractures in childhood?Diagnosis and management in acute and chronic cases. Eur J Trauma. 30(6):361–370

Kraus R (2013 Oct 15) The pediatric vs. the adolescent elbow. Some insight into age-specific treatment. Euro J Trauma Emerg Surg 40(1):15–22, Springer, Berlin Heidelberg

Kraus T, Tauber S, Linhart W (2013 Jan 11) Posttraumatic complications on children's elbows. Orthopade 42(1):57–70

Kumar K, Sharma VK, Sharma R, Maffulli N (2000 Oct) Correction of cubitus varus by French or dome osteotomy: a comparative study. J Trauma 49(4):717–721

Lädermann A, Ceroni D, Lefèvre Y, De Rosa V, De Coulon G, Kaelin A (2007 Aug 29) Surgical treatment of missed Monteggia lesions in children. J Child Orthop Springer-Verlag 1(4):237–242

Laer von L (1986) Frakturen und Luxationen im Wachstumsalter. © Georg Thieme Verlag Stuttgart · New York, Stuttgart, New York

Laer von L, Pirwitz A, Vocke AK (1997 Dec) Post-traumatic problem cases involving the elbow in children. Orthopade 26(12):1030–1036

Laer von L, Pirwitz A, Hasler CC (2000 Mar 1) Late missed Monteggia fractures. Tech Orthop 15(1):27

Letts M, Locht R, Wiens J (1985 Nov) Monteggia fracture-dislocations in children. J Bone Joint Surg Br 67(5):724–727

Linhart WE, Kraus T (2008 Nov 16) Reconstruction of Humeroradial joint. Orthop Traumatol 20(4–5):396–408

Marzi I (2009) Kindertraumatologie, 2nd edn. Springer, Berlin, p 1

Marzi I, Schmittenbecher PP, Ploss C, Frank J Spezieller Teil Kinder- … 2016

Morrey BF, Sanchez-Sotelo J (2009) The elbow and its disorders. Saunders Elsevier, Philadelphia

Olney BW, Menelaus MB (1989 Mar) Monteggia and equivalent lesions in childhood. J Pediatr Orthop [Internet] 9(2):219–23. Available from: https://journals.lww.com/pedorthopaedics/abstract/1989/03000/monteggia_and_equivalent_lesions_in_childhood.21.aspx

Raney EM, Thielen Z, Gregory S, Sobralske M (2012 Apr) Complications of supracondylar osteotomies for cubitus varus. J Pediatr Orthop 32(3):232–240

Ring D, Waters PM (1996 Sep 1) Operative fixation of Monteggia fractures in children. J Bone Joint Surg Br 78-B(5):734–739

Slongo TF (2008 Nov 16) Correction osteotomy of neglected "Monteggia" lesion with an external fixator. Orthop Traumatol 20(4–5):435–449

Stoll TM, Willis RB, Paterson DC (1992 May 1) Treatment of the missed Monteggia fracture in the child. Bone Joint J 74-B(3):436–440

Tajima T, Yoshizu T (1995 May) Treatment of long-standing dislocation of the radial head in neglected Monteggia fractures. J Hand Surg Am 20(3 Pt 2):S91–S94

Usui M, Ishii S, Miyano S, Narita H, Kura H (1995 Jan) Three-dimensional corrective osteotomy for treatment of cubitus varus after supracondylar fracture of the humerus in children. J Shoulder Elb Surg 4(1 Pt 1):17–22

Weinberg AM, Reilmann H (2000) Frakturen der Diaphyse im Kindesalter Teil II: Obere Extremität. Unfallchirurg

Weinberg AM, Marzi I, Günter SM, Wessel L, Riedel J, Laer von L (2002 Feb 19) Die suprakondyläre Oberarmfraktur im Kindesalter – eine Effizienzstudie Ergebnisse der multizentrischen Studie der Sektion Kindertraumatologieder Deutschen Gesellschaft für Unfallchirurgie – Teil I: Epidemiologie. Effektivitätsprüfung und Klassifikation Der Unfallchirurg 105(3):208–216

Weise K, Schwab E, Scheufele TM (1997 Apr 17) Ellenbogenverletzungen im Kindesalter. Der Unfallchirurg Springer-Verlag 100(4):255–269

20 Secondary Reconstruction of the Forearm and Wrist

20.1 Epidemiology

Most fractures in this anatomical region result from falls (20%) and sport injuries (15%). Fractures of the distal radius account approximately for 15%, forearm fractures for 10% of people below the age of 18 years. Even this is a very high number only in a very limited number of corrective osteotomies are needed (less than 0.1%). However, centers with a high frequency (>2000 cases a year) of trauma in young people and children should see between 5 and 10 post—trauma—deformities, which might need a corrective procedure.

20.2 Deformities of the Forearm

Fractures of the forearm result very quickly, if not addressed appropriate, in loss of function. Since the radial and ulna bone are connected at both ends with a bi-condylar swivel joint, the distal and proximal radio-ulnar-joint, every anatomical mal-alignment (axis, length, rotation) has a potential to impair ROM. Therefore, conservative treatment is very limited and operative treatment preferred to avoid a deformity, and reconstruct the original bone dimensions including the axis of rotation between the center of the radial head and the ulna fossa. Due to these facts indications for correction are:

- Malalignment of the axis
- Reduced Rotation
- Impairment of PRUJ and elbow function
- Impariment of DRUJ and wrist function

Therapy

Basics

In most cases of deformities at the forearm level they result in a limitation of rotation. Problems at the elbow level are due to monteggia-like lesions with various impairment including flexion and extension. Therefore, this topic is addressed in the this chapter, secondarty reconstruction of the elbow. Also wrist problems might occur due to forearm fractures, especially luxation's of the DRUJ (Galeazzi-like lesions), resulting in limited rotation. Further deformities—especially length discrepancies—are addressed later in this chapter.

Corrective Procedures

Pre-Operative Preparation

Most deformities seem to be very obvious in the forearm region. However in any case a precise analysis of the anatomic situation should be performed. This includes usual x-ray pictures to address the following points:

- Location of the deformities
- Elbow-joint including PRUJ
- Wrist-joint including DRUJ

I. Marzi et al., *Pediatric Skeletal Trauma*, https://doi.org/10.1007/978-3-030-93685-3_20

- Determination of length, axis and rotation
- Evaluation of possible synostosis
- Complete clinical evaluation with measurements of ROM

At the elbow and wrist level deformities of the radial and ulna bone, of the joint surfaces and/or neo-joints need to be searched for, as well as possible congenital or long lasting early deformities or even luxations (Fig. 20.1). The determination of length, axis and rotation could be very demanding requiring further diagnostic. If plain x-ray pictures are used the axis of the ulna and radial bone can be evaluated as described by various authors. In some cases the exact location and characteristics of the deformity in its three dimensions might not be clear. Therefore, a CT in low dose technique with 3D-reconstruction is very helpful to visualize the complete forearm in different ankles with comparison to the healthy other side (Fig. 20.2). If this is not enough most centers are able to perform a 3D-print helping to understand the problem and also to demonstrate it to the patient and the family (Fig. 20.3). Using standardized scan protocols one can also have industrial partners to provide such prints. Some of these commercial companies are even able to print tools for the operative procedure based on these data. These are very well established in maxilla-facial surgery.

Especially in rotational impairment one has to carefully evaluate the forearm for synostosis (Fig. 20.4). In such cases a successful reconstruction of complete rotation is limited, as well as the rate of recurrence very high. Various operative techniques have been suggested, including interposition of de-epithelialized skin, various flaps or biomaterials. However, none of these techniques have proven to be reliable to preserve function in long term.

Operative Techniques

Depending of the preoperative analysis, osteotomy of the ulna and/or radial bone is needed. Sometimes length discrepancy is obvious and a multi-staged procedure necessary e.g. bone lengthening and final adjustment with definitive stabilization (Fig. 20.5). For such procedures various external fixators are available followed by a method of secondary osteosyn-

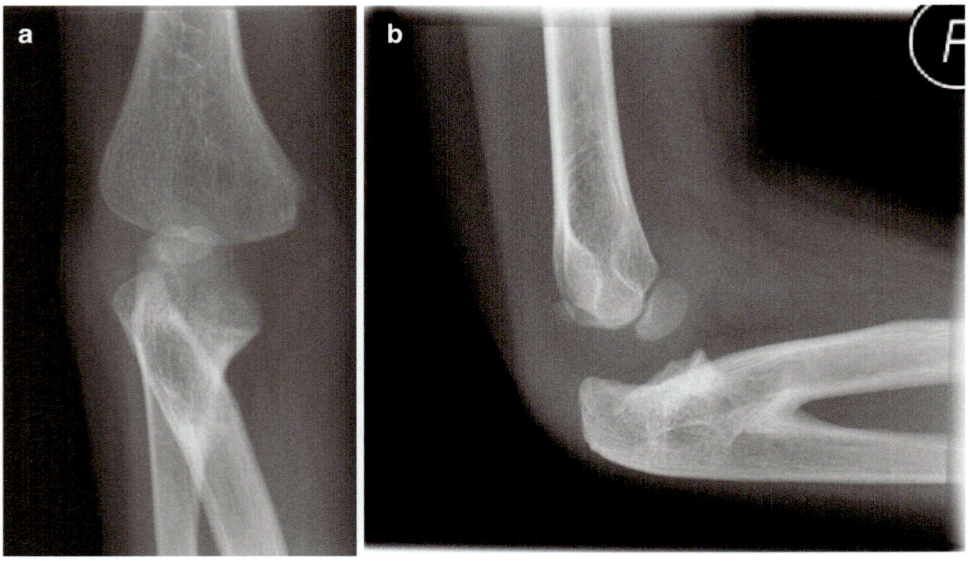

Fig. 20.1 Example for a long lasting/or congenital deformity at the elbow level, (**a**) A.P. view, (**b**) Lateral view

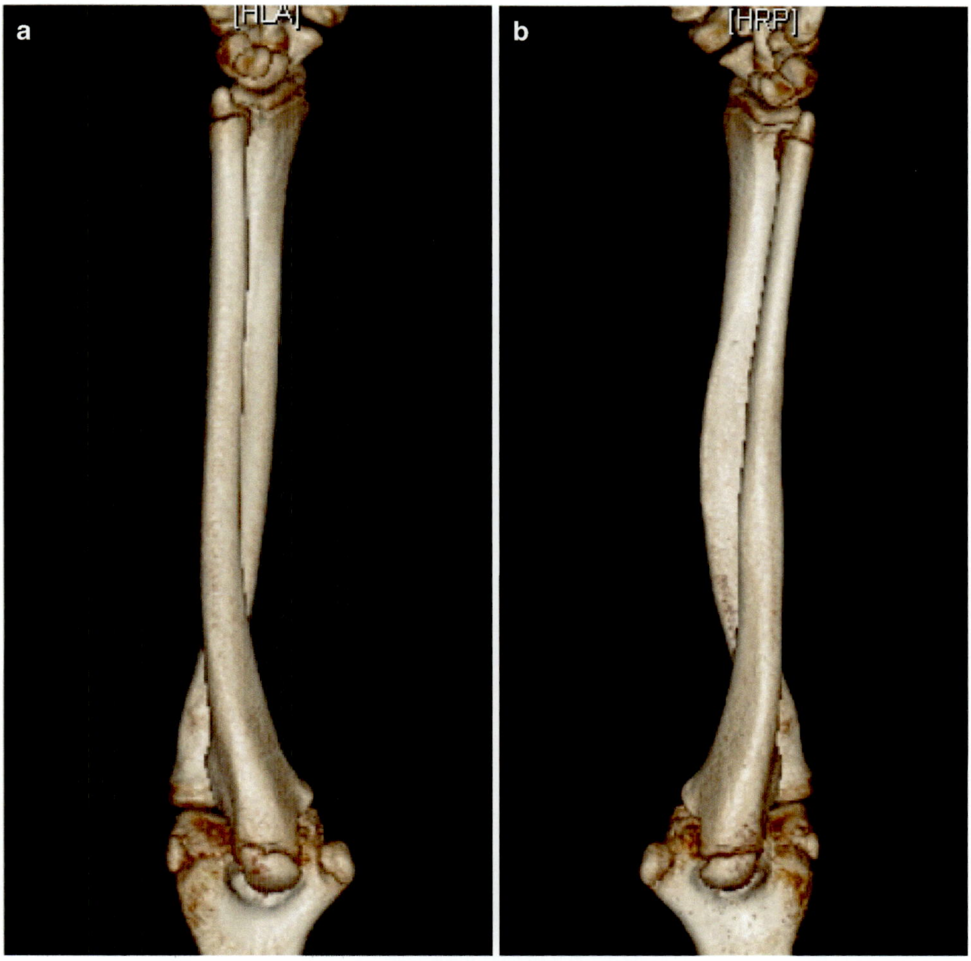

Fig. 20.2 Appearance of a forearm deformity after low dose CT-scan and 3D-reconstruction (**a**) Normal (**b**) Deformity

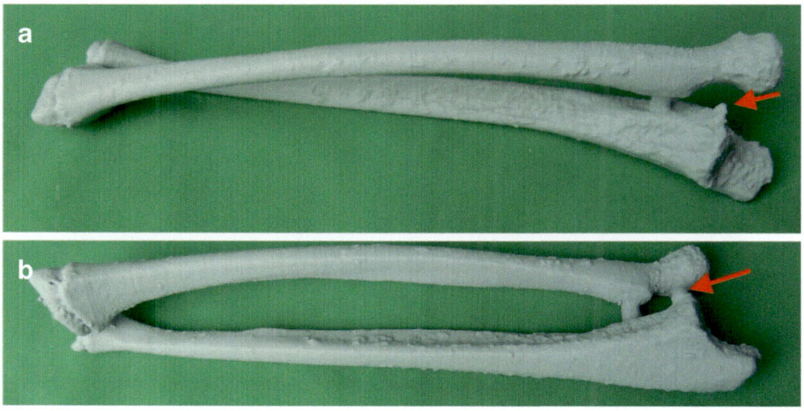

Fig. 20.3 3D-model to analyze a forearm deformity. No significant bone deformity was obvious aside the luxation and proximal dislocation of the radial bone. At the ulna side the old ligamentous lesion is marked due to the bony extension, different views (**a**, **b**). Due to the long standing dislocation and free function no correction was performed

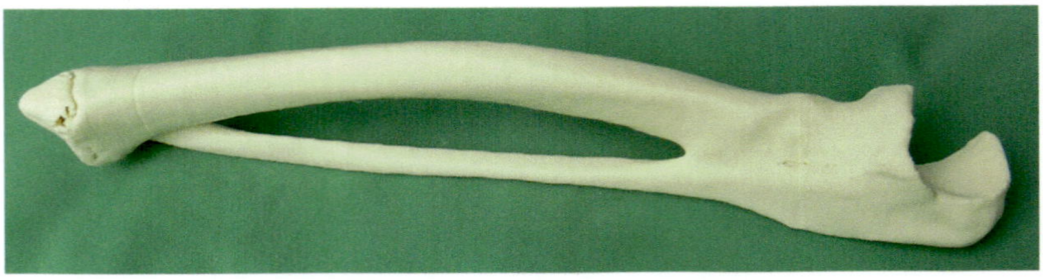

Fig. 20.4 3D-model of a synostosis

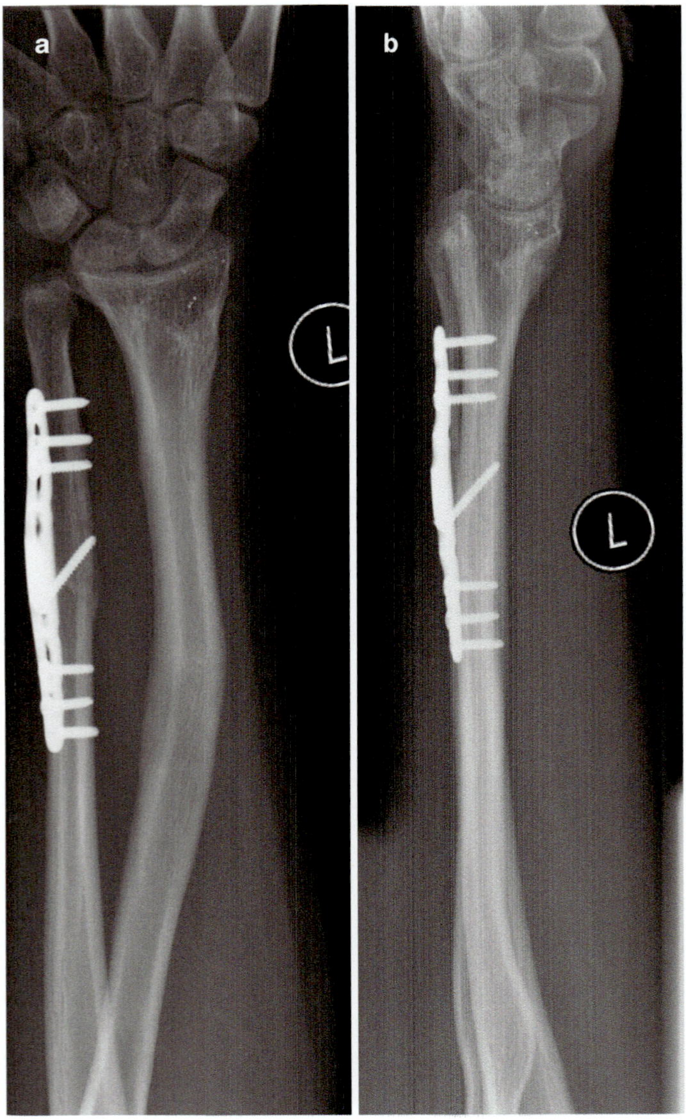

Fig. 20.5 Final adjustment at the wrist level using ulna shortening and plate osteosynthesis (**a**) A.P. view (**b**) Lateral view

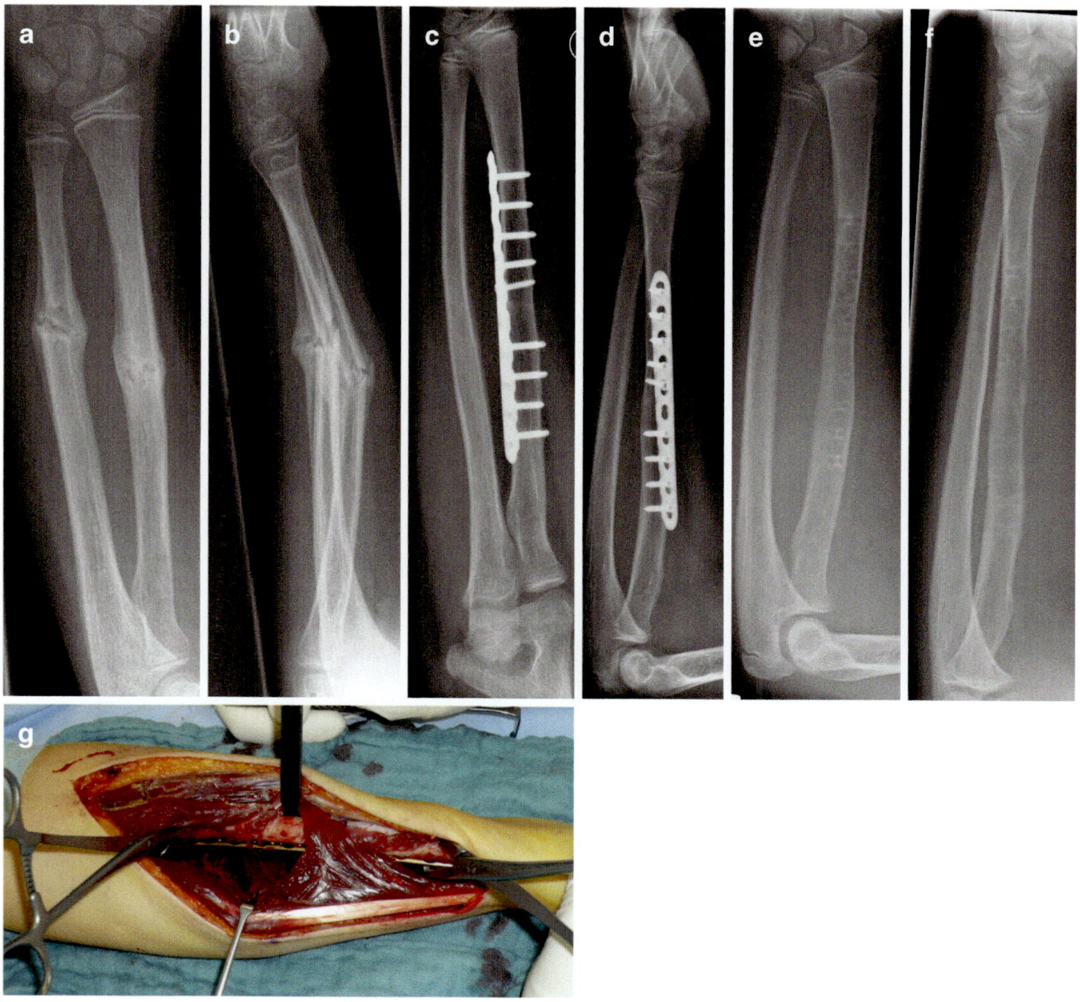

Fig. 20.6 Corrective osteotomy of the radial bone in a 10 year old boy, (**a**) Deformity A.P. view, (**b**) Deformity lateral view, (**c**) Correction with plating A.P. view, (**d**) Lateral view, (**e**) Final picture after hardware removal A.P. view, (**f**) Lateral view, (**g**) Intraoperative picture of a radial bone correction through a Henry-approach

thesis. Mostly this type of correction is needed in adolescents and therefore following osteotomy stabilization with plate(s) advised (Fig. 20.6). However, in young patients a fixation is very well possible with ESIN (Fig. 20.7).

Postoperative Care

Depending on the procedure, after definitive stabilization a long arm cast is needed around 2 weeks for pain control. After this period of time movement of the arm and joints is encouraged to regain function or to avoid restriction due to bone or scare formation. Weight bearing takes in most of the cases longer compared to fracture healing and is limited to less than 1 kg for 3–4 month. Also, in difficult cases physiotherapy is advised to support functional recovery, especially if a synostosis was removed.

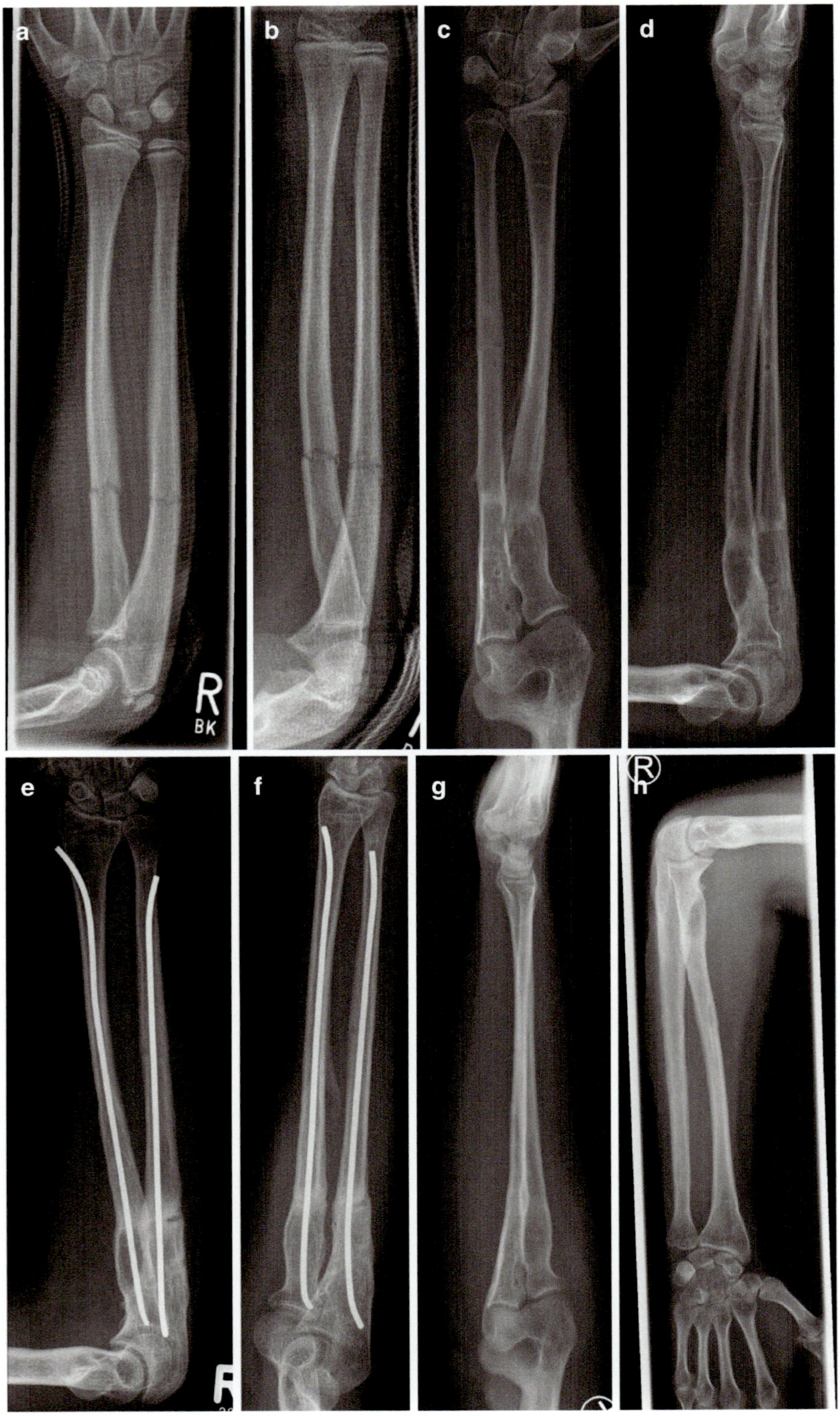

Fig. 20.7 Corrective osteotomy of the forearm in a 11 year old girl and stabilization with ESIN, (**a**, **b**) 2 Plane view of the forearm after initiation of conservative treatment, (**c**, **d**) 2 Plane view of the deformity at the proximal forearm, (**e**, **f**) 2 Plane view after correction with ESIN, (**g**, **h**) Views after hardware removal

20.3 Deformities at the Wrist Level

Due to the fact, that distal radial fractures are one of the most common fractures, deformities after such fractures are the most common and appear in up to 25% after conservative treatment. However, problems at the distal end after fractures in younger people especially younger than 10 years are rare, due to the growth potential at this level. The potential of remodeling must be taken into consideration and valued against an early corrective procedure (Fig. 20.8). This might be difficult at the level of the metaphysis where a deformity up to 30° might be corrected at this young age. Between at the age of 10 and 12 years a more anatomic reduction should be aimed. A significant problem which is relatively rare, but needs more often a correction is growth arrest at the physis and might need a long ongoing reconstruction at a level where simple ulna shortening is not an option (Fig. 20.9).

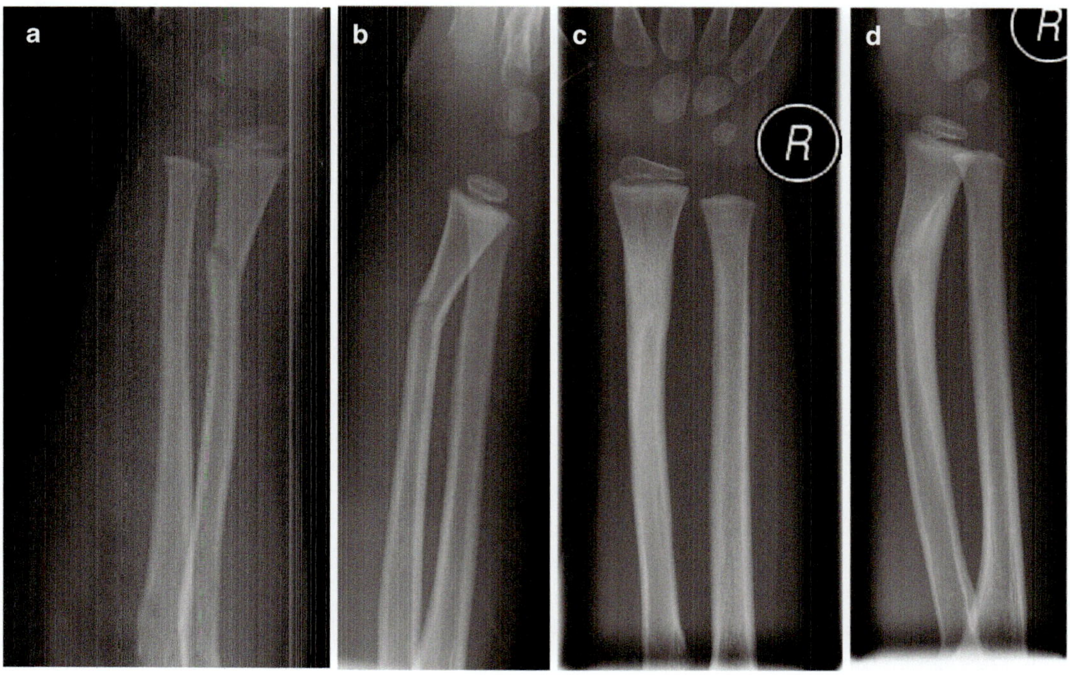

Fig. 20.8 Forearm fracture of a 5 year old boy, (**a**) A.P. view, (**b**) Lateral view, x-ray picture at the day of injury, (**c**, **d**) X-ray picture 3 month later, demonstrating a spontaneous correction

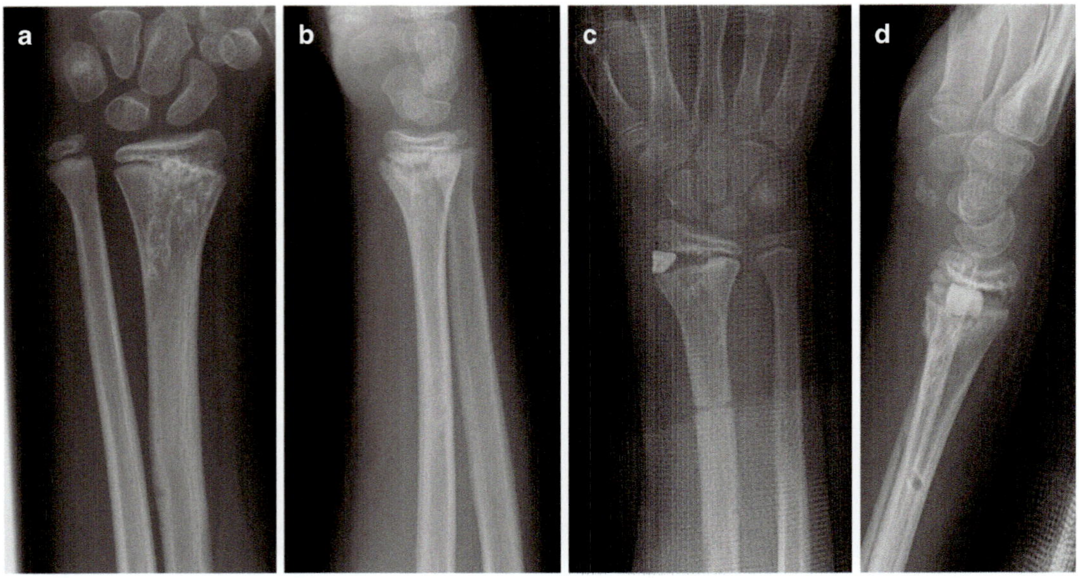

Fig. 20.9 Closure of the distal radius growth plate due to a traumatic epiphysiolysis in a 9 year old boy, (**a**) A.P. view, (**b**) Lateral view, (**c**) A.P. view, (**d**) Lateral view after epiphysiolysis and resection of the bridging callus with bone cement interposition

Treatment

Underlying Principles

The treatment modality depends on the type of deformity (Table 20.1). In children the age of the child and the correction potency of the physis is very important as well as the exact location of the deformity (Table 20.2). In cases of dislocations in the sagittal level less dislocations (about 20°) should be tolerated compared to the frontal level. In a few cases the joint surface is directly involved. In such a case an anatomical reconstruction should be achieved as soon as possible and as in all cases a follow up program initiated. Such patients are at high risk of growth plate lesions which will end in shortening of the involved bone due to partial or complete preliminary closure of the physis. Common complications of such deformities are:

Table 20.1 Post-trauma deformities of the distal forearm

Deformities	
Deformity of the joint axis	Radial inclination Dorsal/Palmar dislocation
Shortening	Ulna/radial bone due to lesion of the physis Bone defects
Rotation deformity	
Incongruency of the joint line	Radiocarpal joint Distal radioulnar joint

Table 20.2 Potential of correction after fractures of the distal forearm

Anatomical location	Age/angle of correction potential
Metaphysis	<8 years >30° 8–12 years >25° >12 years >10°
Epiphysis	<8 years >50° 8–12 years > 30° >12 years > 10°

- pain
- reduced range of motion
- loss of strength
- osteoarthritic changes
- instabilities of the carpal bones
- nerve irritation
- cosmetic appearance/mal alignement of the hand

Operative Therapy

Preoperative Preparation

The first preparation step is to analyze the deformity precisely, measuring deviation, axis and all joint surfaces including the DRUJ. The deformity should also be evaluated with respect to the clinical function of the upper extremity, including an intense discussion with the parents and the child about the prognosis, changes of spontaneous correction and expected limitations. The procedure might be explained in detail using figures, as well as possible complications and changes of the therapy and/or additional operative procedures. It is not easy to explain the down-sides if the deformity is neglected. Possible risks can be given accordingly a few reliable studies in adults. A dorsal dislocation of more than 20° could result in more than 60% of the patients in osteoarthritic changes along with the development of carpal problems within weeks. Also, if a fracture results in a relative lengthening of the ulna bone already measurable functional deficiency could be measured starting at 2 mm. A step in the joint could induce arthritic deformities above 1 mm.

Therefore, at the distal forearm the following points for a corrective procedure can be outlined:

- young patients
- pain and loss of function
- ulna shortening >4 mm
- expected long lasting deformity of more than 20° in sagittal/frontal plane
- secondary carpal instability
- articular displacement >1 mm
- cosmetic deformities
- no significant arthritic changes

Operative Methods

Angulation-Deformity

Due to the above-mentioned variety the exact operative techniques vary depending on the actual deformity. Angulation-Deformities are usually a straight forward procedure and preoperative planning is relatively simple (Fig. 20.10). For orientation the epiphyseal plate or the joint line can be used to outline the amount of correction. After the correction in most cases plates can be used to stabilize the correction. A simple method is to approach the Deformity directly, dorsal deformities from dorsal and palmar deformities from palmar. However, some authors prefer dot perform a correction independent from the dislocation from palmar. One should be aware, that even with the intention to avoid extensor tendon irritation also flexor tendon lesions after palmar plating is an issue. Usually, it will not lead to major complications, like tendon ruptures. However, the extensor pollicis tendon is at risk at any approach. So it might be wise in cases of dorsal dislocations to expose this tendon and perform a transposition to reduce the risk of rupture to a minimum. Also, External fixation can be used to stabilize a corrective osteotomy at the distal forearm. However, this method is mostly used in complex cases where bone lengthening is needed. In any case the implants need to be adjusted to the bon size, usually the plate will have a dimension between 2.3 and 2.7 mm (Figs. 20.11 and 20.12) and the epiphyseal plate must be preserved.

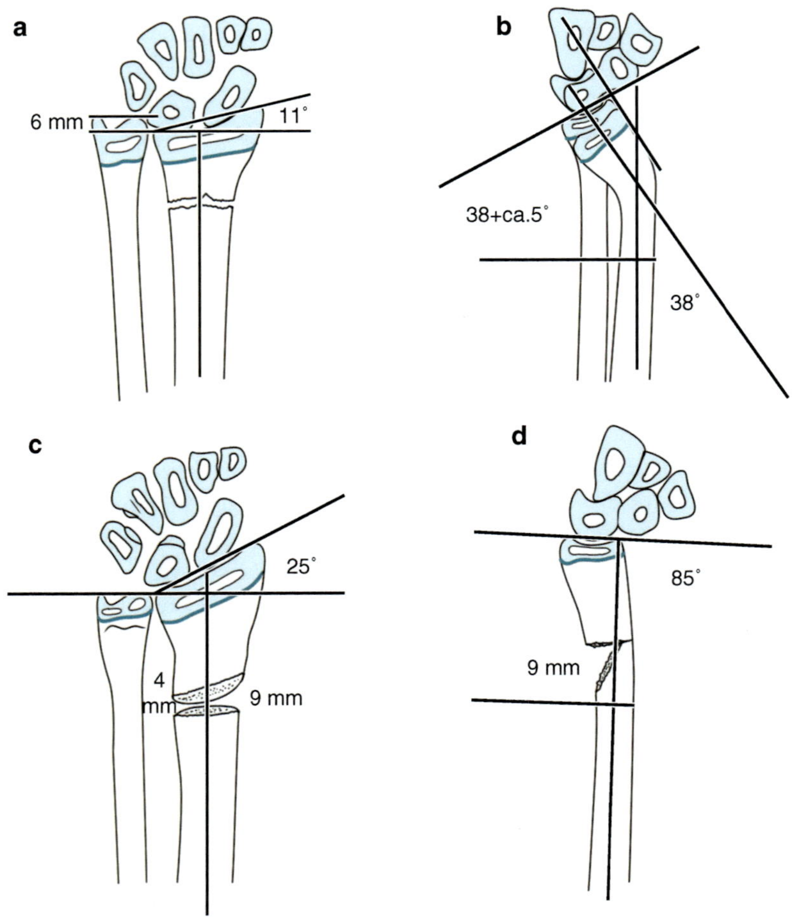

Fig. 20.10 Planning and principles for a corrective osteotomy of the distal radial bone, (**a**) A.P. view of the deformity, (**b**) Lateral view of the outlined deformity with measurements, (**c**) A.P. view of the correction, (**d**) Lateral view of the correction

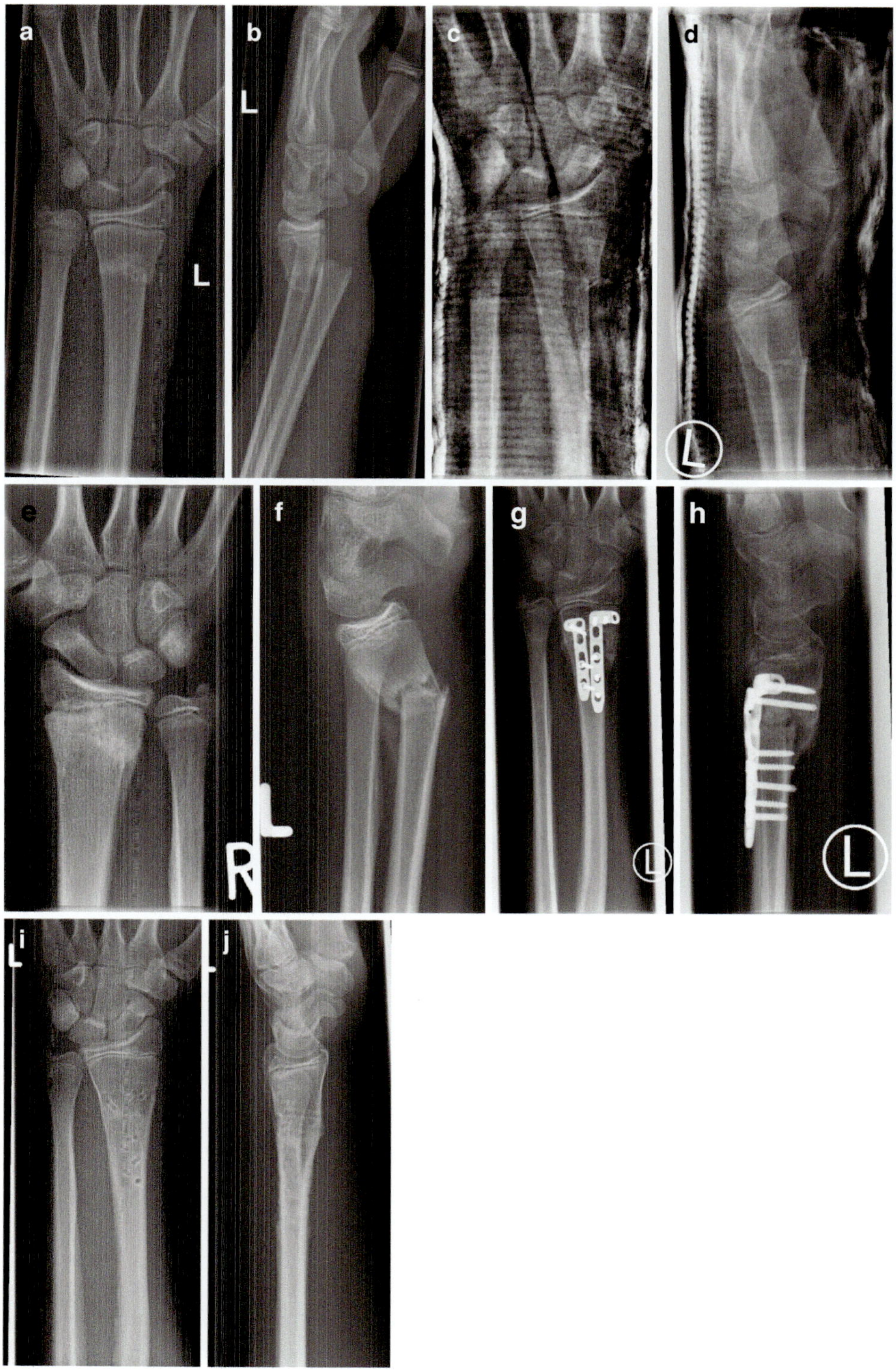

Fig. 20.11 Distal forearm fracture of a 13 year old boy, (**a**) A.P. view, (**b**) Lateral view of the fracture at the day of injury, (**c**) A.P. view, (**d**) Lateral view of the early reduction an cast immobilization, (**e**) A.P. view, (**f**) Lateral-view of the deformity with angulation and limited forearm rotation, (**g**) A.P. view, (**h**) Lateral-view after the operative correction, (**i**) A.P. view, (**j**) Lateral-view of the final result after hardware removal

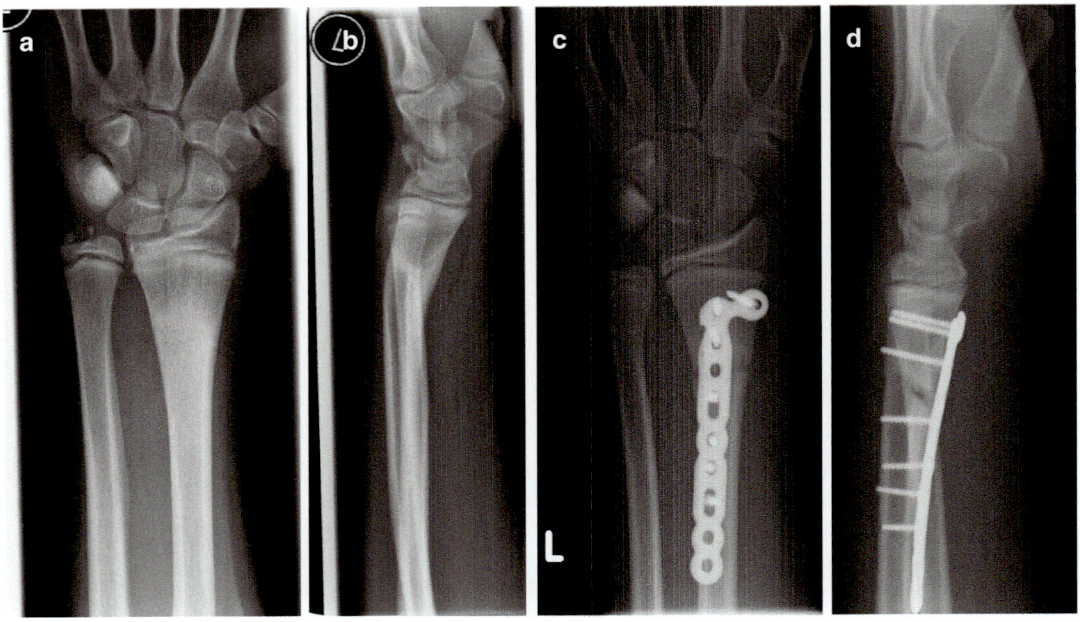

Fig. 20.12 Deformity after a distal forearm fracture with palmar angulation and limited rotation in a 12 year old boy, (**a**) A.P. view, (**b**) Lateral-view, (**c**) A.P. view and (**d**) Lateral view after corrective osteotomy

Compared to adults in children very seldom bone grafting is needed, therefore an unstable osteosynthesis in corrective osteotomies must be avoided, which is much more likely if K-wires are used. If a defect seems to be getting to big bone lengthening should be considered before the final adjustment or I less extensive defects local callus or bone can be used according to the method described by Watson and Castle, (Fig. 20.13).

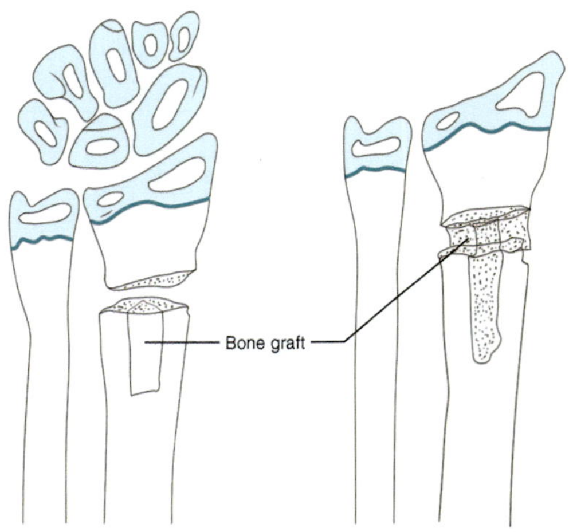

Fig. 20.13 Alternative bone grafting for corrective osteotomies to avoid taking bone from the ilica crest

Growth-Arrest

Fractures involving the physis might end up in shortening of the radial/or ulna bone due to growth arrest. Some might involve only a part of the growth plate with minor deformity. If function and alignment of the hand and carpal bones is preserved a correction can be performed to achieve anatomical alignment after growth has finished (Fig. 20.14). If there is a significant loss of function and secondary changes can be expected to the carpal structures leveling and joint congruency should be aimed earlier. Some cases might not need bone lengthening and can be solved at once (realignement of the radio-

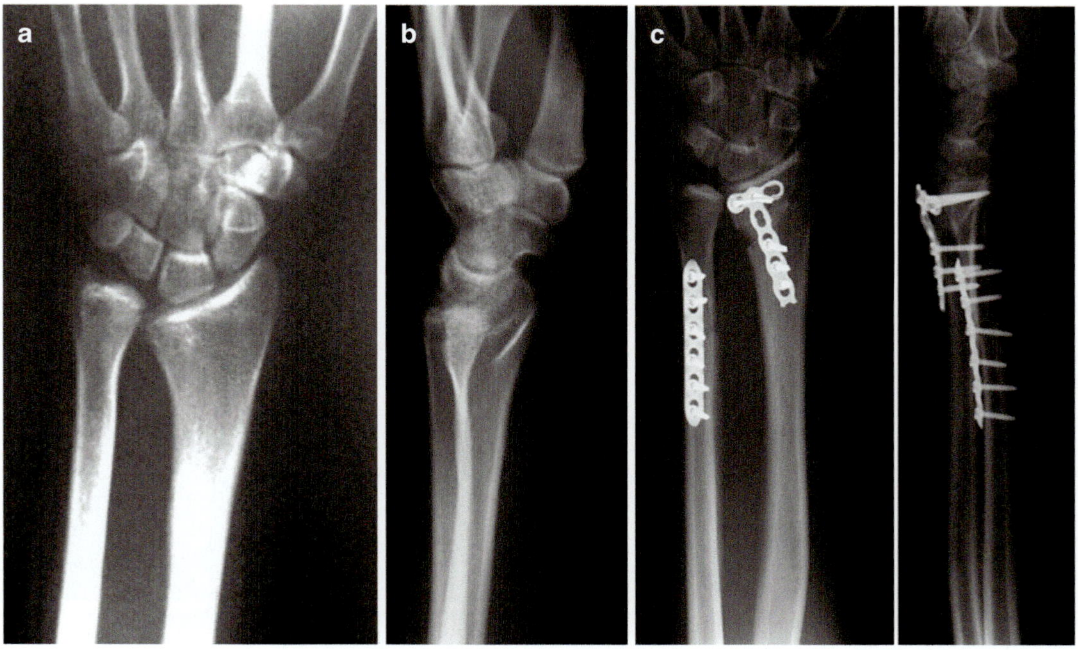

Fig. 20.14 Twenty-year-old woman after partial closure of the ulna-sided radial growth plate due to a wrist fracture, (**a**) A.P. view, (**b**) Lateral view of the deformity, (**c**) A.P. view and lateral-view after correction and realignment of the carpal bones

carpal and distal radio-ulnar joint, Fig. 20.15). In other cases, bone lengthening with an external fixation is recommended. To improve comfort till bone callus is mature and stable enough, secondary plating is an option (Fig. 20.16). If the bone stock is very fragile (defects, pseudarthroses) a combination of plating and external fixation might help to adjust the wrist joint. An option to ovoid ulna overgrowth might be screw epiphysiodesis. One should be aware that the implant will violate an intact triangular fibrocartilage, especially if big crew heads or washers are used. Smaller crews might not slow down the growth enough. Therefore, a secondary ulna shortening can be chosen as an additional procedure. This is also advised if an impaction syndrome persists (Figs. 20.5, 20.16, and 20.17). In disaster cases it might be helpful to avoid a summarization of complications to break the correction down into multiple steps (Fig. 20.18):

1. Alignment of the wrist, avoidance of major secondary deformities, acute pain management
2. Leveling e.g. bone lengthening
3. Optimization of function and maximal joint congruency

However, if secondary changes are significant (e.g. joint lines, osteoarthritic changes) only instability or painful joints should be addressed with the usual rescue procedures, knowing that there will never be no long-lasting satisfaction with a normal functioning and weight bearing joint (Table 20.3 and Fig. 20.19). In a few cases it might be worth performing osteochondral transplantations especially if there is a partial osteochondral defect of the radio-carpal joint surface. In such cases this might be done in young adults after growth persists, (Fig. 20.20).

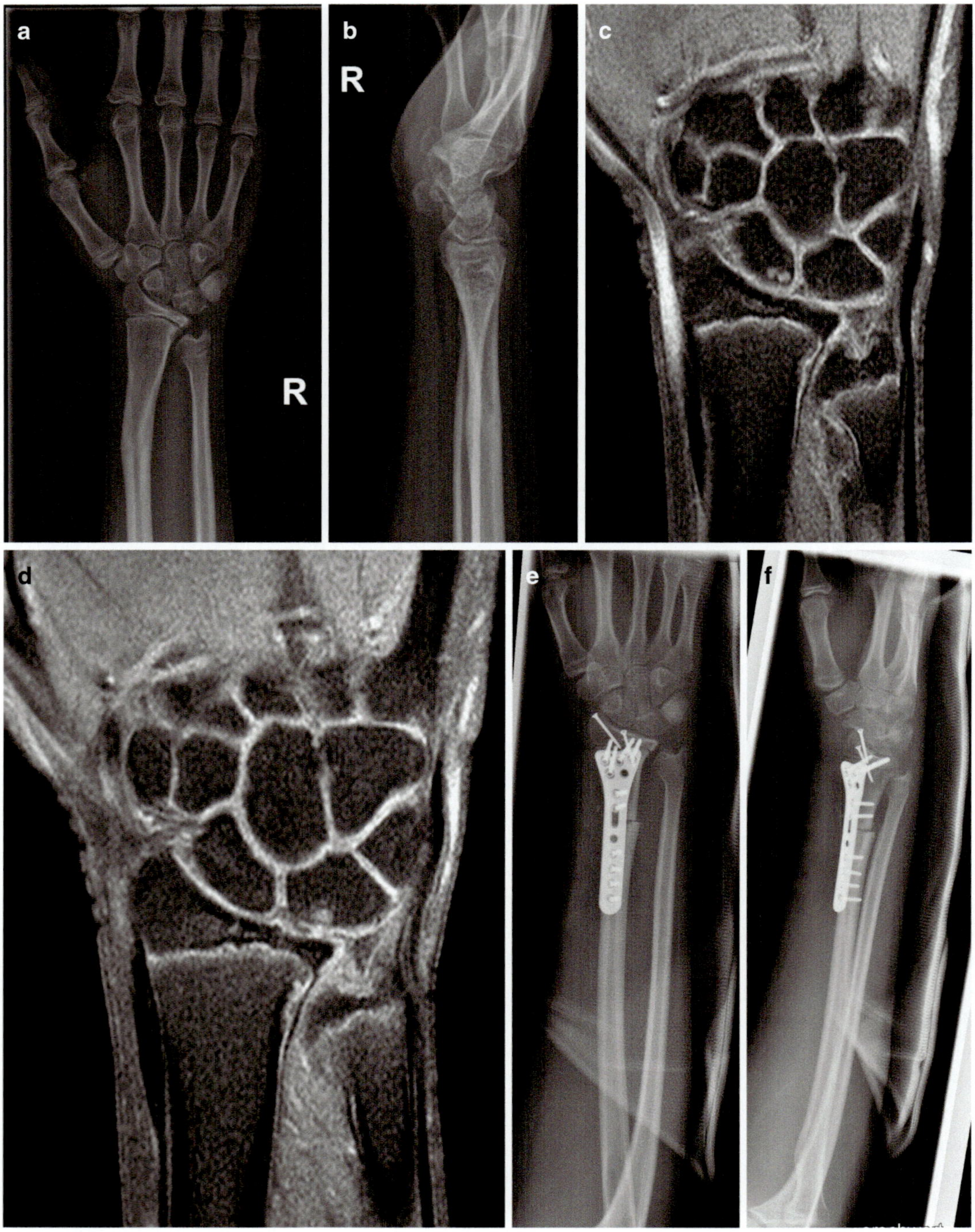

Fig. 20.15 Deformity of the forearm in a 15 year old boy with limited rotation and ulnar deviation, (**a**) A.P. view, (**b**) Lateral-view of the deformity, (**c**, **d**), MRI-pictures of the joint levels and deformities, (**e**) A.P. view and (**f**) Lateral-view after the correction with radial shortening and reduction of radial inclination to improve hand position, 2 screws are inserted through the growth plate area to avoid any further radial growth

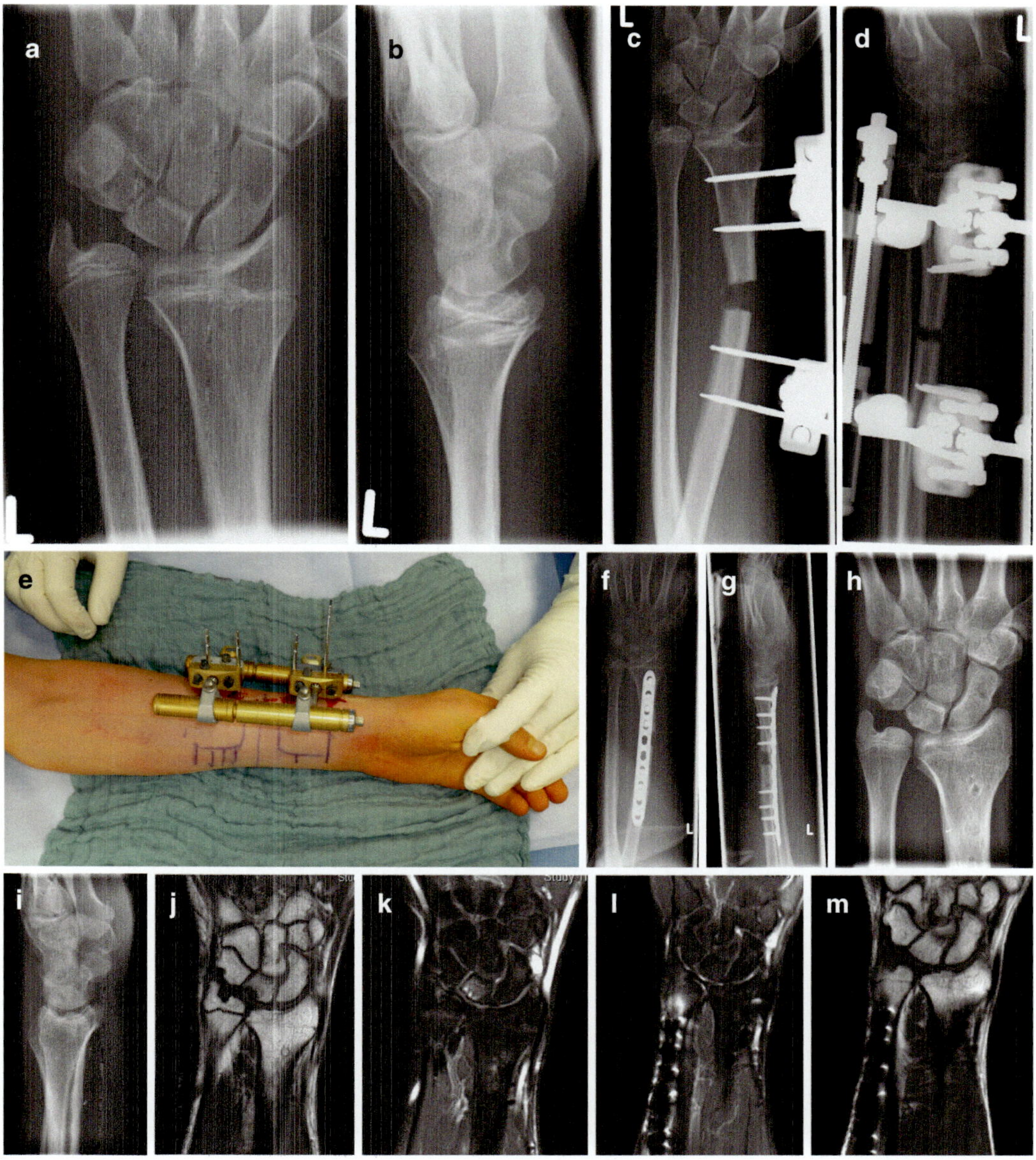

Fig. 20.16 Growth arrest of the distal radius after lesion of the physis in a 14 year old boy, (**a**) A.P. view, (**b**) Lateral-view before reconstruction with bone lengthening, (**c**) A.P. view, (**d**) Lateral-view demonstration the x-ray views during bone lengthening, (**e**) Intraoperative view at the time of external fixation application, (**f**) A.P. view, (**g**) Lateral-view of plate stabilization after external fixateure removal during bone consolidation, (**h**) A.P. view, (**i**) Lateral-view of persisting relative ulnar plus with impaction syndrome, (**j**, **k**) MRI-pictures demonstration the impaction syndrome at the ulna side of the lunate, (**l**, **m**) Resolution of the impaction syndrome after ulna shortening, MRI one year later

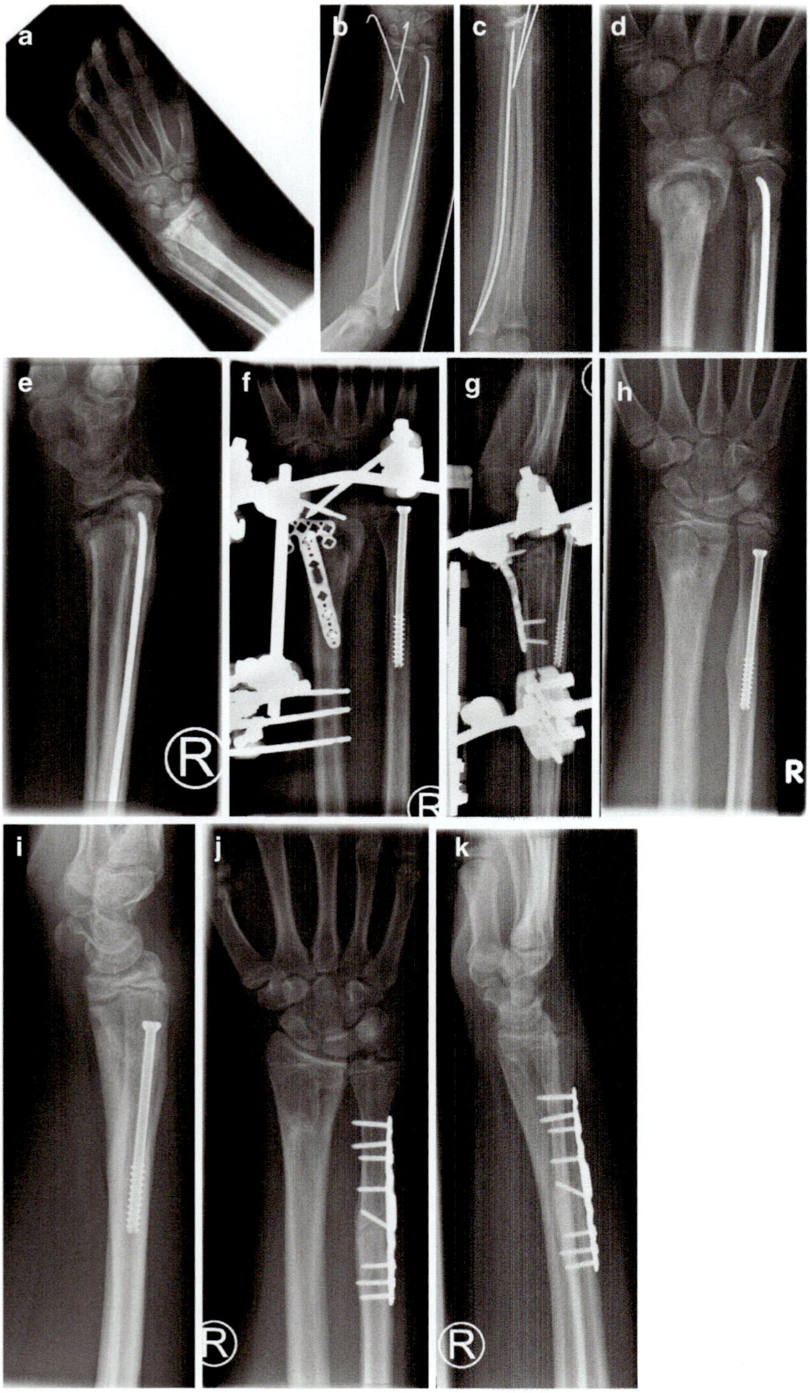

Fig. 20.17 Severe wrist fracture of an 11 year old boy, (**a**) X-ray picture after the injury, (**b**) A.P. view, (**c**) Lateral view after primary stabilization of the radius with k-wires and the distal ulna with an ESIN, (**d**) A.P. view, (**e**) Lateral-view post-trauma deformity with shortening of the radial bone and increase angulation of the distal epiphyseal portion of both bones, (**f**) A.P. view, (**g**) Lateral-view of the revision of this deformity, due to the unstable distal fragment a plate and an additional external fixation was chosen and the expected overgrowth of the ulna limited by screw epiphysiodesis, (**h**) A.P. view, (**i**) Lateral-view after good consolidation of the radial bone, however the screw was not able to avoid overgrowth of the ulna, (**j**) A.P. view, (**k**) Lateral-view of the forearm after final alignment of both forearm bones by ulna shortening

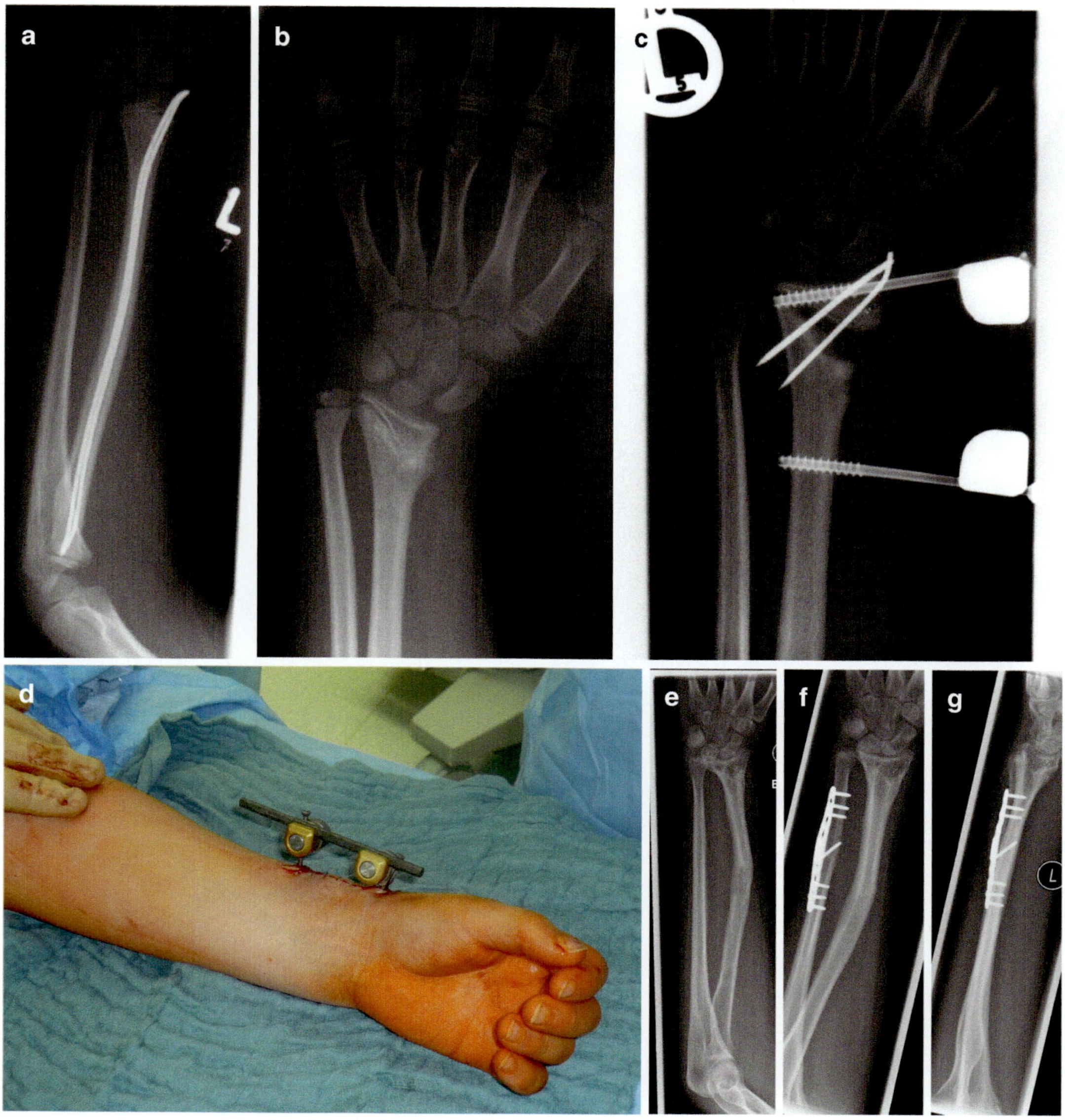

Fig. 20.18 ESIN-stabilization of a distal radius fracture in a 11 year old boy (**a**) Healed fracture with 2 ESIN to stabilize the radial bone, (**b**) Radial closure of the growth plate, (**c**) Release of the growth plate with external fixation using cannulated screws for better intraoperative placement to avoid additional iatrogenic lesions, (**d**) Intraoperative picture with good alignment of the hand and free rotation of the forearm, (**e**) X-ray picture of the forearm after bone lengthening at the age of 16 years, (**f**) A.P. view, (**g**) Lateral-view of the wrist after final adjustment at the age of 19

Table 20.3 Various rescue operative procedures to improve function and reduce pain at the distal forearm level

Radio-carpal joint	Distal radio-ulnar joint
Radio-Scapho-lunate fusion	Darrach resection
Wrist fusion	Bowers Hemiresection
Osteochondral Transplantsation	Watson adjusted resection
Interpositon-arthroplasty (fascia lata, biologicals)	Sauvé-Kapandji procedure

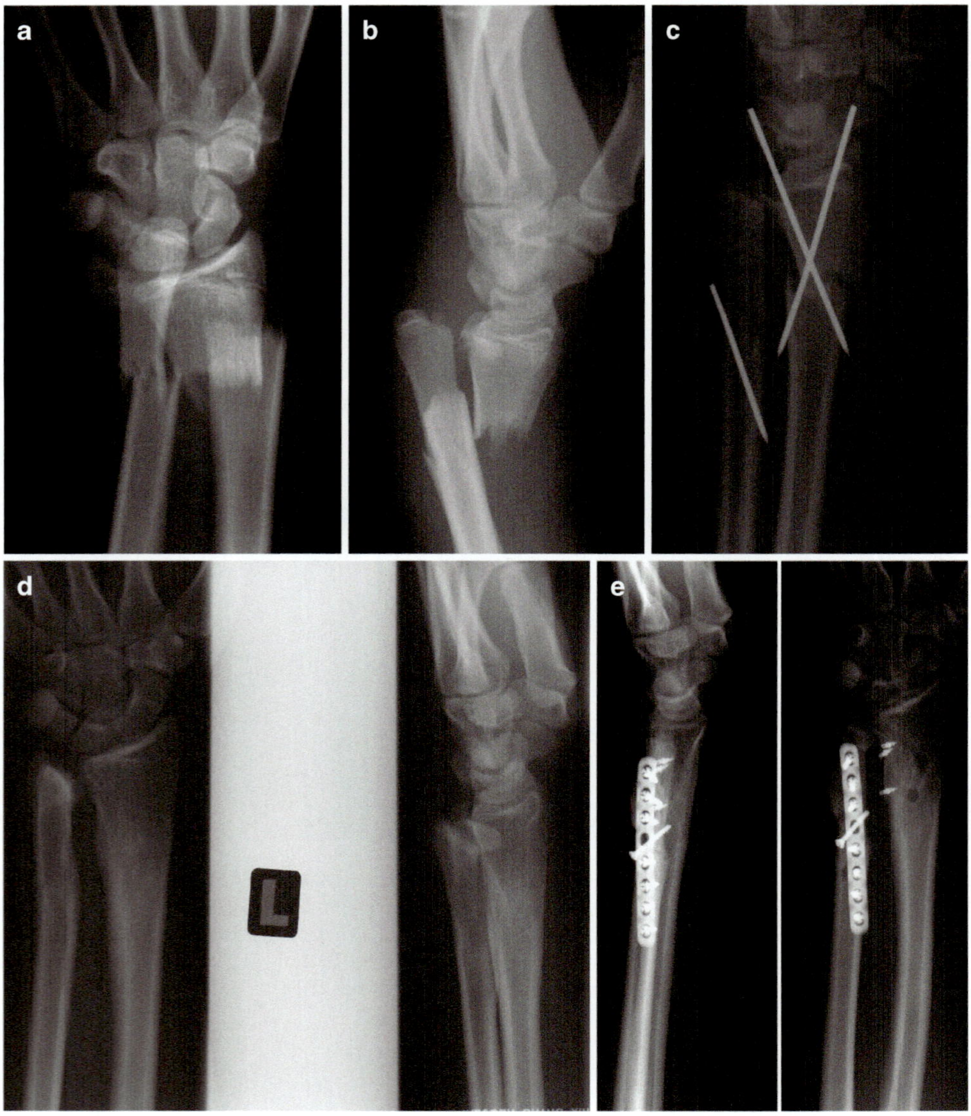

Fig. 20.19 Forearm fracture in a 12-year-old boy (**a**) A.P. view, (**b**) Lateral-view of the fracture, (**c**) Stabilization with k-wires, (**d**) Deformity of the DRUJ with instability and palmar dislocation of the radial bone, (**e**) Corrective osteotomy and stabilization with palmaris longus described by Scheker

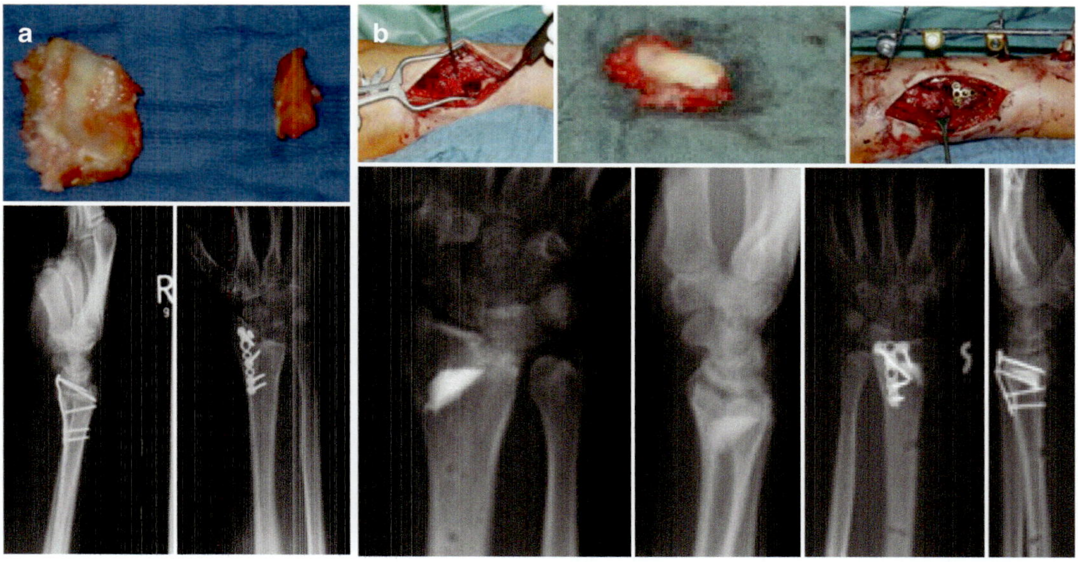

Fig. 20.20 Joint reconstruction of the distal radial bone with osteochondral transplantation, (**a**) Reconstruction of the fossa scaphoide in a 22 year old woman, (**b**) Reconstruction of the fossa lunata in a 26 year old man

20.4 Complications

Corrective interventions at the distal forearm are seldom and usually done early on before the therapy is finished, since most patients and parents will recognize the deformity and the loss of function. Even this area is exposed surgically routinely, there are acute complications that are obvious immediately, like nerve lesions (ulnar-, median-nerve, superficial radial branch) or tendon ruptures (mostly EPL). If the growth plate is intact and damaged throughout the corrective procedure a delay in growth will be seen after month. Depending on the stabilization technique, re-fractures or re-malalignment is a significant complication. This is also true for correction in the more proximal forearm area. Especially pseudarthrosis due to the osteotomies in the diaphysis. The surgical exposure is also much more demanding and therefore the complications more likely, however the same as in acute fracture care:

- Hematoma formation, Compartment Syndrome
- Tendon lesions (EPL, FPL)
- Vascular lesions
- Nerve lesions
- Malalignment
- Loss of function
- Pseudarthrosis
- Infections
- Scar formation

20.5 Conclusions

Operative therapy of posttraumatic deformities at the forearm and wrist is characterized be a very mixed pattern, starting at simple angular deformities mostly limiting forearm rotation and easy to be corrected. Complex deformities at the diaphysis need to be analyzed very carefully and weighted against the actual impairment, risk of a corrective procedure and expected improvement. Dramatic deformities, involving the growth plate might need multiple steps to achieve correction and therefore the surgeon and family must be aware of changes necessary throughout the treatment course. In some cases, it must be explained that sometimes only partial goals can be meet and some limits in ROM will persist as well as pre- arthritic deformations, which might end up in further operative procedures late in live.

Recommended Literature

Albert M, McCaig LF (2014 May) Injury-related emergency department visits by children and adolescents: United States, 2009–2010. NCHS Data Brief NCHS Data Brief 150:1–8

Amadio PC, Botte MJ (1987 Nov) Treatment of malunion of the distal radius. Hand Clin 3(4):541–561

Aro HT, Koivunen T (1991 May) Minor axial shortening of the radius affects outcome of Colles' fracture treatment. J Hand Surg Am 16(3):392–398

Bowers WH (1985 Mar) Distal radioulnar joint arthroplasty: the hemiresection-interposition technique. J Hand Surg Am 10(2):169–178

Cooper C, Dennison EM, Leufkens HG, Bishop N, van Staa TP (2004, Dec 1) Epidemiology of childhood fractures in Britain: a study using the general practice research database. J Bone Miner Res 19(12):1976–1981. John Wiley & Sons, Ltd

Darrach W (1913) Partial excision of the lower shaft of the ulna for deformity following Colles fracture. Ann Surg 57:764–765

Flynn JM, Sarwark JF, Waters PM, Bae DS, Lemke LP (2003) The surgical management of pediatric fractures of the upper extremity. Instr Course Lect Instr Course Lect 52:635–645

Forward DP, Davis TRC, Sithole JS (2008 May) Do young patients with malunited fractures of the distal radius inevitably develop symptomatic post-traumatic osteoarthritis? J Bone Joint Surg Br 90(5):629–637

Jayakumar P, Jupiter JB (2014 Sep) Reconstruction of malunited diaphyseal fractures of the forearm. Hand (N Y) 9(3):265–273

Joeris A, Lutz N, Wicki B, Slongo T, Audigé L (2014 Dec 20) An epidemiological evaluation of pediatric long bone fractures – a retrospective cohort study of 2716 patients from two Swiss tertiary pediatric hospitals. BMC Pediatr BioMed Central 14(1):314–311

Knirk JL, Jupiter JB (1986 Jun) Intra-articular fractures of the distal end of the radius in young adults. JBJS. J Bone Joint Surg Am 68(5):647–659

Makhni EC, Ewald TJ, Kelly S, Day CS (2008 Oct) Effect of patient age on the radiographic outcomes of distal radius fractures subject to nonoperative treatment. J Hand Surg Am 33(8):1301–1308

Mann D, Schnabel M, Baacke M, Gotzen L (2003 Feb) Results of elastic stable intramedullary nailing (ESIN) in forearm fractures in childhood. Unfallchirurg 106(2):102–109

Mehin R, Giachino AA, Backman D, Grabowski J, Fazekas A (2003 Mar) Autologous osteoarticular transfer from the proximal tibiofibular joint to the scaphoid and lunate facets in the treatment of severe distal radial fractures: a report of two cases. J Hand Surg Am 28(2):332–341

Miyake J, Murase T, Oka K, Moritomo H, Sugamoto K, Yoshikawa H (2012 Oct 17) Computer-assisted corrective osteotomy for malunited diaphyseal forearm fractures. J Bone Joint Surg Am 94(20):e150

Miyake J, Oka K, Kataoka T, Moritomo H, Sugamoto K, Murase T (2013, Jul 1) 3-dimensional deformity analysis of MalunitedForearm Diaphyseal fractures. J Hand Surg Am 38(7):1356–1365. Elsevier Inc

Morrey BF, Schneeberger AG (2002 Nov 1) Anconeus arthroplasty: a new technique for reconstruction of the Radiocapitellar and/or proximal radioulnar joint. J Bone Joint Surg Am 84(11):1960–1969

Murase T, Oka K, Moritomo H, Goto A, Yoshikawa H, Sugamoto K (2008 Nov 1) Three-dimensional corrective osteotomy of Malunited fractures of the upper extremity with use of a computer simulation system. J Bone Joint Surg Am 90(11):2375–2389

Nishida K, Iwasaki N, Minami A (2009 Aug 12) Anconeus muscle flap for the treatment of soft tissue defects over the olecranon after total elbow arthroplasty. Journal of Hand Surgery (European Volume) 34(4):538–539

Price CT, Knapp DR (2006 Mar) Osteotomy for Malunited forearm shaft fractures in children. J Pediatr Orthop 26(2):193–196

Prommersberger K-J, Kalb K, van Schoonhoven J (2007 Feb) Mal-united fractures of the distal radius--biomechanics and operative treatment options. Handchir Mikrochir Plast Chir 39(1):9–18

Prommersberger K-J, Pillukat T, Mühldorfer M, van Schoonhoven J (2012 May) Malunion of the distal radius. Arch Orthop Trauma Surg 132(5):693–702

Randsborg P-H, Gulbrandsen P, Saltytė Benth J, Sivertsen EA, Hammer O-L, Fuglesang HFS et al (2013 Apr 3) Fractures in children: epidemiology and activity-specific fracture rates. J Bone Joint Surg Am 95(7):e42

Rikli DA, Babst R, Jupiter JB (2007 Feb) Distal radius fractures: new concepts as basis for surgical treatment. Handchir Mikrochir Plast Chir 39(1):2–8

Rubin G, Rozen N, Bor N (2013 Mar) Gradual correction of congenital radioulnar synostosis by an osteotomy and Ilizarov external fixation. J Hand Surg Am 38(3):447–452

Ruffing T, Danko S, Danko T, Henzler T, Winkler H, Muhm M (2016 Aug) Injuries in children and adolescents in emergency services. Unfallchirurg 119(8):654–663

Sauvé L, Kapandji M (1936) Nouvelle technique de traitement chirurgical des luxations recidivantes isolfies de l'extremite inferieure du cubitus. J Chir 47:589–594

Scheker LR, Ozer K (2004 Dec) Ligamentous stabilization of the distal radioulnar joint. Tech Hand Up Extrem Surg 8(4):239–246

Schmittenbecher PP, Dietz HG, Uhl S (1991 Apr) Late results of forearm fractures in childhood. Unfallchirurg 94(4):186–190

Short WH, Palmer AK, Werner FW, Murphy DJ (1987 Jul) A biomechanical study of distal radial fractures. J Hand Surg Am 12(4):529–534

Taleisnik J, Watson HK (1984 May) Midcarpal instability caused by malunited fractures of the distal radius. J Hand Surg Am 9(3):350–357

Voth M, Lustenberger T, Auner B, Frank J, Marzi I (2017) What injuries should we expect in the emergency room? Injury. Elsevier 0(0):640–645

Watson HK, Castle TH (1988 Nov) Trapezoidal osteotomy of the distal radius for unacceptable articular angulation after Colles' fracture. J Hand Surg Am 13(6):837–843

Watson HK, Ryu JY, Burgess RC (1986 Nov) Matched distal ulnar resection. J Hand Surg Am 11(6):812–817

21 Secondary Reconstruction of the Lower Leg: Femur, Tibia and Ankle

21.1 Epidemiology

Injuries to the lower extremity in children account for 30% of the injuries, mostly as a result of falls or impact injuries. As they grow older and activity increases outside the household, along with more sport activities the ankle and knee are more involved (10%). Fractures of the lower extremity in children are mostly seen in the foot (8%) and ankle (6%). The tibia and femur suffer due to a fracture in 3% of the cases. Even the knee needs some attention (minor injuries, soft tissue), however fractures are very seldom, less than 1%.

Differential Diagnosis

Most importantly in trauma care related to children pathological fractures should be discovered and a long-term treatment protocol established. Depending on the lesion referral to a specialized center is advised.

A reduced resilience of the bone could be due to local or systemic reasons. In cases of local lesions benign, mostly bone cysts, and malignant processes have to be differentiated. In such cases the different sarcomas have to be considered and further diagnostic is needed before operative treatment. Sometimes a bowing is obvious without a fracture and typical for large pathological processes like fibrous dysplasia (Table 21.1).

Table 21.1 Reasons for pathological fractures/deformities to be considered

Localized reasons	Systemic reasons
Bone cysts	Brittle bone disease
Giant cell tumor	Rickets, vitamin D deficiency
Enchondroma	Osteoporosis
Chondrosarcoma, osteosarcoma, Ewing sarcoma	M. Gaucher, Stüve-Wiedemann-syndrome
Fibrous dysplasia	Parathyroid gland disorder
Osteomyelitis	Osteopetrosis

21.2 Deformities of the Femur

The first step to address deformities of the femoral bone is to differentiate to normality and calculate possible increasing problems like leg length discrepancy (LLD). Also, possible spontaneous corrections must be considered. Rotational or varus/valgus deformities which need to be corrected are seldom, since most of the time an acceptable reduction is achieved using the outlined therapeutic strategies and stable osteosynthesis techniques. Significant problems would result in fractures near the femoral head causing bone necrosis or at the distal femur, if the growth plate is involved, resulting possibly in a significant valgus/varus deformity. A rotational malalignment might result in an ante- or retroversion of the femoral neck. A correction of an antever-

I. Marzi et al., *Pediatric Skeletal Trauma*, https://doi.org/10.1007/978-3-030-93685-3_21

sion might be considered around 50° at the age of 12 years, however most of these cases are not trauma related at the proximal femur.

Therapy

Basics

Especially treating deformities of in the lower extremity, including the femoral bone, it is important to evaluate the whole musculoskeletal system to exclude secondary deformities or oversee system or local diseases. One should not forget or evaluate the Spine and the pelvis, there might already secondary deformities, due to the adaption to the primary malalignment. For the femur rotational deformities below 20° are well tolerated and length discrepancies must be carefully evaluated, since physiological differences up to 1.5 cm are possible and a significant shortening of the fractured femur might be compensated due to growth stimulation, especially during the first year after injury. It is common to follow up for this period of time before a corrective procedure is performed, especially in younger children (2–10 years). If the problem persists the following deformities represent an indication for corrective procedures:

1. Varus deformity >5°
2. Valgus deformity >10°
3. Malrotation >10°
4. Deformity of curvaton >15°
5. Side-to-Side mal-alignment >15 mm
6. LLD > 20 mm

Corrective Procedures

Pre-Operative Preparation

According to the location of the deformity the amount of deformity needs to be measured as well as remaining growth. Therefore, the following diagnostics are advised:

1. Bilateral full Leg View in standing position to evaluate bone length discrepancy, axis deformity and to calculate further leg length discrepancy, remaining growth, timing of angular correction or epiphysiodesis (Fig. 21.1)
2. MRI to evaluate rotational deformity. Also, it is possible to calculate the rotational deformity with CT-scans, however, in children unneeded x-ray exposure should be avoided (Fig. 21.2)

After the analysis of the deformity is finished, the options and the treatment plan must be discussed with the child and the parents. Especially possible complications should be mention and their resolution. In cases were sequential operative procedures during growth are needed, this should be explained. Also, the devices used should be shown, especially external fixators, to reduce concerns and fear after the operative procedures is done. This includes postoperative care and handling.

Today most of the planning can be done with the help of applications used on a smart phone. This allows to avoid a time-consuming analysis of tables and difficult calculations (e.g. The Multiplier, Rubin Institute for Advanced Orthopedics, Sinai Hospital of Baltimore).

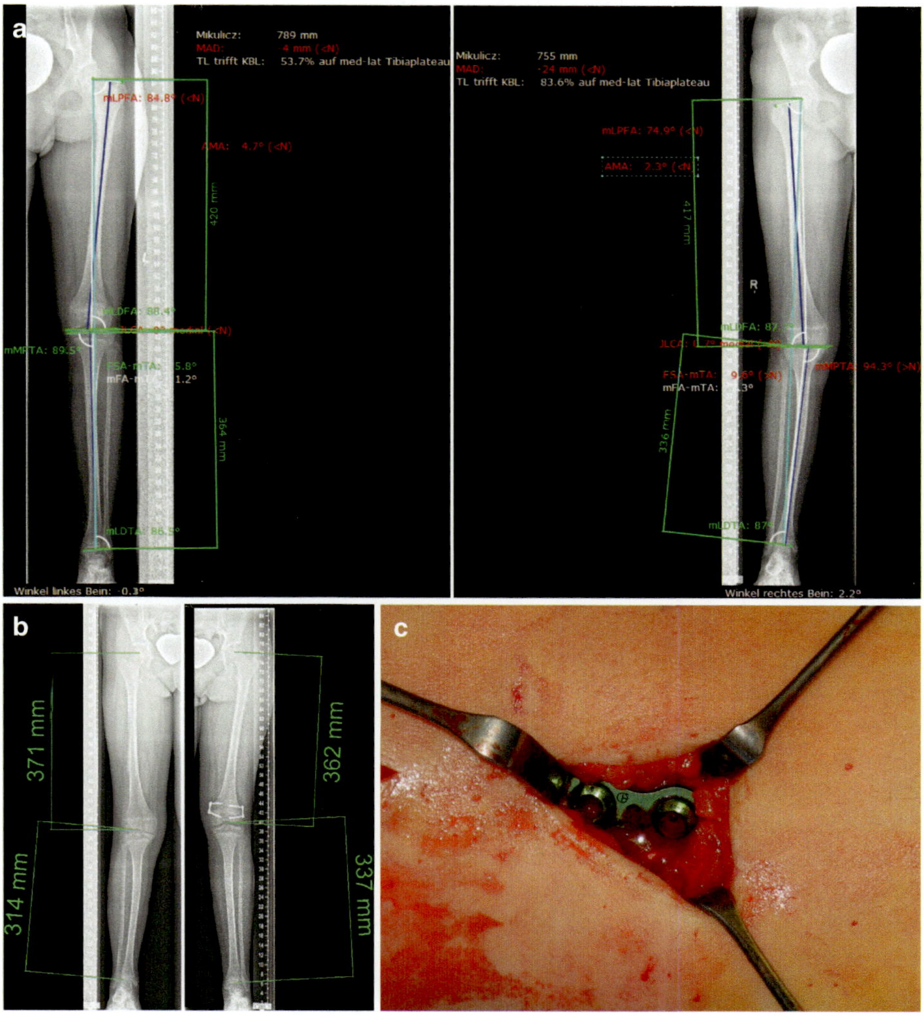

Fig. 21.1 (**a**) Example to evaluate leg length discrepancy in a 10-year-old girl and correction with temporary epiphysiodesis on the left distal femur with eight-plates, (**b**) Angular deformity analysis one year later after temporary epiphysiodesis. For the angular deformity, the timing is calculated to perform a temporary epiphysiodesis medially at the distal femur and proximal tibia, (**c**) Clinical picture during 8-plate application at the proximal tibia

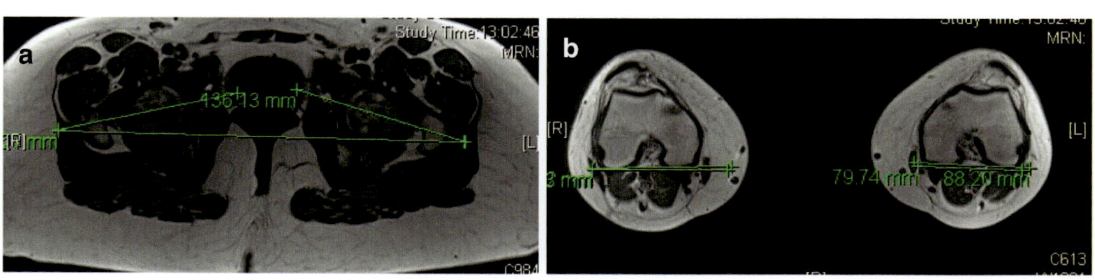

Fig. 21.2 MRI to evaluate rotational deformities of the femur. In children MRI is preferred to avoid significant x-ray exposure. Calculation can be performed using the proximal femur (**a**) and the distal femur (**b**)

Operative Techniques

Depending of the preoperative analysis, and consideration about the condition, age and possibly underlying disease the correction is planned. In the case of bone length discrepancy with open growth plates either temporary or near growth completion definitive epiphysiodesis could be performed at the longer leg (Fig. 21.1). If the result would be a significant loss of bone length, distraction osteotomy is performed. This would be most common achieved preserving the growth plate with an external fixation device. Therefore, two technique principals need to be considered at this anatomic region. A stabile and precise lengthening could be achieved with a ring system. Today systems are available which allow permanent adjustment during the lengthening procedure using a computerized system. This is provided by the various companies mostly based on web access. Ring systems are not very comfortable for the patients on the femur (Fig. 21.3). Due to these circumstances a unilateral system might be preferred. The disadvantage might be the tendency to push the distal femur in a varus position. However, this could be helpful in cases where a valgus deformity and a short femur coexist (Fig. 21.4). Whatever type of external fixation might be used, a change of procedure should be calculated. It might be more comfortable for the patient, to change to a angle stable plate after the desired bone length is achieved, because callus maturation might need quite a long time. This will allow to review the planning and perform a final adjustment during the procedure (e.g. angle corrections). In younger children more lengthening periods are needed and could be combined with hardware removal and reapplication of the lengthening device.

Much easier is the methods of guided growth performing a temporary epiphysiodesis. This could be performed with various methods (clamps, plates or screws). Percutaneous screw epiphysiodesis has become more popular in the last years, due its relatively simple technique and minimal invasive attitude (Fig. 21.5). For a temporary percutaneous screw epiphysiodesis it is recommended to use cannulated screws. Therefore, the K-Wire can be placed just before the growth plate und the position proved in appropriate AP-view and exact lateral-view to ensure the correct position. Using this method, the screw can be inserted with no need of further corrections and the trauma to the growth plate will be minimal.

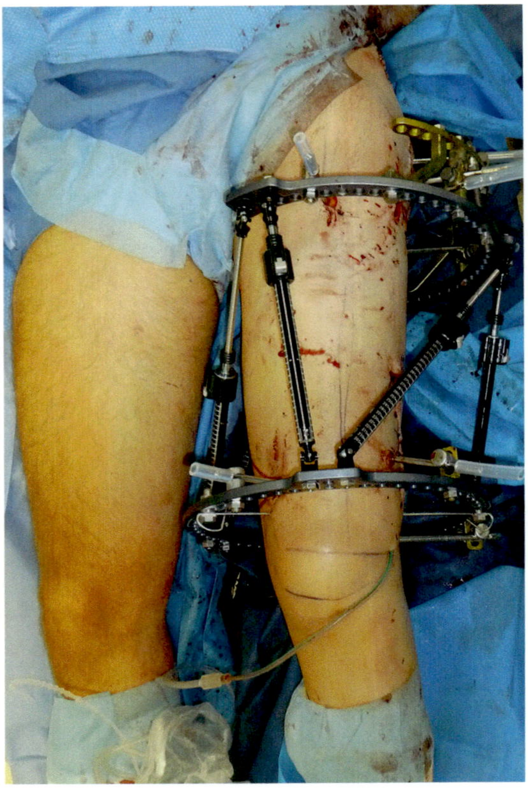

Fig. 21.3 Clinical picture after application of external ring device on the left femur (Maxframe, DepuySynthes)

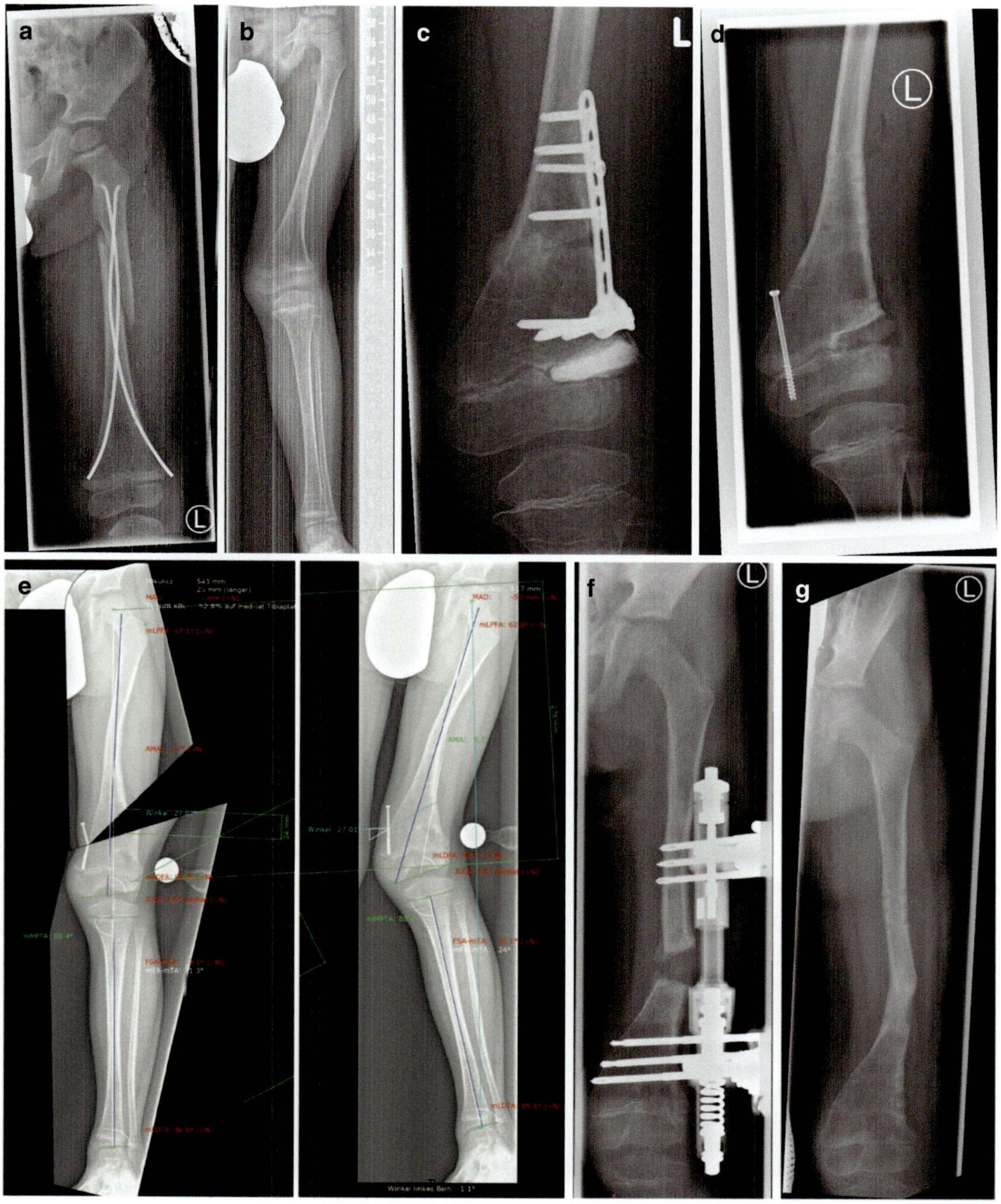

Fig. 21.4 Growth arrest and angular deformity after a femur fracture in a 5 year old boy, (**a**) Primary fracture care with ESIN, (**b**) Growth arrest and valgus deformity of the distal femur due to osseous bridging of the growth plate, (**c**) Resection of the bone-band and bone cement interposition together with a corrective osteotomy to compensate the deformity, (**d**) To achieve a final realignment a temporary screw epiphysiodesis was performed at the medial distal growth plate to achieve an alignment, (**e**) Due to growth arrest and increased valgus deformity bone lengthening including correction was planned, (**f**) This could be achieved with a unilateral external fixation device—it must be considered that with this method it is very likely to induce a varus, which in this case is an advantage, (**g**) Final appearance of the distal femur, growth calculation reveal, that there might be two more lengthening episodes needed till growth ends and an epiphysiodesis at the opposite side might be discussed close to the end of the growth to avoid more demanding bone lengthening and preserve an acceptable position of the joint line in both legs

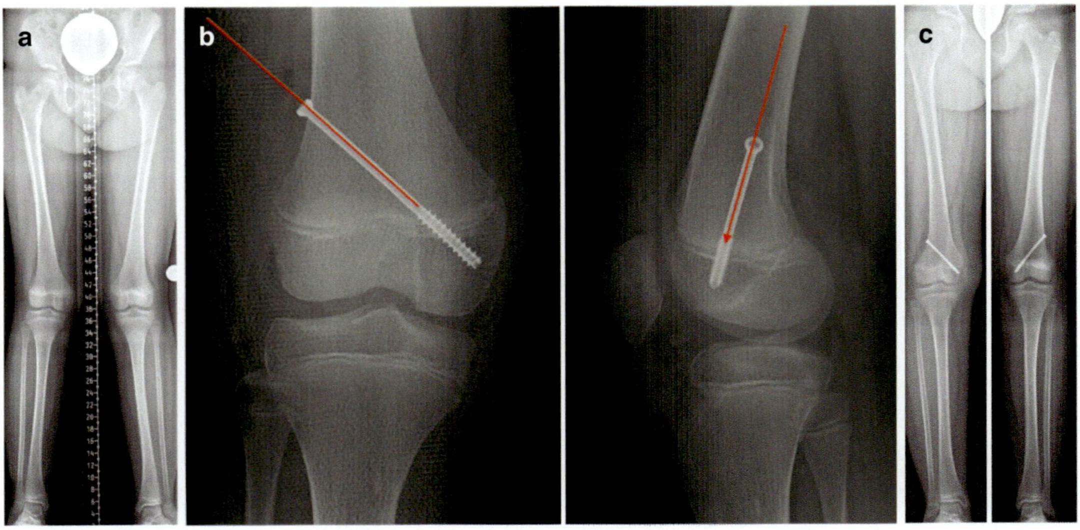

Fig. 21.5 Angular correction in a 10 year old boy with repetitive luxation of the patella at the right leg, (**a**) Preoperative planning, (**b**) Method of screw insertion, the red line illustrates the K-wire positioning before drilling through the growth plate to ensure the exact position in both planes (A.P. view; lateral view) and avoid multiple perforations of the physis causing damage and possibly growth arrest, (**c**) Final alinement of the legs with some overcorrection on the right side. No relaxation of the patella appeared

However, sometimes a combination of growth guidance and corrective osteotomy might be successful or could lead to significant complications with further deformities or infections as some of the worst-case scenarios (Fig. 21.6). Therefore, it is very helpful if all these problems are discussed in advance, as well as the possible procedures needed to surpass this complicated situation.

Sometimes due to the underlying disease and additional fractures a corrective procedure is not possible, however the osteosynthesis might be modified to enable a correction later, after the fracture is healed (Fig. 21.7).

Postoperative Care

Depending on the situation and the operative procedure performed the instruction are very different. In a simple epiphysiodesis reduced movement and weight bearing is only needed till the wounds are healed. Complex deformity corrections might need a maximum weight reduction. If an external fixature is applied instructions for pin care need to be provided to avoid pin track infection and a regular control is recommended to prove the constructs stability and avoid loosening (e.g. weekly). Depending on the amount of disability caused by the device, including limitations of joint movement, physiotherapy might be necessary through the treatment period, this is more important in cases of bone lengthening, since the tension on the soft tissues might cause discomfort and consequently limitations in the range of motion. If guided growth is intended a regular clinical evaluation of leg axis and length is recommended (e.g. every 4–6 weeks.). Some cases might correct much faster as calculated and an overcorrection should be avoided.

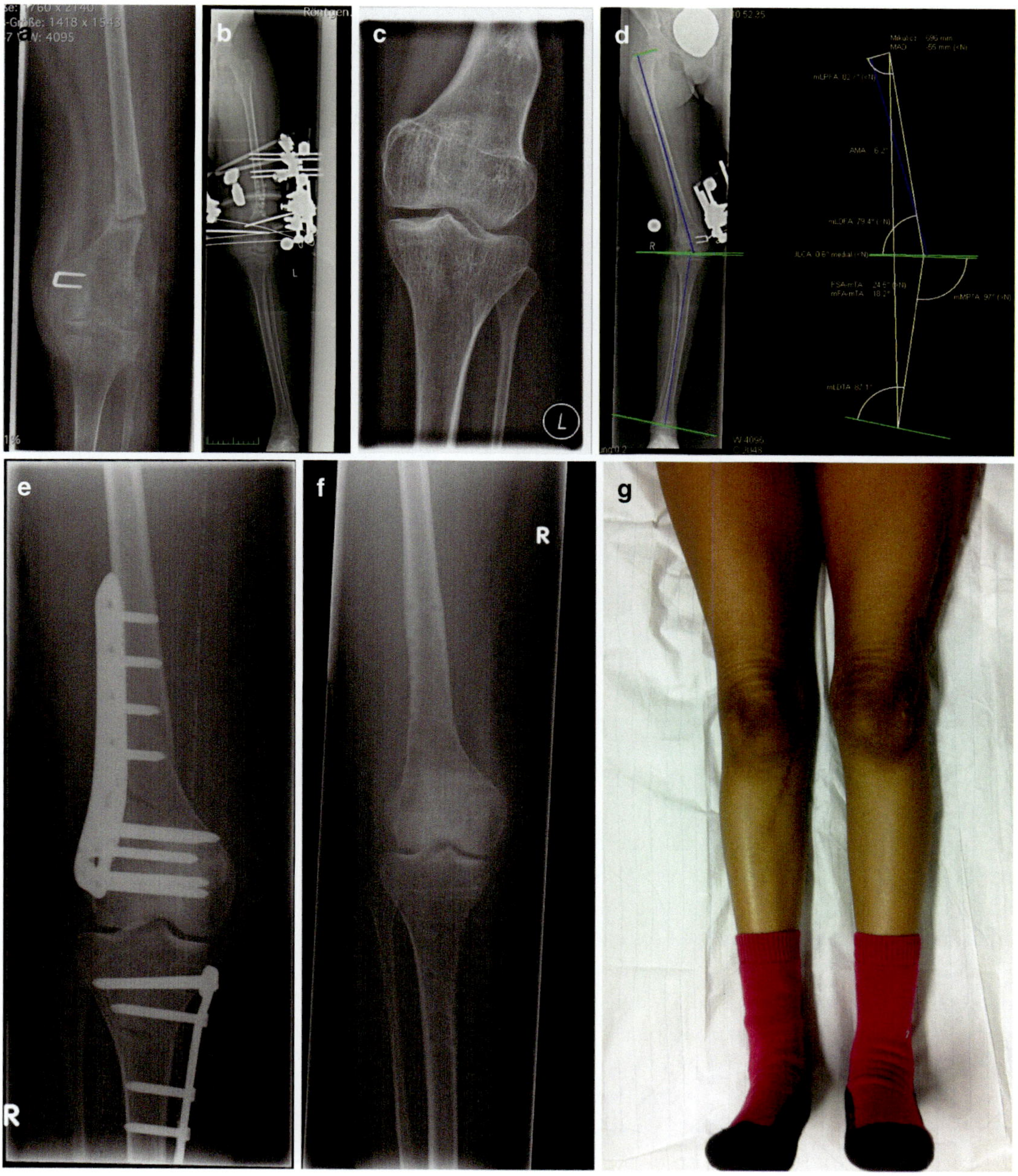

Fig. 21.6 Infected pseudarthrosis after corrective osteotomie and guided growth at the distal femur in a 14 year old girl, (**a**) Appearance before revision surgeries, (**b**) Correction and healing at the distal femur could be achieved with an external fixation device, (**c**) Appearance after bone healing, (**d**) The deformity on the right leg was analyzed, (**e**) Correction was performed with double osteotomy, (**f**) X-ray of the right leg after bone healing and removal of the implants, (**g**) Clinical appearance of the both legs at the end of treatment

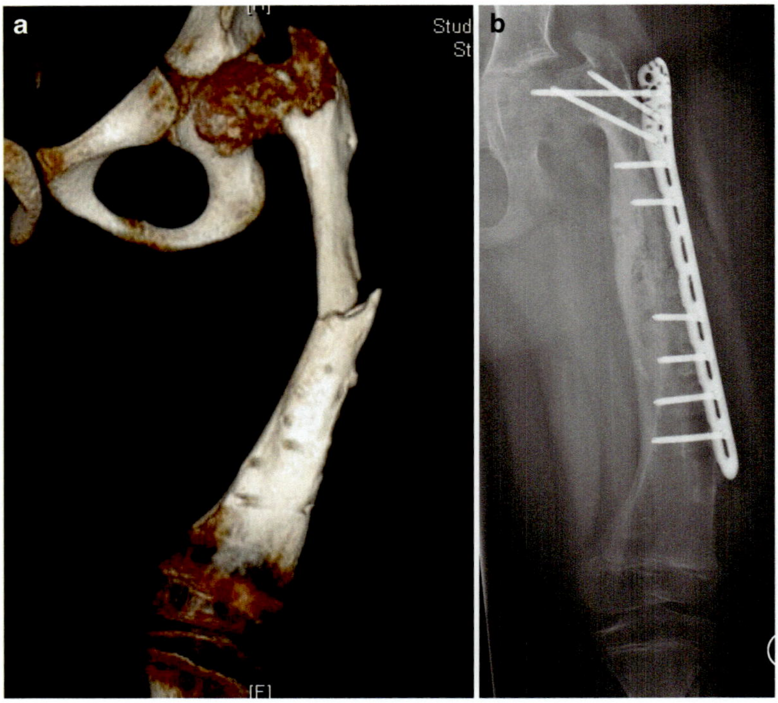

Fig. 21.7 Fracture of the lateral femoral neck in a 12 year old boy with short femur syndrome, (**a**) Appearance of the factures at the proximal femur and the shaft, (**b**) A corrective procedure together with this type of fractures seemed to be to risky, therefore a plate was adjusted to allow a intertrochanteric correction later

21.3 Deformities of the Tibia and Ankle

Deformities after a tibia shaft fracture are rare and therefore the knowledge of the age-related distribution of the angles, still considered to be in a normal range, must be reviewed for each individual case. After birth in most individual a varus is present which will change to a valgus, sometimes more than 10°, in the second year. This will decrease again passing the age of 12 years. Also, there is no torsion at birth. The child develops, compared to the axis of the thigh, a lateral torsion of the foot between 10 and 20° around the age of 12 years.

Other lesions like epiphyseal necrosis or pseudarthrosis are rare, however lesions of the physis will result in significant deformities. More often deformities will result due to a non-anatomic reduction of a fracture or a dislocation of the epiphyses not well realigned. At the proximal tibia a deformity due to partial stimulation of the growth plate is typical and will result in a valgus deformity, as well as partial closure of the physis is more common after a injury to the distal physis with a bridging and consequently varus deformity.

Therapy

Basics

In most cases of deformities at the lower leg a complete evaluation of the musculoskeletal system is needed as proposed for the femur. Deformities of the foot need to be considered especially for distal tibia deformities. With the correction of the lower leg an additional procedure might be needed to align established secondary deformities distally if they could not be controlled by conservative measures.

The following parameters represent an indication for corrective procedures at the lower leg:

1. Varus deformity >7°
2. Valgus deformity >10°
3. Malrotation >15°
4. Deformity of curvaton >10°
5. LLD > 20 mm

Corrective Procedures

Pre-Operative Preparation

The lower leg can be evaluated more easily clinically as the femur. With the child sitting on the examination couch with lower leg hanging of the corner and the foot extended to a neutral position a rotational mal-alignment could be easily evaluated. Also a length discrepancy could be clinically evaluated, aside standing on standardized boards examining the joint lines, hip and spine alignment. Therefore, the child could be brought in a prone position and the knees bend 90 degrees. A significant length difference will be obvious with examining the sole of the foot. The same could be performed in a supine position at a 90 degree flexion of the hip and knee to clinically compare the femur to the tibia in cases of LLD.

As mentioned before, also for the lower leg the following diagnostics are advised:

1. Bilateral full Leg View in standing position to evaluate bone length discrepancy, axis deformity and to calculate further leg length discrepancy, remaining growth, timing of angular correction or epiphysiodesis.
2. MRI to evaluate rotational deformity. Also, it is possible to calculate the rotational deformity with CT-scans, however, in children unneeded x-ray exposure should be avoided.

After the analysis of the deformity is finished, the options and the treatment plan must be discussed with the child and the parents. Especially possible complications should be mention and their resolution. In cases were sequential operative procedures during growth are needed, this should be explained. This is very true in cases of valgus deformities after proximal tibia fractures or growth arrest at the distal physis. In such cases more often multiple procedures are necessary to solve the problem. Of course, it is helpful to visualize as well the needed fixation devises, especially external fixators, to assure more postoperative acceptance. The postoperative course, treatment plan and upcoming additional procedures should be explained in advance.

Operative Techniques

There is no doubt, addressing the growth plate to perform a correction with guided growth has a risk to cause damage with a result of secondary deformity. Some might consider to perform the correction away from this region. However, this might result in a recurrence of the deformity, especially at the proximal tibia. However, if explained to the parents and the child, this is an option to improve the clinical situation and perform a temporary or permanent epiphysiodesis closer to the completion of growth (Fig. 21.8). Some deformities are very complex and might not be easy to be planned in advance. Problems with at the Tibia shaft with a malalignment in multiple planes are easier to be corrected with an external fixation device allowing multiple axial correction designed as a hexapod ring fixation device (e.g. Maxframe, DePuySynthes; Taylor Spatial Frame, Smith & Newphew). Due to the complex correction procedure a software assistance for planning and correction is needed. Most of these are web-based allowing continues recalculations throughout the corrective process (Fig. 21.9). However, this is a time-consuming method and corrective procedures in one or two plane—as well as segmental transfers or simple bone lengthening - can be managed with standard external fixation or external ring fixation systems. Treating such problems are mostly complicated with pseudarthrosis and need sometimes a consequent change to such systems, even if intramedullary nailing or plates are much more comfortable (Fig. 21.10). Compared to the problems at the proximal tibia and distal tibia most of these cases are relatively simple, since there is no growth plate involved.

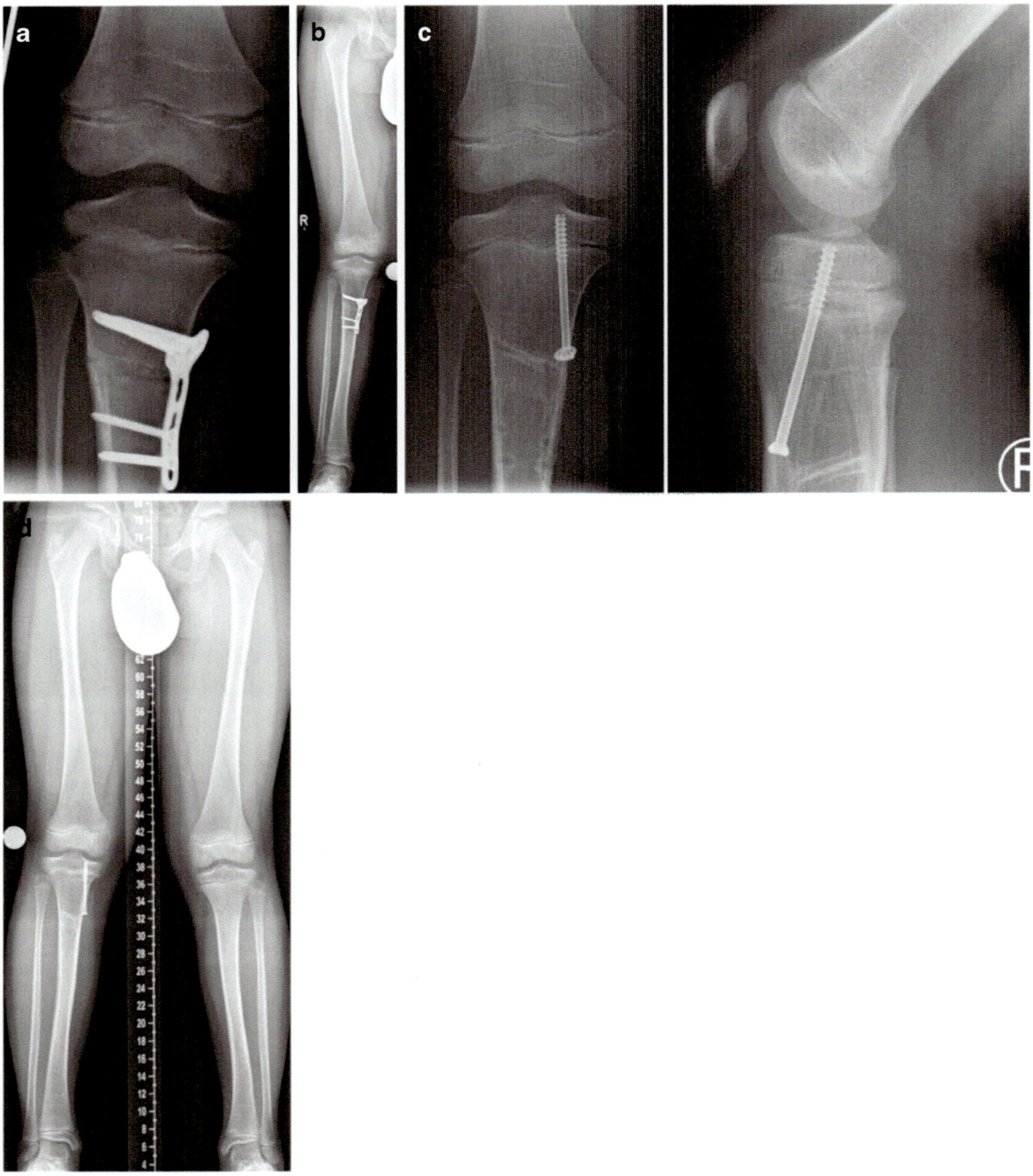

Fig. 21.8 Correction of a valgus deformity after a proximal tibia fracture in a 9 year old boy, (**a**) A overcorrection was performed using a plate to compensate for recurrency of the valgus deformity, (**b**) The reappearance of the valgus deformity could not be avoided, (**c**) After 3 years with an acceptable angulation a guided growth correction was performed with an transcutaneous screw epiphysiodesis, (**d**) Achieving a well aligned leg

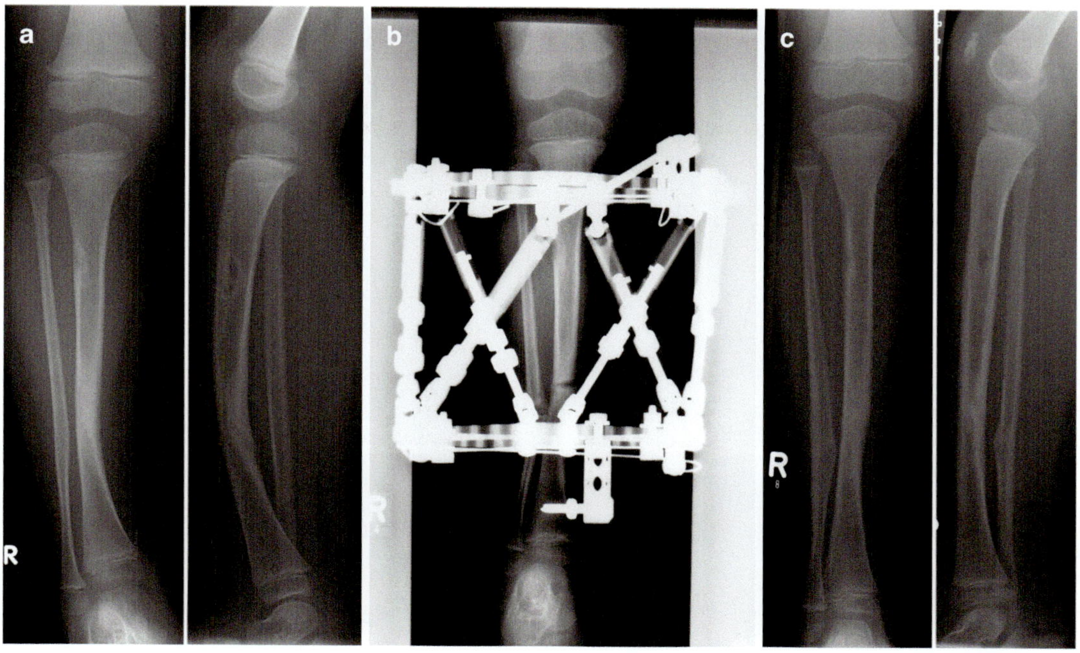

Fig. 21.9 Posttraumatic deformity of the tibia in a 5-year-old boy, (**a**) The mid-shaft fracture resulted in a varus, antecurvation and internal rotation deformity, (**b**) The correction was performed with a hexapod ring fixation device, (**c**) Final result after removal of the device

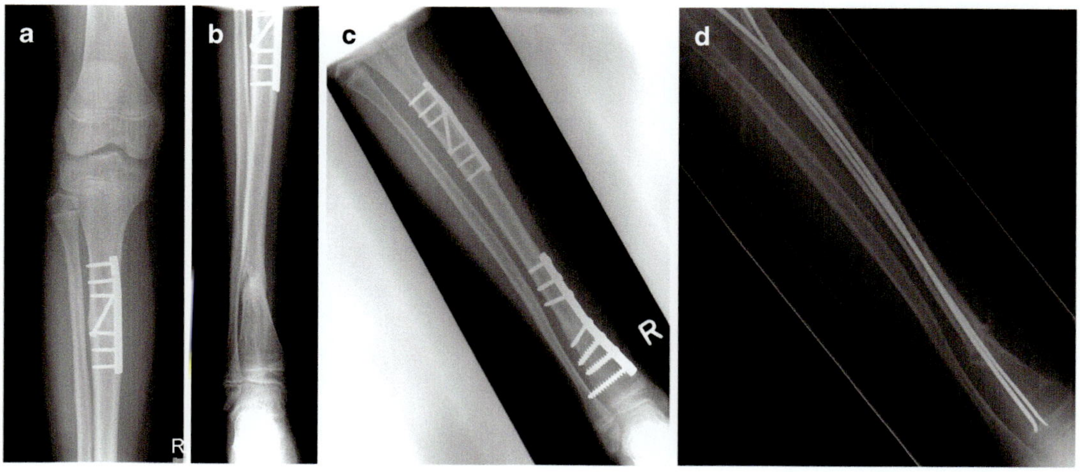

Fig. 21.10 Medical course of a boy suffering a proximal tibia fracture at the age of 12, (**a**) Stabilization of the facture with plating, (**b**) One year later he suffered of a distal tibia fracture, (**c**) This fracture was plated as well, (**d**) 9 Month later the plates were removed, however healing at the distal fracture side was not be achieved, therefore intramedullary nailing was performed, (**e**, **f**) Due to persistent pseudarthrosis a revision was performed with plating, (**g**) After plate removal refracture occurred and (**h**) Anther plate application did not resolve the problem, (**i**) To solve the problem 4 years after the appearance of the tibia fracture the pseudarthrosis was removed, resulting in a 2 cm shortening with a preexisting shortage of the leg of 2 cm and a ring fixation device applied, (**j**) With the device a segmental transport to treat the pseudarthrosis was performed, as well as a bone lengthening of 4 cm, (**k**) Final x-ray after healing and (**l**) Clinical appearance of the leg

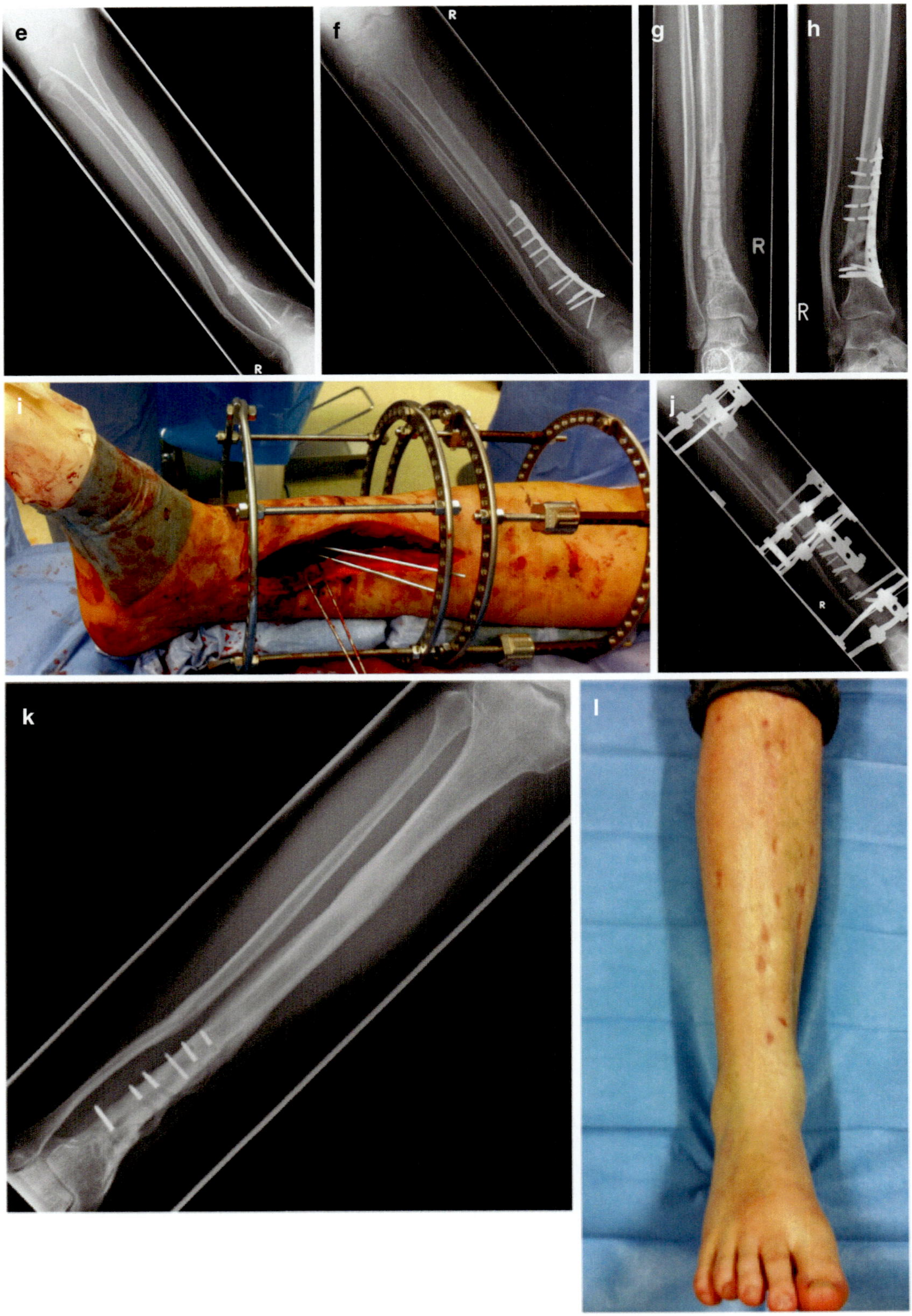

Fig. 21.10 (continued)

At the level of the ankle lesions of the physis on the tibia can be very demanding and difficult to control. Especially partial closure of the physis might need more procedures due to the high recurrence rate (Fig. 21.11). The various techniques for resection of the bony bridge or band are sometimes not as successful as expected. Various optionsn (e.g. free fat, bone cement) could be considered to fill the defect after the resection of the bone crossing the growth plate.

Contrary to the difficulties, which might occur at the distal tibia fractures of fibula appearing with significant malalignment can be left alone in most cases, due to the fact, that the realign very well with time. It will just need some time to explain this to the patients, family and referring colleagues (Fig. 21.12).

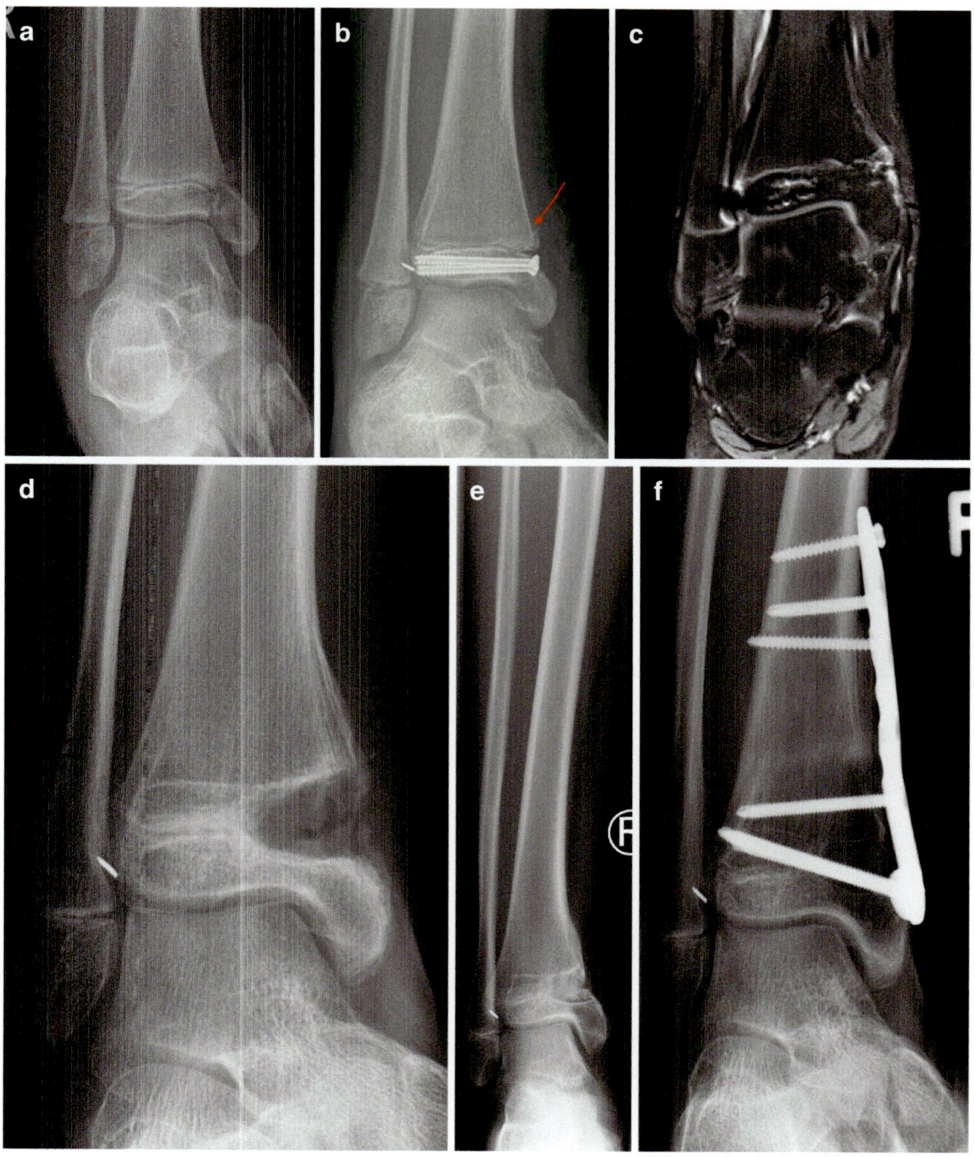

Fig. 21.11 Fracture of the distal epiphysis of the tibia in a 10 year old girl, (**a**) X-ray of the fracture, (**b**) Delayed screw fixation, callus formation is already visible (arrow), (**c**) Partial closure of the physis with varus deformity seen here on the MRI, (**d**) Resection of the medial ossified physis did not resolve the problem and (**e**) Recurrence of the deformity appeared, (**f**) Close to the definitive closure of the physis at the end of the child's growth

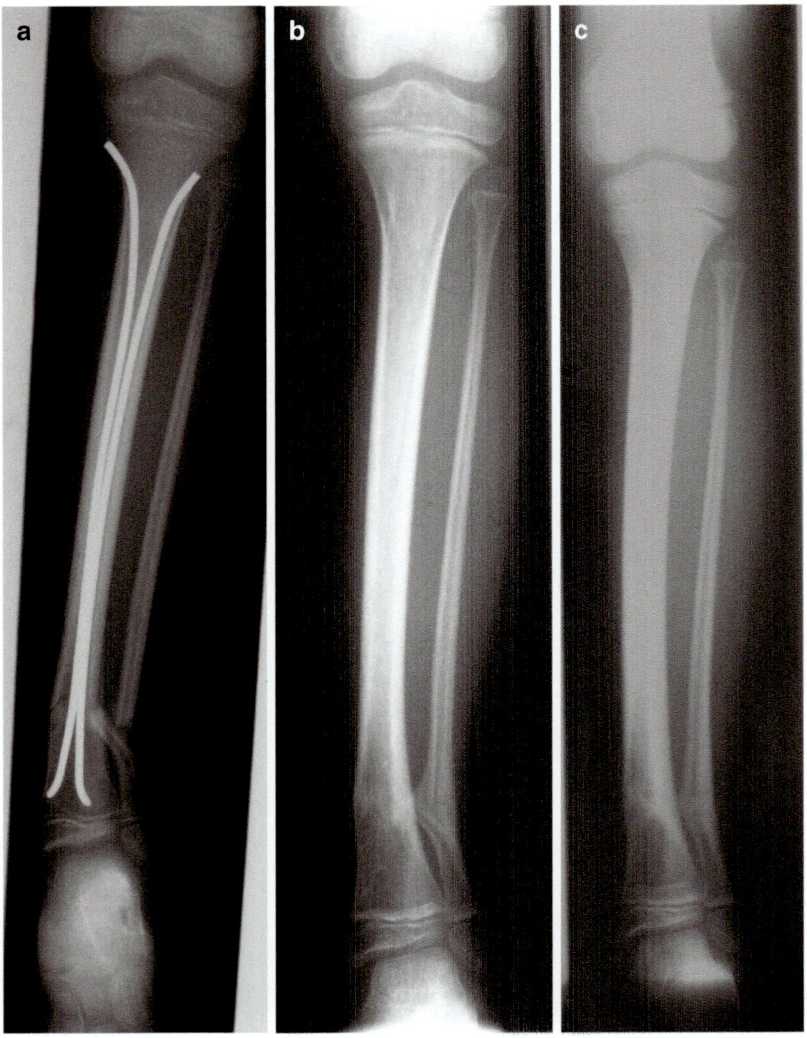

Fig. 21.12 Valgus deformity due to a distal tibia and fibula fracture in a 11 year old girl, (**a**) The tibia was stabilized with ESIN, (**b**) Spontaneous correction is obvious and well seen already after 6 month and (**c**) 9 Month

Postoperative Care

Depending on the procedure, after definitive stabilization.

Depending on the situation and the operative procedure performed, the instruction are very different. In a simple epiphysiodesis reduced movement and weight bearing is only needed till the wounds are healed. Complex deformity corrections might need a maximum weight reduction. If an external fixature is applied instructions for pin care need to be provided to avoid pin track infection and a regular control is recommended to prove the constructs stability and avoid loosening (e.g. weekly). Depending on the amount of disability caused by the device, including limitations of joint movement, physiotherapy might be necessary through the treatment period, this is more important in cases of bone lengthening, since the tension on the soft tissues might cause discomfort and consequently limitations in the range of motion. If guided growth is intended a regular clinical evaluation of leg axis and length is recommended (e.g. every 4–6 weeks.). Some cases might correct much faster as calculated and an overcorrection should be avoided.

21.4 Complications

Corrective interventions at the lower extremity are characterized by a number of risks, especially the critical soft tissue coverage of the lower leg and foot. Therefore, the same complication might appear as in acute fracture care and sometimes, due to the previous operative procedures and deformity, the circumstances at start might be worse. The following complications must be considered:

- Hematoma formation
- Compartment Syndrome
- Tendon lesions (reduced toe and ankle function)
- Vascular lesions
- Nerve lesions
- Malalignment
- Pseudarthrosis
- Infections
- Scar formation

21.5 Conclusions

The operative therapy of posttraumatic deformities at the lower extremity can be very complex. As all deformities they need to be analyzed very carefully and weighted against the actual impairment, risk of a corrective procedure and expected improvement. Dramatic deformities, involving the growth plate might need multiple steps to achieve correction and therefore the surgeon and family must be aware of changes necessary throughout the treatment course. In some cases, it must be explained that sometimes only partial goals can be achieved and some limits in ROM will persist as well as pre-arthritic deformations, which might end up in further operative procedures later during live. If the decision is made to perform a correction, the family and the patient should be informed and educated with respect to the complete treatment plan and possible variations and complications as early as possible.

Recommended Literature

Albert M, McCaig LF (2014 May) Injury-related emergency department visits by children and adolescents: United States, 2009–2010. NCHS Data Brief NCHS Data Brief 150:1–8

Cooper C, Dennison EM, Leufkens HG, Bishop N, van Staa TP (2004, Dec 1) Epidemiology of childhood fractures in Britain: a study using the general practice research database. J Bone Miner Res 19(12):1976–1981. John Wiley & Sons, Ltd

Ghanem I, Karam JA, Widmann RF (2011 Feb) Surgical epiphysiodesis indications and techniques: update. Curr Opin Pediatr 23(1):53–59

Gottliebsen M, Shiguetomi-Medina JM, Rahbek O, Møller-Madsen B (2016 Dec) Guided growth: mechanism and reversibility of modulation. J Child Orthop 10(6):471–477

Joeris A, Lutz N, Wicki B, Slongo T, Audigé L (2014 Dec 20) An epidemiological evaluation of pediatric long bone fractures - a retrospective cohort study of 2716 patients from two Swiss tertiary pediatric hospitals. BMC Pediatr BioMed Central 14(1):314–311

Langenskiöld A (1981) Surgical treatment of partial closure of the growth plate. J Pediatr Orthop 1(1):3–11

Paley D (2002) Principles of deformity reconstruction. Springer, Berlin, New York

Randsborg P-H, Gulbrandsen P, Saltytė Benth J, Sivertsen EA, Hammer O-L, Fuglesang HFS et al (2013 Apr 3) Fractures in children: epidemiology and activity-specific fracture rates. J Bone Joint Surg Am 95(7):e42

Ruffing T, Danko S, Danko T, Henzler T, Winkler H, Muhm M (2016 Aug) Injuries in children and adolescents in emergency services. Unfallchirurg 119(8):654–663

Ruzbarsky JJ, Goodbody C, Dodwell E (2017 Feb) Closing the growth plate: a review of indications and surgical options. Curr Opin Pediatr 29(1):80–86

Wagner P, Standard SC, Herzenberg JE (2017 Apr/May) Evaluation of a Mobile Application for Multiplier Method Growth and Epiphysiodesis Timing Predictions. J Pediatr Orthop 37(3):e188–e191. https://doi.org/10.1097/BPO.0000000000000805.

Vogt B, Schiedel F, Rödl R (2014 Mar 15) Guided growth in children and adolescents. Orthopade 43(3):267–284

Voth M, Lustenberger T, Auner B, Frank J, Marzi I (2017 Oct 1) What injuries should we expect in the emergency room? Elsevier Ltd 48(10):2119–24.

GPSR Compliance

The European Union's (EU) General Product Safety Regulation (GPSR) is a set of rules that requires consumer products to be safe and our obligations to ensure this.

If you have any concerns about our products, you can contact us on ProductSafety@springernature.com

In case Publisher is established outside the EU, the EU authorized representative is:

Springer Nature Customer Service Center GmbH
Europaplatz 3
69115 Heidelberg, Germany

Batch number: 10756382

Printed by Printforce, the Netherlands